ALLERGIC DISEASES

Diagnosis and Management

Contributors

Donald W. Aaronson, M.D.

Bernard Hess Booth III, M.D.

Walter W. Y. Chang, M.D.

Richard D. DeSwarte, M.D.

Angelo E. Falleroni, M.D.

Jordan N. Fink, M.D.

Thomas M. Golbert, M.D.

Arnold A. Gutman, M.D.

John D. Holloman, M.D.

James D. Lakin, PH.D., M.D.

Phillip L. Lieberman, M.D.

Howard L. Melam, M.D.

Terumasa Miyamoto, M.D., PH.D.

Roy Patterson, M.D.

Jacob J. Pruzansky, PH.D.

Raymond G. Slavin, M.D.

Alice Solar-Mills, M.D.

Dale B. Sparks, M.D.

James I. Tennenbaum, M.D.

Isaac Weiszer, M.D.

ALLERGIC DISEASES

Diagnosis and Management

Edited by

ROY PATTERSON, M.D.

Ernest S. Bazley Professor
Chief, Section of Allergy and Immunology
Associate Chairman
Department of Medicine
Northwestern University, Chicago

J. B. Lippincott Company
Philadelphia • Toronto

ISBN 0-397-50291-5

Library of Congress Catalog Card Number 70-173258

Printed in the United States of America
3 2 1

Library of Congress Cataloging in Publication Data

Patterson, Roy, 1926–
    Allergic diseases.

    Includes bibliographies.
    1. Allergy—Addresses, essays, lectures.   I. Title.
[DNLM: Hypersensitivity—Diagnosis.   2. Hypersensitivity—Therapy.
WD300 P318a 1972]
RC584.P37   616.9'7   70-173258
ISBN 0-397-50291-5

Contributors

DONALD W. AARONSON, M.D.
Attending Physician; Lutheran
General Hospital; Assistant Pro-
fessor of Medicine; Northwestern
University Medical School; Chicago,
Illinois

BERNARD HESS BOOTH III, M.D.
Clinical Assistant Professor of
Medicine; University of Mississippi;
Jackson, Mississippi

WALTER W. Y. CHANG, M.D.
The Chock-Pang Clinic; Honolulu,
Hawaii

RICHARD D. DeSWARTE, M.D.
Assistant Professor; Northwestern
University Medical School; Chi-
cago, Illinois; Allergist, Rockford
Clinic; Rockford, Illinois

A. E. FALLERONI, M.D.
Associate in Medicine; North-
western University Medical School;
Chicago, Illinois

JORDAN N. FINK, M.D.
Associate Professor of Medicine;
Chief, Allergy Section; Medical
College of Wisconsin; Milwaukee,
Wisconsin

THOMAS M. GOLBERT, M.D.
Chief, Section of Allergy (Denver
General Hospital); Denver De-
partment of Health and Hospitals;
Assistant Clinical Professor of
Medicine; University of Colorado
School of Medicine; Denver,
Colorado

ARNOLD A. GUTMAN, M.D.
Associate in Medicine; North-
western University Medical School;
Chicago, Illinois

JOHN HOLLOMAN, M.D.
Associate in Medicine; North-
western University Medical School;
Chicago, Illinois

JAMES D. LAKIN, PH.D., M.D.
Department of Internal Medicine;
University of Michigan Medical
Center; Ann Arbor, Michigan

PHILLIP L. LIEBERMAN, M.D.
Assistant Professor; Chief, Section
Allergy; University of Tennessee
Medical School; Memphis,
Tennessee

HOWARD L. MELAM, M.D.
Instructor; Northwestern University
Medical School; Chicago, Illinois

TERUMASA MIYAMOTO, M.D., PH.D.
Research Associate; University of
Tokyo, School of Medicine; Tokyo,
Japan

ROY PATTERSON, M.D.
Bazley Professor of Medicine;
Chief, Section of Allergy and Im-
munology; Associate Chairman of
Medicine; Northwestern University
Medical School; Chicago, Illinois

JACOB J. PRUZANSKY, PH.D.
Associate Professor Microbiology;
Northwestern University Medical
School; Chicago, Illinois

RAYMOND G. SLAVIN, M.D.

Associate Professor Internal Medicine; Director of the Section of Allergy and Immunology; St. Louis University School of Medicine; St. Louis, Missouri

ALICE SOLAR-MILLS, M.D.

Associate, Department of Medicine; Northwestern University Medical School; Chicago, Illinois

DALE B. SPARKS, M.D.

Assistant Clinical Professor of Medicine; Riverside General Hospital; University Medical Center; Riverside, California

JAMES I. TENNENBAUM, M.D.

Associate Professor of Medicine; Director, Division of Allergy; Ohio State University Hospitals; Columbus, Ohio

ISAAC WEISZER, M.D.

Clinical Instructor in Medicine; George Washington University Medical School; Washington, D.C.

Preface

This book covers those clinical problems that are commonly seen in the daily practice of the speciality of Allergy. Because of the high incidence of hypersensitivity disease of the immediate type in the general population, reagin-mediated disease is responsible for the majority of clinical immunologic problems seen in medical practice. The theoretical and practical aspects of these IgE-mediated diseases are discussed in detail. Diseases that have clinical manifestations similar to the reagin-mediated reactions but are probably not IgE-mediated are included, because they are commonly referred to the specialist in Allergy. These diseases may include certain types of asthma, urticaria and rhinitis. The complex problem of drug reactions, most of which are probably not IgE-mediated, is discussed in detail, because it is a common and growing problem in the clinical practice of allergy.

The remarkable advances made in basic and clinical immunology in the past 15 years have extended the range of diseases now considered to be of immunologic origin. We have decided not to attempt to review the basic and clinical information relating to the immunology of hematology, nephrology, rheumatology, transplantation, infectious diseases and other major areas of current interest. The consultant in the specialty of Allergy and Immunology must be familiar with these problems, but detailed information regarding them is already available in a variety of recent texts and reviews. The comprehensive practice of modern clinical allergy requires knowledge and training separate from immunology because of the importance of such aspects as pulmonary physiology in asthma, the pharmacology of therapeutic agents, and the botany and aerobiology of antigenic materials. These areas, relevant to the common allergic diseases seen in practice are reviewed in some detail because they are less frequently encountered in recent texts dealing primarily with nonreaginic immunologic diseases.

It is the opinion of many practitioners and teachers in the field of allergy that the recent advances in basic and clinical immunology must not lead to a decline in emphasis on the common allergy problems, if only because of the high incidence of allergy and the lack of appropriate care patients may receive.

This book has been written by a group of authors, who have worked together, either during their training period in Allergy, or as faculty members of the Allergy-Immunology Section of the Department of Medicine at Northwestern University Medical Center. Although they were selected because of their unified approach to teaching and clinical care in allergy, they have either trained or are currently working in other medical centers; so their opinions and approaches are not restricted to those of one small group.

Fifteen of the authors of this book have been supported in whole or in part during periods of research or clinical training by United States Public Health Service training or research grants to Northwestern University Medical Center. The Allergy Immunology Section has been supported in addition by the Ernest S. Bazley Grant to Chicago Wesley Memorial Hospital and Northwestern University Medical Center.

ROY PATTERSON, M.D.

Acknowledgments

We are grateful to the following pharmaceutical manufacturers for their generous support in helping to defray the cost of the color plates appearing in this book: Parke, Davis and Co.; Smith, Kline and French Laboratories; Schering Corp.; Hollister-Stier Laboratories; Center Laboratories, Inc. and Greer Laboratories.

Furthermore, we are indebted to MEDCOM, Inc., for permission to base certain paragraphs in some of our chapters upon material originally prepared for the MEDCOM UPDATE SERIES.

Contents

Contents

In Memory of
ERNEST S. BAZLEY

1

Classification of Hypersensitivity Reactions

James D. Lakin, PH.D., M.D.

The rapid expansion of the immunologic literature has been apparent to immunologists and to interested clinicians who have found this area relevant to their own fields of interest. It is the purpose of this chapter to review briefly some of the more recent and significant findings of immunology and immunochemistry as they relate to the subject of clinical hypersensitivity phenomena. Obviously such a broad subject does not permit detailed examination, and throughout this discussion the reader is referred to a number of excellent review articles which have recently appeared.

Clinical allergy or hypersensitivity processes embrace a wide range of disease states including such diverse entities as bronchial asthma, a number of dermatologic disorders, the connective tissue syndromes, transplantation, tumor and auto-immunity. However, throughout this seeming potpourri of clinical and pathological entities, a common denominator of pathophysiology must be either objectively demonstrable or reasonably inferred: allergy or hypersensitivity is immunologically mediated, through interaction of antigen, of exogenous or endogenous origin, with specific humoral antibodies or specifically sensitized lymphocytes. The consequences of this interaction may be quite diverse, accounting for a variety of clinical manifestations.

Historically the definition of allergy has been based on the acquisition by the individual of an altered reactivity to a normally innocuous substance. This older concept has been shown not to be strictly applicable to clinical observation. For example, allergic rhinitis due to reaginic antibody against ragweed pollen is an immunologically mediated disease. However, a very similar clinical picture occurs in vasomotor rhinitis due to increased reactivity of the microvasculature to cold temperatures. In the first instance the reaction is immunologic; in the second, idiosyncratic. In other situations the differentiation of the immunologic from the nonimmunologic may be even more difficult. Indeed with increasingly sensitive techniques for the detection of immunoglobulin and antibody activity, a number of diseases, such as ulcerative colitis, pernicious anemia and some forms of hepatitis, are being associated with the presence of immunoglobulin (presumably antibody) deposits in the area of pathology. In some cases, however, these presumed auto-allergic processes are results rather than causes of the basic lesion of the disease, merely representing a secondary response of the immune system to tissue breakdown. The classification of hypersensitivity diseases has often proved to be as problematic as the differentiation of the allergic from the nonallergic. The traditional subdivisions of immediate and delayed allergy are inadequate to encompass the quite diverse reactions accepted as manifestations of hypersensitivity. Classification according to antigen type, as in drug allergy, or according to organ involvement has produced the grouping of rather dissimilar conditions in common company.

As more basic immunologic data has been correlated with clinical experience, a workable system of general classification has been produced.[30] It is based on four general reaction types originally proposed by Gell and Coombs. Type I hypersensitivity is mediated by reaginic antibody which is predominately, if not exclusively, of the IgE class in man (anaphylaxis and allergy). Type II hypersensitivity reactions are produced by reaction of antibody with cell-bound antigen followed secondarily by complement fixation. Type III reactions are effected by soluble antigen-antibody complex deposition at a reaction site (toxic-complex reactions). Following complex formation, complement fixation occurs mediating many of the biologic consequences of Type III reactions. Type IV reactions (delayed or cellular hypersensitivity) refer to that group of allergic disorders caused by the reaction of specifically sensitized small lymphocytes with antigen. The remainder of this chapter will be devoted to a more detailed examination of these reaction types.

TYPE I OR ANAPHYLACTIC REACTIONS

The first type of hypersensitivity reaction considered in the Gell and Coombs classification is termed anaphylactic hypersensitivity. This reaction group is also referred to as immediate type hypersensitivity (atopy or allergy) or reaginic hypersensitivity. The clinical conditions in which Type I hypersensitivity appears to play a role include extrinsic bronchial asthma, seasonal allergic rhinitis or hayfever, some cases of urticaria, certain food and drug allergies, reactions to stinging insects, systemic anaphylaxis and possibly atopic dermatitis or eczema. The mediation of these reactions is accomplished by a distinct group of antibodies termed reagin, or skin-sensitizing antibodies. The work of Ishizaka and others has demonstrated that the majority, if not all reaginic activity in humans is confined to a class of immunoglobulins separate from the better characterized IgG, IgM, IgA and IgD categories. Antibody of this immunoglobulin class, IgE, has been shown to possess the classic characteristics of reagin.[39] Reagin can circulate in serum or bind to certain cells including those of the respiratory or gastrointestinal mucosa or circulating leukocytes. Unlike most other antibodies, its biologic activity is destroyed upon heating to 56° C. It does not cross the placental barrier. When cell-bound reagin combines with antigen, it initiates the characteristic events of immediate type allergy within minutes. Histamine, slow reacting substance and possibly kinins (discussed in succeeding sections) are thought to be released by human reagin-bearing cells causing vasodilation, increased capillary permeability and smooth muscle contraction. This in turn leads to the clinical manifestations of urticaria, angioedema, hypotension, bronchospasm, spasm of gastrointestinal musculature or uterine contractions, depending on the location and severity of the reaction.

The IgE class of immunoglobulins which possess reaginic activity has been found to have a molecular weight of approximately 200,000 and a sedimentation coefficient of 8S. With the discovery of the IgE type of myeloma, structural studies of the protein have been possible. Prior to the availability of these IgE myelomas, the normal concentrations of IgE of from 6 to 780 nanograms per ml. had technically precluded such investigations.[43, 66, 34] In common with the other immunoglobulins, IgE molecules are composed of two light chains of either kappa or lambda type. Its heavy chains are antigenically unique to IgE, being termed epsilon chains. IgE is a glycoprotein, its epsilon chain containing a very large amount of the sulfur-containing amino acids, methionine and cystine. Although IgE can sensitize both human and monkey skin, it will not sensitize guinea pig skin. Complement fixation by IgE antibodies has not been detected, consistent with the lack of complement fixation and anaphylatoxin formation observed in Type I reactions. Further structural studies have revealed that the Fc portion of the IgE molecule contains the structures essential for attaching to the cell sites. Binding of reaginic antibody to cells has been shown to be inhibited by pretreatment of the cells with Fc fragment.

The IgE molecule has been show to contain two antigen binding sites, and thus IgE is divalent in analogy to IgG. However, it has been further noted that two IgE molecules are required for the formation of skin reactive complexes. It has been suggested that induction of skin reactive properties by the formation of cell-bound, antigen-antibody complexes may involve interaction between the IgE antibody molecules, structural changes in the molecules or both. The induction of this allosteric phenomenon by combination with antigen may effect the cell membrane in some manner, leading to the release of effector molecules (histamine, slow reacting substance etc.).[78]

In clinical practice, correlation of specific IgE type antibody with atopic disease has been suggested in a number of instances.[44, 74] It has been observed that IgE fixes to basophilic leukocytes and mast cells that can release mediators of inflammation upon exposure to specific antigen. A number of investigators have speculated regarding a protective function for IgE. In intestinal parasitic infestations markedly elevated levels of IgE have been documented although their significance is not known.[38, 45] A protective function for IgE in the respiratory tree has been suggested (10); however, more recent reports have failed to support a relation between increased susceptibility to sinopulmonary infection and a deficiency of IgE.[75] Indeed, IgE deficiency has been documented in a 28-year-old female in good health.[56] Further studies of the relation of IgE to the immune defenses are necessary before meaningful conclusions can be made.[34]

TYPE II OR CYTOTOXIC REACTIONS

The second major type of hypersensitivity reaction described in the classification of Gell and Coombs is termed cytotoxic or cytolytic. Alternately, this reaction group is referred to as complement dependent cytotoxicity. This should not be confused with Type IV reactions which also result in cytotoxicity, although by quite a different mechanism. Also, the distinction between Type II and Type III reactions should be stressed, each reaction pattern involving secondary complement fixation, after different primary reactions. The distinctive primary event of Type II reactions is that of antibody combining with an antigenic determinant which is present on tissue cells. The antigen may be part of the internal structure of the cell involved or it may be an exogenous antigen or hapten which is absorbed on or combined with tissue cells. Complement usually, but not always, is necessary to produce cellular damage.

The Complement System

It may be surmised that complement is an important effector system in vivo. It is involved in Type II reactions after combination of cell-bound antigen with antibody has occurred and in Type III reactions after deposition of antigen-antibody complexes at the reaction site has occurred.

The biologic consequences of the interaction of antigen, antibody and the complement system are diverse. Phenomena which have been described in vitro include immune adherence, anaphylatoxin production, leukocyte chemotaxis, and phagocytosis. Complement-dependent reactions in vivo include phagocytosis, immune hemolysis, nephrotoxic nephritis, serum sickness arteritis and nephritis and experimental immune vasculitis.

The complement system is composed of a group of serum proteins which, when reacting in combination, have the capacity of causing cell lysis. In addition to lysing erythrocytes, the classic laboratory model, complement may lyse a variety of mammalian and bacterial cells. Complement is also capable of participating in a number of non-cytolytic processes which may lead to indirect cell injury.[64]

The morphology of complement-dependent cytolysis is striking. Drastic changes resulting in cell death occur rapidly after introduction of antibody and fresh complement. Electron microscopy has revealed that the cell surface sustains "membrane holes" measuring 80 and 100 Ångstrom units in diameter. The production of these breaks in membrane integrity has been correlated with the light microscope findings of cell lysis.[13]

The definition of the biochemical events leading to these phenomena has been the result of investigation over much of this century, beginning with Ehrlich and Bordet. At least 11 different serum proteins have been shown to comprise the complement system. The majority of these factors have been isolated from serum and have been shown to comprise a group of molecules of relatively large size, their molecular weights ranging from 60,000 to 400,000. Electrophoretic mobility varies from fast alpha-globulin to slow gamma-globulin.[63] The complement components participating directly in immune hemolysis are denoted numerically, with the letter C preceding each. Thus, in the order of reaction, the C components are designated,

$$\text{C1qrs, C4, C2, C3, C5, C6, C7, C8, C9.}$$

C4 is the second reactant in sequence rather than C2, the first four complement components being numbered before their reaction sequence was known.[4] The first component of human complement is composed of three distinct subcomponent protein molecules to which the names C1q, C1r, and C1s have been given. Although the three subcomponents are separate proteins, they function as a unit occurring as a macromolecular complex in vivo, held together by calcium ions. In a Type II reaction, after combination of complement-fixing antibody with the specific antigenic determinant of the target cell membrane, C1 in turn combines with a receptor site on the antibody molecule. The site of combination of C1 (specifically C1q) with antibody is on the Fc portion of the heavy chain. The different immunoglobulin classes vary in their ability to fix C1q and, consequently, initiate immune cytolysis.[40] IgM is most effective on a molar basis, IgG being less so. IgA in monomer and polymer state appears not to fix C1q in any significant amount. Among the subclasses of IgG, IgG1, IgG3 and, to a lesser degree, IgG2 fix complement, while IgG4 does not.[41] Thus, C1q constitutes the functional link between antibody and the other complement components.

After attachment to antibody, C1s is converted from a proesterase to an enzymatically active esterase capable of activating the subsequently reacting complement components C4 and C2. The conversion of C1 esterase to its active form is regulated by another serum protein, C1 esterase inhibitor. The congenital absence of this functional regulator protein has been demonstrated to be associated with the clinical entity of hereditary angioneurotic edema.

Using standard nomenclature where A represents antibody; E, erythrocyte; S, a site of complement fixation, the reaction may thus far be written,

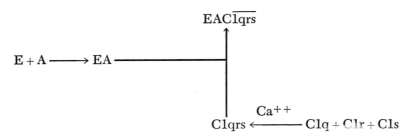

The bar placed over the affected components represents the acquisition of enzymatic or other biologic activity. The fourth component of complement attaches directly to the cell membrane after being activated by the esterase activity of C1s in its bound, activated form. Alternatively, if C4 does not collide with and bind to a suitable acceptor site on the cell membrane after its activation, C4 will spontaneously lose its state of activation with a rapid decay rate. Once inactivated, C4 is no longer a suitable substrate for C1 esterase and therefore cannot become reactivated. This is diagrammed, where the subscript i represents the loss of a defined activity by a complement component. After C4 is bound to a separate site, S, from that of AC1qrs, C2 is transferred from the fluid phase to the cell surface and activated by C1 esterase. C2 appears to be enzymatically cleaved in the process. A $\overline{C4,2}$ complex forms on the cell surface. With magnesium ion, this complex can activate C3, the next complement component.

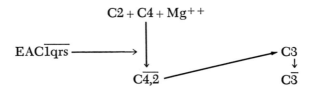

The active complex $\overline{C4,2}$ is in a dynamic equilibrium with C4 and C2 and with inactive C2. This may be represented,

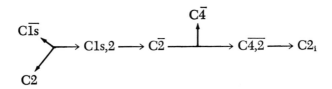

The conversion of C3 and $\overline{C3}$ entails a structural conversion enabling it to react with seperate cell membrane receptors. Thus, activated C3 is bound directly to the cell membrane and not to cell-bound $\overline{C4,2}$ which mediates its activation. $\overline{C3}$ will rapidly decay to C3i if membrane binding is not achieved. This is summarized,

$$\begin{array}{ccc} & \overline{C4,2} & \quad C3_i \\ & \downarrow & \nearrow \\ C3 \longrightarrow & \overline{C3}< \\ & & \searrow \\ & & S\overline{C3} \end{array}$$

One $\overline{C4,2}$ complex may catalyze the conversion of a number of C3 molecules, resulting in the circumferential distribution of SC3 sites about a single $\overline{C4,2}$ focus on the cell membrane.

The three following complement components, C5, C6, C7, react as a functionally interdependent unit. C5,6,7, acts on the erythrocyte membrane without being permanently bound. It is hypothesized that C5,6,7, after being activated by $\overline{C4,2,3}$, interacts with the cell surface causing chemical modification of a membrane site. The modified site is susceptible, to attack by the two lysis-producing components of complement, C8 and C9. In addition to being necessary reactants prior to lysis, C5,6,7 in the fluid phase has been shown to exert a strong chemotactic influence.[84]

Cells which have reacted with C1-7 still retain membrane integrity, lysing only after reaction with C8.[60] In causing membrane rupture, C8 reacts directly with the cell surface. C9 combines with C8, apparently enhancing the lytic effect of the latter. It is of interest that C9 may be substituted by the simple organic compounds phenanthroline and bipyridine in this function.[36] Both C8 and C9 are trace proteins in human serum.

Although cytolysis is the end result of the C1-9 reaction sequence, a number of other biologic phenomena are produced by intermediate complexes in the sequence of reactions. One such phenomenon, the elaboration of a chemotactic factor, has already been mentioned. This appears to be of significance in vivo in the pathogenesis of Type II and, as will be discussed later, Type III reactions. The action of leukocyte lysosomal enzymes on substrate tissue and on the kinin system described further on in this chapter, leads to target cell injury.[86]

Complement intermediates can also mediate histamine liberation, apparently through a biochemical process distinct from the histamine liberation produced by Type I reactions. When $\overline{C4,2}$ acts on C3, histamine liberators are formed, presumably representing split products of native C3. This split product of C3 also has been shown to have chemotactic properties in addition to acting as an opsonin, enhancing phagocytic activity. In a similar fashion, C1,4,2,3 has been shown to cleave a fragment from C5 in the process of the latter's activation. This C5 split product has histamine-liberating and permeability-enhancing activity in addition to chemotactic activity distinct from that of the trimolecular C5,6,7 complex. These C3 and C5 split products, designated C3a and C5a, respectively, have been shown to be identical to anaphylatoxin. The latter substance is known to produce systemic reactions in laboratory animals closely mimicking Type I systemic anaphylaxis mediated by IgE. C3a can be produced from C3 by trypsin and plasmin, in addition to C1,4,2 (C3 convertase).[15]

The clinical significance of the complement system in normal body defense mechanisms has recently been demonstrated in the reports of several patients deficient in functional complement components. Alper et al.[2] have described a patient with Kleinfelter's syndrome with a defect in C3 stability resulting in low serum concentrations of C3 with increased $C3_i$. Clinically the patient presented with repeated infections, primarily with pyogenic organisms, from the first year of life. All known aspects of immunity were intact except for those mediated by the complement system. Miller and Nilsson have related a familial deficit of the phagocytosis-enhancing activity of serum to a dysfunction of the fifth component of complement.[61] Members of this family with increased susceptibility to gram negative bacteria and coagulase positive staphylococci in local and systemic infections were shown to have deficiency of phagocytosis enhancement correctable by highly purified C5.

Clinical Examples of Type II Reactions

Of the diverse clinical entities which appear to have Type II reactions as a basis for their pathophysiology, two subgroups may be distinguished. In the first group, complement-fixing antibody is directed against an antigenic determinant on the cell membranes of various tissues in the patient. In the second group, the antigenic determinant is exogenously introduced, becoming intimately associated with the patient's tissue. In this way, the exogenous antigen acts as a hapten in combining with complement-fixing antibody. Included in the first group are transfusion reactions due to antibody reacting with red cells, white cells and platelets. The clinical consequences of intravascular hemolysis, pyrogen release and febrile reactions are well known. Hemolytic disease of the newborn and iso-allergic neonatal thrombocytopenia are other Type II reactions involving antepartum transfers of cytolytic maternal antibody into the neonate's circulation. Also complement-dependent in its pathogenesis is auto-immune (or auto-allergic) hemolytic anemia. This may be observed clinically as an isolated entity or as a secondary manifestation of systemic auto-allergy as in systemic lupus erythematosus (SLE). In SLE both Type II and Type III reactions appear to be occurring in the diverse target organs involved in the active case. The etiologic or pathophysiologic significance of this is still not completely clear, however. Other auto-allergic diseases seem to be at least in part produced through Type II reactions. For example, in chronic thyroiditis in the human and experimentally induced thyroiditis in the monkey antibodies to antigen located in the microsomal fraction of the cytoplasm of the epithelial cells lining the follicles have been characterized. These antibodies are cytotoxic and are thought to be involved in tissue destruction in vivo.

Acute poststreptococcal glomerulonephritis has long been considered by some to be an example of Type II auto-allergy to renal glomerular basement membrane. One current theory maintains that nephritogenic strains of Group A beta-hemolytic streptococci possess antigenic determinants which cross react with those present on human glomerular basement membrane. Antibody produced in response to the invading streptococci is thought to react with the patient's glomeruli, producing a linear distribution of antibody on the basement membrane. The antibody in turn fixes complement, leading to the characteristic inflammatory reaction.[1] This type of nephritis should be distinguished from that involving accumulation of antigen-antibody complexes in an irregular distribution along the basement membrane in a Type III reaction, described below.

The role of humoral antibodies in human allograft rejection has received recent attention with current widespread activity in transplantation. Early work in transplantation immunology had led investigators to conclude that homografts were relatively resistant to humoral antibodies and that graft destruction was primarily mediated by Type IV, delayed hypersensitivity. The rather extensive experience of the past decade in kidney transplantation has tended to support this view in the majority of instances. However, it has occasionally been noted that destruction of grafted kidneys in man may occur within hours or even minutes of transplantation. This type of rejection has been related to the presence in the recipient of humoral antibody capable of reacting with donor tissues, presumably in a complement-fixing reaction with antigens of the vascular endothelium resulting in acute vasculitis.[42] Reexamination of long term renal allografts has also suggested that Type II and III reactions involving humoral antibodies may be operative in chronic rejection, superimposed on a longstanding reaction of delayed hypersensitivity.

In cardiac transplantation, acute rejection occurring from 7 to 18 days after grafting has been thought to involve circulating antibodies, perhaps acquired through presensitization. Delayed hypersensitivity is also operative in cardiac rejection.[59]

Type II reactions stimulated by an exogenous antigenic determinant appear to occur in some instances of drug allergy. It is thought that a number of pharmacologic agents, in attaching themselves to the formed elements of the blood, act as haptens in inducing formation of complement-fixing lytic antibodies. Subsequent cell lysis then produces the clinical pictures of thrombocytopenic purpura, hemolytic anemia, agranulocytosis, or pancytopenia. For example, a Coombs-positive hemolytic anemia is occasionally seen as a side effect of the administration of the anti-hypertensive agent alpha-methyldopa. After withdrawal of the drug, which is thought to bind to red cell membrane as a hapten, the anemia usually resolves.

TYPE III OR TOXIC-COMPLEX REACTIONS

The third major type of hypersensitivity is the toxic-complex reaction. This category of allergic phenomenon is alternatively termed soluble-complex- or immune-complex hypersensitivity. In each instance the term "complex" refers to the antigen-antibody aggregates which are the mediators of Type III reactions. Experimental and clinical examples include the Arthus reaction, experimental and clinical serum sicknesses, certain of the glomerulonephritides and some drug reactions.[25] The basic mechanism of toxic complex disease involves the introduction of antigen either locally or systemically in relatively large quantities (in contrast to Type I reactions which may require exquisitely small amounts of antigen in a highly sensitive individual). Antibody is produced, or is preexistent in such proportion as to form soluble antigen-antibody complexes upon reaction with antigen. These complexes in turn fix complement which induces PMN migration, phagocytosis and release of permeability factors and protease from the PMN. The clinical picture of an acute inflammatory reaction, often a vasculitis, results.

The Quantitative Precipitin Reaction

Essential to the understanding of complex formation is consideration of the quantitative precipitin reaction. A precipitin is a general term for any antibody mixture which, upon incubation with antigen, forms a precipitate. If increasing amounts of antigen are added to test tubes containing a constant amount of antibody-containing antiserum and the total mass of the resulting precipitate is measured, a curve such as is depicted in Figure 1-1 is generated by plotting total mass of precipitate as a function of amount of antigen added. Initially, as increasing antigen is added, all of the antigen and increasing amounts of the antibody precipitate. This region of the curve is termed the zone of antibody excess. Finally, a point is reached where all antibody is brought down into the precipitate in combination with all of the antigen. This maximum on the curve is termed the zone of equivalence. However, as more antigen is added to the system, increasing the ratio of antigen to antibody, the amount of observable precipitate decreases. This region of the curve is termed the zone of antigen excess. If the supernatants of these test tubes in antigen excess are examined, it is found that soluble antigen-antibody complexes with a high ratio of antigen to antibody are present. The lattice theory of Marrack has been utilized to explain this phenomenon (Fig. 1-2). Whereas most precipitable antigenic proteins and polysaccharides contain multiple reactive antigenic

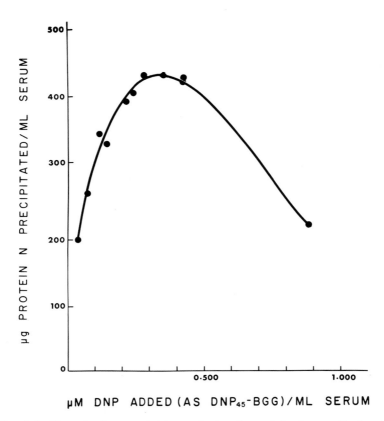

Fig. 1-1. Quantitative precipitin analysis of precipitating antibody obtained from rhesus monkeys immunized to dinitro-phenol (DNP). The antigen used in the test system is dinitrophenyl-bovine gamma globulin (DNP_{45}-BGG). (Reprinted from Lakin, J. D., Patterson, R. and Pruzanski, J. J.: Immunoglobulins of the rhesus monkey *(Macaca mulatta)* I. J. Immunol., 98:745, 1967 by permission of The Williams & Wilkins Co.).

determinants on the surface of the molecule, the majority of antibody is bivalent, containing only two antigen-combining sites per molecule. Indeed, most precipitin-containing hyperimmune sera are composed of IgG type antibody, which is entirely bivalent. In a region of equivalent quantities of antigen and antibody, the formation of multiple bridges by antibody from antigen to antigen molecule is accomplished with ease, creating a relatively large and consequently precipitable crystaloid aggregate. In antigen excess, relatively few bivalent antibody molecules are available for bridging polyvalent antigen molecules to each other. This is thought to decrease the extent of crystalloid formation, creating

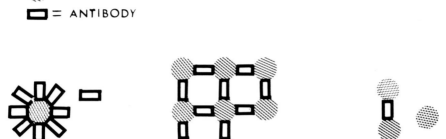

= ANTIGEN

= ANTIBODY

ANTIBODY
EXCESS

EQUIVALENCE

ANTIGEN
EXCESS

Fig. 1-2. The lattice theory of Marrack is graphically presented, depicting antigen-antibody complexes in antibody excess, equivalence and antigen excess. See text description, The Quantitative Precipitin Reaction.

smaller, more hydrophilic antigen-antibody complexes. The precipitin reaction and lattice theory are more fully explained in standard texts of immunology.[14, 46]

Activities of Antigen-Antibody Complexes in Vivo

The in vivo behavior of these antigen-antibody complexes is significant in that complexes formed in antibody excess and at equivalence are rapidly cleared from the circulation by the phagocytes of the reticulo-endothelial system (RES). In contrast, the smaller, soluble antigen-antibody complexes formed in antigen excess persist longer in the circulation, since they are less readily phagocytized by the RES. In consequence, localization of complexes at the glomerular basement membrane or other target organs may occur. These localized complexes are capable of fixing complement in the sequence described in the discussion of Type II reactions. C3 and C5 split products and trimolecular C5,6,7 are generated. These molecules in turn exert a number of biological influences including kinin activation, chemotaxis, increase of vascular permeability and histamine release.

There has been some speculation that complement and, perhaps, soluble antigen-antibody complexes themselves activate the kallikrein–kinin system in the course of the pathogenesis of some Type II and Type III reactions. The kallikrein system is considered to be the final common pathway effector system in a variety of inflammatory reactions both immunologic and nonimmunologic.[76] The end product effector molecules, kinins, are a family of structurally similar octapeptides to decapeptides having the common property of inducing vasodilation, increased vascular permeability, pain and hypotension. Kinins are released from alpha-2-plasma globulin (kininogen) through the action of a proteolytic enzyme present in serum, kallikrein. Like blood coagulation, the kinin-generating system is initiated by activation of factor XII (Hageman factor). Active factor XII then converts plasma kallikreinogen (or prekallikrein) into the active enzyme. Kallikrein then cleaves kininogen to release the vasoactive polypeptide, bradykinin. This reaction sequence is normally regulated at each step by clearance of Hageman Factor, inactivation of kallikrein by its plasma inhibitor which appears to be identical to plasma C1 esterase inhibitor, and destruction of kinin by kininase, respectively.[18] Although the precise mechanism by which the humoral immune mechanism interacts with the kallikrein system remains to be elucidated, it seems that antigen-antibody complexes might directly activate it through Hageman factor and that C1-7 may also act on the kinin-releasing mechanism.[47]

Polymorphonuclear leukocyte infiltration is indispensable to the production of immune-complex mediated tissue injury. After being attracted to the site of a Type III reaction, infiltrating PMN's have been shown to ingest complexes, degranulate and release the contents of their lysosomal granules. These in turn act as even more powerful chemotactic agents and mediators of increased vascular permeability. The most destructive components released are proteolytic enzymes which directly attack tissue involved in the reaction.[35] It may be concluded that immune complexes may induce intense inflammatory reactions through the initiation of a complex and incompletely understood chain of biochemical events producing a number of effector molecules.

Experimental Type III Reactions

The classic laboratory example of Type III reactions is the Arthus reaction. It was originally observed by Arthus and Breton that repeated injection of horse serum into rabbits over a period of several days leads to a reaction at subsequent injection sites characterized by infiltration, edema, sterile abscess and, in severe reactions, gangrene. Microscopically, arteriolar contraction occurs followed by massive infiltration of PMN's which clump in, and eventually occlude, arteriolar lumina. Endothelial necrosis which follows may extend through the vessel wall. Fluid and blood cell exudation into the surrounding tissue results. Necrosis may occur due to microinfarction mediated by PMN clumping. Thus a picture of hemorrhagic necrosis results.

Consistent with the proposed mechanism of Type III reactions, precipitating antibody present in the animal's circulation was found to be an essential requirement for the Arthus reaction. Large amounts of antigen injected locally intensified the reaction by driving the local precipitin reaction into antigen excess. Injection of preformed soluble immune complexes will also lead to the characteristic local Type III reaction.[14]

The systemic analogue of the local Type III reaction of the Arthus phenomenon is experimental serum sickness.[25] It may be produced in rabbits by repeated injection of large amounts of an appropriate antigen, e.g., heterologous serum proteins. After injection of a suitably tagged heterologous protein, the foreign material will be gradually eliminated from the circulation by the RES, following a period of equilibration. This is reflected in the initial gradual downslope of the antigen concentration curve in Figure 1-3.*

Immune elimination of the antigen is shown by a sudden increase in the down slope of the antigen concentration curve in Figure 1-3. After all antigen is eliminated from the circulation, free antibody can be detected. This is preceded by a period of several days during which antigen is being rapidly eliminated and circulating antigen-antibody complexes are detectable in serum.

For many animals the period of "immune elimination" is benign. Complexes in such animals are found to be composed predominately of antibody on a molecular basis. This is analogous to those complexes precipitated in the zone of antibody excess in the quantitative precipitin reaction. However, some animals will demonstrate signs of systemic toxicity with inflammatory lesions being observed in the heart, arteries, kidneys and joints. The onset of this process correlates with the appearance of circulating soluble immune complexes. These circulating complexes differ from those of asymptomatic rabbits in that they are composed predominately of antigen and are thus analogous to those antigen-antibody complexes found in the supernatant in the antigen-excess zone of the quantitative precipitin reaction in vitro. Localization of antigen, antibody and complement has been demonstrated in the heart, correlating with endocardial, myocardial and epicardial inflammation. Their deposition in arterial endothelium is also observed with focal inflammation and fibrinoid necrosis resulting. On the kidney basement membrane irregular antigen-antibody-complement deposition causes a glomerulonephritis manifested by endothelial proliferation of the glomerular capillaries and basement membrane thickening. Immune-complex deposition in synovial tissue leads to focal inflammatory infiltrates, edema and fibrinoid formation.[32]

---

* Although the graph shown in Figure 3 is taken from work done in our laboratories with rhesus monkeys, its form is quite similar to that seen with the rabbits used in the classical experimental serum sickness model, and is therefore presented.

From these studies of experimental immune-complex disease it has become apparent that exogenous or perhaps endogenous circulating antigen-antibody complexes may result in severe and extensive systemic toxicity. The environmental and/or genetic factors operative in the predisposition to this state of altered reactivity remain to be defined.

Clinical Type III Reactions

The pathogenesis of serum sickness in the human is considered to be similar to that of the experimental model described. The entity in its classic form is observed much less frequently today than in former times when the use of heterologous serum, such as equine tetanus antitoxin, was more prevalent in clinical practice. The four cardinal manifestations of this disease are skin lesions, fever, joint symptoms and lymphadenopathy. Similar symptoms occur in certain cases of drug allergy. For example, in some instances of pencillin allergy, it has been suggested that the drug may be acting as a serum protein-bound hapten, in this capacity eliciting a Type III allergic response. A similar reaction presenting the characteristic features of a generalized hypersensitivity angiitis [10] has been reported with the use of pertussis vaccine.

A number of clinicopathologic entities are associated with necrotizing angiitis. Speculation has been made that a Type III auto-allergy may be operative in such diseases as allergic granulomatous angiitis, rheumatic arteritis, periarteritis nodosa and temporal arteritis.[16] Although these inferences may appear consistent with the pathologic processes observed in these conditions, no conclusive statements can be made.

A number of diseases possibly related to toxic complexes are in the category of connective tissue disorders. It should be stressed that the etiology of such diseases as systemic lupus erythematosus, polyarteritis nodosa and rheumatoid arthritis are unknown. A great deal of presumptive evidence has accumulated, however, suggesting at least a partial role for immune mechanisms in their pathogenesis. One of the major entities in this group with respect to clinical prevalence and clinical investigation is systemic lupus erythematosus (SLE). The syndrome characteristically involves multiple systems. Nephritis, arthritis, serositis, dermatitis and blood cytopenias are variably observed.[16] Death in these patients is usually secondary to nephritis and chronic renal insufficiency. Numerous studies of the histopathology of lupus nephritis have demonstrated the microscopic picture of chronic nephritis involving glomerular capillary loops and basement membranes associated with irregular desposition of anti-nuclear protein antibody, nucleoprotein and complement.[48, 49]

Anti-nuclear antibodies have been detected with frequency in systemic rheumatic disease and scleroderma. These factors have been

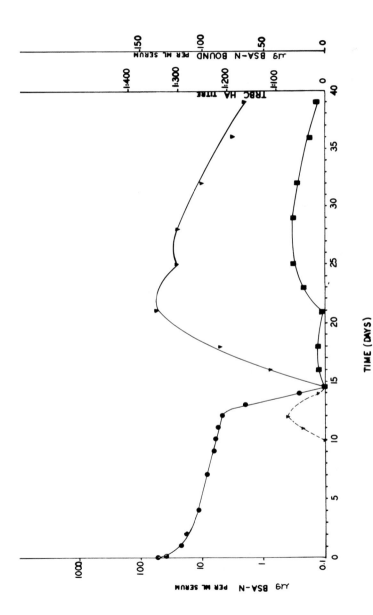

Fig. 1-3. The primary response of a rhesus monkey to the injection of bovine serum albumin (BSA). Serum concentration of BSA (●—●), circulating BSA; anti-BSA antigen-antibody complexes (▲--▲), anti-BSA hemagglutinating antibody titers (■—■) and BSA-binding activity (▲—▲), a measure of total serum antibody activity, are plotted as a function of time. (Reprinted from Lakin, J. D., Patterson, R., and Pruzansky, J. J.: Immunoglobulins of the rhesus monkey (*Macaca mulatta*) IV. J. Immunol., *103*:577, 1969; by permission of the Williams & Wilkins Co.).

shown to be present in four classes of immunoglobulins: IgG, IgA, IgM and IgD. Their significance in pathogenesis of these phenomena is the subject of current investigation.[70]

A renal picture similar to that of SLE has been noted in nephrosis accompanying quartan malarial infection and in some cases of subacute and chronic glomerulonephritis and membranous glomerulonephritides of adults and children. Irregular deposition of antigen, antibody and complement on the basement membrane appears to be a common denominator of their pathophysiology.[26]

Finally, in the field of renal allograft rejection, recent reports have indicated that the hyperacute form of rejection may involve an Arthus-like reaction in the renal parenchymal arterioles.[65] This is in contrast to the Type II and IV mechanisms of allergic reactivity operative in the acute and chronic renal rejection processes.

TYPE IV OR CELLULAR HYPERSENSITIVITY

The fourth major category of allergic reactions is that of "delayed" or "cellular" hypersensitivity. These two synonymous terms are derived from two unique attributes of this type of reaction. First, a twenty-four to seventy-two hour delay occurs in onset of the reaction after exposure of a sensitized individual to specific antigen. Second, delayed hypersensitivity is not mediated by the conventional circulating antibodies previously considered in the discussion. Rather, specifically "sensitized" small lymphocytes are the agents which directly interact with antigen and effect the characteristic reaction. The ontologic development of "these" lymphocytes appears to be thymus dependent.

Delayed hypersensitivity is involved in a diversity of clinical phenomena, including contact dermatitis, tuberculin hypersensitivity, allograft transplantation [9] and tumor immunity.[31] In spite of the importance of cellular hypersensitivity in immunologic phenomena, knowledge of the cellular and molecular mechanisms involved in this process have only recently been forthcoming.[51] Therefore, many of the current conclusions regarding cellular hypersensitivity are tentative.

Morphology

The gross morphology of a delayed reaction is rather undistinguished. After intradermal injection of antigen into a sensitized host, no reaction is visible for 5 to 24 hours. Erythema and induration of the site then supervene, usually reaching maximum intensity by 16 to 72 hours. The degree of induration is indicative of the extent of cellular infiltration occurring within the skin. Induration is considered to be the most characteristic process of this reaction type. More intense reactions may be accompanied by regional lymphadenopathy with or without necrosis at the site of antigen injection. Systemic reaction may occur with fever, generalized lymphadenopathy and lymphopenia.

The histopathology of delayed hypersensitivity is generally characteristic in its sequence of development. Similar reaction patterns are noted in skin or parenchymous organs although temporal and morphologic relations vary with different antigens, their dosage and local conditions. The prototype of this phenomenon is the delayed reaction to tuberculin purified protein derivative or tubercle bacilli. When either of these materials is introduced into the skin of a sensitive recipient, no reaction is observed for as long as 24 hours, aside from a variable accumulation of fluid and polymorphonuclear leukocytes. These cells may phagocytize antigen, but they are not bactericidal to viable tubercle bacilli. By 24 hours the PMN's are replaced in the main by mononuclear cells, predominately macrophages or monocytes with occasional small lymphocytes. This process of macrophage accumulation may persist for 6 to 12 days or more, creating a diffuse round cell infiltrate. Coalescence of macrophages to form giant cells is characteristic of tuberculin reactivity. In severe reactions necrosis of the central portion of the lesion may be seen in several days, with variable degrees of caseation or liquefaction supervening.[82]

Antigen Interaction

A variety of substances can act as antigens in elicitation of delayed hypersensitivity much as in the case with circulating humoral antibodies. Proteins, polysaccharides, mucopolysaccharides and simple organic chemicals have all been documented participants in this reaction pattern. It is presumed that low-molecular weight simple organic chemicals must combine with a protein or polysaccharide carrier before becoming immunogenic. The carrier molecule may be of exogenous origin, as in experimental systems, or endogenous origin, as, for example, skin proteins in contact dermatitis. A covalent bond with proteins present in the skin must be formed before such a hapten-like substance may be immunogenic.[27] Using such hapten-carrier conjugates it has been demonstrated that the immunological specificity of delayed hypersensitivity is directed not only to the hapten but to the adjacent portions of the carrier molecule.[77] In contrast, Arthus and passive cutaneous anaphylaxis reactions do not demonstrate this great a degree of carrier protein reactivity. It seems then that the site on the serum antibody molecule which combines with antigen reacts with a smaller area of the antigen molecule than does the analogous site in cellular hypersensitivity reactions.[6] Although it is known that the degree of specificity in a reaction of antigen and circulating antibody is determined by the structure of the antigen-combining site on the immunoglobulin molecule, the identity and characteristics of the combining site on the small lymphocyte in delayed reactions are not as well described.[37]

Immunochemistry

The cellular and molecular events operative in the production of delayed hypersensitivity reactions have been the subject of considerable recent investigation.[54] Much of the resultant information has been obtained from the study of in-vitro correlates of the classic in-vivo delayed reaction. These include lymphocyte blast transformation, transfer factor, macrophage inhibition and cytotoxic reactions in vitro.[55]

The initial cellular event observed when thymus-dependent small lymphocytes from an individual demonstrating delayed hypersensitivity are incubated with specific antigen is "blast" or "lymphocyte" transformation. Morphologically, the small lymphocyte transforms into a larger lymphoblast identical in appearance to the pyroninophilic lymph node cells which appear after antigen stimulation in vivo. Correlating with these morphologic alterations, an increased rate of histone acetylation occurs, followed by increase in the rates of protein, RNA and DNA synthesis leading to mitosis of the transforming lymphocyte.[67]

Although it was initially claimed that blast transformation closely correlated with the cellular but not the humoral immune response, further investigation has shown that specific lymphocyte transformation activity may be detected in the circulating cells of immunized animals with no apparent delayed hypersensitivity.[57] Likewise, the lymphocytes of patients with immediate (Type I) allergy to a variety of antigens will exhibit similar blast transformation activity with or without concomitant in vivo delayed hypersensitivity.[33] Furthermore, lymphocyte transformation may be nonspecifically induced by a variety of stimulants including phytohemagglutinin, staphylococcal filtrate and streptolysin S.

The mechanism of blast transformation may not be identical in immunospecific and nonspecific reactions.[67] It has therefore been assumed that blast transformation occurs in both cellular and humoral responses.[8] It does appear that those lymphocytes engaged in the synthesis of circulating antibody are more pluripotent in their capacity to form multiple immunoglobulin classes and allotypic specificities than are antibody-producing plasma cells. The suggestion has been made that "uncommitted" lymphocytes may be even less differentiated in that they may participate in either cellular reactions or circulating antibody synthesis.[68]

Transfer Factor. Although the cell population which produces the small lymphocyte of delayed hypersensitivity is not clearly defined, once that lymphocyte is committed to the delayed reaction, metabolic activity is accelerated. There is uncertainty regarding the exact events occurring during this period of increased cellular activity; however, several substances result as consequences of the delayed-type response. The biologic activities of these various effector molecules have in part been characterized.

One of the first of these materials to be described in association with the acquisition of specific hypersensitivity by the small lymphocyte was "transfer factor." This material was originally studied by Lawrence who reported that delayed cutaneous hypersensitivity can be transferred in man using the cell free extract of disrupted leukocytes obtained from an individual with cellular hypersensitivity to PPD.[52] Lawrence's transfer factor is unaffected by ribonuclease (RNase), deoxyribonuclease (DNase) or trypsin; is stable at $-20°C$ for five months; is dialyzable; and has a molecular weight of less than 10,000. In vitro transfer of sensitivity to cells in leukocyte cultures has been produced using a similar substance.[53]

Subsequently, a variety of transfer factors have been described which differ from the original material.[69] Baram, et al. have reported a dialyzable polynucleotide transfer factor with a 10,000 molecular weight and a second transfer factor with a 150,000 molecular weight consisting of protein and nucleic acid.[5] Thor and Dray have studied a high molecular weight RNA capable of converting "nonsensitive" human lymph node cells to "sensitive" cells as assayed by migration inhibition of human lymph node cells. This factor is sensitive to RNase.[79]

The mechanism by which these nucleotides or nucleoproteins might confer sensitivity is still at the level of speculation. One theory suggests that the RNA extract acts as a messenger, which codes for polypeptide synthesis. The resultant protein is hypothesized to be immunospecific for the antigen which originally induced the donor cells. While this would be feasible for a 150,000 molecular weight RNA, the smaller 10,000 molecular weight ribonucleotides could only code for 5 or 6 amino acids. Alternatively, the RNA transfer factors may not be informational molecules but, rather, may act as "adjuvants," functioning as carriers for "processed" antigen which could act as a highly potent immunogen capable of inducing nonsensitized cells.[69]

The system described above is thought to be analogous to the hypothesised role of RNA in cell-to-cell transfer of the capacity for humoral and antibody synthesis. RNA extracts from cells actively producing antibody have been shown to induce the synthesis of immunoglobulin in other, nonsensitized cells.[17, 29] Antigenic fragments have been variably reported in these extracts, it being equally unclear as to the informational or adjuvant nature of RNA extracts in the transfer of humoral antibody synthesis.[20, 22]

Macrophage Inhibiting Factor. The percentage of sensitized small lymphocytes in a delayed reaction is quite small, comprising as little as 2.5 per cent of the total cell population.[22] The bulk of cells appear to be nonspecific monocytes or nonsensitized lymphocytes. Presumably, it is these nonsensitized cells which comprise the majority of the infiltrate in the inflammatory reaction. The means by which a relatively small number of sensitized small lymphocytes might induce a massive cellular infiltrate at a given site following their contact with specific antigen has been the subject of considerable study.[20]

As early as 1932, it was reported that migration of cells from explanted fragments of spleen and bone marrow from tuberculin sensitive animals was inhibited by tuberculin. Over the ensuing years either destruction or stimulation of sensitive cells in the presence of antigen was reported in a variety of systems.[50] Quantitative study of the phenomenon was made possible by the development of a technique whereby migration from a capillary tube of peritoneal exudate cells obtained from sensitive donors could be measured. Originally, peritoneal macrophages were obtained from guinea pigs by injection of mineral oil into the abdominal cavity with collection of the resultant exudate several days later. The cells, when placed in a small bore capillary tube, were found to migrate out from its end forming a fanlike pattern. However, if tuberculin or other antigen to which the cell donor guinea pig had been sensitized was placed in the medium surrounding the capillary tube, the migration of the macrophages was inhibited. This was reflected by a decrease in the amount of fanning from the tip of the capillary tube.[21, 23]

The phenomenon of "macrophage inhibition" has been shown to be an in-vitro correlate of in-vivo delayed hypersensitivity.[24] The sensitive cell causing the inhibition of macrophage migration has been shown to be the lymphocyte.[11] These sensitized guinea pig lymphocytes in the presence of specific antigen produce a soluble factor which causes inhibition of migration of normal as well as sensitized guinea pig macrophages. This migration inhibiting factor is referred to as MIF. The relevance of MIF to human delayed hypersensitivity has been demonstrated by the finding that human peripheral blood lymphocytes, when incubated with specific antigen in vitro, also produce a soluble factor which inhibits the migration of normal guinea pig peritoneal exudate cells.[80] This has been shown to be a reproducible assay for delayed hypersensitivity in man. Its specificity for delayed hypersensitivity appears to be greater than that of blast transformation.[71]

The detection of MIF produced by human lymphocytes in response to antigen may prove to be a useful clinical tool. For example, it has been found that lymphocytes from patients with chronic mucocutaneous candidiasis and anergy fail to produce MIF when stimulated by *Candida* antigens. Antigen uptake into the patients' cells was normal.[71] Lymphocyte responses in-vitro of patients with immunologic deficiency diseases have further demonstrated the correlation of production of MIF with delayed hypersensitivity. Lymphocytes from agammaglobulinemic patients with normal delayed type hypersensitivity respond to specific antigenic challenge by the production of MIF. However, lymphocytes from patients who fail to manifest delayed hypersensitivity in vivo fail to produce MIF in response to challenge with antigen in vitro. Included in this latter group are patients with congenital thymic aplasia who regain their ability to produce MIF after thymic transplant.[72] Variations of the technique have been described [58] and their application to the measurement of homograft immunity has been described.[28] Also, tumor rejection has been associated with MIF production in certain cases.[54] Cellular immunity to fibroma virus correlates with the capacity of infected cell homogenates to inhibit migration of peritoneal exudate cells from fibroma-virus infected rabbits.[81]

The accumulation of macrophages at the site of an in vivo cellular hypersensitivity reaction appears to have its molecular basis in the elaboration of MIF. The same mechanism may be operative in the localization and massive diapedesis of mononuclear cells at the site of homograft reactions, contact dermatitis and experimental Type IV in vivo reactions such as auto-allergic encephalomyelitis and thyroiditis.[83] After localization by MIF, whese mononuclear cells then exert their cytotoxic effect, completing the reaction of cellular immunity.[73]

Cytotoxicity. This leads us to the final process in the chain of events producing Type IV reactions: cytotoxicity. Cell destruction by lymphoid cells occurs, in such diverse in vivo phenomena as homograft rejection, tumor immunity and autoimmune disease. Yet the study of the mechanism by which this is accomplished has been dependent on the development of in vitro systems. These have involved the culture of monolayers of so-called target cells, which are observed in their interaction with sensitized mononuclear cells.[62]

It has been noted that immunospecific cytolysis is composed of a sequence of distinct cellular events involving cell-to-cell adherence followed by biosynthesis and culminating in target cell lysis. First, adherence of sensitized lymphocyte effector cell membrane to target cell membrane has been observed to be a prerequisite for the reaction. In a suspension of fibroblasts and lymphoid cells obtained from a donor animal possessing delayed hypersensitivity to fibroblast antigens, lymphoid cells are noted to adhere in clusters to target (fibroblast) cells. The fibroblasts swell. Their motility decreases and the cell membrane ruptures. The most striking destruction is seen after 24 to 48 hours of incubation. The lymphoid cells mediating the reaction are mostly small and medium sized lymphocytes.

Many studies with various tumor-specific antigen systems have confirmed this selection of target cells by sensitized lymphocytes to be immunologically specific. The means by which specificity is obtained appears to be through selectivity in membrane attachment. For example, it has been observed that cytolysis is prevented by the addition of immune isoantiserum to cultures of sensitized lymphocytes and target cells, presumably by blocking antigenic sites on target cells.[28] The nature of the receptor site on the lymphocyte membrane which specifically reacts with the antigenic determinant on the target cell membrane is unknown. The suggestion that it is a cell-bound antibody or antibody-like structure is a longstanding one, although not uncontroversial.[7, 19] Target cell-lymphocyte adherence may be nonspecifically induced by the mitogen, phytohemagglutinin. Once this nonspecific membrane adherence is achieved, cytolysis may ensue.

After membrane adherence has occured, the lymphocyte engages in active biosynthesis resulting in the elaboration of materials causing cytolysis. Consistent with this is the observation that cellular integrity of the lymphocyte is necessary for a period of time after target cell attachment for cell lysis to occur. It appears that the events after attachment are not immunologically specific, specificity residing in the prior act of cell attachment.

It should be stressed that the cytolysis resulting from Type IV reactions is not complement dependent in contradistinction to Type II reactions. Rather, it is a quite distinct biologic process.[28]

Summary

To briefly summarize what has been said of the mechanisms of delayed hypersensitivity, contact of lymphocytes with antigen leads to blast transformation. Biosynthetic events leading to the creation of a "sensitized lymphocyte" ensue. A diversity of nucleic acid-antigen fragment agglomerates capable of transferring this sensitivity has been described. Upon recurrent contact with antigen, sensitized cells recruit other mononuclear cells to the reaction site through MIF production. Cytolysis of antigen-bearing cells may then occur through adherence of sensitized cells and elaboration of lytic factors. Immunologic memory for Type IV reactions appears to reside in a sub-class of small lymphocytes that are quite long-lived. These long-lived lymphocytes appear to retain for many years the ability to initiate the above described series of immunologic events upon contact with antigen.[31] Many gaps in our knowledge of this sequence of events are apparent and much of what has been presented should be regarded as hypothesis.[12]

REFERENCES

1. Adams, D. D.: A theory of the pathogenesis of rheumatic fever, glomerulonephritis and other autoimmune diseases triggered by infection. Clin. Exp. Immun. 5:105, 1969.
2. Alper, C. A., Abramson, N., Johnston, R. B., Jandl, J. H., and Rosen, F. S.: Increased susceptability to infection associated with abnormalities of complement-mediated functions and of the third component of complement (C3). New Eng. J. Med., 282:349, 1970.
3. Ammann, A. J., Cain, W. A., Ishizaka, K., Hong, R., and Good, R. A.: Immunoglobulin E deficiency in ataxia-telangiectasia. New Eng. J. Med., 281:469, 1969.
4. Austen, K. F., et al.: Nomenclature of complement. Int. Arch. Allerg., 37:661, 1970.
5. Baram, P., Yuan, L., and Mosko, M. M.: Studies on the transfer of human delayed-type hypersensitivity. I. Partial purification and characterization of two active components. J. Immun., 97:407, 1966.
6. Benacerraf, B., and Gell, P. G.: Immunological specificity of delayed and immediate hypersensitivity reactions. *In:* Grabar, P., and Moscher, eds.: Mechanisms of Cell and Tissue Damage Produced by Immune Reactions (Second International Symposium on Immunopathology). P. 136. Basel, Benne Schwabe and Co., 1962.
7. Benacerraf, B.: Cytophilic immunoglobulins and delayed hypersensitivity. Fed. Proc., 27:46, 1968.
8. Benezra, D., Gery, I., and Davies, A. M.: The relationship between lymphocyte transformation and immune responses. II. Correlations between transformation and humoral and cellular immune responses. Clin. Exp. Immun., 5:155, 1969.
9. Billingham, R. E.: The passenger cell concept in transplantation immunology. Cellular Immunology, 2:1, 1971.
10. Bishop, W. B., Carlton, R. G., and Sanders, L. L.: Diffuse vasculitis and death after immunization with pertussis vaccine. New Eng. J. Med., 274:606, 1966.
11. Bloom, B. R., and Bennett, B.: Migration inhibitory factor associated with delayed type hypersensitivity. Fed. Proc., 27:13, 1968.
12. Bloom, B. R. and Glade, P. R.: In Vitro Methods in Cell-Mediated Immunity. New York, Academic Press, 1971.
13. Borsos, T., Dourmasnkin, R. R., and Humphrey, J. H.: Lesions in erythrocyte membranes caused by immune hemolysis. Nature, 202:251, 1964.
14. Boyd, W. C.: Fundamentals of Immunology. ed. 4. New York, Interscience Publishers, 1966.

15. Budzko, D. B., and Muller-Eberhard, H. M.: Anaphylatoxin release form the third component of human complement by hydroxylamine. Science, *165*:506, 1969.
16. Christian, C. L.: Immune-complex disease. New Eng. J. Med., *280*:878, 1969.
17. Cohen, E. P.: Conversion of non-immune cells into antibody-forming cells by RNA. Nature, *213*:462, 1967.
18. Colman, R. W., Mason, J. W., and Sherry, S.: The kallikreinogen-kallikrein enzyme system of human plasma. Assay of components and observations in disease states. Ann. Intern. Med., *71*:763, 1969.
19. Daguillard, F., and Richter, M.: Cells involved in the immune response, XVI. The response of immune rabbit cells to phytohemaggulutinin, antigen and goat anti-rabbit immunoglobulin antiserum: J. Exp. Med., *131*:119, 1970.
20. David, J. R.: Macrophage migration. Fed. Proc., *27*:6, 1968.
21. David, J. R., Al-Askari, S., Lawrence, H. S. and Thomas, L.: Delayed hypersensitivity *in vitro*. I. The specificity of inhibition of cell migration by antigens. J. Immun., *93*:364, 1964.
22. Daivd, J. R., Lawrence, H. S., and Thomas, L.: Delayed hypersensitivity *in vitro*. II. Effects of sensitive cells on normal cells in the presence of antigen. J. Immun., *93*:274, 1964.
23. David, J. R., Lawrence, H. S., and Thomas, L.: Delayed hypersensitivity *in vitro*. III. The specificity of hapten-protein conjugates in the inhibition of cell migration. J. Immun., *93*:279, 1964.
24. David, J. R., and Schlossman, S. F.: Immunochemical studies on the specificity of cellular hypersensitivity. The *in vitro* inhibiting of peritoneal exudate cell migration by chemically defined antigens. J. Exp. Med., *128*:1451, 1968.
25. Dixon, F. J.: Experimental serum sickness. *In:* Samter, M., ed.: Immunological Diseases. p. 162. Boston, Little, Brown, and Co., 1965.
26. Dixon, F. J.: The pathogenesis of glomerulonephritis. Amer. J. Med., *44*:493, 1968.
27. Eisen, H. N., Orris, L., and Belman, S.: Elicitation of delayed allergic skin reactions with haptens: the dependence of elicitation on hapten combination with protein. J. Exp. Med., *95*:473, 1952.
28. Falk, R. E., Thorsby, E., Moller, E., and Moller, G.: *In vitro* assay of cell-mediated immunity: The inhibition of migration of sensitized human lymphocytes by HL-A antigens. Clin. Exp. Immun., *6*:445, 1970.
29. Fishman, M., and Adler, F. L.: Antibody formation initiated *in vitro*. II. Antibody synthesis in x-irradiated recipients of diffusion chambers containing nucleic acid derived from macrophages incubated with antigen. J. Exp. Med., *117*:595, 1963.
30. Gell, P. G. H. and Coombs, R. R. A., eds.: *Clinical Aspects of Immunology*. ed. 2. Philadelphia, F. A. Davis Co., 1969.

31. Gowans, J. L. and McGregor, D. D.: Immunologic activities of lymphocytes. Progr. Allerg., 9:1, 1965.

32. Germuth, F. G.: A comparative histological and immunologic study in rabbits of induced hypersensitivity of the serum sickness type. J. Exp. Med., 97:257, 1953.

33. Girard, J. P., Rose, N. R., Kunz, M. L., Kobayashi, S., and Arbasman, C. E.: *In vitro* lymphocyte transformation in atopic patients induced by antigens. J. Allerg., 39:65, 1967.

34. Gleich, G. J., Averbeck, A. K., and Swedlund, H. A.: Measurement of IgE in normal and allergic serum by radioimmunoassay. J. Lab. Clin. Med., 77:690, 1971.

35. Golub, E. S., and Sprotznagel, J. K.: The role of lysosomes in hypersensitivity reactions: tissue damage by polymorphonuclear neutrophil lysosomes. J. Immun., 95:1060, 1965.

36. Hadding, U., and Muller-Eberhard, H. J.: The ninth component of human complement: Isolation, description and mode of action. Immunology, 16:719, 1969.

37. Hill, W. C.: The antigen receptor in delayed-type hypersensitivity. I. and II. J. Immun., 106:414 and 421, 1971.

38. Hogarth-Scott, R. S., Johansson, S. G. O., and Bennich, H.: Antibodies to *Toxicara* in the sera of visceral larva migrans patients: The significance of raised levels of IgE. Clin. Exp. Immun., 5:619, 1969.

39. Ishizaka, K. and Ishizaka, T.: Biologic function of gamma-E antibodies and mechanisms of reaginic hypersensitivity: Clin. Exp. Immun., 6:25, 1970.

40. Ishizaka, T., Ishizaka, K., Borsos, T., and Rapp, H.: Complement fixation by human isoagglutinins: fixation of C'l by gamma G and gamma M but not by gamma A antibody. J. Immun., 97:716, 1966.

41. Ishizaka, T., Ishizaka, K., Salmon, S., and Fudenberg, H.: Biologic activities of aggregated gamma-globulin. VIII. Aggregated immunoglobulins of different classes. J. Immun., 99:82, 1967.

42. Jeannet, M., V. W., Flax, M. H., Winn, H. J., and Russell, P. S.: Humoral antibodies in renal allotransplantation in man. New Eng. J. Med., 282:111, 1970.

43. Johansson, S. G. O., and Bennich, H.: Immunologic studies of an atypical (myeloma) immunoglobulin. Immunology, 13:381, 1967.

44. Johansson, S. G. O., Bennich, H., Berg, T., and Hogman, C. F.: Some factors influencing the serum IgE levels in atopic diseases. Clin. Exp. Immun., 6:43, 1970.

45. Johansson, S. G. O., Mellbin, T., and Vahlquist, B.: Immunoglobulin levels in Ethiopian preschool children with special reference to high concentrations of immunoglobulin E (IgND). Lancet, 1:1118, 1968.

46. Kabat, E. A., and Mayer, M. M.: Experimental Immunochemistry. ed. 2. Springfield, Illinois, Charles C. Thomas, 1961.

47. Kellermeyer, R. W., and Graham, R. C., Jr.: Kinins—possible physiologic

and pathologic roles in man. New Eng. J. Med., *279:*754, 802, 859, 1968.

48. Krishnan, C., and Kaplan, M. H.: Immunopathologic studies of systemic lupus erythematosis. II. Antinuclear reaction of gamma-globulin eluted from homogenates and isolated glomeruli of kidneys from patients with lupus nephritis. J. Clin. Invest., *46:*569, 1967.

49. Koffler, D., Agnello, V., Carr, R. I., and Kunkel, H. G.: Variable patterns of immunoglobulin and complement deposition in the kidneys of patients with systemic lupus erythematosus, Amer. J. Path., *56:*305, 1969.

50. Lawrence, H. S. ed.: Cellular and Humoral Aspects of Hypersensitivity States. New York, Hoeber Medical Division, Harper & Bros., 1959.

51. Lawrence, H. S.: *In vitro* correlates of delayed hypersensitivity: introductory remarks. Fed. Proc., *27:*3, 1968.

52. Lawrence, H. S.: Some biological and immunological properties of transfer factor *In:* Wolstenholme, G. E. W., and O'Connor, M. ed.: CIBA Foundation Symposium: Cellular Aspects of Immunity. pp. 243-271. Boston, Little, Brown & Co., 1959.

53. Lawrence, H. S.: Transfer factor. Advances Immun., *11:*195, 1969.

54. Lawrence, H. S.: Transfer factor and cellular immune deficiency disease. New Eng. J. Med., *283:*411, 1970.

55. Lawrence, H. S., and Landy, M., eds.: Mediators of Cellular Immunity. New York, Academic Press, 1969.

56. Levy, D. A., and Chen, J.: Healthy IgE-deficient person. New Eng. J. Med., *283:*541, 1970.

57. Loewi, G., Temple, A., and Vischer, T. L.: The immunologic significance in the guinea pig of *in vitro* transformation of lymph node, spleen and peripheral blood lymphocytes. Immunology, *14:*257, 1968.

58. Lolekha, S., Dray, S., and Gotoff, S. P.: Macrophage aggregation *in vitro:* A correlate of delayed hypersensitivity. J. Immun., *104:*296, 1970.

59. McPhaul, J. J., Dixon, F. J., Brettschneider, L., and Starzl, T. E.: Immunoflourescent examination of biopsies from long-term renal allografts. New Eng. J. Med., *282:*412, 1970.

60. Manni, J. A., and Muller-Eberhard, H. J.: The eighth component of human complement (C8): isolation, characterization and hemolytic efficiency. J. Exp. Med., *130:*1145, 1969.

61. Miller, M. E., and Nilsson, U. R.: A familial deficiency of the phagocytosis-enhancing activity of serum related to a dysfunction of the fifth component of complement (C5). New Eng. J. Med., *282:*354, 1970.

62. Morton, D. L., Holmes, E. C., Eilber, F. R., and Wood, W. C.: Immunological aspects of neoplasia: a rational basis for immunotherapy. Ann. Intern. Med., *74:*587, 1971.

63. Muller-Eberhard, H. J.: Chemistry and reaction mechanisms of complement. Advances Immun., *8:*1, 1968.

64. Muller-Eberhard, H. J., Nilsson, U. R., Dalmasso, A. P., Polley, M. J.,

and Calcott, M. A.: A molecular concept of immune cytolysis. Arch. Path., *82*:205, 1966.

65. Myburgh, J. A., *et al.*: Hyperacute rejection in human kidney allografts —Schwartzman or Arthus reaction? New Eng. J. Med., *281*:131, 1969.

66. Ogawa, M., Kochwa, S., Smith, C., Ishizaka, K., and McIntyre, O. R.: Clinical aspects of IgE myeloma. New Eng. J. Med., *281*:1217, 1969.

67. Oppenheim, J. J.: Relationships of *in vitro* lymphocyte transformation to delayed hypersensitivity in guinea pigs and man. Fed. Proc., *27*:21, 1968.

68. Oppenheim, J. J., Rogentine, G. N., and Terry, W. D.: The transformation of human lymphocytes by monkey antisera to human immunoglobulins. Immunology, *16*:123, 1969.

69. Paque, R. E., Kniskern, P. J., Dray, S., and Baram, P.: In vitro studies with "transfer factor": Transfer of the cell migration inhibition correlate of delayed hypersensitivity in humans with cell lysates from humans sensitised to histoplasmin, coccidioidin or PPD. J. Immun., *103*:1014, 1969.

70. Ritchie, R. F.: Antinuclear antibodies, their frequency and diagnostic association. New Eng. J. Med., *282*:1174, 1970.

71. Rocklin, R. E., Meyers, O. L., and David, J. R.: An in vitro assay for cellular hypersensitivity in man. J. Immun., *104*:95, 1970.

72. Rocklin, R. E., Rosen, F. S., and J. R.: In vitro lymphocyte response of patients with immunologic deficiency diseases. Correlation of production of macrophage inhibiting factor with delayed hypersensitivity. New Eng. J. Med., *282*:1340, 1970.

73. Rosenau, W.: Target cell destruction. Fed. Proc., *27*:34, 1968.

74. Sadan, N., *et al.*: Immunotherapy of pollinosis in children: investigation of the immunologic basis of clinical improvement. New Eng. J. Med., *280*:623, 1969.

75. Schwartz, D. P., and Buckley, R. H.: Serum IgE concentrations and skin reactivity to anti-IgE antibody in IgA-deficient patients. New Eng. J. Med., *284*:513, 1971.

76. Sherry, S.: The kallikrein system: a basic defense mechanism. Hosp. Practice, *5*:75, 1970.

77. Slavin, S. B., and Smith, R. F.: The specificity of allergic reactions. III. Contact hypersensitivity. J. Exp. Med., *114*:185, 1961.

78. Stansworth, D. R.: Immunochemical mechanisms of immediate-type hypersensitivity reactions. Clin. Exp. Immun., *6*:1, 1970.

79. Thor, D. E.: Human delayed hypersensitivity: an in vitro correlate and transfer by an RNA extract. Fed. Proc., *27*:16, 1968.

80. Thor, D., Jureziz, R. E., Veach, S. R., Miller, E., and Dray, S.: Cell migration inhibition factor released by antigen from human peripheral lymphocytes. Nature, *219*:755, 1968.

81. Tompkins, W. A. F., Adams, C., and Rawls, W. E.: An in vitro measure of cellular immunity to fibroma virus. J. Immun., *104*:502, 1970.

82. Uhr, J. W.: Delayed hypersensitivity. Physiol. Rev., *46*:359, 1966.

83. Wasksman, B. H.: Discussion: in vitro correlates of delayed hypersensitivity. Fed. Proc., 27:45, 1968.
84. Ward, P. A., Cocharane, C. G., and Muller-Eberhard, H. J.: Further studies on the chemotactic factor of complement and its formation in vivo. Immunology, 11:141, 1966.
85. Willams, G. M., DePlanque, B., Graham, W. H., and Lower, R. R.: Participation of antibodies in acute cardiac allograft rejection in man. New Eng. J. Med., 281:1145, 1969.
86. Willoughby, D. A., Coote, E., and Turk, J. L.: Complement in acute inflammation. J. Path., 97:295, 1969.

2

Immunologic and Cellular Aspects
of Immediate Hypersensitivity

Jacob Pruzansky, PH.D.

The original designation of immediate hypersensitivity was applied to anaphylaxis, the first pathologic reaction found to be antigen-antibody mediated. With further study, it was found that anaphylaxis was only one of several inflammatory manifestations of the antigen-antibody reaction. The characteristics of these reactions were sufficiently distinct to allow subdivision into the first 3 classes of hypersensitivity described in the preceding chapter. This discussion will be limited to Type I reactions and to allergy in particular. The term "allergy" will be restricted to clinical hypersensitivity mediated by reaginic (IgE) antibody. Both allergy and anaphylaxis are elicited by a common mechanism and are included in the same group. The purpose of this chapter is to outline briefly some basic immunology relevant to allergy and to try to explain in this context the mechanisms which produce clinical symptoms and which underlie the benefits of therapy.

The immunologic nature of allergy is apparent from several observations. Prausnitz and Küstner first showed that the characteristic cutaneour wheal and flare reaction may be transferred by serum from an allergic to a nonallergic individual.[22] This is the Prausnitz-Küstner or P-K reaction. In addition, systemic passive sensitization was accomplished inadvertently by transfusion of blood from atopic donors to nonatopic recipients during the ragweed season. The nonatopic recipient transiently developed typical symptoms of ragweed hayfever. The serum factor responsible for either cutaneous or systemic transfer of sensitivity had the characteristics of an antibody. It was not present in serum before exposure to an antigen, was detected after exposure and reacted specifically with the eliciting antigen. Subsequent study has shown that it is a very distinct kind of antibody.

31

ANTIBODIES AND IMMUNOGLOBULINS

ANTIBODIES INVOLVED IN ALLERGY

Even before current studies which demonstrated the diverse nature of antibody molecules, it was recognized that there were two antibodies in man with different biologic activity but the same specificity for antigens (allergens) commonly associated with allergy.[4] These were reagin and blocking antibody.

Reagin

The passively transferable serum factor responsible for P-K reactivity and allergic reactions in man has been variously termed reagin, skin sensitizing antibody (SSA), homocytotropic antibody and mastocytotropic antibody. It was found to be unstable at 56°C and failed to precipitate with antigen. SSA has an affinity for mast cells, but all of the early indications were that it was only for mast cells of the same mammalian species. It was shown later that human reagin also passively sensitizes blood basophils of about 20 percent of nonatopic individuals. SSA is present in the serum of allergic individuals as a consequence of environmental exposure to antigens and is the antibody involved in the production of the clinical symptoms of allergy.

Blocking Antibody

Parenteral immunization of atopic or nonatopic individuals with an allergen such as ragweed results in production of a circulating antibody which is heat stable, does not induce or transfer sensitivity and actually inhibits the P-K reaction by competition with SSA for allergen. This factor has been termed blocking antibody and is produced during clinical immunotherapy. It is thought by some investigators to be partially responsible for clinical relief from symptoms. The relationship of SSA and blocking antibody to each other and to other antibodies was unknown until quite recently. The nature of these and other antibodies will therefore be discussed in the next section.

CURRENT KNOWLEDGE OF THE NATURE OF ANTIBODY

Understanding of the structure of antibodies has been gained by advances in physico chemical and immunologic techniques and by recognition of the relationship between myeloma proteins and antibodies. Immunoelectrophoresis of serum [7] was a primary tool in the differentiation of normal gamma globulin into the three major immunoglobulin classes, IgG (γG); IgA (γA) and IgM (γM). These immunoglobulins were related immunologically and structurally to the three different pathologic proteins (M proteins) of multiple myelomas G and A and of Waldenströms macroglobulinemia.

Ultracentrifugation of whole sera showed that most antibody activity in mammalian sera was associated with proteins having a sedimentation coefficient of 7S with an approximate molecular weight of 160,000 but some activity was attributable to 19S protein corresponding to a molecular weight near 1,000,000. After separation of immunoglobulins was accomplished, serum IgG was found to be 7S, IgA was 7S to 11S and IgM was 19S.

Antisera specific for the three original immunoglobulins were made and used to type myeloma proteins. An M protein was discovered which did not precipitate with the typing sera and a new class of immunoglobulin with a counterpart in normal serum was established as IgD. A fifth immunoglobulin IgE, was isolated by Ishizaka from atopic sera and shown to be immunologically distinct from the other immunoglobulins.[8] Two myeloma patients were subsequently found who produced M proteins of this class. This substantiated the existence of the new class of immunoglobulin. There is the possibility that other immunoglobulins will be found but unless they are associated with unique biologic activity they will be discovered as untypable M proteins. The absence of verified reports of new immunoglobulins to the present time suggests that the possibility is remote.

The five classes of immunoglobulin in man have all been shown to be heterogeneous. Four subclasses of IgG have been established, and IgA and IgM have also been subdivided immunologically. Even within each subclass there is heterogeneity at the molecular level which is genetically controlled. One obvious demonstration of molecular heterogeneity is the large range of antigenic specificities of antibody present in any immunoglobulin class or subclass. Heterogeneity of structure also exists apart from the combining site. In contrast to normal immunoglobulins, M proteins are extremely homogeneous since they are made by a single genetic line of cells. Most of the structural analysis of immunoglobulins has therefore been carried out with M proteins.

Figure 2-1, center, is a schematic representation of the basic but incomplete structure of the immunoglobulin molecule. It is consistent with the known properties of the immunoglobulins and the fragments derived from them. Four polypeptide chains, 2 heavy (molecular weight about 50,000 each) and 2 light (molecular weight about 20,000 each), are bound together by disulfide bonds to form a bivalent antibody molecule with two antigen combining sites.

Partial proteolytic digestion with papain in the presence of a sulfhydryl reducing agent produces three fragments (Fig. 2-1, left). Two are similar and each, called Fab piece, contains one of the two antigen-

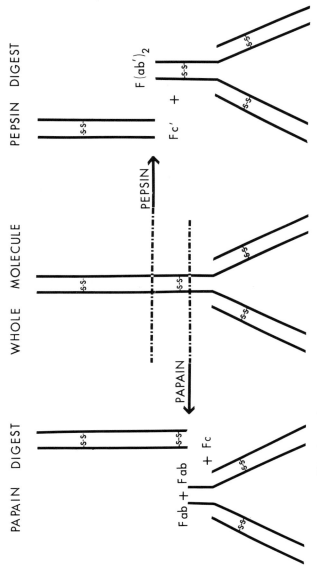

Fig. 2-1. Schematic representation of the basic structure of the immuno-globulin molecule. Fragments derived from papain (*left*) and pepsin (*right*) digestion are shown. Reductive cleavage results in splitting the interchain S-S bonds of the intact molecule or the fragments of pro-teolytic digestion. These products may be readily visualized but have not been drawn.

combining sites of the original whole molecule. The remaining fragment, Fc piece, has no capacity for antigen recognition but has structural groups characteristic of its own immunoglobulin class.[21] An antiserum against Fc piece of one immunoglobulin does not react with any other immunoglobulin. Antiserum against Fab from any immunoglobulin reacts with all immunoglobulins, and this reaction is a requisite for classifying a protein as an immunoglobulin.

Digestion with pepsin (Fig. 2-1, right) results in two major fragments.[17] One is similar to Fc piece but is somewhat smaller and is called Fc'. The other is like Fab but is bivalent and is therefore designated $F(ab')_2$. If this fragment were split symmetrically in half by a mild reducing agent, it would become univalent $F(ab')$ and would correspond to the Fab piece produced by treatment with papain, except that it would be slightly larger. It should be noted that the light chains are contained solely in the $F(ab')$ fragments.

The interchain disulfide bonds may be broken by sulfhydryl reducing agents to separate the chains. Alkylating agents combine with the SH groups produced and are used to keep the S-S bonds from reforming by oxidation after the reducing agent is removed. Although oxidation may be prevented, reassociation of chains by noncovalent bonding occurs. It is nevertheless possible to separate the chains by gel filtration in the presence of organic acids. Light chains alone derived from a specific antibody have negligible antigen binding capacity and heavy chains alone have a small but definite affinity for specific antigen while a mixture of separated light and heavy chains has still greater activity. Mixtures, however, are never as active as Fab piece or intact antibody. This and other information suggests that both light and heavy chains and a definite spatial relationship between them are required for optimal activity of the combining site of the antibody. Light chains exist in two forms, distinguishable immunologically, called κ and λ. Both light chains in any given immunoglobulin molecule are the same, and in normal immunoglobulins about two thirds are κ and one third λ. In M proteins the light chains are either all κ or all λ. Bence Jones proteins, found in the urine of some myeloma patients, are light chains and exist in any one urine as either κ or λ. Antisera to them may be used for typing and to determine whether an immunoglobulin is present, since light chains are common to all classes of immunoglobulin.

Although the five known immunoglobulins have the same basic structure, the differences in biologic activity, size, stability and other properties indicate considerable variation in structural detail. One example of this is the five-fold greater molecular weight of IgM. A roughly circular disposition of five single units has been suggested to form a pentamer. It is also known that serum IgA may exist as a dimer or trimer. In all polymeric forms a new chain called J chain has been found and is thought to function in joining monomers. Another extra chain has been isolated from IgA of secretions but not of serum, which was called T component because it was postulated to be required for transport of IgA. This polypeptide has also been referred to as S, for secretory piece, since its function in transport has not been demonstrated. It is known that the carbohydrate content of IgG is only one fourth that of the other immunoglobulins analyzed. The greater carbohydrate content and its localization in IgM is believed to be responsible for a decreased susceptibility to limited proteolytic cleavage of IgM into Fab and Fc pieces. At about 60° C, trypsin cleaves IgM into an Fab and a polymeric Fc which indicates a basic structural unity for the immunoglobulins despite the variations which exist.

From the standpoint of antibody-mediated hypersensitivity the part of the immunoglobulin molecule that determines the type of reaction is the Fc piece. The Fab piece of each class of immunoglobulin is of course essential in determining specificity and in the activation of any immunologically determined reaction, but all Fab fragments of the same specificity are basically indistinguishable. It is the Fc piece which is responsible for such properties as complement fixation and activation and cytotropic activity which determine the nature of the biologic reactions subsequent to combination of antigen with antibody. Table 2-1 shows some of the known properties of the immunoglobulins.

TABLE 2-1
Some of the Known Properties of the Immunoglobulins

Ig	MOLECULAR WEIGHT	CARBO- HYDRATE %	SERUM CONC. MG. %	RE- PORTED SUB- CLASSES	CROSSES PLA- CENTA	BIOLOGIC ACTIVITY
G	140,000	2.9	1000	4	+	CF, opsonin, pre- cipitin, blocking
A	170,000 (Monomer)	7.5	250	2	–	Secretory Ig
M	900,000	11.8	125	2	–	CF, agglutination
D	200,000	14.8	1	0	–	Unknown
E	200,000	10.7	0.03	0	–	Homocytotropic

ANTIBODY PRODUCTION

Since allergy is an immunologic disease mediated by antibody, knowledge of the process by which antibody is formed is of importance. Although most of the information regarding antibody production has been obtained with respect to IgG and IgM the basic mechanisms would also pertain to IgE and the other immunoglobulins. Antibody is synthesized as a result of activation of cells directly or indirectly by antigen.

Antigens and Allergens

Proteins acting as antigens have not one but many different distinct regions of the molecule which elicit antibody production. These antigenic determinants are approximately the size of six amino acids and 20 or more different ones may coexist on a single protein. An antiserum to such a protein might therefore consist of antibodies of 20 or more different specificities, since each antibody molecule can be specific for only one determinant. Whether a given region of an antigen will act as a determinant is dependent on the animal being immunized. A rabbit may respond to one structural entity among many others on horse serum albumin while a horse probably will not react to any and a second rabbit might not react to that determinant but to others. A rabbit immunized with horse serum albumin may produce antibodies that also react with bovine serum albumin and rat serum albumin but to a lesser extent than with horse albumin. The reason is that some of the determinants on all of the mammalian albumins are the same even though the majority are structurally different. This is one basis for cross reactivity between short and giant ragweed, among various pollens, among various molds and such as is exhibited by the precipitation of canine IgA with rabbit anti-human IgA.

Whether a particular antigen will elicit antibody production and the nature and quantity of the antibody synthesized depends on the quantity and structure of the antigen, its route of entry and the genetic makeup of the individuals immunized. Antigens which initiate production of and react with reagins are called allergens.

There are substances of low molecular weight comparable in size to a single antigenic determinant. They can react with specific antibody but are incapable of stimulating the formation of antibody. If they are combined chemically with a protein, however, they may also stimulate antibody production. Such substances are called haptens and some environmental chemicals and drugs belong to this category. These may be of sufficient chemical reactivity to combine with body proteins to produce complete antigens or allergens. They may therefore initiate hypersensitive reactions of Type I, II, III or IV.

Allergens important clinically are most frequently airborne in the form of fine particles such as pollen grains, dusts, animal danders and mold spores. Ingested proteins and those injected for therapeutic reasons such as foreign sera or polypeptide hormones may be allergenic. Drugs capable of combining with body proteins in vivo are capable of stimulating formation of antibodies including reagin. Proof that most drugs, which are responsible for immediate type hypersensitivity reactions, cause reaginic (IgE) sensitization is lacking, since the natural carrier protein is neither identified nor isolated and available for study. It is also possible that immunoglobulins other than IgE are involved in drug anaphylaxis.

Cells

Antibody production is a process involving sequential action of more than one type of lymphoid cell. The specific details are still obscure but the mechanism is undergoing intensive investigation. It is known that the antibody producing cell is the plasma cell which is a differentiation form of the small lymphocyte. By sensitive techniques it has been demonstrated that a small proportion of lymphocytes in experimental animals have surface receptors for a radiolabeled hapten prior to immunization. Possibly these are the cells that are stimulated by this hapten to become plasma cells which produce antibody. Other lymphocytes are presumably specific for other antigenic determinants. Injected antigen does not appear to stimulate these cells directly, however. The largest concentration of antigen after immunization is in macrophages. RNA complexes which contain antigen have been extracted from these cells and used to stimulate antibody production in lymphocyte-rich cell populations of nonimmunized rats. It is possible to speculate that antigen is first processed by macrophages to a form which activates specific lymphocytes to divide, differentiate and produce antibody. The process as described is not fully substantiated and is not complete.

All small lymphocytes are not alike in origin, and at present two types can be distinguished by specific plasma membrane antigens. One population is bone marrow-derived and seems to be the precursor of the plasma cell. The other is the thymus-derived lymphocyte which seems most important in cellular immunity and Type IV hypersensitivity. These may also have a stimulating or helper effect on antibody production. Antibody production therefore involves the interaction of at least two and possibly three separate cells or their products in a sequence which is still being elucidated.

Plasma cells that produce one immunoglobulin presumably do not produce any other, although there have been sporadic reports to the contrary. The antigenic specificity is also unique for each cell. The immunoglobulin produced and its specificity is genetically determined. After primary stimulation by antigen the pool of lymphocytes which recognize that antigen (memory cells) is increased. This results in the production of larger quantities of antibody in a shorter period of time after secondary stimulation.

MEASUREMENT OF ANTIBODY

In order to study antibodies involved in allergy, methods for their measurement must be available. The classical method of immunology, the precipitin reaction, is not useful because IgE antibodies do not precipitate with antigen owing to the small quantity present and possibly for structural reasons. In addition, most of the other general procedures now in use for antibody detection and determination do not discriminate between immunoglobulin classes. It is apparent, however, that such discrimination is the specific requirement for determination of antibodies important in allergy. Reaginic (IgE) antibody must be measured separately from the other immunoglobulins of the same specificity which act as blocking antibody.

A biologic system has evolved which can be adapted to measure several parameters of interest in allergic disease. It was discovered by Katz and Cohen in 1941 that after incubation of blood from an allergic donor with antigen, cellular histamine was released into the plasma. The leukocytes were subsequently found to be the histamine carrier. This reaction was studied experimentally and clinically, but its usefulness was not fully appreciated until Lichtenstein and Osler [13] washed the leukocytes to determine the role of serum and other components. The procedure for histamine release from washed human leukocytes has been subjected to variations which make it possible to estimate quantitatively reaginic antibody, blocking antibody and the dose response to antigen of basophils from allergic patients (cellular sensitivity). These applications will be described in greater detail.

Reaginic Antibody

Until recently the only procedure available for SSA determination had been P-K titration. Intradermal injections of dilutions of test serum into a nonallergic human or monkey recipient sensitizes the cutaneous sites of the recipient to subsequent challenge with a constant quantity of antigen. The highest dilution of serum giving a standard reaction is the titer. This has the inherent limitations of bioassay plus the risk of hepatitis in a human recipient.

Sensitization of human basophils from nonatopic donors for specific release of histamine is an analog in vitro of the P-K reaction.[19] Dilutions of test sera are incubated with separate aliquots of donor leukocytes. The cells are then washed and incubated with antigen at a preselected optimal concentration. A plot of histamine release versus serum concentration is made, and the concentration that results in release of 50 percent of the cellular histamine is the index of reaginic activity.

The detection of significant quantities of reaginic antibody to individual allergens [29] has been accomplished by a radioallergosorbent test (R.A.S.T.). The allergen is chemically linked to an insoluble dextran matrix, and a predetermined quantity is mixed with an aliquot of the serum or other test fluid. After incubation and washing the immunosorbent, radioactive antihuman IgE is added to the matrix. Unattached antibody is removed by washing and the separated sorbent is counted. A count of two to five times the control is called 1+; greater radioactivity is designated 2+. In this system all classes of antibody to the allergen are bound to the allergen, which has been rendered insoluble. The radioactive anti-IgE will only be immunosorbed if IgE antibody is present.

Blocking Antibody

Blocking antibody can be measured biologically by its inhibition of the P-K reaction. Several methods of titration in human skin are available. One method is to inject a constant quantity of a known atopic serum intradermally in a number of sites on a nonatopic recipient. The serum to be tested is heated at 56° C for 4 hours to destroy reagin. After 24 hours a preincubated mixture of a constant amount of the test serum with an increasing quantity of antigen is used for intradermal challenge of the sensitized sites. More antigen will be required in the serum plus antigen series to elicit a definite urticarium than in controls in which antigen was preincubated with normal human serum or saline. The magnitude of the difference in antigen required is a measure of the blocking antibody. Other modes of assay have been used but they all involve the competition for antigen of the serum and sensitized cells. This assay in vivo has all the inherent disadvantages of the P-K reaction itself.

An analog in vitro of the procedure just described is the inhibition of histamine release from sensitized human leukocytes.[19] Equal aliquots of cells from an atopic donor are incubated with mixtures of increasing quantities of antigen which had been preincubated with a constant amount of the test serum. The controls are preincubated with antigen and nonatopic serum instead of test serum. Histamine released from and remaining in the cells is determined. Plots of percent histamine release versus log antigen added are made and the difference between the antigen required for 50 percent release in test, and control is related to the quantity of antigen neutralized by the quantity of test serum used.

The total antibody to ragweed antigen may be measured.[23] Since reagin is present only in very small amounts in serum, this is also a good estimate of blocking antibody, particularly during hyposensitization therapy. The method involves adding increasing quantities of ^{125}I ragweed antigen E to a constant amount of the human serum. Following incubation either ammonium sulfate (at 40 percent saturation) or rabbit antihuman immunoglobulin serum is added, and a second incubation is made to separate free from antibody-bound ragweed. Counts of the supernatant and precipitate are made. The antibody content may be expressed as the quantity of antigen bound per ml. in slight antigen excess or may be calculated in extreme antigen excess on the assumption that the molecular formula of the ragweed-antibody complex is ragweed $_2$ antibody $_1$.

IgE Content of Human Serum

Since the total IgE content of a human serum is low, sensitive radioactive methods must be used. The most accurate procedure is similar to the radioimmunoassay of insulin and other hormones.[6] Purified human IgE labeled with ^{125}I, rabbit antiserum to the Fc piece of IgE and guinea pig antirabbit gamma globulin are prepared. The highest dilution of anti-IgE which will bind about 3 nanograms of human IgE in slight antigen excess is established. Three nanograms of [125]I IgE, the predetermined quantity of anti-IgE and increasing quantities of from 3 to 40 nanograms of IgE from a human serum of known IgE content are incubated. Antirabbit immunoglobulin is then added to precipitate all of the rabbit gamma globulin. This will separate the bound from the free IgE, since the bound IgE will be in the precipitate. The distribution is readily established by counting the radioactivity in the precipitate and the supernatant. As the quantity of standard serum added increases, the percent of labeled antigen bound decreases. A plot of percent antigen bound against log antigen added will produce a standard curve. Unknown sera or dilutions are run in the same way as the standards and the IgE content is determined from the standard curve and the serum dilution factor.

Another means of performing essentially the same determination [9] has been called the radioimmunosorbent assay (R.I.S.A.). Anti-IgE is chemically linked to insoluble dextran and mixtures of a fixed quantity of radioactive IgE, and increasing quantities of test serum or fluid are added. After incubation the washed sorbent is counted. If the test material contains IgE it will competitively reduce the binding of labeled IgE. The extent of the reduction compared to that of a standardized IgE preparation determines its IgE content. The curves are prepared just as in the double antibody method above.

IgE may also be estimated by radiographic modifications [1, 27] of single gel diffusion as described by Mancini. Agar gel containing an empirically established dilution of rabbit anti-IgE is layered on a glass slide or a plate just as is commercially available for assay of other immunoglobulins. Standards and unknowns are placed in small cylindrical wells punched out of the agar and allowed to diffuse for several days. A ring of precipitate will form but will be invisible because of the small quantity of reactants present. The zone of precipitate may be visualized in several ways. The anti-IgE incorporated in the agar may be labeled with [125]I. Washing the slide will remove all serum components except the IgE-anti-IgE precipitate. The antibody in the ring of precipitate is radioactive and will therefore be detected by exposure to and development of X-ray film. Variants of this procedure employ ^{125}I antirabbit globulin or [125]I IgE to bind to the unlabeled invisible precipitate. The precipitate is again detected as a circle on x-ray film. To process these plates for quantitative assay the agar is dried and the plate placed on x-ray film for several days to 2 weeks. The circular zone of precipitate will appear after development of the film. The outer diameter of circles formed in this way is proportional to the IgE content. A plot of the diameters of the standards against their IgE content, usually in the range of 100 to 800 nanograms per ml., gives a curve from which the IgE content of the unknowns may be read. This technique is less accurate and less sensitive than using inhibition of coprecipitation.

Biologic Activity of Antibody

Many different reactions are known to result from antigen-antibody combination. These include the hypersensitivity reactions (Types I, II and III) and more biologically useful responses such as phagocytosis and the lysis of infectious agents. Antibody of each class of immunoglobulin that has been studied extensively has been shown to act in some but not all of these situations. Since the Fab portion or combining site of all immunoglobulins directed against a single antigenic determinant is essentially the same, differences in reactivity of different immunoglobulins of the same specificity must reside in the Fc portion of the molecule. The nature and extent of most of these reactions is determined by the ability of the Fc piece to combine with certain cellular or serum components before or after combination with antigen and the quantities of antigen, antibody and tissue components present.

Complement Fixation

Serum complement is fixed and activated by antigen-antibody complexes which contain IgM or three of the four subspecies of IgG antibody. Complexes formed with IgA and IgE antibody do not fix complement and will not initiate certain processes described under Types

II and III hypersensitivities. Under certain conditions, not well defined, complexes which fix complement in vivo will generate anaphylatoxins. Two of these are known, one related to the third component (C3) and one to the fifth component (C5) of complement. Injection of these substances in sufficient quantity will cause anaphylactic reactions presumably due to histamine release. It is therefore possible that a Type III reaction such as serum sickness, which is produced by complement fixing antigen-antibody complexes, will also result in some symptoms of Type I hypersensitivity.

Cytotropic Activity

Antibodies may attach themselves to cells. Molecules of IgE and a very limited number of subspecies of IgG have an affinity for mast cells and basophils. There are specific receptor sites on the plasma membranes of these cells for these immunoglobulins. Mast cells of atopics and non-atopics alike will bind IgE but in atopics some of the IgE will be specific for allergens to which the donor is sensitive. If the specific allergen comes in contact with a sensitized cell the interaction results in the release of certain pharmacologic agents from the cells. This is the essence of the allergic reaction which will be discussed later in greater detail.

Human IgE does not passively sensitize guinea pig mast cells for anaphylaxis, but human IgG antibody does. The general rule is that IgE-type antibody is homocytotropic and only transfers sensitivity to mast cells of the same species and IgG antibody is heterocytotropic and sensitizes only mast cells of other species. There are exceptions. Notably in some rodents, a subspecies of IgG antibody is homocytotropic. Since most of the major immunoglobulins in man have been found to have analogs in other mammalian species, it is also likely that findings in other mammals will have relevance to man. It is therefore possible that under appropriate conditions the injection of some antigens into man will induce formation of homocytotropic IgG antibodies and subsequent injections will result in Type I reactions. The antibody generally considered to be responsible for spontaneous human allergy, however, is IgE. There have been some reports of human reagins which are not IgE, but unequivocal proof is lacking. There have also been indications that human reagin sensitizes rat peritoneal mast cells to undergo morphologic changes after incubation with specific antigen. The nature of this reaction is unclear at present and it stands in contrast to the failure of human allergic serum to transfer cutaneous sensitivity to the rat and other species.

The possibility that cytotropic antibodies other than those of the IgE class cause Type I hypersensitivity in man must be kept in mind although it has not yet been demonstrated conclusively that they do. It has recently been shown that while IgE is the only detectable immunoglobulin on the surface of human basophils, IgG is found exclusively on blood neutrophils and monocytes. This is a further example of the selective affinity of the Fc portion of immunoglobulins for cells, but as yet no manifestation of hypersensitivity in man has been associated with "sensitized" neutrophils or monocytes.

Blocking Activity

Blocking antibody, mentioned previously, is an operational designation used for antibody produced in both atopic and nonatopic individuals by immunization with common allergens. Stated simply, the amount of allergen available to react with a sensitized cell will be reduced by reaction with antibody that combines with the allergen but cannot sensitize cells. The intensity of the reaction of the sensitized cells which is dependent on allergen concentration will therefore also be reduced. This inhibitory activity is called blocking and the antibody responsible for it is called blocking antibody. Some have considered it to be IgG antibody of the same specificity as the IgE antibody the reactivity of which it inhibits by competition for antigen. There is no theoretical reason to restrict blocking activity to one class of immunoglobulin. Any antibody which is not mastocytotropic or basophilotropic can block reagin of the same antigenic specificity. As currently understood, blocking is a function of the Fab pieces and not of the Fc piece of the immunoglobulin molecule. The same general phenomenon of inhibition by competition for antigen is observed in any instance in which a mixture of antibody classes is present and only one of them has an Fc piece required for a particular reaction. For example, complement fixation by γG antibody of the three competent subclasses would be reduced in the presence of antibody of the same specificity which is non-complement fixing. An analogous situation occurs when precipitation of an antigen by a precipitating antibody is blocked or inhibited by the presence of antibody of the same specificity which is incapable of precipitating that antigen (nonprecipitating antibody).

It is apparent from the preceding discussion that the immunoglobulin class and amount of antibody as well as the availability of other tissue components are important in determining the occurrence and the nature of a hypersensitivity reaction. Type I reactions require mast cells sensitized by IgE antibody. Antigen which is part of, or bound to, a cell membrane is the requisite for a Type II hypersensitivity. Where cell lysis occurs in Type II reactions the antibody must be IgM or one of the IgG subspecies that fix complement and a source of complement must be readily available. For Type III reactions complement fixing antibody is obligatory as well as neutrophils and sufficient amounts of immune complex in antigen excess.

MEDIATORS OF ALLERGIC SYMPTOMS

Most of the symptoms observed in allergic disease may be very closely approximated in nonatopic individuals by appropriate exposure to histamine. Other naturally occurring agents which have pharmacologic activity similar to that of histamine have been associated with Type I hypersensitivity in various mammalian species. These substances are serotonin, slow reacting substance (SRS) and bradykinin.

Histamine

It was recognized long ago that histamine produced symptoms in guinea pigs that were very similar to the symptoms of anaphylaxis in that species. It was later shown to be released during anaphylactic reactions in vitro and in vivo.

Histamine is a product of the action of histidine decarboxylase on the naturally occurring amino acid histidine. The enzyme and substrate are present in most tissue suggesting that histamine has normal biologic functions but interestingly these functions have not yet been conclusively established.

Histamine is widely distributed in mammalian tissues, mostly in mast cells but also in blood basophils and platelets and in other cells of the intestinal tract. In mast cells, basophils and platelets it has been localized to granules which contain heparin or a similar polysaccharide and a basic protein. The exact structure of the granular matrix is unknown but it has been suggested that histamine is bound electrostatically to the negatively charged sulfate groups of the polysaccharide or to the negative carboxyl groups of the protein. This kind of structure, if correct, is essentially an ion exchanger and positively charged histamine should be displaced by any other positive ion such as Na^+. Isolated rat peritoneal mast cell granules have been shown to exchange Na^+ for histamine. Histamine can be released from some cells by certain basic molecules such as morphine, some antihistamines and by a synthetic polymer, compound 48/80. This has also been cited as evidence of ionic linkage. It has been stated by some that the whole granule is expelled from the cell and histamine is then released by ion exchange. Others have found little or no evidence of extracellular release of monkey or human mast cell or basophil granules during specific immunologic activation of these cells.

Histamine causes contraction of some smooth muscles including those of the bronchioles and of large blood vessels. It also causes dilatation of small venules. As a result of the opposing actions on vessels, histamine produces hypertension in some mammals such as the cat and hypotension in others such as man, depending on the balance of these effects. The action appears to be independent of innervation. Capillary permeability is also increased by histamine resulting in edema. Intradermally a "triple response" is elicited by histamine. First, there is an immediate erythema at the site of injection; second, edema is produced locally surrounding the site and third, the erythema is extended beyond the edematous wheal. These events also occur in a positive skin test with allergen. Histamine has been identified as a major mediator of anaplylaxis in guinea pig, dog and man.

SRS

A substance was found in perfusates of guinea pig lung during anaphylactic shock which caused a sustained contraction of guinea pig ileum that was slow in onset and was not antagonized by antihistamines. It is not present in lung before immunologic or enzymatic activation. Phospholipase A, present in cobra venom, or specific antigen released SRS from guinea pig lung.

Available quantities of SRS have been insufficient to allow definition of its chemical structure. It is a lipid and is acidic, but not much more of its chemistry is presently known. SRS is present in precursor form in peritoneal mast cells and neutrophils of the rat. Its cellular distribution in man is unknown.

SRS contracts human but not guinea pig bronchioles and only a few other smooth muscle preparations. It is released from human lung tissue pretreated with IgE and challenged with anti-IgE. Its importance in human allergy is suggested by its pharmacologic action and by the observed inability of antihistamines to alleviate the symptoms of human asthma. The properties of SRS are consistent with pharmacologic requirements in asthma but direct evidence of causality is lacking.

Serotonin

Serotonin release from rabbit platelets after a specific immunologic reaction indicated that it was of potential significance in anaphylaxis and allergy. Serotonin is produced enzymatically by a two-step reaction of the natural amino acid tryptophan involving hydroxylation and decarboxylation. In man, 90 percent of the serotonin is found in the intestinal tract and the rest mostly in the platelets and the brain. In most mammalian species it is not found in mast cells.

Serotonin is a stimulator of smooth muscle and nerves. It causes dilatation of blood vessels in skeletal muscle and increased capillary permeability in some rodents but not in man. Contraction of human bronchial muscle is produced but tachyphylaxis occurs rapidly. Because of its distribution and pharmacologic properties it appears unlikely that serotonin participates in producing the symptoms of allergy or anaphylaxis in man. It is important in some rodents.

Bradykinin

Many proteolytic enzymes act on an $a2$ globulin in blood to produce a hypotensive agent. Plasma itself contains a protease in inactive form whose activation is accomplished in the same way as the activation of Hageman factor of the clotting system. The enzyme was called kallikrein; the substrate was named kallidinogen; and the vasoactive nonapeptide produced in the reaction was termed kallidin. Bradykinin is the current designation of one of the active peptides. In anaphylaxis in animals, plasma kinins have been identified, and a reduction in kallidinogen has been reported. This suggests the possible participation of bradykinin in allergy and anaphylaxis.

Bradykinin causes vasodilatation and increased capillary permeability, which produces hypotension in vivo. Guinea pig ileum contracts slowly in its presence. A stimulatory action of bradykinin on nerve endings results in the sensation of pain. Kinin activity is inhibited by aspirin, and its generation is prevented by the naturally occurring polypeptide trasylol, which inhibits the enzymatic activity of kallikrein and other proteases.

In hereditary angioneurotic edema, a natural inhibitor of kallikrein which has been identified as C1 esterase inhibitor is absent. A variety of stimuli should then be capable of causing kinin formation and symptoms, but the exact progression of events is not established. In rhinitis and asthma in man histamine and probably SRS are the important mediators of symptomatology. In systemic manifestations of allergy and anaphylaxis, bradykinin may prove to be an additional participant.

THE ALLERGIC CELL

As previously indicated, the symptoms of allergy may be attributed to histamine or other pharmacologic agents. Identification of the cells which contain these mediators, their storage form and the processes which induce their release are therefore of great significance. The discussion which follows will be concerned only with histamine as it has been studied most extensively, but some observations may also pertain to other mediators.

The marked biological activity of histamine is not normally manifested because it is bound intracellulary in mast cell granules which contain a matrix of heparin or a similar poly anion and protein. These cells have receptor sites, which are surface structures on the plasma membranes capable of binding the Fc portion of IgE molecules. If the IgE which becomes attached to the receptors is specific for antigen, the cell becomes sensitized to that antigen. This process occurs in atopics as a result of natural exposure to environmental antigens with subsequent active production of IgE antibody and in nonatopics or in suspensions of their cells by passive transfer of serum from hypersensitive patients.

Combination of allergen with mast cell-bound IgE antibody activates the cell for histamine release. More than one antibody molecule must be present on each adequately sensitized mast cell. It has been shown that one antigen molecule must "bridge" or combine with at least two antibody molecules on the cell to be effective in vivo.[10] This potentially imposes rigid restrictions on Type I hypersensitivity reactions. A protein allergen contains many determinants, probably all different from each other. The distance between them is fixed within the limit of molecular flexibility. The spacing of IgE reagin, of two or more different specificities, on the surface of the mast cell must conform to that of the determinants on the allergen for bridging to occur. If only a small number of IgE receptors were present, the probability of proper alignment resulting in a reaction would be small. The observation of widespread reactivity of cells in vivo and in vitro tends to indicate therefore that a large number of receptor sites are located on mast cell membranes.

Integration of the known facts suggests that a cell which is adequately sensitized for specific release of its stored histamine is one which has a sufficient number of IgE molecules with the correct specificity for determinants located at the proper distance from each other.

Sensitized cells react with specific antigens to release histamine. Of experimental interest is the fact that antihuman IgE and compound 48/80 also activate these cells to release histamine whether or not they are antigen-sensitive. Evidence from animal experiments and studies of isolated cells and tissues indicates that the cells must be viable, that Ca^{++} and Mg^{++} must be present in the medium, and that a temperature near 37° C and pH near 7 must be maintained for optimal activity. Several studies including inhibition of histamine release by various agents suggest that a chymotrypsinlike enzyme [2] and possibly phospholipase A are activated by the antigen-antibody reaction on the cell surface. These enzymatic activities have not been demonstrated directly, but this is difficult to accomplish experimentally.

Other information relates to possible metabolic pathways required for mediator release. Iodoacetate and some other inhibitors of glycolysis have prevented histamine release in vitro. Activators of β-adrenergic mechanisms have also prevented histamine release. The pattern of inhibition by various adrenergic agents and direct measurements of cyclic AMP suggest that an increase in the latter is associated with reduced histamine release from isolated cells and tissue. There is no good evidence yet that a decrease in cyclic AMP causes histamine release. These and other imaginative approaches to cellular mechanisms are being made but definitive answers require further investigation.

Human leukocytes are a readily available source of cells, the basophils, which resemble mast cells in several respects. They are the only leukocytes which have staining characteristics similar to mast cells, contain histamine in granules, may be sensitized with IgE antibody and which release their histamine upon challenge with specific antigen. Much has been learned from study of these cells about cellular reactions in human allergy and the changes resulting from immunotherapy. Some of the studies mentioned above have been done with leukocytes, some on mast cells and some in both. In mediator release from leukocytes, it has been shown that the reaction occurs in at least two stages. In the first step, antigen combines with the cells in the absence of Ca^{++} and Mg^{++}. Unbound antigen may be washed from the leukocytes. If the cells are suspended in physiologic buffer containing Ca^{++} and Mg^{++}, histamine will be released in the second stage.[24] While many studies have used the whole buffy coat, laboratory procedures are available to obtain basophil-rich preparations where needed for certain investigations.[26]

ANIMAL MODELS OF ALLERGY

Elucidation of the mechanism of the allergic reaction is important in itself and is necessary for a rational approach to evaluating conventional therapy and to suggesting new means of treatment. It is difficult to study the allergic reaction in man because of limitations with regard to safety and the availability of patients. Fortunately, the allergic state occurs in other mammalian species. Pulmonary function, electrocardiography, arterial and venous pressures, histamine and heparin release, clotting factors, platelet function and anatomic changes are among the many simultaneous or sequential measurements possible in sensitized experimental animals undergoing controlled challenge with antigen. Changes in any or all of these parameters may also be determined after administration of various drugs or pharmacologic agents. As in other areas of medicine, animal models of disease are invaluable aids in basic science and in clinical research.[20]

The animal with naturally occurring pollinosis which is most useful in experimental investigation is the dog. First reported as an interesting observation, atopic dogs have since been collected and intensively studied to yield valuable information on allergic mechanisms. The dog may be sensitive to the pollen antigens important in human allergy although the clinical manifestations are mainly dermatologic. Artificial exposure to aerosols of pollen extracts in higher concentration than obtained by environmental exposure will produce respiratory symptoms with some similarity to those of human asthma. Hypersensitivity to ascaris antigen is also prevalent in dogs and exists in many animals that are not pollen-sensitive. This increases the availability of subjects for experimental study. The use of passive sensitization by transfer of serum from actively sensitized animals to nonsensitive recipients also enhances the investigative pool. The antibody responsible for symptoms in the allergic dog and for passive transfer to nonsensitive recipients is analogous to IgE in man.

More recently monkeys have been passively sensitized with serum from allergic patients. This brings the model much closer to man with a greater likelihood that results may be extrapolated from experimental observation to clinical significance. The monkey also reacts to ascaris antigen although ascariasis appears to be uncommon in this primate. Sensitivity to ascaris is probably produced by infestation with other nematodes which have antigens related to ascaris antigen. Most monkeys seem to be cutaneous reactors to this antigen but some are much more sensitive than others. In a series of monkeys studied, 3 of 23 were sufficiently sensitive to react with respiratory symptoms after inhalation of an aerosol of ascaris antigen. Their reactivity to controlled delivery of antigen was quite reproducible over a 24-month period and measurements of respiratory function and other physiologic parameters have been made. They could be the counterpart of the atopic patient, since they have persistent sensitivity and develop respiratory symptoms and eosinophilia after aerosol challenge with antigen or with anti-IgE. Animals of this type are valuable for studying the effect of pharmacologic agents on a condition resembling extrinsic asthma in man. Serum from these monkeys could be used for passive transfer of sensitivity to unreactive animals, but the reproducibility of symptoms in the actively sensitized animals and the limited number of respiratory reactors available as blood donors make this a less useful model.

IMMUNOLOGIC PARAMETERS IN ALLERGIC PATIENTS

Immunotherapy is the prevalent treatment for allergic disorders uncontrolled by antihistamines or bronchodilators or where these agents are not well tolerated by the patient. Injection of antigens should be expected to result in antibody production and might cause other biologic changes. For this reason several groups of investigators have measured various serum and cellular factors before, during, and after immunotherapy.

ANTIBODIES IN ATOPIC PATIENTS

The earliest immunologic measurements made in allergic patients were reaginic antibody by P-K titration and blocking antibody by titration of the inhibition of P-K activity. These continue to be primary parameters in ragweed pollenosis and newer methods of analysis, described above, are now available. The development of the symptoms of allergy is an involved process. Reagin is bound to cell receptors on the mast cell. Allergen is extracted from a complex solid such as a pollen grain and transported across a mucosal membrane and through mucosal and intercellular fluids containing blocking antibody. Some of the allergen combines with mast cell bound reagin to activate the release of mediators. It is not surprising, therefore, that the clinical state of the patient is not defined solely by the quantities of blocking and reaginic antibody in his plasma. Their role is nevertheless crucial and will be discussed later.

HISTAMINE RELEASE

Antigen added to anti-coagulated blood of an allergic individual results in release of cellular histamine into the plasma. Since the histamine is present in leukocytes the system was simplified by removing the erythrocytes. Further improvement was obtained by suspension of washed leukocytes in buffered saline. This allowed delineation of the factors required for histamine release. Ca^{++} and Mg^{++} were shown to be necessary, and the limits of temperature and pH were established. Dose response curves of antigen-induced histamine release from leukocytes of most atopics studied were of similar shape, but the minimum amount of antigen necessary for a significant release of histamine varied over a nearly thousandfold range. It was subsequently observed that the clinical sensitivity of untreated patients correlated well with the dose response of their leukocytes to antigen.[12] The most sensitive patients had leukocytes which reacted with the lowest concentrations of antigen, and the leukocytes of the least sensitive patients required large concentrations of antigen for significant release of histamine. It had been shown earlier that after immunotherapy a higher concentration of antigen was required to initiate histamine release from whole blood than before treatment. This inhibition was mostly due to antibody, presumably blocking antibody, but there was a suggestion of cellular desensitization. Examination of the latter possibility could only be made with washed leukocytes. By this means it has been established that after high dose immunotherapy leukocytes from patients who had previously been reactive no longer released histamine at the highest concentration of antigen tested.[25] This observation has been confirmed in several laboratories.

Serum IgE

With the changes already recorded during immunotherapy it is also valuable to determine the serum IgE content of patients undergoing therapy. These data are being gathered by several groups of investigators and will show whether treatment will reduce production of IgE generally as well as of specific reagins. The measurement of cell bound IgE and cell bound reaginic antibody is not presently possible but would be most important in defining the immune system of the allergic cell.

Reverse Histamine Release

Another dimension of cellular reactivity is currently under study. Leukocytes of many individuals react with anti-IgE serum to release histamine. This is because IgE is cytotropic for mast cells and basophils which contain histamine. Cells of both atopics and nonatopics have IgE attached to their surfaces. Interaction of anti-IgE with the cell-bound IgE sets off the histamine release mechanism and should be independent of the antigenic specificity of the IgE. The dose response of white cells to anti-IgE in normal patients and in atopics before and after treatment may aid in understanding how they become unresponsive to antigen.

Nonimmune Histamine Release

An additional measure of cellular response which has not yet been sufficiently investigated to determine its potential utility in allergy research is the reaction to compound 48/80. Mast cells are degranulated by this substance with loss of intracellular histamine. It may be a valuable tool, because cells may be activated by nonimmunologic means, and this may provide an indication of the metabolic state of the cell subsequent to initiation of release by the antigen-antibody reaction. Although histamine is released from human leukocytes by 48/80, the concentration of 48/80 necessary to initiate histamine release from the basophils is cytotoxic. Thus the usefulness of this system is questionable. Perhaps other agents will be found which are more suitable for activation of basophils in a manner similar to allergen and reagin.

CORRELATION OF IMMUNOLOGIC CONSEQUENCES OF IMMUNOTHERAPY WITH CLINICAL RESULTS

It has been established in several studies that there is a significant decrease in clinical symptoms in patients receiving hyposensitization by injections of allergen. Ultimately this is the consideration that determines the efficacy of any treatment. In seasonal allergy the evaluation of therapy is extremely difficult for a number of reasons. Symptoms may occur for a short period of time each year and grading of severity by the patient may vary from year to year. The relative degree of environmental exposure differs each year and even within a single season. One individual may be more perceptive of discomfort than another. Attempts to maximize objectivity such as symptom scores based on daily diaries are only partially successful. In spite of these difficulties, careful studies have substantiated the value of immunotherapy. It occurred to us and to others that if any of the immunologic parameters described in the previous section were correlated with the clinical state of the patient then these objective measurements might be used in the future to assess clinical results with current or newly devised treatments.

A very recent study has shown that the earliest changes that could be measured during immunotherapy with ragweed extract were increases in ragweed-binding antibody (blocking antibody). This was related temporally with reduction in clinical symptoms. Several groups have found that binding or blocking antibody to ragweed increased during treatment and severity of symptoms declined but that the correlation was imperfect. Patients with the highest levels of blocking antibody were not necessarily those with greatest relief from symptoms. It was also noted that some individuals had good relief of symptoms prior to substantial increases in serum antibody. Attempts to correlate the quantity of blocking antibody in respiratory secretions with improvement in symptoms were similarly unsuccessful. It has been demonstrated on the other hand [3] that autologous blocking antibody delivered to the respiratory tract has substantial protective value in proportion to the quantity delivered. These apparently contradictory findings may be explained by the following considerations. Blocking antibody can only competitively reduce but not abolish exposure of sensitized cells to antigen because increasing the antigen concentration sufficiently can partially or completely nullify the effect of any given concentration of blocking antibody. If the concentration of aeroallergen during natural exposure is often high relative to the quantities of blocking antibody developed in most individuals during treatment, the effect of blocking antibody can easily be missed. Relief from symptoms due to blocking antibody might only be obvious at lower environmental allergen concentrations when all groups, high- and low sensitivity and treated and untreated, would tend to have fewer symptoms. Differences due to blocking antibody in treated patients, might therefore be obscured. A study using delivery of graded concentrations of aerosolized antigen below antibody saturation, in which each individual is his own control, might establish the efficacy of actively produced blocking antibody.

In summary it is quite likely that blocking antibody contributes to clinical improvement and that this will be demonstrated in the future, but factors such as innate cellular sensitivity, the degree of antigenic exposure or other unknown factors are quantitatively more important. The current tendency of some to dismiss the role of blocking antibody in clinical improvement seems premature.

Histamine release from washed leukocytes of atopic individuals has shown good correlation with clinical results of immunotherapy. First, it is known that in untreated patients the greater the intensity of clinical symptoms the lower the concentration of antigen necessary to induce release from peripheral cells. After treatment at relatively high doses of antigen (above 100,000 PNU) given within a few months, 10 of 11 patients studied in our laboratory no longer released a significant proportion of cellular histamine in the presence of antigen. This finding has been confirmed in at least some patients in other similar investigations. The peripheral leukocytes are therefore a relatively good index of clinical sensitivity, since there is generally a good correlation between dose response of specific histamine release from these cells and severity of clinical symptoms before, during and after treatment.

The mechanism by which cells are rendered insensitive to antigen subsequent to intensive immunotherapy is not clear. Among the possibilities are inhibition of synthesis of reagin, alteration of the surface of the mast cells such that it no longer binds the Fc piece of IgE and alteration of the metabolic activity of the cell so that antigen-antibody reaction on the cell surface does not trigger histamine release.

The high degree of correlation between decreased cellular sensitivity and decreased symptoms is easy to understand. A patient whose cells are no longer responsive to antigen will be symptom-free at any level of antigen exposure as long as the peripheral cells reflect the sensitivity of the respiratory mast cells. This contrasts with the effects of blocking antibody, which are allergen-dose dependent as discussed above.

After immunotherapy the titers of SSA may be reduced. This usually occurs following several years of treatment but may be seen earlier when high doses of antigen are administered frequently. How the modest reductions in reagin concentration which have been reported are sufficient to account for complete cellular insensitivity and complete absence of clinical symptoms seems difficult to explain.

One possible explanation is the apparent stereo-specificity of the IgE binding sites, discussed above, which would require large amounts of reagin to insure reactivity. A lower serum reagin content must at least contribute to the clinical benefits obtained from hyposensitization.

There are preliminary indications that leukocytes of treated individuals no longer release histamine when incubated with anti-IgE as well as with specific allergen, but this has not yet been established. If this turns out to be a general observation and if serum IgE were essentially unchanged it would support the idea of an alteration in either surface structure or in metabolic activity of mast cells and basophils brought about by immunotherapy. The effect of treatment on concentration of serum IgE, cell-bound IgE and the dose response of cells to anti-IgE and possibly to nonimmune triggers of basophils such as 48/80 are being investigated, but published results are not yet available. When the studies are completed, some of the questions about the mechanism by which leukocytes are desensitized may be answered.

WHAT IS THE ATOPIC STATE?

Atopy is a genetically determined state but is apparently not the result of simple Mendelian inheritance. One possibility is that atopic individuals are genetically better IgE producers. There is evidence for this, although the levels of serum IgE in hayfever and asthma patients are generally not markedly higher than those of the normal population and there is considerable overlap. In certain regions of the world and in patients with atopic dermatitis the serum IgE is very high. These observations suggest the importance of environmental factors and the difficulty in identifying atopic individuals by measurement of serum IgE.

It may be that the specificity of the IgE antibody response to antigens (in addition to or rather than the magnitude of the response) is genetically controlled. A recent animal study indicated that homocytotropic antibody was produced better at low concentrations of antigen and further that only certain genetic strains responded at all under these conditions.[11] Atopics may simply be those individuals whose IgE antibody capacity is directed against those common environmental antigens such as pollens which are associated with hayfever and extrinsic asthma. If other antigens were commonly airborne and in sufficient concentration it is possible that individuals not now considered atopic would have these symptoms. Bakers' asthma might be a case in point since some of these individuals do not react to common allergens. The ability to induce sensitivity of the immediate-type to ascaris antigen in most individuals may reflect a universal specificity of IgE for parasitic antigens resulting from natural selection.

An interesting suggestion has been made that the genetic variable in atopy is an enhanced permeability of bronchial membranes to allergen. Immunization with aerosols of ribonuclease or dextran resulted in higher levels of SSA in atopics than in normals. The evidence is consistent with altered permeability of mucosal surfaces but is incomplete. It is also indirect in that serum antibody was measured and not the actual permeability of antigen. Differences in antigen processing and/or reagin producing capacity rather than permeability could have accounted for the results. A definitive answer must await further study.

Another concept of the genetic basis for atopy is a blockade of the β-adrenergic receptors.[28] In its most advanced form this theory encompasses not only asthma but all manifestations of atopy including increased production of reagin. No evidence has been produced to show a genetically induced blockade in atopics. The only models available require environmental agents such as endotoxin or infection to accomplish blockade. It is not within the scope of this discussion to elaborate further on this concept or its strengths and weaknesses. It is appropriate, however, to mention the view that in extrinsic asthma the mediators released from mast cells upset the normal balance of contraction and relaxation of the bronchial smooth muscle. Restoration of normal tension might ordinarily be accomplished by adrenergic mechanisms but in beta blockade, such as that produced by infection, homeostatic control would be inhibited. This would mean that β-blockade where present does not initiate the asthmatic attack but that it hinders its resolution. Exogenous β-adrenergic agents would help restore the normal homeostatic balance in ordinary extrinsic asthma. Where asthma is complicated by infection and resultant β-blockade, epinephrine could be helpful, ineffective or even harmful depending on the extent of blockade. The concept that a β-adrenergic blockade exists in asthmatics and even in atopics has at least provided an approach which has stimulated new areas of investigation.

There must be a structural complementariness of the surface of mast cells or basophils and the Fc piece of the IgE of an allergic individual. The low failure rate in the P-K reaction means that there is an almost universal acceptance of reagin by human cutaneous mast cells. Passive sensitization of leukocytes with reagin on the other hand has only been reported to be demonstrable in 20 percent of nonatopic donors. This suggests a difference in mast cell surface structure in different tissues of the same individual and the possibility that changes in structure may be influenced by environmental factors including therapy.

In summary, the atopic individual appears genetically predisposed to produce IgE antibody upon environmental exposure to the common allergens. The nature of expression of the genetic trait is not known presently but most probably involves enhanced qualitative and/or quantitative response to these antigens. The series of events which occurs when IgE is bound to mast cells and the sensitized cells react with antigen to release the mediators of allergic symptoms is similar in both atopics and nonatopics. Passive transfer of these reactions to nonatopic individuals with serum from atopics indicates that the crucial difference between them is the presence or absence of reagin after sufficient exposure to allergen.

NEW APPROACHES TO THERAPY

ADJUVANTS

With the current availability of quantitative procedures for measuring various immunologic parameters it is possible to objectively evaluate new forms of therapy. Earlier attempts to improve immunotherapy suffered from lack of these methods and, in the case of emulsion therapy, from use of materials not meeting standards acceptable for human administration.

Extraction of ragweed pollen in pyridine followed by alum precipitation was suggested and is now offered commercially. Some experiments in animals showed a reduction in antigenicity of this material and others implied that it maintained its potency. Good clinical results have been reported with this material, but caution is advised in evaluating this or any other treatment because of the subjective factors previously discussed. Alum precipitates of aqueous extracts are also being evaluated with preliminary indications of efficacy. Other adjuvants have been and will continue to be developed and tested.

ALLERGOIDS

Since one of the deterrents to immunotherapy is the occurrence of systemic reactions, attempts have been made to modify the capacity of the allergen to trigger mediator release while maintaining its ability to elicit blocking antibody and/or reduce reactivity of mast cells to antigen. If one could alter or destroy the antigenic determinants which combine with the IgE antibody bound to the surface of the sensitized cells while leaving intact or exposing other determinants a valuable tool would be available. This molecule could induce formation of a blocking antibody without the danger of systemic reactions. It could not desensitize mast cells with specific reagin bound to its surface, however. Treatment of pollen antigens with formaldehyde analogous to treatment of bacterial toxins with this agent results in a product called allergoid. If the properties of allergoid were also analogous to toxoid this would be an advance in treatment. Several allergoids are being used in new experimental treatments which are still in the evaluation stage.[15]

OTHER IMMUNOLOGIC APPROACHES

Aside from traditional immunotherapeutic approaches there are other possibilities. If a fragment were derived from an allergen which could still react with reagin but was insufficient in size to trigger the sensitized mast cell it would effectively desensitize these cells. It would also combine with circulating reagin and render it inactive even after it became cell-bound. Blocking antibody might or might not be produced depending on size and structure. Sporadic attempts have been made to isolate or degrade allergenic fragments without notable success. Recently a low molecular weight grass pollen antigen has been isolated from extracts [14] and claims of efficacy in blocking antibody production and inhibition of reagin formation have been made, but insufficient data are available for a complete evaluation of the general clinical applicability of such materials.

New Drugs

The mechanisms discussed in the section on the allergic cell suggest a systematic approach to therapy. Drugs may be found which intervene in each of the sequential processes which ultimately produce clinical symptoms. If these steps are subdivided in the future, new agents may be found to inhibit at these points.

The Antigen-Antibody Reaction

There are no chemical agents known which are relatively nontoxic and are capable of destroying or neutralizing allergens, preventing reagin production or inhibiting the combination of allergen with reagin. In cases resistant to other forms of therapy, steroids are used, and they may act in part by inhibiting the formation of reagin. They are best avoided, however, because of their side effects. Immunosuppressive agents would also be expected to be effective but would not be used for obvious reasons.

Activation of Cells for Mediator Release

If there are no good ways of preventing antigen and antibody from appearing or from reacting, the next possible attack might be the inhibition of the specific activation of the mast cell.

Hetrazan *, an antihelminthic agent, appears to selectively inhibit the release of SRS from activated tissue.[18] This compound was originally claimed to be effective in suppressing asthmatic symptoms in patients receiving the drug to combat parasitic infestations. Interestingly the original investigator has recently withdrawn this claim.

Chlorphenesin, a fungicide, inhibits release of histamine from leukocytes of atopic patients. Its clinical value in asthma is not currently known.

An agent currently being tested for its antiasthmatic activity, disodium cromoglycate, inhibits release of histamine and SRS from monkey mast cells but does not affect histamine release from basophils of allergic

* Trademark, Lederle Labs.

patients. It appears to be effective clinically in reducing steroid dosages but does not result in complete remission from symptoms.[5] Final judgment of its full clinical value is yet to be made.

Trasylol, a polypeptide obtained from bovine adrenal medulla, inhibits the proteolytic activity of kallikrein and therefore prevents bradykinin formation.

The area where this small series of drugs operates is to prevent mediator release from activated cells. This is the most promising area in which new antiallergic agents can be developed. Mediator release from leukocytes has been divided into two phases, but useful inhibitors of the second stage have not been described.

Pharmacologic Action of Mediators

Prevention of the pharmacologic action of the mediators histamine, SRS and bradykinin is also possible. Many antihistamines are known and in general use (See Chapter 6). Drugs effective against the actions of SRS are not currently available for clinical use but will probably be developed. Aspirin is an antagonist of bradykinin action but its clinical usefulness for this purpose is not known. Beta adrenergic agents do not directly antagonize the actions of histamine and other mediators but do reverse their action. Further knowledge of adrenergic mechanisms may provide better drugs in this area.

REFERENCES

1. Arbesman, C. E., and Ito, K.: A new method of measuring IgE. J. Allerg., 47:85, 1971.
2. Austen, K. F., and Humphrey, J. H.: In vitro studies of the mechanism of anaphylaxis. Adv. Immun., 3:1, 1963.
3. Connell, J. T., and Klein, D. E.: Protective effect of nasal sprays containing blocking antibody in hay fever. J. Allerg., 45:115, 1970.
4. Cooke, R. A., Barnard, J. H., Hebald, S., and Stull, A.: Serological evidence of immunity with co-existing sensitization in a type of human allergy (hay fever). J. Exp. Med., 62:733, 1935.
5. Cox, J. S. C., et. al.: Disodium cromoglycate (Intal). Adv. Drug Res., 5:115, 1970.
6. Gleich, G. J., Averbeck, A. K., and Swedlund, H. A.: Measurement of IgE in normal and allergic serum by radioimmunoassay. J. Lab. Clin. Med. 77:690, 1971.
7. Grabar, P., and Williams, C., Jr.: Method of immuno-electrophoretic analysis of mixtures of antigenic substances. Biochim. Biophys. Acta, 17:67, 1955.
8. Ishizaka, K., and Ishizaka, T.: Identification of γE antibody as a carrier of reaginic activity. J. Immun., 99:1187, 1967.

9. Johansson, S. G. O., Bennich, H., and Wide, L.: A new class of immunoglobulin in human serum. Immunology, *14:*265, 1968.
10. Levine, B. B., and Redmond, A. P.: The nature of the antigen-antibody complexes initiating the specific wheal and flare reaction in sensitized man. J. Clin. Invest., *47:*556, 1968.
11. Levine, B. B., and Vaz, N. M.: Effect of combinations of inbred strain, antigen and antigen dose on immune responsiveness and reagin production in the mouse. A potential mouse model for immune aspects of atopic allergy. Int. Arch. Allerg., *39:*156, 1970.
12. Lichtenstein, L. M., Norman, P. S., and Winkenwerder, W. L.: Clinical and in vitro studies on the role of immunotherapy in ragweed hay fever, Am. J. Med., *44:*514, 1968.
13. Lichtenstein, L. M., and Osler, A. G.: Studies on the mechanisms of hypersensitivity phenomena: IX. Histamine release from human leukocytes by ragweed pollen antigen. J. Exp. Med., *120:*507, 1964.
14. Malley, A., and Perlman, F.: Timothy pollen fractions in treatment of hay fever. I. Clinical and immunologic response to small and higher molecular weight fractions. J. Allerg., *45:*14, 1970.
15. Marsh, D. G., Lichtenstein, L. M., and Campbell, D. H.: Conversion of Group I rye pollen antigens to "allergoid" by mild formalin treatment. J. Allerg., *43:*179, 1969.
16. Melam, H., Pruzansky, J., Patterson, R., and Singer, S.: Clinical and immunologic studies of ragweed immunotherapy. J. Allerg., *47:*262, 1971.
17. Nisonoff, A., Wissler, F. C., Lipman, L. N., and Woernley, D. L.: Separation of univalent fragments from the rabbit antibody molecule by reduction of disulfide bonds. Arch. Biochem. Biophys., *89:*230, 1960.
18. Orange, R. P., Valentine, M. D., and Austen, K. F.: Inhibition of the release of slow-reacting substance of anaphylaxis in the rat with diethylcarbamazine. Proc. Soc. Exp. Biol. Med., *127:*127, 1968.
19. Osler, A. G., Lichtenstein, L. M., and Levy, D. A.: In vitro studies of human reaginic allergy. Adv. Immun., *8:*183, 1968.
20. Patterson, R.: Laboratory models of reaginic allergy. Prog. Allerg., *13:*332, 1969.
21. Porter, R. R.: The hydrolysis of rabbit γ globulin and antibodies with crystalline papain. Biochem. J., *73:*119, 1959.
22. Prausnitz, C., and Küstner, N.: Studien über die Ueberempfindlichkeit, Zbl. Bakt., *68:*160, 1921.
23. Pruzansky, J. J., and Patterson, R.: Binding of I[131]-labeled ragweed antigen by sera of ragweed-sensitive individuals. J. Allerg., *35:*1, 1964.
24. Pruzansky, J. J., and Patterson, R.: The interaction of antigen with leucocytes of allergic individuals. J. Immun., *97:*854, 1966.
25. Pruzansky, J. J., and Patterson, R.: Histamine release from leukocytes of hypersensitive individuals: II. Reduced sensitivity of leukocytes after injection therapy. J. Allerg., *39:*44, 1967.

26. Pruzansky, J. J., and Patterson, R.: Histamine in human leucocytes. Localization of histamine and beta glucuronidase in human leucocytes. Int. Arch. Allerg., 37:98, 1970.
27. Rowe, D. S.: Radioactive single radial diffusion. A method for increasing the sensitivity of immunochemical quantification of proteins in agar gel. Bull. W.H.O., 40:613, 1969.
28. Szentivanyi, A.: The beta adrenergic theory of the atopic abnormality in bronchial asthma. J. Allerg., 42:203, 1968.
29. Wide, L., Bennich, H., and Johansson, S. G. O.: Diagnosis of allergy by an in vitro test for allergen antibodies. Lancet, 2:1105, 1967.

3

Diagnosis of Immediate Hypersensitivity

Bernard Hess Booth III, M.D.

Immediate type hypersensitivity is one of the explanations for conjunctivitis, rhinitis, or wheezing dyspnea. In addition, it is possibly responsible for some cases of eczema. There are, however, many other etiological explanations of each of these symptoms. Consequently when a patient has been troubled enough with one of these conditions to consult a physician, it is necessary to perform a complete medical evaluation.

First it must be determined whether the symptoms are allergic in origin or whether they have another etiology. Then if the symptoms are considered to be allergic, more specific diagnostic evaluations must be completed. This more specific diagnosis must be made by identifying the antigen or antigens that are clinically significant. In addition, a number of other variable factors must be evaluated. The degree of sensitivity to an antigen may vary as may the degree of exposure to a clinically significant antigen. Many patients are sensitive to multiple antigens, and cumulative effects of exposure to several antigens may be important. The influence of nonimmunologic phenomena on these symptoms must also be evaluated. Infection, inhaled irritants, fatigue and emotional problems may be significant independently or cumulatively and may fluctuate widely in degree of significance. Considering the large number of variables that must be considered, it is not surprising that the most important portion of any clinical evaluation is an expertly taken history.

Many techniques have been utilized in obtaining a history such as forms filled out by the patient or the interviewer. (An example of an Allergy Survey Sheet is shown, p. 64.) These may be useful but they can only facilitate and not replace the careful inquiries of a skilled historian. Though the significant information can sometimes be obtained with relative ease, in the usual case adequate information can be obtained only after a considerable investment of time and energy.

63

ALLERGY SURVEY SHEET

Name—————————————————   Age——— Sex——— Date———

  I. Chief complaint:

 II. Present illness:

III. Collateral allergic symptoms:

Eyes:	Pruritus———— Burning———— Lacrimation———— Swelling———— Injection———— Discharge————
Ears:	Pruritus———— Fullness———— Popping ———— Frequent infections————
Nose:	Sneezing———— Rhinorrhea———— Obstruction———— Pruritus———— Mouth breathing———— Purulent discharge————
Throat:	Soreness———— Post-nasal discharge———— Palatal pruritus———— Mucus in the morning————
Chest:	Cough ———— Pain ———— Wheezing ———— Sputum ———— Dyspnea ———— Color ———— Rest ———— Amount ———— Exertion ————
Skin:	Dermatitis ———— Eczema ———— Urticaria ————

 IV. Family Allergies:

  V. Previous allergic treatment or testing:

Prior skin testing:

Drugs:	Antihistamines	Improved ————	Unimproved ————
	Bronchodilators	Improved ————	Unimproved ————
	Nose drops	Improved ————	Unimproved ————
	Hyposensitization	Improved ————	Unimproved ————
	Duration ————		
	Antigens ————		
	Reactions ————		
	Antibiotics	Improved ————	Unimproved ————
	Steroids	Improved ————	Unimproved ————

VI. Physical agents and habits:

Bothered by:

Tobacco for —— years	Alcohol ———— Air cond. ————
Cigarettes ———— packs/day	Heat ———— Muggy weath. ——
Cigars ———— per day	Cold ———— Weath. chngs. ——
Pipe ———— per day	Perfumes ———— Chemicals ————
Never smoked ————	Paints ———— Hair spray ————
Bothered by smoke ————	Insecticides —— Newspapers ——
	Cosmetics ——

VII. When symptoms occur:
  Time and circumstances of 1st episode:
  Prior health:
  Course of illness over decades: progressing——— regressing———
  Time of year:
    Perennial———   Exact dates
    Seasonal———
    Seasonally exacerbated———
  Monthly variations (menses, occupation):
  Time of week (weekends vs weekdays):
  Time of day or night:
  After insect stings:

VIII. Where symptoms occur:
  Living where at onset:
  Living where since onset:
  Effect of vacation or major geographic change:
  Symptoms better indoors or outdoors:
  Effect of school or work:
  Effect of staying elsewhere nearby:
  Effect of hospitalization:
  Effect of specific environments:
  Do symptoms occur around:
  old leaves——— hay——— lakeside——— barns———
  summer homes——— damp basement——— dry attic———
  lawnmowing——— animals——— other———
  Do symptoms occur after eating:
  cheese——— mushrooms——— beer——— melons———
  bananas——— fish——— nuts——— citrus fruits———
  other foods (list)————————————————————
  Home: city ——————rural —————————
      house ————— age —————————
      apartment ——— basement ——— damp——— dry———
      heating system ———
      pets (how long) ——— dog——— cat——— other———

Bedroom:	Type	Age	*Living Room:*	Type	Age
Pillow	——	——	Rug	——	——
Mattress	——	——	Matting	——	——
Blankets	——	——	Furniture	——	——
Quilts	——	——			
Furniture	——	——			

  Anywhere in home symptoms are worse: ————————————

IX. What does patient think makes him worse: ————————————

X. Under what circumstances is he free of symptoms: —————————

XI. Summary and additional comments:

The history not only provides most of the information necessary for diagnosis but it is necessary before further diagnostic tests can be selected that will be of value and will not be dangerous to a patient with an extreme degree of sensitivity.

GENERAL HISTORICAL CHARACTERISTICS OF IMMEDIATE TYPE HYPERSENSITIVITY

The history of the patient is taken as an ordinary medical history is taken. The patient is asked to state his chief complaint and to describe his symptoms. During the history the presence or absence of symptoms of nonallergic conditions must be determined and evaluated. Certain details of the allergic history are so characteristic that they should be elicited early. Is there a history of atopic disease in the parents, grandparents, siblings, aunts, uncles, cousins or children of the patient? Most allergic patients will have a positive history in this respect.

Are there other symptoms in addition to the presenting complaint that may be allergic in origin? The presence of urticaria, other skin eruptions, pruritus, sneezing, rhinitis, eye irritation, intermittent hearing loss, wheezing dyspnea or cough should always be determined. Several allergic symptoms frequently exist in one patient even though he has not associated them with a common cause. If several of these symptoms are present, then it is likely that they all will have an allergic etiology. Conversely rhinitis without associated nasal pruritus probably is not allergic. Unilateral ocular, nasal or chest symptoms also suggest the presence of nonallergic conditions.

Are the symptoms continuous or intermittent? Allergic symptoms are usually intermittent and even in those cases in which they are continuous there are usually intermittent exacerbations.

A good response to previous antihistamines or other symptomatic therapy tends to substantiate an allergic etiology, while failure to obtain even partial relief makes one consider other illnesses.

IDENTIFICATION OF SPECIFIC ETIOLOGICAL AGENTS

Usually the general physician can and is required to determine if an allergic disease is present, and he usually initiates appropiate therapy. To arrive at a more specific diagnosis of the antigens responsible for the illness a detailed allergic history is mandatory. The purpose of the detailed allergic history is to obtain the information necessary to allow a correlation of symptoms with the known time and place of occurrence of various antigens.

The decision to pursue a more specific diagnosis depends on several factors. If the disease is mild, produces no disability and responds to symptomatic therapy, an elaborate investigation may not be indicated. Conversely severe discomfort or disability would make a complete evaluation mandatory. Becasuse asthma is a potentially lethal illness every asthmatic patient should have an evaluation.

Whether the general physician performs the more detailed evaluation or consults an allergist for this depends upon his own interest, the severity of the patient's illness and the availability of a competent allergist.

Characteristics of Antigens

Detailed information about clinically significant antigens is given in Chapters 4 and 5. Some general characteristics of the antigens responsible for allergic illnesses must be appreciated however before an adequate clinical history can be obtained or interpreted.

Foods. Though **foods** may have a major importance in cases of infantile eczema, urticaria, angioedema or anaphylaxis, they are relatively unimportant in most cases of allergic conjunctivitis, allergic rhinitis or allergic asthma.

The antigens most important in these conditions are usually airborne. There are several different groups of these aeroallergens that are of major clinical significance including the pollens, fungi, house dust and animal danders.

Pollen. The grains of **pollen** from flowering plants are among the most important antigens that cause clinical sensitization. Most flowering plants produce pollen that is rich in protein and consequently potentially antigenic. Whether or not a specific pollen causes symptoms regularly depends upon several factors. The pollens that routinely act as significant antigens usually fulfill three criteria. They are produced in large quantity by a plant that is common. The pollens depend primarily upon the wind for their dispersal and the pollen itself is antigenic.

Many plants produce pollens that are large, thick and waxy. Under natural conditions transfer of the pollen between plants is accomplished chiefly by insects. These pollens are not widely dispersed in the air and therefore are rarely significant. Goldenrod which is popularly considered a cause of hay fever has little significance for this reason. Its pollen rapidly falls from the air before it can be widely dispersed and reach the patient with hay fever. In contrast the ragweed plant pollenates at the same time and its pollen is small, light and widely dispersed by the wind. In addition it grows in abundance in many areas.

In the United States most trees and grasses and many weeds produce large quantities of highly antigenic, windborne pollen. The seasonal occurrence of tree, grass and weed pollens varies with the geographical location. Even though many factors may alter the total amount of pollen produced in any year, the season of pollenation of a plant remains remarkably constant in any one area from year to year. The physician treating allergic problems must know which windborne pollens are abundant in his area and their seasons of pollenation (See Chaps. 4 and 5). Because the major clinically significant pollens do vary with geographic location some companies have designed regional skin test kits that contain only the pollens that are prevelant in a specific area.

Many thousands of different **fungi** or molds exist. The role of most of them in the production of allergic symptoms is speculative, but some species have been definitely implicated. Because they can colonize almost every possible habitat and because they reproduce spores prolifically, the air is never free from fungus spores. Consequently they are very important in some patients with perennial symptoms. However, seasonal or local situational influences can greatly alter the number of airborne spores.

A period of warm weather with relatively high humidity allows optimal growth. If this period is then followed by hot, dry, windy weather, the spores often become airborne in large concentrations. Consequently in large portions of the United States there may be a maximal peak between late June and early September. Mold-sensitive patients may therefore have major difficulty between the grass and weed pollen seasons. A frost may produce a large amount of dying vegetation which provides a suitable media for the growth of fungi. If in addition, there is a period of warm weather with high humidity in the late fall, mold-sensitive patients may have significant difficulty well after the normal weed pollen season. Snow not only covers dying vegetation but the decreased temperature may reduce the rate of growth of fungi during cold winter months. In contrast, spring may provide the relative warmth, humidity and adequate substrate necessary for the growth of fungi.

High local concentrations of mold spores are also frequently encountered. Deep shade may produce high humidity because of condensation of water on cool surfaces. High humidity may occur in areas of water seepage such as basements, or in refrigerator drip trays or in garbage pails. Food storage areas, dairies, breweries, air conditioning systems, piles of fallen leaves or rotting wood, barns or silos with hay and other grains may provide nutrients as well as high humidity and may therefore have high concentration of mold spores.

Persons who have symptoms when molds are inhaled may also occasionally have difficulty after ingesting foods that contain molds or their products. Cheeses and fermented drinks, usually beer or wine, are the most common offenders. Occasionally other foods such as those prepared with a large amount of yeast, buttermilk, mushrooms or dried fruits or vinegar may be implicated.

House Dust. The most common cause of perennial allergic rhinitis or asthma is probably an allergy to house dust. Allergy to house dust may represent sensitivity to a large group of antigens all of which are probably the breakdown products of organic matter. The mechanical and chemical trauma of use probably causes a breakdown of the cellulose fibers of fabrics and converts them into antigens. For example, extracts made from new cotton are not antigenic for dust sensitive patients but extracts from old cotton stuffing may give positive reactions in the same patients.

Animal danders may contribute to the antigenicity of dust. Not only household pets but the presence of horse, cattle or hog hair in stuffed chairs, couches, mattresses, or rug mattings may be significant. The products of certain microscopic mites have also been implicated as a source of potent antigens. Regardless of the exact nature of the antigen, after use and aging, rugs, bedding, furniture stuffing and a variety of fabrics commonly found in the home may be sources of clinically potent antigens.

Dust-sensitive patients have perennial symptoms though they may be somewhat better during the summer months or when the patient is outside. There may be a history of sneezing, rhinorrhea, lacrimation or mild asthma whenever the house is cleaned or the beds made. With the onset of cool weather the house may be closed, and the heating system may stir up the house dust and produce an exacerbation of symptoms. This is much more likely to occur if there is a forced air heating system and less likely if there is radiant heat. In many dust-sensitive patients the history is not so obvious and the presence of perennial symptoms is the only suggestive feature.

Animal Dander. Particles of the fur, the skin and the dried saliva of animals can act as potent antigens. When pets live inside a home, these products can reach high concentration and completely permeate the furniture, bedding, rugs and air of a home. Household pets are frequently entirely responsible for severe disabling asthma. A short-haired pet does not eliminate this hazard. Though cats and dogs are most frequently involved, a large number of other animals are occasionally responsible. A remarkable number of homes have hamsters, gerbils, rabbits, parakeets, parrots, or mice. Certain occupational groups such as laboratory workers, veterinarians, ranchers, or farmers may have exposure to an unusual variety of animal danders.

A patient with clinical sensitivity to a household pet may have a history similar to that of dust sensitive individuals. In addition the patient may have a rapid, marked symptomatic improvement when he leaves his home or is hospitalized. Many patients may give a history of having a wheal and erythema reaction at a skin site that the animal scratched or bit. Animal sensitivity should always be suspected when a patient develops fairly severe asthma as an adult.

A patient with an inhalant allergy may respond well to treatment for many months only to have a sudden increase in symptoms. Frequently this may be due to the introduction of a pet into the home. If the physician is unaware of this he will completely misinterpret these symptoms and may embark upon an incorrect therapeutic regimen.

TYPE AND SEQUENCE OF CLINICAL MANIFESTATIONS

Knowledge of the commonly significant allergens allows the physician to use the detailed allergic history to confirm the differential diagnosis of allergic disease and to provide clues to the specific diagnosis. The course of the disease over decades should be determined. Age of onset, geographical location of the patient throughout life, health during the patient's school years, the nature and place of employment, any change in symptoms with puberty or pregnancy should be recorded. It should be determined if the disease has progressively improved or worsened over the years.

It is very important to determine when the patient does or does not have symptoms. The yearly seasonal variations are significant. Even if perennial symptoms are present a seasonal variation may be superimposed. It is necessary to elicit the dates of exacerbations as exactly as possible. There may be significant differences in springtime symptoms that occur in early April and those that occur in late May.

Fluctuation in symptoms during the week are sometimes common and suggest the importance of antigens that are encountered in the home, school or work environment. Variations in symptoms during the day are less helpful because nasal congestion increases during recumbency and asthma tends to occur at night. This does not necessarily indicate allergy to something in the bedroom.

Next it is necessary to determine where the patient does or does not have symptoms. Did his symptoms change when he moved from one place to another? Are any places regularly associated with an increase in symptoms such as barns, damp basements, a weekend or summer home, fields, or factories? Is he better indoors or outdoors? Was he better when on vacation in other locations? Does he improve rapidly in the hospital or at the homes of friends? It is frequently useful to ask the patient what agents he believes cause his difficulty.

A detailed survey of the patient's home, work or school environment is also useful. Are there pets in the house? What are the ages and types of home furnishings? Specific questions regarding his mattress, pillows, rugs, drapes and upholstered furniture are frequently relevant. What type of heating, air conditioning and air filters are in the home? Is there a damp basement or dry attic? When and how is the home cleaned? A detailed survey of his work environment is also necessary. Knowing that the patient is an accountant may be meaningless, since he may sit in an air conditioned office or he may take inventory in damp, dusty warehouses.

Specific information about previous therapy is useful. Determine if there was a good response or if previous therapy was harmful in terms of drug allergy or prolonged use of nose drops. Antihistamines and sympathomimetic amines may alter physical findings or interfere with skin tests.

Certain nonimmunologic factors so frequently make the allergic patient worse that they should always be evaluated. Primary irritants such as tobacco smoke, paint or gas fumes or more generalized air pollution need to be identified. The effects of infection on the patient's disease should be noted. The effects of weather and of psychic conflicts must be evaluated.

PHYSICAL EXAMINATION

Every patient should have a complete physical examination. Particular attention obviously must be paid to the more common sites of allergic disease. These findings are reviewed in detail in the chapters dealing with each specific entity.

Conjunctivitis. Physical findings of allergic conjunctivitis are hyperemia and edema of the conjunctiva. Occasionally a pronounced chemosis occurs associated with a clear watery discharge. Periorbital edema may be present and, rarely, a bluish discoloration may occur about the eyes. If chemosis is severe, acute allergic conjuctivitis might be confused with epidemic kertoconjunctivitis. In these cases the examination should include staining the secretions for eosinophils and observing the effectiveness of eye drops containing sympathomimetic amines or antihistamines.

Rhinitis. The examination of the nose requires good exposure and adequate light. A head mirror and nasal speculum provide this effectively. In a patient with allergic rhinitis the inferior turbinates usually appear to be swollen and may actually meet the septum. They may have a uniform bluish or pearly gray discoloration, but more frequently there may be adjacent areas where the membrane is red, giving a mottled appearance. Polyps may or may not be seen within the nose.

The skin of the nose and particularly the upper lip may show irritation and excoriation produced by the nasal discharge and continuous nose wiping. Transillumination of the paranasal sinuses may be of occasional value if concomitant infection is suspected. In patients with nasal allergic disease the ears should be examined for evidence of acute or chronic otitis media either serous or infectious in nature. Nasal secretions may also be observed draining into the posterior pharynx.

For many years certain structural characteristics of the face have been considered to be the result of chronic nasal congestion and mouth breathing. The characteristics of these "allergic faces" are a pointed chin, a narrow, highly arched palate with an elongated upper jaw and a marked overbite. Such facial structure is definitely seen in many but not all allergic children. It is also seen in children with no allergic disease. The questions of whether "allergic faces" are more common in allergic children and whether they have any common etiological factors are unanswered. In any case, the presence or absence of such a facial structure has no specific diagnostic significance.

Asthma. Physical findings in asthmatic patients are highly variable not only between patients but in one patient at different times. The rapidity with which both symptoms and physical findings can appear or disappear is one of the characteristic features of the illness.

During an acute attack of asthma the patient usually uses his accessory muscles of respiration. Mechanically, these muscles are more effective if the patient stands or sits and leans slightly forward. During an acute attack the patient will rarely lie down unless he is severely exhausted. Intercostal, subcostal and supraclavicular retraction as well as flaring of the ala nasi may be present with inspiratory effort.

Physical findings attributable to hyperinflation of the chest may be present. The chest may be held continuously in the mid-inspiratory position, and there may be increased resonance to percussion. In addition percussion may reveal that the diaphragms are in a low position and have limited respiratory excursion.

On auscultation, musical wheezes may be heard during both inspiration and expiration, and the expiratory phase of respiration may be prolonged. In uncomplicated asthma these auscultatory findings tend to be uniformly present throughout the lungs. Asymmetry of auscultatory findings might be caused by concomitant disease such as pneumonia or by a complication of the asthma itself such as plugging a large bronchus with a mucus plug.

In severely ill patients extreme bronchial plugging and loss of effective mechanical ventilation may be associated with a disappearance of wheezing and a marked decrease in all audible breath sounds. In these patients, alveolar ventilation has almost disappeared, and the patient may be cyanotic.

In less severe, uncomplicated acute cases, cyanosis seldom occurs and the patient is afebrile. A tachycardia is regularly present during acute attacks.

When the asthmatic patient is not having an acute attack there may be no demonstrable physical abnormalities. In many patients asthma is chronic and wheezes may be heard even while the patient is feeling subjectively well. In some patients wheezes will not be heard during normal respiration but will appear if the patient exhales forcefully.

Atopic Eczema. The findings of physical examination of a patient with atopic eczema can vary as widely as those of an asthmatic. The symptoms are dependent upon the stage of the disease. When it first appears in a small child or infant 4 to 6 months of age, the initial manifestation is usually erythema and edema. Initial lesions are most likely to occur on the cheeks, in the antecubital fossae or popliteal spaces or about the neck and ears. Generalized skin involvement may then occur and any area of the body can be involved. After the initial erythema, a finely papular rash may appear. The papules then may form vesicles and as these vesicles rupture there may be oozing and crusting. Different areas of the skin may show erythema, papules, vesicles or oozing indicating that there are multiple lesions in varying stages of development. Regardless of the stage of development there are almost always excoriations from scratching. Secondary bacterial infection is frequently present.

In the chronic form lichenification of the skin is the predominant lesion. The skin appears thickened, coarse and dry. There may be moderate scaling and alteration in pigmentation. Pruritus may not be as severe as during the acute phases but is still present. The cosmetic effects of the chronic form are often very distrubing to the patient.

ROUTINE LABORATORY STUDIES

Complete Blood Counts. Abnormalities of red cells or of the sedimentation rate are not associated with atopic disease. If such abnormalities are present, other illnesses or complications should be suspected.

The differential white blood cell count is usually normal with the frequent exception of eosinophilia that may range from 3 to 7 percent. Eosinophilia of 12 to 20 percent is seldom present in allergies to extrinsic antigens unless an infection is also present. In nonreagenic asthma it is more common. Eosinophilia greater than 25 percent is not ordinarily seen in atopic diseases and suggests other diagnoses.

Urinalysis. The urine of all patients should be examined routinely in order to help rule out other nonallergic dieases.

Stool Examination. Stools should be examined in patients with pronounced peripheral blood eosinophilia or unexplained urticaria to help exclude parasitic infestations.

X-ray Examination. A chest x-ray should be obtained in every patient with asthma. This is necessary to exclude other illnesses. X-rays of the mastoids and paranasal sinuses are frequently indicated.

Examination of Secretion. Both gross and microscopic examination of nasal secretion can be of great value. The easiest way to collect nasal secretions is to have the patient blow his nose on a piece of wax paper. The secretions can be examined grossly then transferred to a microscope slide, air dried and stained. Wright stain is adequate, but with commercially available Hansel's stain, eosinophiles can be easily distinguished from neutrophils by their intensely eosinophilic granules.

In allergic rhinitis the nasal secretions are usually watery and completely clear on gross examination. Microscopically large number of eosinophils are commonly seen and may account for 30 to 90 percent of all the cells. With infection of the nose or paranasal sinuses yellow or green mucoid secretions may be present and microscopically many neutrophils and bacteria may be seen. Moderate eosinophilia may be present with infection however, so their presence or absence alone cannot completely exclude either diagnosis. The nasal secretions in vasomotor rhinitis are usually relatively acellular.

Eosinophils may also be seen in the sputum of asthmatic patients, and rarely Curschmann's spirals, Charcot-Leyden crystals or Creola bodies are present during acute episodes. Sputum gram stains, cultures and cytology may at times aid in differentiating purely atopic asthma from infectious or malignant conditions.

TESTS FOR EVALUATION OF RESPIRATORY FUNCTION

Quantitative tests of ventilation can be of great value. They may yield some insight into the type and severity of the functional defect and more importantly provide an objective means for assessing changes in these parameters that may occur with time or be induced by treatment. These tests will be described in detail in Chapter 7. It must be remembered that single sets of values describe conditions at designated points in time only and conditions such as asthma have rapid pathophysiological changes.

SKIN TESTING

General Considerations

At the present time no reliable test in vitro for atopic sensitization is clinically available. Most testing is dependent upon the production of an allergic reaction on a small scale by the intentional exposure of the patient to a minute amount of antigen. The organ tested may be the conjunctiva, nasal or bronchial mucosa, or the skin. Because the skin is readily accessible and easily observed this is the site chosen for most allergic tests.

Three types of direct skin tests are widely used in clinical practice, and each has its relative merits. All involve the production of the immediate wheal and erythema reaction that is characteristic of atopic sensitization.

With the scratch test, the antigen is applied to a superficial scratch that penetrates the outer cornified area of the skin. The prick test is performed by pricking the skin with a needle through a drop of the antigen solution. These tests can be performed with a mimimum of equipment and with relatively crude antigens. The insensitivity of these two methods as compared with intracutaneous testing accounts not only for their major value but also their major limitation. There is relatively little risk of a general constitutional reaction and even extreme sensitivity to an antigen can usually be determined without a significant hazard to the patient. On the other hand, scratch or prick tests may not be sufficiently sensitive to demonstrate significant atopic sensitization unless very concentrated antigens are used.

Intracutaneous testing is performed by injecting a small amount of antigen into the superficial layers of the skin. Because there is a risk of a systemic reaction either preliminary scratch or prick tests with the same antigen are advisable or else the initial intracutaneous tests must be performed with very dilute solutions of antigen. In the same patient the concentration of an antigen solution required to elicit a positive reaction in the scratch test may be 100 times or more as great as that needed in the intracutaneous test. If the scratch test shows an unusually large reaction, then intracutaneous tests should be avoided since they would be unnecessary and potentially dangerous. Nonspecific reactions at control sites are much less common than with the prick or scratch tests; therefore positive reactions are more clearly apparent.

The number and variety of prick tests performed depends upon clinical aspects of the particular case. The antigens used also vary because of the prevelance of a particular antigen in any geographic location. Satisfactory information can usually be obtained with less than 30 tests if they are carefully chosen.

Intracutaneous tests are chosen from the list of antigens giving negative or equivocal results on scratch testing. Many allergists feel that intracutaneous testing with foods produces so many nonspecific reactions that they have little value.

Techniques of the Prick or Scratch Test

Antigen extracts for diagnostic skin tests and hyposensitization can be obtained commercially from various pharmaceutical houses. The extracts can be purchased singly or in prepared diagnostic kits that include the major antigens prevalent in a specific geographic location.

The skin tests can be placed on the back or on the volar surface of the forearms. The patient should be placed in a comfortable position before the testing is begun. The skin should be properly cleansed with alcohol and air dried. Small drops of the test antigens and a drop of a glycerine-saline solution to serve as a control are then placed on the skin. Several rows of antigen may be used. Because large reactions at adjacent test sites might coalesce, the test sites should be at least 4 or 5 cm. apart. It is useful to mark the location of the drops with a marking pencil. Though various scarifying instruments are available, a sharp darning needle is adequate. After the antigen has been placed the needle can be used to puncture the skin (prick test) or to scratch the skin for two millimeters (scratch test). This procedure should lightly abrade the skin but not draw blood. The needle should be wiped free of antigen after each scratch with an alcohol sponge.

The tests should be read in 20 to 30 minutes, but if a large wheal reaction occurs before that time the test site should be wiped free of antigen.

Intracutaneous Testing

One-milliliter tuberculin syringes with 26-gauge needles are adequate. If disposable syringes and needles are not used, great care must be taken to be certain that glass syringes are not contaminated with previously used antigens. They must be meticulously cleaned and autoclaved and probably marked in a manner that permits a single syringe to always be used with a particular antigen. Because of these difficulties disposable syringes are frequently used.

The test sites are marked and cleaned with an alcohol sponge. The skin is held tense, and the needle is inserted almost parallel to its surface just far enough to cover the beveled portion. The injection of 0.02 ml. of the antigen extract as superfically as possible is then performed.

Because of the increased sensitivity of this method more dilute solutions of the antigen are used than were used for prick testing. For example 1:1000 or 1:5000 dilutions would be used only if the preliminary scratch or prick test had been negative.

The patient should be kept under observation until the tests are read in 20 minutes.

Many systems for grading positive reactions have been devised. A simple, adequate system consists of grading the reactions from negative to 4-plus (4+). A 4-plus reaction consists of erythema and a wheal with pseudopod formation. A 3-plus reaction (3+) would consist of erythema and wheal formation without pseudopods. A 2-plus (2+) reaction would consist of an area of erythema larger than a nickel in diameter (21 mm.). A 1-plus (1+) reaction is characterized by an area of erythema smaller than a nickel in diameter. A negative skin test (–) would have no reaction or a reaction that was no different from the control.

In cases of dermographism there may be reactivity at the control site. This should be noted when the results of the tests are recorded. Interpretation of the tests is then more difficult.

A skin testing sheet used in the Northwestern University Medical Center Allergy Service for cutaneous tests is shown. Intracutaneous tests for the inhalant allergens may be done if indicated.

SKIN TESTS

SCRATCH:

TREE	Reaction:	WEED (*Cont.*)	Reaction:
White Ash	————	Lambs Quarter	————
Common Cottonwood	————	True Marsh Elder	————
Elm	————	Rough Redwood Pigweed	————
White Hickory	————	Giant Ragweed	————
Maple, Hard	————	Short Ragweed	————
Oak—White	————	Western Ragweed	————
Eastern Sycamore	————	Russian Thistle	————
Black Walnut	————	White Prairie Sagebrush	————
Black Willow	————	Common Sagebrush	————
		Sheep Sorrel	————
GRASS		Western Water Hemp	————
Bermuda Grass	————		
Canada Blue Grass	————	MOLDS	
June Grass	————		
Orchard Grass	————	Aspergillus Mix	————
Red Top	————	Botrytis Cinerea	————
Timothy	————	Chaetomium Sp	————
		Dematiaceae Mix	————
WEED		Fusarium Vasinfectum	————
Bitter Dock	————	Monilia Sitophila	————
Burweed Marsh Elder	————	Mycogone Nigra	————
Cocklebur	————	Paecilomyces Varioti	————
English Plantain	————	Penicillium Mix	————
Kochia	————	Phycomycetes Mix	————

SKIN TESTS (*Cont.*)

SCRATCH:

HOUSE DUST		FOODS (*Cont.*)	Reaction:
Control General	———	Beef	———
Control Mold	———	Carrot	———
		Chicken	———
NONSEASONAL		Chocolate	———
INHALANTS		Cod Liver	———
		Corn	———
Acacia Gum	———	Egg White	———
Karaya Gum	———	Egg Yolk	———
Tragacanth Gum	———	Halibut	———
Cat Hair	———	Lamb	———
Cattle Hair	———	Milk—Cow	———
Dog Hair	———	Milk—Goat	———
Goat Hair	———	Oat	———
Hog Hair	———	Orange	———
Horse Dander	———	Pea	———
Horse Serum	———	Peach	———
Rabbit Hair	———	Peanut	———
Sheep Wool	———	Pear	———
Cottonseed	———	Pineapple	———
Feathers—Mix	———	Pork	———
Flaxseed	———	Potato	———
Glue—Animal	———	Prune	———
Kapok	———	Rice	———
Orris Root	———	Rye	———
Pyrethrum	———	Salmon	———
Tobacco—Smoke	———	Soy-Bean	———
		Spinach	———
FOODS		String Bean	———
Apple	———	Tomato	———
Apricot	———	Tuna Fish	———
Banana	———	English Walnut	———
Barley	———	Wheat	———

Passive Transfer Test

A similar reaction consisting of a wheal and erythema can be produced by injecting the serum of an allergic patient into the skin of a non-allergic individual and challenging the sensitized site later with the specific antigen.

A positive passive transfer Prausnitz-Küstner test is specific for the presence of skin sensitizing antibody specifically directed against an antigen. The major reasons it is not a widely used clinical test are because the test is time consuming and it involves the considerable dangers inherent in transferring serum from one individual to another.

If the donor gives a history of hepatitis, or unexplained jaundice or if Australia antigen is demonstrated in the donor serum, then the risk of transmitting hepatitis prohibits the use of this technique. Donor sera should also be screened with adequate serological tests for syphilis. The blood must be obtained from the donor and the serum separated using sterile equipment and technique in order to avoid bacterial contamination.

The recipient must be carefully chosen. Because some normal individuals are unsatisfactory recipients it is best to test each donor with a serum known to contain specific skin sensitizing ability. In addition it is mandatory that the recipient have negative reactions to direct skin testing with the antigens to be evaluated. The drugs which interfere with direct skin testing will also interfere with passive transfer testing and must be omitted.

The test is performed by injecting the recipient with 0.1 or 0.05 ml. of serum intradermally. If a quantitative estimate of reaginic antibody is desired, serial dilutions of serum can be injected and the P-K titer can be expressed as the reciprocal of the highest dilution giving a positive response.

After 24 to 48 hours, 0.02 ml. of the antigenic extract is injected intradermally precisely into the pretreated site. The skin is then observed for 20 minutes for wheal and erythema, and reaction can be graded by the same criteria used to grade direct tests.

Passive transfer testing is less sensitive than direct testing but produces almost no false-positive reactions if adequate controls are negative. It has almost no clinical application at the present time but it has remained one of the important investigative tools in experimental work.

Interpretation of Skin Tests

Both false-negative and false-positive skin tests may occur because of improper technique or materials. Improperly prepared or outdated extracts may lose their potency and produce false negative tests. Poorly prepared extracts may also contain nonspecific irritants or they may not be physiological with respects to pH or osmolarity and therefore produce false positive tests. The injection of an excessive volume can result in mechanical irritation of the skin and false positive tests.

Antihistamines, epinephrine, ephedrine, aminophylline and other sympathomimetic amines may interfere with skin testing. Corticosteroids have no effect on immediate skin tests. The skin of young infants or the very elderly may give smaller reactions than those seen in older children or adults of comparable sensitivity.

Even after false-positive and false-negative tests have been eliminated, the proper interpretation of results requires a thorough knowledge of the history and physical findings. A positive skin test alone does not indicate clinical sensitivity to a substance. With inhalent antigens a correlation of positive skin tests with a history suggestive of clinical sensitivity may strongly incriminate an antigen. Conversely a negative skin test and a negative history strongly suggests that the antigen is not clinically significant.

Interpreting skin tests that do not correlate with the clinical history or physical findings is much more difficult. If there is no history suggesting sensitivity to an antigen and if the skin test is positive, the patient can be reexamined during a period of maximal exposure to the antigen. If there are no symptoms or physical findings of sensitivity then the skin test may be ignored. The greatest dilemma is the presence of a negative skin test with a history strongly suggestive of clinical sensitivity to an antigen. The patient should be requestioned and all possibility of a false negative skin test should be excluded. If the discrepancy still exists, periodic examination and observation of the patient may allow more insight. At times provocative nasal or bronchial challenge with the antigen may be useful.

Particular caution must be used when interpreting skin tests to foods. These tests are much less reliable than tests with inhalent allergens. Most allergists use only a limited number of food skin tests or eliminate them entirely.

OTHER DIAGNOSTIC PROCEDURES

Ophthalmic Tests

The conjunctiva can be readily observed and tested for the presence of reaginic antibody. Either dried pollen or aqueous allergenic extracts can be instilled into the eye. The patient is seated and instructed to look upward. With his head tilted forward a lower eyelid is retracted and a small amount of dry pollen is tapped into the conjunctival sac from the flat side of a toothpick or a drop of an aqueous extract is added. If a dried material is used, dried pine pollen can function as a control if dropped in the other eye. If aqueous extracts are used, the diluent can serve as a control in the opposite eye. Aqueous extracts should be used in about the same concentrations as used for intracutaneous testing. The patient keeps his eye closed for a few moments; then it is observed for redness. After 20 minutes, or as soon as a positive reaction occurs, the eye should be washed with saline. Epinephrine eye drops, 1:5000, can be added if a response has occurred.

Conjunctival testing seems to have almost no advantage over skin testing. When the two methods have been compared, intracutaneous tests have required less concentrated extracts, and scratch tests have required more concentrated extracts than opthalmic tests to obtain positive responses.[7, 17] Although a few cases to the contrary have been reported, it is very unusual to obtain a positive conjunctival response when the intracutaneous test to the same antigen in a reasonable concentration has been negative.[1, 17] Some investigators feel that positive ophthalmic tests do correlate better with the clinical history than do intracutaneous tests.[1, 7]

In contrast to the minimal diagnostic value the disadvantages of the tests are numerous. It is impossible to evaluate the tests if there is preexisting inflammation. The tests are time consuming and only one antigen can be evaluated at a time. If a positive reaction occurs further testing must be postponed until another day.

Nasal Tests

A nasal response in allergic individuals can be observed after antigens are introduced directly into the nose. Methods to introduce the antigens have been numerous and have included blowing powder through a cone, insufflating powder from the blunt end of a toothpick, spraying aqueous extracts with an atomizer, or placing cotton pledgets soaked in aqeous extracts in the nose. A positive response would consist of the subjective phenomena of itching and sneezing and the objective criteria of a change in the appearance of the nasal mucous membranes. Even though the response may be immunologically specific the techniques for its evaluation are very crude. Methods for measuring resistance to nasal air flow have been reported and may add some degree of objectivity to the testing procedure [19]. Though the procedure might be of some value if the history and skin tests are vague, all of the advantages listed for the conjunctival tests apply also to the nasal tests. In addition there is the distinct disadvantage of having a gross endpoint that is difficult to interpret.

Bronchial Tests

Bronchial tests are performed by nebulizing an antigen extract into the bronchial tree of a test subject and comparing its effects with the effect produced by an appropriate control solution. Numerous techniques have been employed. Most techniques utilize nebulizers that are powered by compressed air or oxygen flowing at a rate of 6 or 7 liters per minute. This power source is usually necessary for the nebulizer to deliver the aerosol with small enough particle size for it to reach the lower respiratory tract. If a Y-tube is placed between the power source and the nebulizer the extract can be conserved and the patient can still coordinate nebulization with his inspiratory effort.

Testing preferably should be performed while the patient is free of symptoms. Antihistamines and sympathomimetic amines should be omitted for at least 18 hours prior to testing. Various dilutions of extracts have been used and markedly sensitive patients may react to very high dilutions. Usually if intracutaneous skin tests with an extract are negative, it will be safe to nebulize the extract in the same strength as that used for the negative skin test. If this produces no response more concentrated extract may be used. A volume of 0.5 to 1.0 cc. can be nebulized over a 5- to 10 minute period. The patient should be kept under constant observation by a physician, and the procedure should be stopped immediately when a positive response occurs. Further testing that day cannot be performed once a positive response has occurred.

Positive responses usually occur during the nebulization or within 15 to 20 minutes, but delayed responses have been reported.[8, 10] Pronounced responses may be appreciated clinically because of subjective respiratory distress or by careful auscultation of the entire chest. More subtle changes may be discerned only through the use of ventilatory function tests. Many different techniques for measuring pulmonary functions have been used. Most investigators have used either total vital capacity (TVC), first second forced expiratory volume (FEV_1), or maximum mid-expiratory flow rate (MMF). More extensive measurements of pulmonary function are not as practical because the frequent intervals at which they must be obtained may fatigue the patient. A reasonable procedure is the measurement of one or all three of these parameters before, immediately after and at 5, 10 and 20 minutes after nebulization of a control solution. The procedure is then repeated with the antigen nebulized. As a routine clinical procedure provocative bronchial tests have limited value for a number of reasons. The tests require the expenditure of a great amount of time by both the patient and the physician. Patient cooperation is essential. If the patient is wheezing or has a cough, results are difficult to interpret. The dose of antigen that actually reaches the patient's respiratory tree is difficult to assess. The occurrence of delayed reactions represents a possible danger to ambulatory patients.

Bronchial testing has continued to be used as an investigative tool. Its role even in this context is not clear. It has its greatest value because many antigens which give positive skin tests in patients do not induce asthma or elicit significant changes in pulmonary function. In this respect these tests have a high correlation with the clinical history. It would be much more useful if the reverse situation were established. Some investigators have failed to obtain positive bronchial responses to any antigen when the skin tests have been negative.[11,15]

Others have reported bronchial reactions in patients with negative skin tests.[5, 6, 16] A bronchial response to an aerosol challenge may be of such low magnitude that it is not clearly a positive or a negative response. At times positive responses are induced only after prolonged inhalation of concentrated extracts. In both these situations it is difficult to exclude the possibility that these are nonspecific responses to an inhaled irritant. Even if specific antigen-antibody induced responses occur during bronchial testing it may be produced in a setting so different from natural exposure that it has no clinical significance.

PROCEDURES FOR INVESTIGATING SUSPECTED FOOD SENSITIVITY

Dietary Procedures

Diet Diary. A diet diary is the best initial approach if a patient has only occasional symptoms. After the symptoms are produced several times it may become apparent to the physician and the patient what foods are involved. If the symptoms occur as often as every week it is probably best to keep a continuous diary of all foods that are eaten as well as a record of any symptoms. If symptoms do not occur that often, it may still be helpful to have the patient retrospectively list all foods eaten for 48 hours prior to the occurrence of symptoms.

Diet Manipulation. If symptoms are occurring continuously, or even several times each week, a diet diary may be confusing. In these instances elimination diets may be used. These diets are discussed in detail in Chapter 14. Some general principles must be observed, however, if this is to be a successful procedure. The elimination diet must be performed at a time when other variables are minimal. Success is dependent upon explicit instructions by the physician and complete patient cooperation. Once an elimination diet has been started improvement usually occurs fairly soon; therefore diagnostic diets should not be continued indefinitely. The occurrence of symptoms on one occasion after the introduction of a food may be coincidental; therefore it should be withdrawn and reintroduced again unless the reaction has been very severe.

Provocative Food Testing. Occasionally when reactions have been severe or when the physician doubts the validity of a reaction, provocative ingestion tests may be indicated. The patient ingests the food while under the direct observation of the physician.

A different type of provocative food testing has been described.[13] A positive result consists of the induction of allergic symptoms by the intradermal injection of concentrated food extracts. It is further claimed that if a reaction occurs it can be promptly relieved by the injection of a more concentrated extract of the same food.[12] Most allergists would agree with the first assumption: that intradermal injection of concentrated food extracts may lead to systemic reactions and anaphylaxis. The second assumption however is not consistent with the known immunological reactions. Consequently, it seems unlikely that an ethical investigator will risk a patient's life in order to confirm the second assumption.

Additional tests for food sensitivity that have been discussed in the literature, and have been discarded, include measuring the peripheral white blood cell count or the pulse before and after the ingestion of a food. Neither of these responses appears to be a reliable index of food sensitivity.

Tests in Vitro

Leukocyte Cytotoxic Tests. A unique type of blood test has been proposed for the diagnosis of food allergy.[4] In some manner extracts of food are mixed with living leukocyte preparations made from peripherial venous blood. Cytological changes are then described as (1) paralysis of ameboid activity, (2) rounding of all contours, (3) vacuolization and cytoplasmic spreading, and eventually cell fragmentation and degranulation.[4] Consideration of currently available immunological knowledge makes it seem highly unlikely that such a test could have validity. Degranulation has been described in sensitized mast cells and basophils, but in the peripheral blood there is evidence that only the basophils are involved in this reaction.[9, 18] Obtaining enough basophils from peripheral blood to perform cytological studies on them would represent a formidable technical accomplishment. Unfortunately the technical aspects of the test cannot be evaluated because the references cited concerning the techniques do not mention the test.[3] Even if the test does overcome these technical difficulties, no readily available studies of its validity as a test for hypersensitivity have been found.

Basophil Degranulation. In contrast, another test in vitro, the basophil degranulation test of Shelley, has been investigated in a reasonable manner.[2, 20, 21] In this test basophils are provided in adequate numbers by using rabbit leukocytes (Buffy Coat) which have a high percentage of easily identifiable basophils. This is mixed with the test serum and a specific antigen. Supposedly in the presence of a specific antigen-antibody reaction, degranulation of rabbit basophils occurs.

Even those investigators who feel that the test is valid indicate that there can be technical difficulty in performing the test. Nonspecific degranulation occurs if the preparation stands too long, and occasionally degranulation occurs in the control specimens.[20]

Other investigators using the same technique were unable to achieve any degree of reproducibility.[2] After extensive double blind studies they concluded that the degranulation of the basophils was a random phenomenon and was not influenced by the presence or absence of specific antigen or antibody in this test system.[2] Even if the test is specific for antigen-antibody reactions, its technical complexities greatly limit its usefulness as a clinical or even an investigative tool.

Histamine Release. One test in vitro appears to be very specific and reproducable. When antigen is added to the blood of a sensitive individual there is a release of histamine (1 hr.). This phenomena is not dependent upon serum antibodies [14] but upon antibodies specifically on circulating basophils.[9, 18] Though this test is not widely applicable as an aid in clinical diagnosis, its application as a research tool has been responsible for much of our recently acquired knowledge of immediate hypersensitivity reactions.

REFERENCES

1. Abram, L. E.: An evaluation of conjunctival testing in extrinsic respiratory allergy. J. Allerg., 20:66, 1949.
2. Bobitt, J. R., Schechter, H., and Pollak, V. E.: A critical evaluation of the indirect basophil degranulation. Proc. Soc. Exper. Biol. and Med., 117:608, 1964.
3. Bryan, W. T. K., and Bryan, M. P.: Cytologic dagnosis in otolaryngology and Trans. Amer. Acad. Ophthal. Otolaryng., 63:597, 613, 1959. Significance of most cells in nasal secretions.
4. Clemis, J. D., and Derlacki, E. L.: Allergy of the upper respiratory tract. Otolaryng. Clin. N. Amer., 3:265, 1970.
5. Colldahl, H.: A study of provocative tests on patients with bronchial asthma: II. The outcome of provocation tests with different antigens. Acta Allerg., 5:143, 1952.
6. DeSwarte, R. D.: Provocative challenge in the etiologic diagnosis of bronchial asthma. Univ. of Mich. Med. Ctr. J., 34:16, 1968.
7. Fineman, A. H.: Studies on hypersensitiveness: XXIII. A comparative study of the intradermal, scratch, and conjunctival tests in determining the degree of pollen sensitivity. J. Immun., 11:465, 1926.
8. Herxheimer, H.: Bronchial obstruction induced by allergens, histamine and acetyl-beta-methylcholine chloride. Int. Arch. Allerg., 3:189, 1952.
9. Ishizaka, K., Tomioka, H., and Ishizaka, T.: Mechanisms of passive sensitization: I. Presence of IgE and IgG molecules on human leukocytes. J. Immun., 105:1459, 1970.
10. Itkin, I. H., Anand, S., Yau, M., and Middlebrook, G.: Quantitative inhalation challenge in allergic asthma. J. Allerg., 34:97, 1963.
11. Juhlin-Dannfelt, C.: On the significance of exposure and provocation tests in allergic diagnostics. Acta Med. Scand., 239 [supp.]:320, 1950.

86 *Diagnosis of Immediate Hypersensitivity*

12. Lee, C. H., Williams, R. I., and Binkley, E. L.: Provocative inhalant testing and treatment. Arch. Otolaryng., 90:173, 1969.
13. Lee, C. H., Williams, R. I., and Binkley, E. L.: Provocative testing and treatment for foods. Arch. Otolaryng., 90:87, 1969.
14. Lichtenstein, L. M., and Osler, A. G.: Studies on the mechanisms of hypersensitivity IX. Histamine release from human leucocytes by ragweed pollen antigen. J. Exp. Med., 120:507, 1964.
15. Lowell, F. C., and Schiller, I. W.: Measurement of changes in vital capacity as a means of detecting pulmonary reactions to inhaled aerosolized allergenic extracts in asthmatic subjects. J. Allerg., 19:100, 1948.
16. Nilsson, H., and Kaude, J.: Inhalation and skin test in the diagnosis of asthma bronchiale. Dis. Chest, 37:535, 1960.
17. Peshkin, M. M.: XI. A dry pollen ophthalmic test in pollen asthma and hay fever patients negative to intracutaneous tests. J. Allerg., 3:20, 1931.
18. Pruzansky, J. J., and Patterson, R.: Histamine in human leukocytes. Int. Arch. Allerg., 37:98, 1970.
19. Seebohm, P. M., and Hamilton, W. K.: A method for measuring nasal resistance without intranasal instrumentation. J. Allerg., 29:56, 1958.
20. Shelley, W. B.: New serological test for allergy in man. Nature, 195:1181, 1962.
21. Shelley, W. B.: Indirect basophil degranulation tests for allergy to penicillin and other drugs. J.A.M.A., 184:171, 1963.
22. Solomon, W. R., Mc Lean, J. A., Cookingham, C., Ahronheim, G., and DeMuth, G. R.: Measurement of nasal airway resistance. J. Allerg., 36:62, 1965.

4

Allergens and Other Factors
Important in Atopic Disease

Arnold A. Gutman, M.D.

With a section on House Dust and Dust Mites by
Terumasa Miyamoto, M.D.

An *allergen* is an antigen that produces a clinical allergic reaction. In the atopic diseases, allergens are antigenic in the sense of being associated with a particular kind of antibody called skin-sensitizing antibody, reagin, or homocytotropic antibody. These antibodies are mostly, or perhaps entirely, of the IgE class. It might then be said that an *atopic allergen* is one that can be demonstrated by means of a wheal and flare reaction obtained by appropriate skin testing methods. This is in contradistinction to certain drug, microbial and other allergens that induce the formation of other types of antibodies, and to contact allergens (or haptens) that induce delayed hypersensitivity reactions.

Allergens most commonly associated with atopic disorders are inhalants and foods. Drugs, biological products, insect venoms and chemical additives may also induce the immediate-type reactions. In practice, however, most atopic reactions involve pollens, mold spores, house dust, animal epithelials and other substances that impinge directly on the respiratory mucosa. The water soluble allergenic molecules are leached out of the particles and react with antibodies to initiate a series of pathophysiologic steps that result in symptoms.

The chemical nature of certain of these allergens has been intensively studied, and though certain facts are known, the precise composition of most is still undefined. Insulin, for example, can act as an allergen and is well-defined. Dialysis, DEAE-cellulose and Sephadex columns for fractionation, and Ouchterlony gel diffusion and immunoelectrophoresis are some of the methods currently used for analysis.[1]

Pollens are complex mixtures of protein, carbohydrate, fat and other natural substances. They are relatively desiccated on leaving the anther, but imbibe water on contact with a moist surface. Since the fats are not involved in immediate-type allergy, they are commonly removed with appropriate solvents before extraction for clinical or investigative use. The traditional method of standardizing and preparing allergens for clinical use is to extract a given weight of defatted pollen in a given volume of fluid. For example, one gram in 100 cc of fluid would constitute a 1% or 1:100 solution. This *weight-by-volume* (W/V) system is still the most commonly used in clinical practice. This solution could then be concentrated or diluted as needed. A unit system has been assigned so that 1.0 cc of a 1:1,000,000 solution contains one *pollen unit* (Noon unit).

The **protein-nitrogen-unit** (PNU) is preferred by some allergists and manufacturers of allergenic materials. It is predicated on the evidence that the allergenic moieties of pollens are proteins and the ratio of protein to dry weight of pollen may vary. In this method, nitrogen is precipitated by phosphotungstic acid and determined by the micro-Kjeldahl technique. One PNU is approximately equal to two pollen units for ragweed, but this varies regionally and annually. *Total nitrogen* is yet another method of standardization, but it offers no advantage and is infrequently used.

THE ANTIGENICITY OF CERTAIN ALLERGENS

The solutions previously described are of practical value, but tell us nothing of what part of the allergen is allergenic. In general, preparations of pollens contain more than one antigen. Of the several antigens in a given pollen, there are usually one or two that dominate in both frequency and intensity of skin reactions in sensitive patients. It is inferred from this that these antigens are the most important clinically. However, not all patients allergic to a certain pollen react to the same antigens. The antigens of tree, grass and weed pollens are immunologically distinct, and this fact agrees with clinical and skin test data. Additional knowledge in this area is particularly desirable, since diagnosis and injection treatment could theoretically be made more effective if highly purified material could be substituted for the crude extracts now in use.

Ragweed

Since atopic humans do not ordinarily make precipitating antibodies to pollen allergens, studies of antigenicity by gel double diffusion analysis must be done with animal sera. Rabbit serum obtained after immunization with ragweed pollen demonstrates seven to eight separate antigens in the crude ragweed extract. This does not necessarily mean that all of these seven to eight antigens in ragweed are pathogenic for humans. Early studies with ragweed extract using dialysis and other chemical methods separated three distinct fractions, 1, 2, and 3. Fraction 1 most consistently produced positive skin tests in patients with ragweed hay fever and was the only antigenic fraction that produced blocking antibody during immunotherapy. Fraction 2 in certain individuals was more potent in inducing positive skin tests and in these individuals was responsible for intolerance to graded doses of extracts used therapeutically.[43] This knowledge has been used by some in the preparation of extracts that might be more active therapeutically without inducing annoying local reactions. Fraction 3 was of only minor importance.

More recently the use of more sophisticated biochemical methods has resulted in the isolation of ragweed fractions of up to 300 times the potency of crude ragweed as measured by the ability to induce positive skin tests in appropriate individuals, and the ability to cause histamine release from their leucocytes in vitro. A number of investigators have studied and purified ragweed antigens. The work of King and Norman [16, 18] will be used as the basis for discussion. Using the techniques of gel filtration and ion exchange chromatography, two allergens, antigen K and antigen E have been isolated. These have certain immunological and chemical properties in common, but differ in molecular weight and biological activities. Antigen K has a molecular weight of 38,200, is a globulin, contains no carbohydrate and comprises about 3% of extractable ragweed protein. It has less biological activity than antigen E in patients allergic to ragweed. Almost all the other "purified" ragweed fractions that have been isolated by other investigators contain large

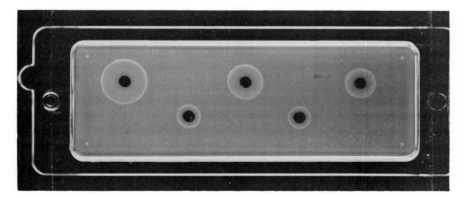

Fig. 4-1. Single radioimmunodiffusion analysis of antigen E by use of antigen E antiserum. Concentration of antigen E antiserum in agar: 1:25. Concentration of antigen E in Wells, mcg./ml.: *(top, left to right)* 200, 100, 50, *(bottom, left to right)* 25, 20 (reference standard). (Center Laboratories, Inc.)

amounts of antigen E, which comprises 90% of the allergenic activity of ragweed pollen. Antigen E is a protein with a molecular weight of 37,800 and accounts for about 6% of the total protein of whole ragweed extract. Quantitative studies of ragweed sensitive patients with antigen E have shown a positive correlation with skin reactivity and leukocyte histamine release, but no correlation with protein nitrogen content in six commercial preparations of ragweed extract.[3] At the time of this writing, one commercial manufacturer of allergy extracts is standardizing ragweed by antigen E assay and this may prove to be a significant advance in assuring uniformity of extracts for clinical and investigational use. It should be added, however, that the few pilot studies done for using antigen E for immunotherapy have not yielded therapeutic results superior to those obtained using crude ragweed extracts. At this time the limited amounts of antigen E available preclude its use for other than experimental purposes.

Grass Pollen

The allergenic and antigenic properties of grass pollens differ in some respects from ragweed, and offer additional immunological perspectives. Rye and timothy grasses have been most extensively studied. Chromatographic analysis originally demonstrated two distinct allergens in rye grass pollen. These are both proteins and are designated Group I and Group II. Group I has a molecular weight of 30,000 and shows skin reactivity in about 95% of grass-sensitive patients. Group II has a molecular weight of 10,000 with skin reactivity in about 70% of grass-sensitive patients. Neither group is dialyzable, and there is no cross antigenicity between the two groups.[20] This is in contrast to ragweed in which there is a cross antigenicity between antigen E and the other antigens. Neither Group I nor Group II cross reacts with antigen E, hence in human atopic disorders grass and ragweed pollinosis represent distinct immunologic entities. This has already been established by clinical observation. Most of the clinically important grass pollens contain both Group I and II allergens, as well as a more recently described Group III fraction.[24]

There are two important exceptions, Bermuda and timothy grass. Bermuda grass contains none of the above antigens, and these studies corroborate the often observed fact that on direct skin testing patients may react to grasses to which they have never been geographically exposed—by virtue of cross-antigenicity—but never to Bermuda grass in this manner.

Timothy grass contains Group I, II and III antigens, but there is weaker cross-antigenicity to rye grass than to other common grasses. Timothy also contains another nondialyzable fraction, antigen B with a molecular weight of about 10,500; and a dialyzable fraction, antigen D, with a molecular weight of 5,000. This latter material can cause positive skin reactions in timothy-sensitive individuals and can inhibit other immunologic reactions in experimental animals.[22, 23] A material of this type has not been found in studies with rye grass pollens. It has been suggested that antigen D has certain properties of a hapten [21] but the significance of this substance is still under investigation.

Individuals allergic to grass pollens may be categorized by their cutaneous reactivity to various fractions of rye, timothy and other grass pollens. The reason for this allergenic specificity of humans is unknown, as is the broader question of why some atopic individuals are sensitive to some pollens and not others; or to other types of inhalant allergens and no pollens.

The best evidence to date invokes a genetic predisposition for both the production of IgE and an antigenic preference. For example, in experiments with inbred mice it was shown that certain strains could be made to produce reaginic antibodies with repeated injections of small doses of antigen, whereas other strains could not. However, all strains that were tested produced reaginic antibodies to a single large dose of injected antigen. Using this as a model for human atopic allergy, it would appear that the ability to synthesize reaginic antibodies is not limited to atopic persons, but the atopic population produces them after a smaller and repeated antigenic stimulus. In the same experiments it was noted that certain strains produced high antibody titers to some antigens and low titers to others.[19]

Tree Pollen

The allergenic fractions of trees have not been as extensively studied as ragweed or grasses. Since a higher degree of specificity exists when patients are skin tested to a number of different tree pollens than does with grass pollens, it may be speculated that there are significant differences among the antigenic determinants.

To summarize the current clinical status of pollen allergens, ragweed is the one that has been most extensively studied. The extract of ragweed pollen is a mixture of allergens of which the major one is antigen E. Antigen E is probably not the only important clinical allergen in ragweed since immunotherapy using antigen E alone has not been as effective as with whole ragweed extract. The therapeutic agent still recommended is whole ragweed extract, and it is anticipated that all future extracts will be standardized by their antigen E content to provide uniformity of extracts. The studies on the groups of grass pollen antigens require further confirmation and clinical studies before their clinical usefulness can be assessed. These studies point out the direction in which investigative and clinical allergy are moving today.

Mold Spores

These have been studied most extensively by Pepys [31] in relation to allergic bronchopulmonary aspergillosis, a disorder characterized by the presence of both reaginic and precipitating antibodies to the fungus, *Aspergillus fumigatus.* Mold-sensitive asthmatics who are allergic to *Aspergillus* show immediate type skin reactions to the same antigens so they are probably also some of the substances responsible for atopic asthma. Though the spores are the causative agents in atopic disorders, mold extracts used clinically and described here are made from culture filtrates and include mycelial antigens. Fifteen to twenty antigens can be demonstrated for *A. fumigatus.* These are predominantly proteins, but some are polysaccharides, glycoproteins and glycopeptides. The major proteins have a negative charge, and on electrophoresis migrate toward the positive pole at a speed similar to the alpha and beta globulins of serum. They are rich in the amino acids serine, threonine and alanine. The polysaccharides are composed largely of mannose, galactose and glucose. Cutaneous tests with polysaccharide antigens are positive in half the patients who react to whole extracts of *A. fumigatus,* but these reactions are much weaker than those obtained with the proteins. Future research should lead to the isolation of one or of a few major allergenic fractions, as was the case with ragweed and those other pollens which have been studied.

AEROALLERGENS

These are airborne particles that can cause respiratory, cutaneous or conjunctival allergy. The water-soluble portion of ragweed pollen, for example, affects the respiratory and conjunctival mucosae, while the fat-soluble allergens may cause a typical contact dermatitis on exposed skin. This *ragweed dermatitis* often occurs in non-atopic individuals and is due to an entirely different immunologic mechanism.

For a particle to be clinically significant as an aeroallergen it must be buoyant, present in significant numbers and be allergenic. Ragweed pollen is archetypical. Pine pollen, by contrast, is abundant in certain regions and buoyant but is not a significant aeroallergen. Mold spores are ubiquitous, highly allergenic, and may exceed the amount of pollen in the air even during the height of the pollen season. The omnipresence of house dust needs no emphasis here. The knowledge of what occurs where and when is essential to the treatment of allergy. The above allergens are emphasized because they are the most commonly encountered and are considered responsible for most of the morbidity among atopic patients.

Aeroallergens, such as the epidermal antigens, feathers and animal danders, may be localized to certain homes. They may be occupational in those who work with animals; farmers who encounter a variety of pollens and molds in hay and stored grains; exterminators who use pyrethrum; dock workers who unload coffee beans and castor beans from the holds of ships; and bakers who inhale flour. Some airborne allergens are geographically narrowly confined such as May fly and caddis fly whose scales and body parts are a cause of respiratory allergy in the eastern Great Lakes area in the late summer. Endemic asthma has been reported in the vicinity of factories where cottonseed and castor beans are processed.

Particle size is important. Airborne pollens are in the range 20-60 μ while mold spores mostly vary between 3-30 μ in diameter or longest dimension. Dust particles are 1-10 μ. Protective mechanisms in the nasal mucosa and upper tracheobronchial passages remove most of the larger particles, so only those of 5 μ reach the alveoli of the lungs. Hence, the conjunctivae and upper respiratory passages get the largest dose of airborne allergens. These are considerations in the pathogenesis of allergic rhinitis, bronchial asthma and hypersensitivity alveolitis (nonatopic) as well as in the effects of chemical and particulate atmospheric pollutants.

Pollens

Pollen grains are living male germinal cells that contain two haploid nuclei (generative and tube), an endoplasmic reticulum, ribosomes and other subcellular architectural structures. There is an internal limiting membrane, the *intine* and a two-layered external coating, the *exine*. The latter is composed of a durable substance called sporopollenin. Mineralization of sporopollenin accounts for the finding of fossilized pollen grains 100 million years old. Morphologic studies of pollens using the scanning electron microscope reveal a fascinating infrastructure.[12] Sporopollenin is primarily a high molecular weight polymer of fatty acids. The intine is cellulose. In addition to protein, fat and carbohydrate, pollen grains contain pigments, vitamins, free amino acids, enzymes and two plant growth hormones, indoleacetic acid and gibberellin.

The morphology of pollen grains varies in relation to size, number of furrows, form and location of pores, thickness of exine and other features of the cell wall. These include spines, reticulations, an operculum in grass pollens and air sacs (bladders) in certain conifers. Ragweed pollen is about 20 microns in diameter; the trees vary from 20 to 60 microns, and the grasses, all morphologically similar are mostly 30 to 40 microns. The identification of pollens important in allergic disease is not difficult and certainly within the capabilities of the physician without special expertise in botany.

Certain plants produce prodigious amounts of pollen. It has been estimated that a single ragweed plant may expel one million pollen grains in a single day; a shoot of hemp (*Cannabis*) may produce five hundred million grains! Trees, especially conifers, may release so much pollen that it is visible as a cloud and may be scooped up by the handful after settling. The seasonal onset of pollination of certain plants, such as ragweed, is determined by the duration of light received daily. The farther north the earlier the pollination, and this is amazingly constant from year to year. In the belt from the Central Atlantic to the North Central States, August 15 is a highly predictable date for the onset of ragweed pollination.

In general, brightly colored flowering plants are of little clinical importance in inhalant allergy since their pollen is teleologically designed to be carried by insects (entomophilous) rather than the wind (anemophilous). These pollens from flowering plants are relatively scant, heavy and sticky. Roses and goldenrod are good examples of plants that are often erroneously thought to cause pollinosis because of the time they bloom. However, in isolated cases the pollens of most entomophilous plants can sensitize and then cause symptoms if exposure is sufficient. Of the anemophilous plants, ragweed pollen has a long range, having been detected 400 miles at sea by sampling methods. The range of tree pollens is shorter. Thus an individual living in the center city is more likely to be affected by weed and grass pollens than by trees. Also, local weed-eradication programs, more often legislated than accomplished, are really quite futile in light of the foregoing information.

POLLEN SAMPLING METHODS

There are two objectives of aerobiologic sampling. These are first, the identification of the pollen grains and the mold spores that occur in a geographic area and second, the determination of the concentration of these aeroallergens by quantitative methods.

The basis of any method of sampling pollen is to provide a sticky surface upon which the grains can adhere and through which they may be microscopically examined. A standard microscope slide coated with soft petrolatum, rubber cement (diluted 1:1 with thinner) or glycerine jelly is satisfactory. Calberla's stain, an alcoholic solution of basic fuchsin, may be added to the glycerine jelly or applied a few minutes before the slides are examined. This expands the pollen grains, colors them red and changes their refractive properties to make pores, furrows and other anatomic features more readily identifiable. A low power objective lens is usually adequate for identification, particularly for an experienced examiner, but a higher power may be helpful. Pollen counts are expressed as grains per square centimeter, and the field can be measured with a hemocytometer, calibrated stage or other device designed for that purpose. Once calibrated for a particular microscope, the examiner knows how many "passes" over a square cover slip need to be examined to constitute 1 cm ^{2}. Since the distribution of particles trapped on the slide may not be uniform, it is more accurate to average the readings of several square centimeters.

The gravity sampler is the method most commonly used because of its simplicity and low cost. The standard device is the Durham Sampler, consisting of a pair of parallel circular plates 3 inches apart. A prepared microscope slide is placed in a holder 1 inch above the lower plate and exposed to the atmosphere for 24 hours. The sampler should be on a rooftop where airflow has free access to the device, i.e., at least 20 feet from any obstruction and 3 feet above the level of the parapets that are present on most rooftops. Air flow rather than gravity is responsible for particle deposition on the slide. It has been shown that the turbulence engendered by the collecting device deflects smaller particles and favors the impingement of larger particles—15 μ or above. However with increased wind velocity, there is increased efficiency in the capture of smaller particles. Orientation of the long axes of the slide with the wind direction also increases particle capture.

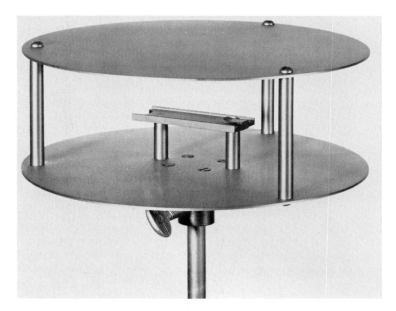

Fig. 4-2. Durham Gravity Slide Sampler. (Wilkens-Anderson, 4525 W. Division Street, Chicago, Illinois 60651.)

Inertial samplers are based on the principles stated above. The impacting surface is rotated to simulate increased wind velocity. The *Rotorod Sampler* employs plastic rods and the *Rotobar Sampler* uses metal bars wound with transparent tape. Both are mechanically rotated and depend on the deposition of particles on a narrow surface. A further refinement of this principle is the *Intermittent Rotoslide Sampler* in which particles are collected on the leading edge of microscope slides that are alternately rotated and protected by metal shields. This allows selective sampling independent of wind velocity.

Inertial suction samplers attempt to stimulate increased wind velocity by suction. The problem with these devices is that disorientation with wind direction and velocity will skew the impaction efficiencies of particles of different sizes. For example, if the wind velocity is less than that generated by the sampler, smaller particles will be collected in greater concentration than exist in ambient air. The reverse is true for greater wind velocities. The *Hirst Spore Trap* is an inertial suction sampler which has a clock mechanism that moves a coated slide at a given rate along an intake orifice. This enables discrimination with regard to diurnal variations of the particulate matter, such as pollens

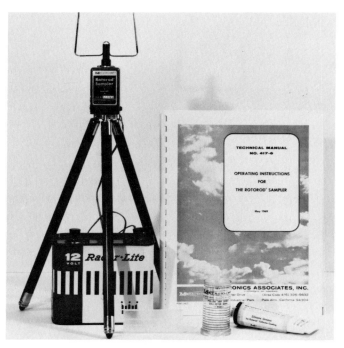

Fig. 4-3. Aeroallergen Rotorod Sampler. (Metronics Associates, 3201 Porter Drive, Palo Alto, California 94304.)

in the air. For the purpose of most clinical allergists the gravity method will yield useful information regarding pollen prevalence. The value of the more sophisticated methods lies in investigative aerobiology.[39]

CLASSIFICATION OF ALLERGENIC PLANTS

The botanical considerations and taxonomic scheme given here are representative rather than exhaustive. The individual plants with both common and botanical names, geographic locations and relative importance in allergy are considered in Chapter 5.

There are a number of excellent sourcebooks for the details of systematic botany, plant identification and pollen morphology.[8, 47]

PLANT ANATOMY

The flower has four fundamental parts:

1. The *pistil*, which consists of an *ovary* at the base, a *style* projecting upward, and a *stigma*, the sticky top surface of the style to which pollen grains adhere. This is the female portion of the plant.

2. *Stamens*, which are variable in number and consist of *anthers* borne on *filaments*. The anthers produce the pollen grains which are released through a longitudinal cleft. These are the male portions of the plant.

3. *Petals*, which are the colored parts of the flower, usually three to five in number.

4. *Sepals*, the green or colorless protective portions of the flower and bud. They usually fall off when the petals appear.

Monoecious plants contain both pistils and stamens and are "perfect" plants. An example is ragweed. *Dioecious* plants are "imperfect" in that pistils and stamens are not on the same plant. An example is the cypress tree.

The *Gymnosperms* are characterized by their anthers and ovules being borne on cones rather than flowers. The families containing the conifers and ginkos are gymnosperms, all trees. Pines, firs, junipers, spruces, yews, hemlocks, savins, red cedars, cypresses and retinisporas are in this category.

The *Angiosperms* are the plants previously described that bear their seeds in closed ovaries. They may be *monocotyledons,* such as grasses, in which the seedlings produce a single leaf (cotyledon); or *dicotyledons,* in which the seedlings produce two cotyledons. Most allergenic plants (except grasses) are dicotyledons, which usually bear sepals and petals in groups of four or five and have leaves with branching veins.

Monocotyledonous flowers generally have sepals and petals in threes, and their leaves have parallel veins. There are other differences between these two classes of plants that are unimportant for this discussion. Fusion of the parts of flowers, resulting in fewer petals and anthers is characteristic of phylogenetic advancement. Hence monocots are higher on the evolutionary scale than dicots.

TAXONOMY

Trees

These may be gymnosperms or angiosperms. *Gymnosperms* include two families, *Ginkgoaceae* and *Coniferae,* the conifers. None of these are of particular importance in allergy, but because of the prevalence of conifers and the incidence of their pollens in surveys, some comments are in order.

CONIFERS are found mainly in temperate climates and have flat, needle-shaped leaves. There are six tribes, but only three are germane to this discussion:

1. *Abietineae*—the pines, spruces, firs and hemlocks.

The *pines* are monoecious evergreens whose leaves are enclosed at their base by a sheath. The pollen grains are 45 to 65 μ in diameter and in addition have two bladders. This pollen has occasionally been implicated in allergy.[30]

The *spruces* produce pollen grains that are morphologically similar to pine pollen, but are much larger, ranging 70 to 90 μ exclusive of the bladders.

The *hemlocks,* depending on species, may or may not have bladders.

The *firs* produce even larger pollens ranging from 80 to 100 μ, not including the two bladders.

2. *Cupressineae*—the junipers, cypresses, cedars and savins. These trees are mainly dioecious and produce large quantities of round pollen grains 20 to 30 μ in diameter, with a very thick intine. The mountain cedar tree is an important cause of allergic rhinitis in certain parts of Texas, and has proliferated where the ecology has been disturbed by over-grazing of the grasslands.

3. *Chamaecyparis*—other cypresses. Lawson cypress in the Pacific Northwest has shown to cause allergic rhinitis and to cross-react with the pollen of mountain cedar.

Angiosperms comprise the bulk of the allergenic trees. The more important botanical families are listed below with the common names of the trees in each family and appropriate notations.

SALICACEA—the willows and poplars. The former are mainly insect-pollinated and are not generally considered allergenic. The poplars, on the other hand, are wind pollinated. Poplar pollen grains are spherical, 27 to 34 μ in diameter, and are characterized by a thick intine. The genus, *Populus,* includes trees commonly known as poplars, aspens and cottonwoods, and is of considerable allergenic importance. It is interesting to note that their seeds are borne on buoyant cottonlike tufts that may permeate the air in June, resembling a localized snowstorm. Patients often erroneously attribute their symptoms to this "cottonwood". The true cause is usually grass pollens.

BETULA—the birches. The various species are widely distributed in North America and produce abundant pollen which is highly allergenic. The pollens are 20 to 30 μ, flattened and generally have 3 pores, though some species have up to 7 pores. The pistillate catkins may persist into winter, discharging small winged seeds.

ALNUS—the alders. These are shrubs and mainly small trees, though the white alder may grow as tall as 75 feet. The pollen grains usually have 4 or 5 pores, all characterized by a bandlike thickening of the exine that extends from pore to pore, and are 19 to 27 μ in diameter. Alders do cause allergic symptoms but are not as important as many other families of trees.

FAGACEAE—the beeches, oaks, chestnuts and chinquapins. This family contains five genera found in North America, of which only the beeches (genus *Fagus*) and oaks (genus *Quercus*) are wind-pollinated and of allergenic importance. The pollens of these two genera are morphologically similar but not identical, 40 μ in diameter, with an irregular exine and three tapering furrows. Both produce prodigious amounts of pollen, and oaks in particular are responsible for a great deal of tree pollinosis in the areas where they abound. There are numerous species of oaks, but their description is not within the scope of this survey.

ULMACAE—the elms and hackberries. There are about 20 species of elm trees in the northern hemisphere, mainly distributed east of the Rocky Mountains. They produce large amounts of very allergenic pollen and continue to be a major cause of the tree pollinosis despite their progressive elimination by Dutch elm disease. Elm pollen is 35 to 40 μ in diameter, has 5 pores and a thick, rippled exine. The hackberries are unimportant for this discussion.

INGLANDACEAE—the walnuts. The walnuts are not important causes of allergy, but their pollen is often found on pollen slides. The pollen grains are about 35 to 40 μ in diameter, contain about 12 pores localized mainly on one surface of the grain, and the exine is smooth.

CARYA—the hickories. These trees, pecan in particular, are important in the etiology of allergic rhinitis in the areas where they grow or are cultivated. The pollen grains are 40 to 50 μ in diameter and usually contain 3 germinal pores. These trees produce prodigious amounts of highly allergenic pollen.

MYRICACEAE—the bayberry family. These trees produce large amounts of wind-borne pollen that closely resemble the grains of the *Betulaceae* (birches and alders). The wax myrtles are thought to cause pollinosis in some areas.

MORACEAE—the mulberry family. Certain members of the genus *Morus* may be highly allergenic. The pollen grains are small for tree pollens, about 20 μ in diameter, and contain 2 or 3 germinal pores arranged without a geometric pattern, i.e., they are not polar or meridial.

PLATANACEAE—the sycamore family. These are sometimes called the plane trees. Their pollen is plentiful and the grains are flattened at the poles (oblately), are about 20 μ in diameter, and contain no pores. There are 3 or 4 furrows on the thin, granular exine. The sycamores may be of significant allergenic importance in some regions.

SIMARUBACEAE—the ailanthus family. Only the tree-of-heaven (A. *altissima*) is of allergenic importance regionally. Its pollen grains have a diameter of about 25 μ and are characterized by 3 germinal furrows and 3 germinal pores.

TILIACEAE—the linden family. Only one genus, *Tilia*, the linden or basswood tree, is of allergenic importance, though pollination is mainly by insects. The pollen grains are distinct, measuring 28 to 36 μ, with germ pores sunk in furrows in a thick reticulate exine.

ACERACEAE—the maple family. There are over 100 species of maples, and many of these are of significant importance in allergy. Maple pollen grains have 3 furrows but no pores. Boxelder is a common species of the genus, *Acer*, and is particularly important because of its wide distribution, prevalence and the large amount of pollen it sheds.

FRAXINUS—the ash family. There are about 65 species in this family, many of which predominate among the allergenic trees. The pollen grains have a diameter of 20 to 25 μ, are somewhat flattened and usually have four furrows. The exine is coarsely reticulate.

Other trees have been implicated in pollen allergy, but the preceding families comprise the most important ones, and most of the tree pollinosis in the United States is the result of the trees described above.

Grasses

The grasses are all angiosperms and monocotyledons. In addition to parallel veined leaves, the stems do not build up layers of cambium and do not have a central core of conducting ducts. The ductal system is spread at random throughout the stem. The pollen grains of monocotyledons characteristically have only one germinal pore. Grasses are in the order *Glumiflorae*, family GRAMINEAE.

The flowers are usually perfect, i.e., they contain both pistils and stamens. The pollen grains of most allergenic grasses range 20 to 25 μ and have one germinal pore or furrow. The intine is thick. Some grasses are self-pollinating and therefore unimportant for allergy. The others are wind-pollinated, but of the over 1,000 species in North America only a few are significant in producing allergic symptoms. But those few are very important in terms of the numbers of patients affected and the high degree of morbidity produced. Most of the allergenic grasses are cultivated and therefore are prevalent where people live.

The grass family contains ten tribes of varying importance to allergists. The most important are:

1. Tribe *Festuceae* contains the bluegrasses, Canada bluegrass (*Poa compressa*), June grass or Kentucky bluegrass (*Poa pratensis*) and orchard grass (*Dactylis glomerata*). These are among the most important allergenic grasses. These pollens are about 30 to 40 μ in diameter.

2. Tribe *Argostideae* includes timothy (*Phleum pratense*) and redtop (*Agrostis alba*), two particularly significant grasses in terms of amount of pollen shed, allergenicity of the pollen, and intensity of symptoms produced. Both are cultivated as forage grasses and timothy is used to make hay. Other species of the genus *Agrostis*, immunologically similar to redtop, are used for the greens of golf courses. Timothy pollens are 30 to 35 μ; redtop, 25 to 30 μ.

3. Tribe *Chlorideae* includes Bermuda grass (*Cynodon dactylon*) which is abundant in all the southern states. It is cultivated for decorative and forage purposes. It pollinates almost all the year and is a major cause of pollen allergy. Its peculiar immunologic properties are discussed on page 90. The pollen grains are 35 μ in diameter.

4. Tribe *Phalarideae* includes sweet vernal grass (*Anthoxanthum ordoratum*), which is an important cause of allergic rhinitis in the areas where it is indigenous. In the total picture of grass allergy, however, it is not as major an allergen as the plants previously mentioned. The pollen grains are 38 to 45 μ in diameter.

Other tribes include *Hordeae* (wheat and wheat grasses), *Aveneae* (oats), *Zizaneae* (wild rice), *Paniceae* (crabgrass), *Andropogoneae* (sorghum) and *Tripsaceae* (corn and sedges). These are of only minor or local importance in allergy since they may be self-pollinating or produce pollen that is not abundant or readily airborne.

Weeds

A weed is a plant that grows where man does not intend it to grow. Hence a rose could be considered a weed if it were growing in a wheat field. What we commonly call weeds are small annual plants that grow wild and have no agricultural or decorative value. All are angio-

sperms and dicotyledons. Those of interest to allergists are wind-pollinated, hence their flowers are not prominent, though some weeds are
quite colorful.

The COMPOSITAE (composite family) is perhaps the most important
weed group from the standpoint of allergy. Sometimes called the sunflower family, it is characterized by multiple flower heads arranged on
a common receptacle. There are many nuances of taxonomy within
this family, but they are unimportant for this discussion. There are
fourteen tribes of COMPOSITAE; only those of allergenic or general interest will be mentioned.

1. Tribe *Helianthe*—includes the sunflower, dahlia, zinnia and black-
eyed Susan. These flowers cause pollinosis mainly among those who
handle them.

2. Tribe *Ambrosiaea*, the ragweed tribe, is the most important cause of
allergic rhinitis and pollen asthma in North America. Other common
weeds included in this tribe are the cockleburs and marsh elders.

Ambrosia trifida is giant ragweed which may grow to a height of
15 feet. The leaves are broad with 3 to 5 clefts. The staminate heads
are borne on long, terminal spikes and the pistillate heads are borne
in clusters at the base of the staminate spikes. The pollen grains, 16
to 19 μ in diameter, are slightly smaller than those of short ragweed.

Ambrosia eliator is short ragweed, which grows to a height of 4 feet.
The leaves are more slender and usually have two pinnae on each side
of a central axis. The pollen grains range from 17.5 to 19.2 μ in diameter
and are almost indistinguishable from those of giant ragweed. There
is no practical reason for distinguishing between the two pollens.

Ambrosia bidentata, southern ragweed, is an annual that grows 1
to 3 feet tall. The pollens are 20 to 21 μ in diameter and resemble
those of giant ragweed.

Ambrosia psilostachya is western ragweed, an annual that grows to a
height of 1 to 4 feet. The pollen grains are larger than the other
ragweeds, ranging 22 to 25 μ in diameter.

Franseria, false ragweed, is found mainly in the south and southwest,
where it may cause allergic symptoms. *Franseria tenuifolia,* slender
ragweed, is the best known species of this tribe.

Xanthium, the cockleburs, are morphologically distinct from the ragweed, but their pollen grains are similar. Except for *Xanthium speciosum,*
the great clotbur, most species produce little pollen and are relatively
unimportant causes of allergic rhinitis. Many patients with ragweed sensitivity also give strong skin test reactions to cocklebur, and this is
probably a cross-reaction.

3. Tribe *Anthemideae*, the mayweed tribe, is important to allergy since
it contains the chrysanthemums. *Pyrethrum* is an insecticide made

from the flower heads of these plants and inhalation of this substance may cause allergic symptoms in ragweed-sensitive patients as well as those who have been sensitized to the pyrethrum itself.

Artemisia includes the sagebrushes, mugworts and wormwoods and is one of the most important of the allergenic weeds. *Artemisia vulgaris* is the common mugwort or sagewort, found mainly on the east coast and midwest. The plant is indigenous to Europe and Asia, and this author found a large number of atopic patients in Afghanistan to be skin test-positive to mugwort. The pollen grains, like those of the other *Artemisias*, are oblately spheroidal, 17 to 28 μ in diameter, with 3 furrows and central pores, a thick exine and essentially no spines. Other very similar species are found on the west coast, southwest, Great Plains and Rocky Mountain areas. *Artemisia campestris candata* is tall wormwood, prevalent in the upper midwest.

Artemisia tridentata is common sagebrush, the most important allergenic plant of this tribe. This plant ranges from 3 to 12 feet in height. It is most prevalent in the Great Plains and Northwest. Overgrazing of the grasslands has increased the presence of sagebrush.

CANNABINACEAE—the hemp family. *Cannabis sativa* is the hemp plant, originally brought into the United States from Asia for its fibers used in the manufacture of rope and other binding materials. It is also the source of marijuana and hashish, and its cultivation is now illegal. However, it grows wild in much of the eastern and midwestern United States, and its pollen may be identified on slides in significant numbers. The grains are oblately spheroid, 25 μ in diameter and contain 3 germ pores. The exine is thin. Though extracts of the pollen are not readily available for routine allergy testing, hemp has been reported in the past as a cause of allergic rhinitis.

POLYGONACEAE—the buckwheat family. The docks, comprising the genus *Rumex* are the only allergic members of this family. *Rumex acetosella* (sheep sorrel), *Rumex crispus* (curly dock) and *Rumex obtusifolius* (bitter dock) are the most important species. However in the whole spectrum of pollen allergy, the docks are of minor significance.

AMARANTHACEAE—the pigweed and waterhemp family. The best known of the Amaranths are *Amaranthus retroflexus* (red-root pigweed), *Amaranthus palmeri* (carelessweed) and *Amaranthus spinosus* (spring amaranth). They are prolific pollen producers and should be considered in the etiology of hay fever in the areas where they abound.

The genus *Acnida* comprises the waterhemps. Western waterhemp (*Amaranthus tamariscina*) is most prevalent in the middle west and is also a potent allergen.

The pollens of the *Amaranths* and the *Chenopods* (to be subsequently described) are so morphologically alike that they are generally described as "chenopod-amaranth" when found in pollen surveys. Though subtle differences exist, it is generally fruitless and impractical to attempt to identify them more precisely. They have the appearance of golf balls and in this respect are unique and easy to identify. Multiple pores give this peculiar surface appearance. The grains are 20 to 30 μ in diameter and spheroidal.

CHENOPODIACEAE—the goosefoot family. The genus *Chenopodium*, comprising the goosefoots is best illustrated by lambsquarters (*Chenpodiaceae album*). Each plant produces relatively small amounts of pollen, but in some areas the abundance of plants may assure a plethora of pollen in the air.

Salsola pestifer or Russian thistle, and *Kochia scoparia* or burning bush, are other members of the CHENOPODIACEAE whose allergenic presence is more significant than lambsquarters. Russian thistle is also known as "tumbleweed," since in the fall the plant separates from its roots and is rolled along the ground by the wind. Burning bush may be easily recognized in the fall by the fire-engine red color assumed by its leaves. For that reason it is often cultivated as an ornamental plant. Originally indigenous to Europe and Asia, these two weeds first became established in the prairie states but have migrated eastward and are now important in the pathogenesis of pollinosis.

Atriplex is the genus of the saltbushes, including the bractscale, wingscale and shadscale. These are of some allergenic significance in the far West and Southwest.

Two crops are numbered among the CHENOPODIACEAE; the sugar beet (*Beta vulgaris*) and spinach (*Spinacea oleracea*). The former has been implicated in allergy in the areas where beet sugar is cultivated.

PLANTAGINACEAE—the plantain family. The only member of this family that is important for allergy is *Plantago lanceolata*, English plantain. It pollinates mainly in May and June, corresponding to the time grasses pollinate. The pollen grains may be distinguished by their multiple pores (7 to 14) and variable size, 25 to 40 μ in diameter. English plantain may be a potent cause of allergic rhinitis which may be confused with grass pollinosis.

Mold Spores

The role of fungi in producing respiratory allergy is established. Initial evidence was presented by several European workers in the mid-1920's, and the independent studies by Prince [35] and Feinberg [13] in the 1930's gave convincing documentation and added much knowledge to this concept. An encyclopedic study of the relation of molds to asthma may be found in Van der Werff's text.[44] Inhalation challenge studies by Itkin [15] and others have presented more direct evidence, and Pepys [31, 32] has shown that two types of immunopathology can result from sensitization to certain molds.

The major clinical problem is the extent to which a mold-sensitive patient's symptoms can be attributed to mold allergy. This is because exposure to molds, like exposure to house dust, is a continuum without definite seasonal end points. Mold spores can be roughly quantitated in the air, and some have their own seasons and ecology. During any season, however, and winters especially, the number and types of spores a patient inhales on a given day are purely conjectural. This is in contrast to pollens that have distinct seasons, or to animal danders for which a definitive history of exposure usually can be obtained. Such a history is sometimes possible for mold exposure, such as raking leaves or being in a barn, but these instances are not daily occurrences for most patients. The *cliché* among allergists, "it must be the molds," to explain some exacerbations of symptoms may be a truth, but one that needs additional evidence.

Fungi are members of the phylum *Thallophyta,* plants that lack definite root, stem and leaf structures. They are separated from the *Algae* in that they do not contain chlorophyll and are therefore saprophytic or parasitic. Almost all of the allergenic molds are saprophytes. The basis of classification is the mode of spore formation, particularly the sexual spore. The *Fungi imperfecti* (here considered a separate class) reproduce asexually by the differentiation of specialized hyphae called *conidiophores* that bear the *conidia,* or asexual spore-forming organs. The subclasses of *Fungi imperfecti,* which include most of the molds of allergenic importance, are differentiated by the morphology of the conidia. The other classes of molds can also reproduce asexually by means of conidia, and some of the imperfect fungi have been shown to be the asexual forms of members of other classes, particularly the *Ascomycetes. Hyphae* are filamentous strands that constitute the fundamental anatomic units of fungi. Yeasts are unicellular and do not form hyphae. The *mycelium* is a mass of hyphae, and the undifferentiated body of a fungus is called a *thallus.*

A practical taxonomic scheme is given below, with annotations of interest to allergists.[9, 10, 14, 23]

Eumycetes—True Fungi

Class *Phycomycetes*

Subclass *Oomycetes.* This subclass is of little allergenic importance but includes the *Phytophtorae* which caused the Irish potato blight of 1845.

Subclass *Zygomycetes.* These are sexual forms characterized by thick-walled, spinous zygospores; and asexually by sporangia. The order

Mucorales includes the genera *Mucor* and *Rhizopus,* both allergenic. The hyphae are non-septate. *Rhizopus nigricans* is the "black bread mold" whose hyphae are colorless but sporangia (visible to the naked eye) are black.

Class *Ascomycetes.* These are the "sac fungi"; their spores are produced in asci, or spore sacs. The powdery mildews and many plant parasites, including *Claviceps,* which produces ergot, are in this class but have not been implicated in human allergy. The two significant microorganisms that cause allergy are *Saccharomyces cerevisiae,* a yeast, and *Chaetomium indicum.* The former, known as "baker's yeast" is most commonly seen in its asexual budding form but under certain culture conditions forms hyphae and asci. *Chaetomium* is unusual among allergenic molds in its ability to digest cellulose. It also produces an antibiotic toxic for certain other molds. The fruiting bodies are formed directly on the mycelium.

Class *Basidiomycetes.* These are the "club fungi" and include mushrooms, toadstools, morels and other nonallergens. The only members of this class occasionally implicated in allergy are *Merulius lacrymans,* the cause of "dry rot" in wood; *Ustilaginales,* the smut fungi; and *Uredinales,* the rust fungi. The latter two are plant parasites of enormous agricultural importance and may cause allergy where wheat is grown or in the vicinity of granaries.

Class *Fungi imperfecti.* Conidia rather than sexual spores characterize the reproductive mechanism and account for further subclassification into the following orders:

Order *Sphaeropsidales.* The conidiophores are grouped in spherical or flask-shaped structures called *pycnidia.* The genus *Phoma* is the only common allergenic mold in this order and frequently gives a positive skin test in patients sensitive to *Alternaria.*

Order *Melanoconiales* is not of allergenic importance.

Order *Moniliales.* The conidiophores are spread over the entire colony. In this order there are three families which account for most of the molds that cause allergy in humans.

MONILIACEAE. This family is characterized by colorless or light-colored hyphae and conidia, and the colonies are usually white, green or yellow. The genera *Aspergillus, Penicillium, Botrytis, Monilia, Mycogone, Paecilomyces, Trichoderma* and *Gliocladium* are "moniliaceous molds."

DEMATIACEAE. This family is characterized by the production of dark pigment in the conidia and often in the mycelium, and is one of the most important from the standpoint of allergy. It contains the genera *Alternaria, Hormodendrum (Cladosporium),* * *Curvularia, Helmintho-*

* *Hormodendrum* is the generic name most firmly entrenched in the allergy literature, though *Cladosporium* is currently preferred by mycologists.

sporium, Spondylocladium, Stemphyllium, Nigrospora, and *Pullularia.* The last is morphologically similar to the yeasts and is sometimes classed with them and called the "black yeast." This group is often called the "dematiaceous molds."

TUBERCULARIACEAE produce a sporodochium, which is a rounded mass of conidiophores containing macro- and microconidia in a slimy substrate. *Fusarium* and *Epicoccum* belong in this family.

CRYPTOCOCCACEAE. This family contains true yeasts, such as *Rhodotorula,* that do not produce hyphae under any known culture or natural circumstances. Rhodotorula produces a characteristic dark pink carotenoid pigment, is frequently cultured on Sabauroud's agar from patients' homes and is antigenic. *Cryptococcus* is a pale yeast sometimes cultured. The differentiation of yeasts is not always possible on a morphologic basis and may require the use of specialized nutrient media.

Mycelia sterilata is the descriptive term for the growth of mycelia on culture plates without fruiting bodies or spores.

The foregoing classification and genera mentioned are not exhaustive but do represent most of the molds found in environmental surveys. The most intensive longitudinal studies in the United States have been

TABLE 4-1   The MMP Molds

PHYCOMYCETES	
Mucor racemosus	
Rhizopus nigricans	
ASCOMYCETES	
Saccharomyces cerevisiae	
Chaetomium indicum	
FUNGI IMPERFECTI	
DEMATIACEAE	MONILIACEAE
Alternaria tenuis	Aspergillus fumigatus
Curvularia spicifera	Aspergillus flavus
Spondylocladium sp.	Aspergillus glaucus
Helminthosporium interseminatum	Aspergillus nidulans
Hormodendrum cladosporoides	Aspergillus niger
Stemphyllium botryosum	Aspergillus syndowi
Nigrospora sphaerica	Aspergillus terreus
Pullularia pullulans	Botrytis cinerea
	Monilia sitophila
OTHER FUNGI IMPERFECTI	Mycogone sp.
	Paecilomyces varioti
Phoma herbarum	Penicillium atramentosum
Fusarium vasinfectum	Penicillium biforme
Rhodotorula glutinis	Penicillium carmino-violaceum
	Penicillium intricatum
	Penicillium luteum
	Penicillium notatum
	Trichoderma viride
	Gliocadium fimbriatum

made by a group, including mycologists, known as the Association of Allergists for Mycological Investigations.[29, 34, 36] For practical purposes in clinical allergy a series of molds known as the "MMP molds" (the initials of three of the members) has been compiled for use in diagnosis and treatment. These are presented here as the framework upon which the individual allergist can build or from which he can delete depending on region or clinical judgment. Most atopic mold allergy is specific to genus, though species differences have been reported. Where more than one species occurs for a given genus, the species are usually mixed together, as in "Aspergillus mixture" or "Penicillium mixture." The MMP Molds are outlined in Table I.

Certain data concerning the prevalence and ecology of these molds make this list less formidable in practice. *Alternaria* and *Hormodendrum* (*Cladosporium*) are the most numerous in almost every survey made of outdoor air. The Pacific Northwest is the exception. These molds are "field fungi" and thrive best on plants on the field and their decaying parts in the soil. They require a relatively high moisture content (22% –25%) in their substrate. They are mainly seasonal, from spring to late fall, and diminish markedly with the first hard frost. In the Chicago area their numbers are reported along with ragweed on the evening television news programs. *Helminthosporium* and *Fusarium* are other common field fungi. The former is the cause of the current corn blight affecting parts of Illinois, and the latter causes flax wilt and has a predilection for melons, peas and bananas. These and certain other molds propagate in the soil and their spores are released in large numbers when the soil is tilled.

Aspergillus and *Penicillium,* on the other hand, are sometimes called "storage fungi," since they are common causes of rot in stored grain, fruits and vegetables. *Aspergillus* in particular will thrive on a substrate with low moisture content (12% to 16%). These are the two molds most commonly cultured from houses, especially basements, crawl spaces and bedding. *Penicillium* is the green "mildew" so often seen on articles stored in basements. *Rhizopus* is the cause of black moldy bread and proliferates in vegetable bins in homes, especially on onions.

The four most common allergenic molds are *Alternaria, Aspergillus, Hormodendrum* and *Penicillium,* based not only on incidence, but on skin test reactivity. Roughly 85 percent of patients allergic to molds will react to one or more of these allergens. However, many react to other molds as well, and some to molds other than these four. It should also be emphasized that the designation "field" and "storage" fungi are not precise, since exceptions are commonplace in surveys of outdoor and indoor air.

The *yeasts* require a high sugar content in their substrates, which limits their habitat. Certain leaves, pasture grasses and flowers exude a sugary fluid which serves as a carbon source for the nonfermentative yeasts, *Pullularia, Cryptococcus* and *Rhodotorula.* Hundreds of millions of yeast colonies may be obtained per gram of leaf tissue. Berries and fruits are other common colonizing sources. The soil is not a good habitat for yeasts unless it is in the vicinity of fruit trees. Yeasts are often cultured indoors, and in the author's experience *Rhodotorula* in particular is more commonly allergenic than documented in the literature.

Green algae have been implicated by several investigators as a cause of human respiratory allergy. The genera *Chlorella, Chlorococcum, Scenedesmus* and *Ankistrodesmus* are disseminated widely in the air. Algae show skin reactivity in some atopic patients and have provoked asthma by inhalation challenge. Animal studies have confirmed their antigenicity.[5] The importance of these organisms as significant allergens requires further study.

The relation of weather to spore dissemination is clinically important since the patients with respiratory allergy are often worse in rainy or damp weather. This has been attributed by some to an increase in the "mold count." Actually absolute mold counts decrease during and after a rainstorm, since the spores are either washed out or made less buoyant, like pollen grains. All of the commonly allergenic molds are of the dry spore type, in which the spores are released by the wind during dry periods. The slime spore molds include the genera *Fusarium, Phoma, Pullularia* and *Trichoderma.* These spores are loosened during wet periods and dispersed by raindrops. However, it is unlikely that these spores are responsible for the mass symptoms that occur during inclement weather. It should be mentioned that high spore counts are found in clouds and mist, and it is reasonable to attribute some of the symptoms encountered during long periods of high humidity to mold allergy. Snow obliterates the outdoor mold count, but the conditions subsequent to thawing predispose to mold growth and propagation.

METHODS OF STUDYING AIRBORNE MOLDS

The gravity slide method is as applicable to molds as to pollens. A microscope slide is coated with an adhesive substance such as petrolatum, diluted rubber cement or glycerine jelly and exposed to the air in a Durham Gravity Slide Sampler or similar device. The adherent spores are usually stained with cotton-blue, a cover glass is applied and the spores are classified and counted. Counting methods are described in the section on enumeration of pollen grains. As with pollens, gravity methods tend to favor collection of the heavier particles since slight turbulence engendered by the apparatus has a greater effect on carrying the lighter spores away from the impacting surface.

Another gravity method consists of simply exposing a Petri dish with appropriate nutrient agar to the air for periods of 5 to 30 minutes, depending on the anticipated growth. The plates are incubated at room temperature for about five days, then inspected grossly and microscopically for the numbers and types of colonies present. Potato-dextrose agar, to which rose bengal may be added to retard bacterial growth and limit spread of fungal colonies, is one of a number of media satisfactory for general mycological use. Specialized media are also available, such as Czepak Agar which favors growth of *Aspergillus* and *Penicillium*.

The advantages of the slide method are that the exposure is usually for 24 hours, giving a more representative sample than a plate exposure of 30 minutes. Also, rusts and smuts do not grow on ordinary nutrient media, and would not be detected by the routine culture technique. The disadvantage is that many spores cannot be morphologically identified without other colony characteristics.

The advantage of the plate method is more positive identification, including the ability to isolate and subculture colonies when in doubt. This is the only significant method for indoor surveys. The disadvantages are a short sampling time, underestimation of numbers of spores (since a microconidium containing many spores will grow only one colony), and underestimation because of mutual inhibition or overgrowth of a single colony. Furthermore, it is difficult to avoid massive spore contamination of the laboratory without elaborate precautions. Detailed mycological investigations are probably best not carried out by mold-sensitive persons unless an isolation chamber and ventilation hood are used.

More recently, attempts are being made to increase the efficiency of mold spore sampling by use of the Anderson Sampler. With this device air passes through a series of six sievelike plates, each containing 400 holes of decreasing diameter. An agar Petri dish is placed beneath each plate. The larger particles impinge on the higher plates and the smaller ones are carried by the airstream to the successively lower plates. It has been found that using only the lowest sieve plate with a hole diameter of 0.01 inch, and orienting the sampler towards the wind improves the efficiency of the device. The Hirst Spore Trap, previously mentioned in connection with pollens, may be used to assay mold spores by the slide method. The advantage is that a clock mechanism exposes certain portions of the slide at given time intervals so that circadian variations can be studied. Details of these and other sampling methods are described in the references cited.[39, 40]

EPIDERMAL ALLERGENS

This category includes animal emanations; dander, hair, feathers and saliva. Although saliva is not an epithelial antigen, antigenic similarity of salvia and dander from the same animal is such that they may be considered in the same class. It is well-known that animals are a common cause of nasobronchial allergy but certain points deserve emphasis and will serve to avoid much of the confusion that exists in this area.

Dander, not hair, is the major allergen. All living animals commonly encountered continually shed and replace epidermal cells. These degenerate and the cell products become part of the amorphous particulate matter in the air. These dander materials contain many water soluble proteins. These have been shown to be highly antigenic and allergenic. The hair itself is more visible but less airborne and less water soluble, therefore less allergenic. Saliva is rich in proteins, including for example, secretory IgA globulins and enzymes. These substances become airborne particularly when dried and are allergenic. The precise chemical nature of the allergens in unknown. It is not uncommon for persons to develop local urticaria at the sites where they have been licked by a cat or dog, or where they have been scratched by claws or teeth.

It follows that a dog may be allergenic whether it sheds hair or not since skin and saliva are continuous emanations. It is important to stress this fact to patients, who tend to equate hair with allergy, and who often insist that their pets cannot be allergenic since "they don't shed," using the French poodle as an example. It is obvious that the closer the contact with an animal, the greater the likelihood of increased symptoms. However, airborne particles travel easily over all the house, particularly with forced-air heating systems so prevalent in modern homes, and permeate furniture, drapes and bedding. They become a part of the house dust of that house.

Processed furs such as coats and collars do not desquamate and therefore do not cause respiratory allergy. Contact dermatitis is sometimes seen from the dyes and mordants used in the fur industry. Wool rugs similarly bear little resemblance to the raw product shorn from sheep, and though some patients react on skin tests to wool, it is the crude material that is used for testing.

Feathers are epidermal appendages that may be significant allergens. Goose and duck down are most commonly used in the manufacture of pillows and with use are pulverized, increasing the access of particles to the respiratory tract. Commercial processing does not remove the soluble portions responsible for allergy. Feather pillows are also suit-

able culture materials for molds and bacteria. Dacron is the most satisfactory substitute, since foam rubber tends to pulverize and support
mold growth. Parakeets, canaries and other birds as household pets are
another source of feather allergens and contain sufficient immunological
uniqueness to warrant individual testing when suspected.

Cats are by far the most highly allergenic animals encountered by most
people. Cat dander, like ragweed pollen, has a clinical importance that
sets it apart from other allergens in its class. Explanations for this are
uncertain. "Cat asthma" is an entity that is self-explanatory. Sudden
rhinitis, conjunctivitis, asthma or urticaria may occur when highly sensitive persons simply enter a room where a cat has been. This type of
exquisite hypersensitivity is seen less commonly with dogs and other
household pets. However, cat allergy need not be dramatic to be
significant.

Dogs are important in the total management of many patients, but are
not often the sole cause of symptoms. In dog owners with perennial
rhinitis or asthma and a positive skin test to dog, removal of the animal
is certainly indicated. Clinical improvement may not occur for several
weeks or even months because of residual dander in the house. But
all too frequently clinical improvement does not occur at all in a multi-
ply allergic patient, so the role played by the dog becomes an unknown quantity. Furthermore patients with purely seasonal symptoms
attributable to pollens may react strongly on skin tests to dog dander,
but are able to live with a dog with impunity. The intent of these
statements is not to minimize the potential significance of dog allergy
or discredit the principle of environmental control, but rather to point
out a need for individual evaluation of patients and further study. Dogs
may have strong emotional impacts on their owners, and an imperative
by the physician forces the patient and family to choose between a
sense of loss or guilt. A trial separation may be helpful, physically and
psychologically. Again the best solution results from evaluation of the
severity of illness and the total problem. A child with severe asthma
may require a different concern than an adult with mild nasal
symptoms.

Horses are like cats in the explosive symptoms that may occur on exposure to their dander, but the clinical situation is less common and
not as difficult to manage primarily because of the absence of horse
dander in the household. Horsehair is used in the manufacture of some
mattresses, furniture and rug pads, but again the allergenic potential
of hair nowhere approaches that of dander. There are antigens common
to horse dander and serum, so patients sensitive to horse dander should
be prophylactically immunized with tetanus toxoid, or given tetanus
antitoxin made from human rather than horse serum.

Allergy to cows, goats, sheep, hogs, rabbits and small rodents may occur under circumstances that need no amplification here. Gerbils, guinea pigs, hamsters, mice and rats are common household pets today. The allergy may also be occupational. Respiratory allergy to human dander or saliva has not been documented.

Avoidance is the treatment of choice for epidermal allergens. Immunotherapy should be reserved for situations where this is not feasible, such as occupational types of allergy, and should be done only after serious consideration. The results are usually disappointing.

HOUSE DUST

A recent thorough and critical review of the allergens in house dust [7] points out the uniqueness of house dust as an allergen. It is not a simple substance, but an accumulation of living and nonliving materials gathered from a particular environment. Moreover, the allergenicity of the dust from a given home, for example, will vary depending on the temperature, humidity and other factors.

If one considers the problems of standardizing and isolating the antigens in a relatively constant, if not homogenous, allergen such as pollen, the magnitude of the difficulty of these determinations in house dust becomes obvious.

The current thinking in chemical terms is that the antigens in house dust are glycoprotein carrier molecules whose allerginicity depends on structural sites—N-glycosidic lysine-sugar linkages. The glycoproteins may come from animal or vegetable sources, and the amount of allergy produced by a given dust sample is related to the number of allergenically active sites on the carrier molecules. Whether these sites are the result of a degradative process, or a proliferative process such as the growth of mites in dust, is a lively topic in allergy today.

It is suggested that the clinical allergist perform skin tests to house dust using preparations from several different sources or manufacturers. In some patients there will be differential reactions.

The question of mites as an important component of house dust allergy has occupied a prominent place in the allergy literature for the past few years. The following section will elaborate on this subject.

HOUSE DUST AND DUST MITES

Terumasa Miyamoto, M.D. , PH.D.

House dust [2, 11, 25-28, 41, 42, 45, 46] is a mixture of materials such as various kinds of fibers, molds, human and animal danders, bacteria and remnants of food. Because of the presence of these multiple materials, it has been uncertain which is the major allergen in house dust. It is known that the allergenic potency of house dust appears to increase when it is stored for several months before an extract is made. For this reason, it has been suspected that viable material is an important antigen in house dust. House dusts obtained from Netherlands, Switzerland, Sweden, Germany, Austria, Poland, Italy, England, the United States and Japan have been found to have similar antigenicity as indicated by skin testing of allergic subjects. Consequently, house dust from various parts of the world was thought to have all of the specific antigens universally distributed in spite of the different sources. Previously, mold antigens or microorganisms were considered by some to be important antigens in house dust or to contribute to deterioration of various kinds of fibrous materials in house dust with resultant production of a potent common antigen. Human dander was believed to be the major antigen in house dust by others. The role of molds, bacteria and dander as important antigens in house dust has been questioned more recently. In a search for specific house dust antigens, studies were extended to consider arthropods such as house flies, mosquitoes, moths, spiders and mites as contributing factors.

The results of studies using extracts of insects and spiders showed that these organisms could not be considered to be the source of major antigens in house dust. The only extracts that were promising and gave intense skin reactions in house dust-sensitive patients were those prepared from mites.

In the early 1920's it was suggested that mites might be an important source of allergens. In 1923, Ancona reported an epidemic of asthma in 21 Italian grain workers. This asthma was found to be due to a mite, *Pyemotes ventricosus*, infesting the grain. Storm van Leeuwen [42] *et al.* described a case of a farmer who suffered from severe asthmatic attacks after inhalation of dust from oats heavily infested with *Acarus siro* and a species of *Glycyphagus*. Dekker [11] considered mites to be one of the most important causes of asthma in Germany. Subsequent to these basic studies, more recent investigations have been focused on mites in house dust to determine whether these mites are the important source of house dust antigens which cause human allergic disease.

The total number of mites found in house dust differs, depending on

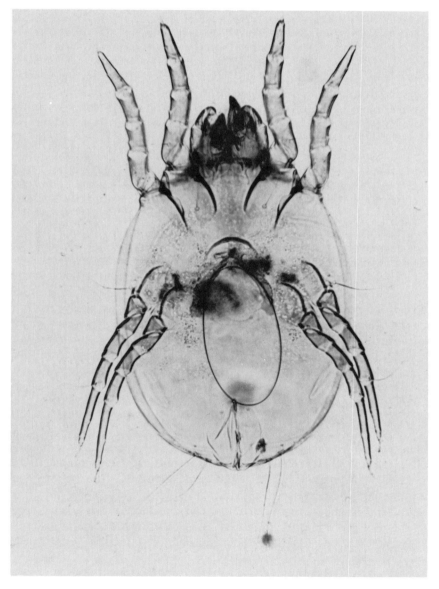

Fig. 4-4. *Dermatophagoides farinae.* Female mite. (T. Miyamoto, M.D.)

the source of the house dust and the method used to identify the mites. As an indication of concentrations, the number of mites was reported to be up to two thousand in one gram of a house dust sample. Current investigations have shown that there are more than 36 species of mites in house dust. In general, the genus *Dermatophagoides* occurs in house dust most frequently.

To analyze the antigenic similarity between house dust and mites, pure cultures of *D. pteronyssinus* and *D. farinae* were used initially. A close correlation between house dust extract and mite extract was found by skin testing. This correlation was that a majority of patients reactive to house dust antigen by cutaneous testing were also reactive to mite antigen. Most patients who were shown to have positive inhalation provocation responses with house dust extract reacted positively to the provocative inhalation challenge with the mite extract.

As a result of these studies, house dust mites were considered to be the antigenic constituent of house dust responsible for these human respiratory responses. Other studies indicated the following: Skin-sensitizing antibody against the mite was detected in sera of patients allergic to house dust. Skin-sensitizing antibody against *D. farinae* extract was almost completely neutralized with house dust extract in both in vivo and in vitro tests. Skin-sensitizing antibody against house dust was largely neutralized by *D. farinae*. Antigenic potency of *D. farinae* was calculated to be 10 to 100 times stronger by weight than house dust from the results of skin tests, inhalation provocation tests, P-K tests and neutralization tests. When house dust and *D. farinae* extracts were fractionated through Sephadex G-50 and G-200, similar fractions of the house dust extract and mite extract contained the most potent antigens as determined by skin reactions in house dust-sensitive subjects. The most active antigen obtained by Sephadex chromatography was evaluated by testing on subjects allergic to house dust and appeared to have a molecular weight larger than 10,000 but smaller than 69,000. The composition of the antigen is probably a protein and polysaccharide conjugate. Cross reactivity of antigens from various mites was found although this cross reactivity was not complete and each species of mite appears to have some individually specific antigens. Among mites, the family *Dermatophagoides* is most closely related to the commercially available house dust antigen preparation obtained from Japan, the Netherlands and England. Bodies of mites had an identical antigenicity with the excreta under the conditions of the experiments. The potency of house dust allergen is largely determined by the number of mites contained in house dust.

These observations are based on results obtained from our experience. Recently, however, there have been many investigations of house dust mites in relation to house dust antigen reported from various countries. The results of most of these other studies were in agreement with our findings, and it can be concluded that the house dust mite is a major antigenic material in house dust. However, it is obvious that house dust is a mixture of various materials and the mite is not a single antigen contained in house dust. Some Japanese allergic patients had strongly positive skin reactions to house dust extract but minimal reactions against mites. These patients were found to be very sensitive to silk antigen. Such patients appear to be uncommon. Some investigators consider that cockreal or air-borne algae are more significant components of house dust allergy. This is not generally recognized.

For the laboratory growth of mites, a temperature of 26° to 27° C and a relative humidity of air of 70 to 75 percent appear to be most suitable. The nutrient for the mites is extremely important, and if suitable foods for mites are available in places in the house with adequate climatic conditions, a dense population can be expected to develop. The most suitable foods differed for different species but most of mites living in house dust utilize food materials with high protein content of animal origin, such as hides of mammals or birds, dander, and remnants of household foods. Yeast and molds are also utilized as nutrient by mites.

House dust mite extract has been used successfully for hyposensitization treatment by several investigators. The initial concentration for hyposensitization therapy should be 100 to 1000 times more dilute than commercial house dust extract. The mite extract is generally more potent than crude house dust extract and may produce a higher incidence of side reactions than house dust extract unless the higher dilutions are used.

In summary, current evidence indicates that mites are the source of the major antigenic component of house dust as it relates to human allergic disease of the immediate type. Further evaluation of this question will likely lead to improved understanding and treatment of house dust allergy.

OTHER IMPORTANT ALLERGENS

In this category are included allergens that are applicable in selected cases and those, such as certain insects, perhaps more significant than hitherto suspected.

Insects as inhalant allergens have been previously mentioned in this chapter in connection with epidemic allergy (May fly and caddis fly) and in the section on house dust. The convincing studies on mites have prompted allergists to reexamine other insects such as cockroaches, carpet beetles, moths, butterflies and locusts. These have been reported in the past to cause symptoms in some patients, based on their presence in the environment and ability to elicit positive skin tests to provoke symptoms by inhalation challenge. With the cockroach, the distinction has been made between allergy to the whole body extract and fecal extract.[6] May fly and caddis fly have been most extensively studied clinically and immunologically. Their larvae are aquatic and they have been described most commonly in the Great Lakes area, particularly Lake Erie; however, worldwide distribution exists adjacent to bodies of water. There is little doubt of their clinical importance in late summer, in certain geographic locations, but their numbers have declined recently in some areas due to water pollution. Fractionation studies have shown that the caddis fly antigen is probably a peptide with a molecular weight of 3,000. An exhaustive discussion of insect allergens may be found in the review article by Shulman.[38]

Hypersensitivity to the salivary secretions of biting insects exists. Local immediate and delayed allergy to the bites of mosquitoes, fleas (papular urticaria), sand flies, deer flies, horse flies and tse-tse flies has been reported. Other case reports have described generalized reactions to multiple bites (deer fly) consisting of fever, malaise and hypotension, associated with antibodies to the offending insect. Experimental sensitization in humans with flea bites results first in the induction of delayed, then immediate wheal-and-flare hypersensitivity on skin testing.

Hypersensitivity to stinging insects is the subject of a different chapter in this text and will not be discussed here.

Seeds may be important causes of asthma and rhinitis. Cottonseed and flaxseed are exceptionally potent antigens and should be used for skin testing only by the scratch method. Deaths have been reported from intradermal tests to both these substances. Extreme caution should be used in skin testing.

Cottonseed is the seed of the cotton plant. After extraction of the oil, which is not allergenic, the seed is ground into meal which may be used for animal feeds or fertilizer. Cottonseed meal and flour are also used in the baking industry for certain cookies, cakes and pan-greasing compounds. Cotton linters are the short cotton fibers that adhere to the seeds after the cotton is ginned. These are separated and used for stuffing mattresses and furniture. Enough of the water soluble cottonseed allergen adheres to these linters to render them antigenic.

Flaxseed (linseed) has the same properties as cottonseed and many of the same general uses in industry and agriculture. Additional uses are found in hair preparations, poultices, electrical wire insulation and for the tough backing material in the manufacture of rugs. Linseed

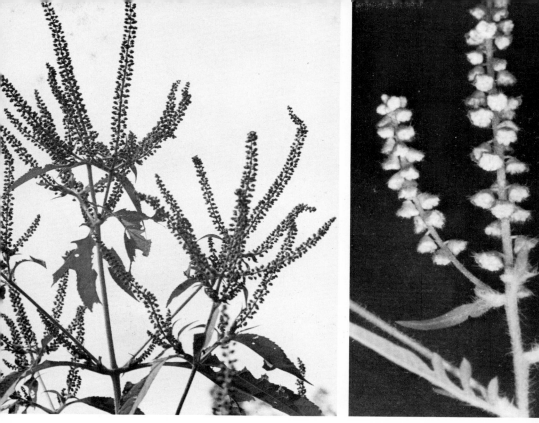

Fig. 4-5. Giant ragweed (*Ambrosia trifida*). Arrangement of staminate heads. (Arnold A. Gutman, M.D.)

Fig. 4-6. Short ragweed (*Ambrosia eliator*). Closeup of staminate head. The anthers are full of pollen just before anthesis. (Arnold A. Gutman, M.D.)

Fig. 4-7. Scanning electron photomicrograph of ragweed pollen. Note the pore on the pollen grain (*lower right*). (D. Lim, M.D. and J. I. Tennenbaum, M.D.)

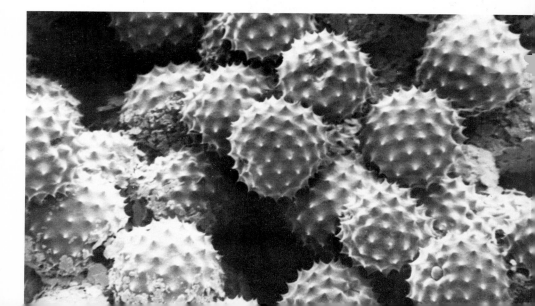

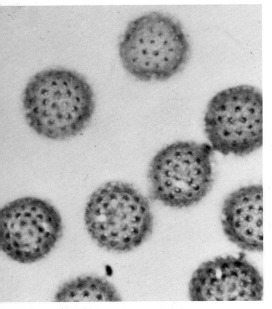

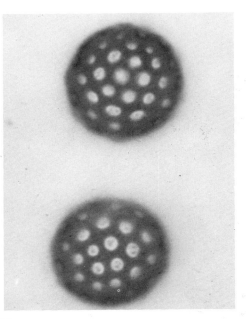

Fig. 4-8. Short ragweed (*Ambrosia eliator*). Average diameter 20μ. Pollen grains have spicules on the surface. (Schering)

Fig. 4-9. Pigweed (*Amaranthus retroflexus*). Average diameter 25μ. The "golf ball" appearance of these pollen grains is characteristic of the chenopod-amaranth groups. (Schering)

Fig. 4-10. Red sorrel (*Rumex acetosella*). Average diameter 21.5μ. These pollens most commonly have four furrows and a thin exine. (Schering)

Fig. 4-11. Common sagebrush (*Artemisia tridentata*). Average diameter 26μ. Three furrows and a thick exine are characteristic of this pollen. (Schering)

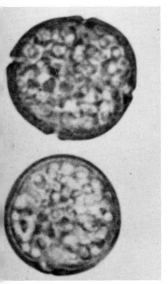

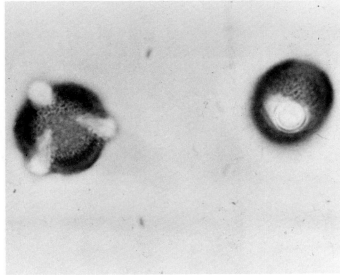

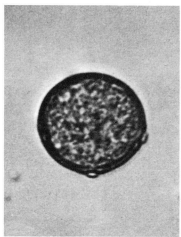
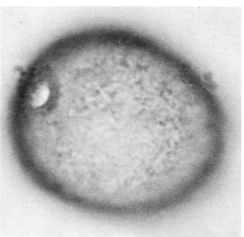

Fig. 4-12. English plantain (*Plantago lanceolata*). Average diameter 27μ. A thin exine and four to seven pores typify this pollen. (Center Labs.)

Fig. 4-13. Johnson grass (*Sorghum halepense*). Average diameter 43μ. This grass is considered a weed in the southern and southwestern states. (William P. Solomon, M.D.)

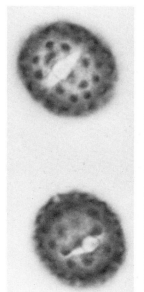
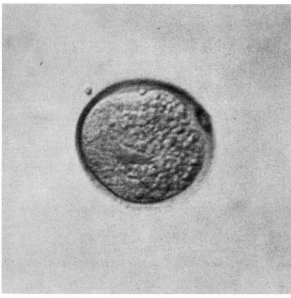

Fig. 4-14. Burweed marsh elder (*Iva xanthifolia*). Average diameter 19.3μ. Three pores are centered in furrows, distinguishing it from ragweed. (Schering)

Fig. 4-15. Timothy grass (*Phleum pratense*). Average diameter 34μ. The grass pollens are all morphologically similar, with a single germinal pore and thin exine. (Center Labs.)

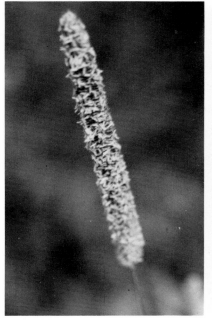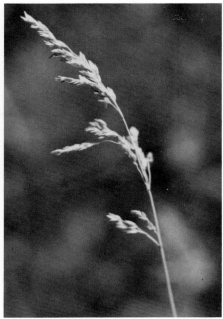

Fig. 4-16. Timothy grass (*Phleum pra-tense*). Morphology of flowering head. (Arnold A. Gutman, M.D.)

Fig. 4-17. June grass or bluegrass (*Poa pratensis*). Morphology of flowering head. (Arnold A. Gutman, M.D.)

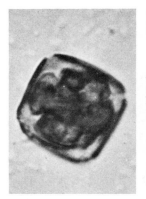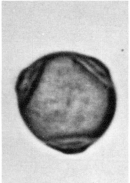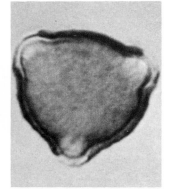

Fig. 4-18. (*left*) Ash (*Fraxinus americana*). Average diameter is 27μ. The pollen grains are square or rectangular, with four furrows. (Center Labs.)

Fig. 4-19. (*center*) Birch (*Betula nigra*). Average diameter 24.5μ. Pollen grains have three pores and a smooth exine. (Center Labs.)

Fig. 4-20. (*right*) Oak (*Quercus sp.*). Average diameter 32μ. Pollens of the various species are similar, with three long furrows and a convex, bulging granular exine. (Center Labs.)

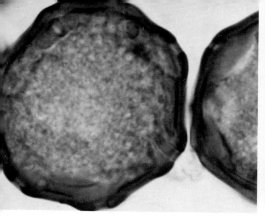

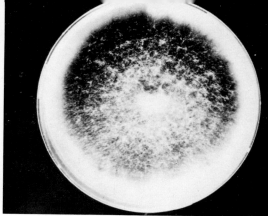

Fig. 4-21. Walnut (*Juglans nigra*). Average diameter 36μ. Grains have multiple pores surrounded by thick collars, arranged in a nonequatorial band. (William P. Solomon, M.D.)

Fig. 4-22. *Alternaria tenuis*. Potato-dextrose agar; culture eight days old. The black pigment is characteristic of, but not peculiar to the *Dematiaceae*. (Schering)

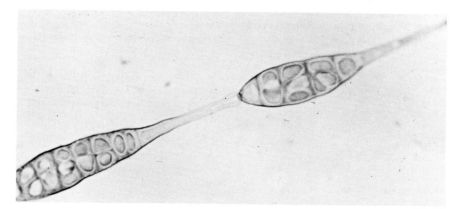

Fig. 4-23. *Alternaria tenuis*. Average spore size 12 × 33μ. Spores are snow-shoe shaped, and contain transverse and longitudinal septae with pores. (Schering)

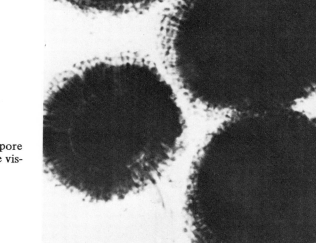

Fig. 4-24. *Aspergillus niger*. Spore masses on stalks, depicted here, are visible to the naked eye. (Schering)

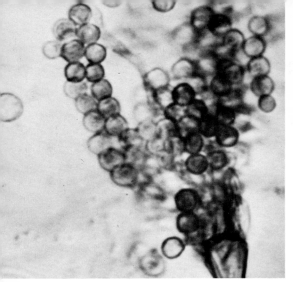

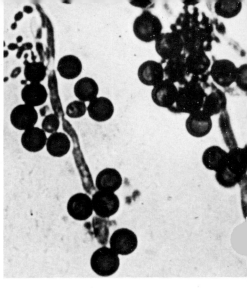

Fig. 4-25. *Aspergillus sp.* Average spore diameter 4μ. The spores are borne in chains and have connecting collars. (Hollister-Stier Laboratories)

Fig. 4-26. *Candida albicans.* This is a yeast and reproduces by budding. The filaments shown here are pseudo-hyphae, actually elongated buds. (Hollister-Stier Laboratories)

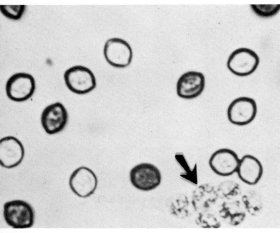

Fig. 4-27. *Chaetomium globosum.* Average spore size is 7 × 11μ. The lemon-shaped spores are released through a pore in an ascus (*see arrow*). (Hollister-Stier Laboratories)

Fig. 4-28. *Curuularia sp.* Average size 10 × 37μ. Curved spores having two to four transverse septae occur on the ends of conidiophores. (Schering)

Fig. 4-29. *Epicoccum nigrum.* Average diameter 20μ. Large spores are borne singly on the ends of conidiophores. They are yellowish brown, rough and have transverse septae when older. (Hollister-Stier Laboratories)

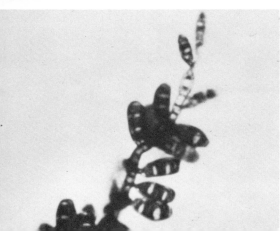

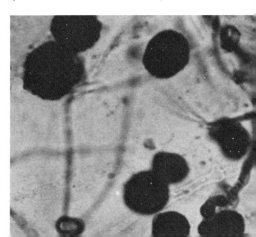

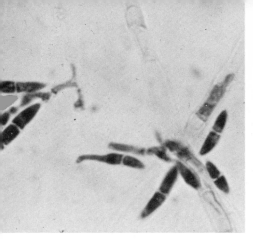

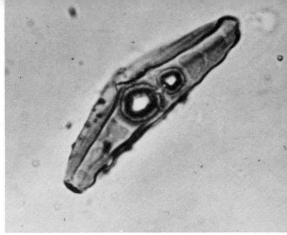

Fig. 4-30. *Fusarium vasinfectum.* Average spore size 4 × 50μ. The most prevalent spore type is the macrospore, which is sickle-shaped, colorless, and contains transverse septae and a point of attachment at one end. (Hollister-Stier Laboratories)

Fig. 4-31. *Helminthosporium sp.* Average spore size is 15 × 75μ. The spores occur in the ends of conidiophores, are large, brownish and have transverse septae. (Schering)

Fig. 4-32. *Hormodendrum (Cladosporium) sp.* Average spore size 4 × 16μ. Spores occur in chains and have small attaching collars at one end. The first spore buds off from the conidiophore, then the spore itself buds to form a secondary spore. (Hollister-Stier Laboratories)

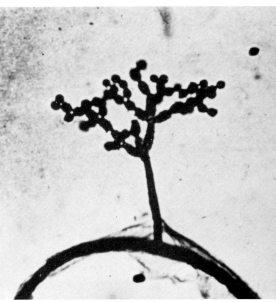

Fig. 4-33. *Monilia sitophila.* The spores (conidia) are formed by budding. In mass they are pink. *Monilia* is the asexual form of *Neurospora,* hence if ascospores (sexual) are found on culture, the organism must be *Neurospora.* (Hollister-Stier Laboratories)

Fig. 4-34. *Mucor sp.* Average spore size 4.5μ. The spores are contained within a sporangium. The hyphae are nonseptate. (Hollister-Stier Laboratories)

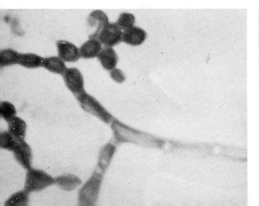

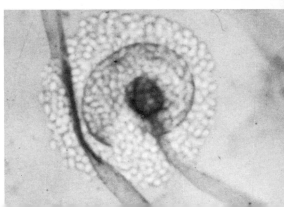

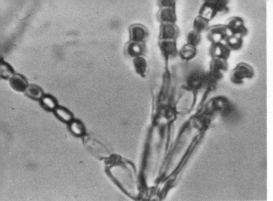

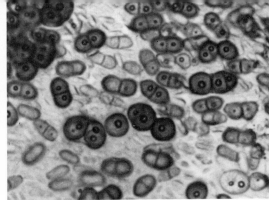

Fig. 4-35. *Penicillium notatum.* Average spore diameter is 2.5μ. The spores appear in unbranched chains on *phia-lides,* the terminal portions of the conidiophores. The appearance of the phialides and chains of spores resemble a brush. (Hollister-Stier Laboratories)

Fig. 4-36. *Pullularia pullans.* The spores characteristically appear as pairs of yeastlike cells with an oil droplet in each cell. As colonies age they form fine, then thick, dark hyphae. (Hollister-Stier Laboratories)

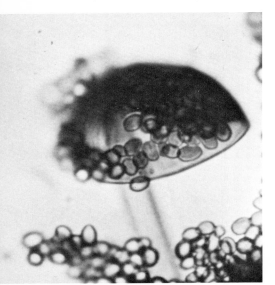

Fig. 4-37. *Rhizopus nigricans.* Average spore diameter is 4.5μ. Spores are being liberated from the *sporangium* which is borne on a nonseptate, filamentous *sporangiophore.* The sporangia are just visible to the naked eye. (Hollister-Stier Laboratories)

Fig. 4-38. *Saccharomyces cerevisiae.* Average cell size is 5μ. This organism is a true yeast and does not form hyphae. Budding is the major, asexual form of reproduction. Notice the presence of a tetrad of sexual haploid spores (*arrow*). (Hollister-Stier Laboratories)

Fig. 4-39. *Stemphyllium sp.* The spores superficially resemble those of *Alternaria* but lack the "tail" appendage. Also they are borne singly rather than in chains. (Schering)

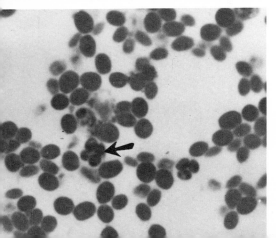

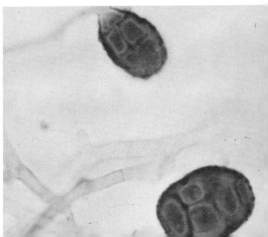

oil is a common household product and is found in furniture polish and printer's ink. This produces contact rather than inhalant allergy.

Coffee bean allergy is largely confined to those who handle the green beans commercially, including longshoremen who unload the sacks from ships. Chlorogenic acid has been considered an allergenic determinant in green coffee beans, castor beans and oranges. This is a simple chemical that presumably acts as a hapten. However, its importance is in question and it is destroyed by roasting and cannot account for allergy from drinking coffee. *Castor bean* allergy is mainly from the pulp and hull that remains after the castor oil is pressed from the bean. This castor pomace is ground into a meal that is used for fertilizer. Thus castor bean allergy is also largely occupational. There are probably allergenic determinants other than chlorogenic acid since low molecular weight protein fractions have been isolated, as well as a toxic substance, *ricin,* which is not allergenic.

Soybean allergy may be more generalized and prevalent because of the increased use of soy flour and meal in commonly encountered products. In addition to its use as an animal feed, it is used for infant feeding, bakery goods, Chinese cooking, cereals, fillers in meat and candy products and in certain topical dermatological preparations.

Kapok was once used as a substitute for feather pillows for certain allergic patients, but is itself allergenic and has been supplanted by synthetic polymers in pillows and other commercial items. Sometimes called Java cotton, most commercial kapok comes from Indonesia and is the fibrous material that is contained within the seed pods of the kapok tree (*Ceiba pentandra*). It is very impervious to water and may still be found as an insulating material in sleeping bags and as a stuffing in cushions for boats.

Pyrethrum is an insecticide derived from the flower heads of the Chrysanthemum group of plants, which like ragweed, are members of the Compositae family. Positive reactions on skin tests are common in patients who react strongly to ragweed, but pyrethrum may be an allergen independently in those who are exposed to insecticides, including many of the common household brands. Its rapid lethality on insects makes it commercially popular.

Orris root is derived from the iris plant and was commonly used in the cosmetic industry, particularly as the base for face powders. Because of its allergenicity it is rarely encountered today except in some imported products.

Glues and *gums* are occasional causes of human allergy. Impure gelatin is the adhesive obtained from the bones and hides of terrestrial animals and fish bones. Other natural glues are made from casein, rubber and gum arabic. The synthetic adhesives have minimized the glue allergy problem in recent years, though the amine hardeners used in the manufacture of epoxies have caused asthma and rhinitis in factory workers. In addition to *gum arabic*, other vegetable gums, *acacia, chicle, karaya* and *tragacanth* have been reported to cause allergy by inhalation or ingestion. These are used in candies, chewing gum, baked goods, salad dressings, laxatives and dentifrices. They are also used as excipients in medications. Their use in hair-setting preparations has been largely replaced by polyvinylpyrrolidone (PVP) which is not allergenic. Parenthetically it might be added here that most cases of chronic pulmonary disease attributed to "hair spray allergy" or "hair spray thesaurosis" have turned out to be sarcoidosis with no basis for attributing the etiology to hair spray.

On the other hand, *toluene diisocyanate* (TDI) used in the manufacture of polyurethane, may cause allergic sensitization and severe asthma in workers where this synthetic resin is made. The consumer who uses the finished product is not affected.

Enzymes used in laundry detergents to enhance cleaning ability of the product may sensitize both the workers where the product is made and the consumer who washes her clothes.[4] The enzyme, subtilin, is proteolytic and derived from *Bacillus subtilis*. It may produce rhinitis, conjunctivitis and asthma, associated with IgE antibodies; or more peripheral alveolar hypersensitivity reactions associated with precipitating antibodies and Arthus-type reactions on skin testing. Because these products are so commonly used today, the physician should increase his awareness of their allergic potential. Many cases reported to date were not atopic individuals.

AIRBORNE SUBSTANCES THAT ARE NOT NECESSARILY ALLERGENS AS CAUSES OF ALLERGIC SYMPTOMS

In this category are respiratory irritants or materials that act by an undetermined mechanism to aggravate or incite symptoms in atopic and nonatopic patients. Air pollution is a prominent topic today and is relevant to the pathogenesis of several disease entities unrelated to asthma and rhinitis. Most pulmonary disease specialists would assign a role to pollutants in producing symptoms in asthmatics (atopic and nonatopic) and patients with rhinitis (allergic and vasomotor), but the primacy, magnitude and mechanism are still unknown. Epidemic asthma has occurred in Yokohama, Japan, and in New Orleans, Louisiana. In the former, pollution has been implicated, but in New Orleans the epidemics have not corresponded with elevated levels of known chemical and particulate pollutants.

New Orleans asthma, originally considered due to air pollution and climatic changes, now appears due to the prevalence of natural inhalant allergens. Hospital admissions for asthma correlate well with high counts of *Ambrosia* pollen and certain mold spores obtained by the use of the automatic intermittent rotoslide sampler.[37]

Sulfur dioxide (SO_2) is a product of soft coal burned for industrial use and is the substance most closely correlated with respiratory and conjunctival symptoms. SO_2 does not come from automobile exhaust. Incompletely oxidized hydrocarbons from factories and vehicular exhaust make up the "smoke" visible in any highly populated or industrial area. These, as well as ozone and nitrates, products of photochemical oxidation, may impair pulmonary ventilation. Carbon monoxide impairs oxygen transport, but its concentration in ambient polluted air is probably important only in patients with marginal respiratory reserve. Traces of lead, arsenic and formaldehyde also occur in polluted air.

REFERENCES

1. Ackroyd, J. F.: Immunological Methods. Philadelphia, F. A. Davis, 1964.
2. Ancona, G.: Asma epidemico da Pediculoides ventricosus. Policlinico Sez. Med.), *30*:45, 1923.
3. Baer, H., et al.: The potency and antigen E content of commercially prepared ragweed extracts. J. Allerg., *45*:347, 1970.
4. Belin, L., et al.: Enzyme sensitization in consumers of enzyme-containing washing powder. Lancet, *2*:1153, 1970.
5. Bernstein, I. L., Villacorte, G. V., and Saffermann, R. S.: Immunologic responses of experimental animals to green algae. J. Allerg., *43*:191, 1969.
6. Bernton, H. S., and Brown, H.: Insect allergy: the allergenicity of the excrement of the cockroach. Ann. Allerg., *28*:543, 1970.
7. Berrens, L.: The allergens in house dust. *In* Kallós, P., and Waksman, B. H., (eds.): Progress in Allergy. vol. 14. Basel, S. Karger, 1970.
8. Brown, G. T.: Pollen Slide Studies. Springfield, Charles C Thomas, 1949.
9. Christensen, C. M.: The Molds and Man. An Introduction to the Fungi. ed 2. Minneapolis, University of Minnesota Press, 1961.
10. Conant, N. F., et al.: Manual of Clinical Mycology. ed 2. Philadelphia, W. B. Saunders, 1954.
11. Dekker, H.: Asthma und Milben. Munch. Med. Wshr., *75*:515, 1928.
12. Echlin, P.: Pollen. Scientific American, *218*:80, 1968.
13. Feinberg, S. M.: Mold allergy: its importance in asthma and hay fever. Wis. Med. J., *34*:254, 1935.

14. Hazen, E. L., and Reed, F. C.: Laboratory Identification of Pathogenic Fungi Simplified. ed 2. Springfield, Charles C Thomas, 1960.
15. Itkin, I. H., *et al.*: Quantitative inhalation challenge in allergic asthma. J. Allerg., *34*:97, 1963.
16. King, T. P., and Norman, P. S.: Isolation studies of allergens from ragweed pollen. Biochemistry, *1*:709, 1962.
17. King, T. P., Norman, P. S., and Connell, J. T.: Isolation and characterization of allergens from ragweed pollen: II. Biochemistry, *3*:458, 1964.
18. King, T. P., Norman, P. S., and Lichtenstein, L. M.: Isolation and characterization of allergens from ragweed pollen: IV. Biochemistry, *6*:1992, 1967.
19. Levine, B. B., and Vaz, N. M.: Effect of combinations of inbred strain, antigen and antigen dose on immune responsiveness and reagin production in the mouse. Int. Arch. Allerg., *39*:156, 1970.
20. Lichtenstein, L. M., Marsh, D. G., and Campbell, D. H.: In vitro studies of rye grass pollen antigens. J. Allerg., *44*:307, 1969.
21. Malley, A., Campbell, D. H., and Heimlich, E. M.: Isolation and immunochemical properties of a haptenic material from timothy pollen. J. Immunol., *93*:420, 1964.
22. Malley, A., and Dobson, R. L.: Isolation of allergens from timothy pollen. Fed. Proc., *25*:729, 1966.
23. Malley, A., and Perlman, F.: Timothy pollen fractions in treatment of hay fever. I. Clinical and immunological response to small and higher molecular weight fractions. J. Allerg., *45*:14, 1970.
24. Marsh, D. G., Haddad, Z. H., and Campbell, D. H.: A new method for determining the distribution of allergenic fractions in biologic materials: its application to grass pollen extracts. J. Allerg., *46*:107, 1970.
25. Miyamoto, T., Oshima, S., and Ishizaki, T.: Antigenic relation between house dust and dust mite (*Dermatophagoides farinae* Hughes, 1961) by a fractionation method. J. Allerg., *44*:282, 1969.
26. Miyamoto, T., Oshima, S., Ishizaki, T., and Sato, S.: Allergic identity between the common flour mite (*Dermatophagoides farinae* Hughes, 1961) and house dust as a causative antigen in bronchial asthma. J. Allerg., *42*:14, 1968.
27. Miyamoto, T., *et al.*: Cross-antigenicity among six species of dust mites and house dust antigens. J. Allerg., *44*:228, 1969.
28. Miyamoto, T., *et al.*: Allergic potency of different house dusts in relation to contained mites. Ann. Allerg., *28*:405, 1970.
29. Morrow, M. B., *et al.*: A summary of airborne mold surveys. Ann. Allerg., *22*:575, 1964.
30. Newmark, F. M., and Itkin, I. H.: Asthma due to pine pollen. Ann. Allerg., *25*:251, 1967.
31. Pepys, J.: Hypersensitivity Diseases of the Lungs Due to Fungi and Organic Dusts. Basel, S. Karger, 1969.

32. Pepys, J., *et al.:* Arthus (Type III) skin test reactions in man. Clinical and immunological features. *In* Rose, B., *et al.* (eds.): Allergology. Amsterdam, Excerpta Medica Foundation, 1968.

33. Pfaff, H. J., *et al.:* The Life of Yeasts. Cambridge, Mass., Harvard University Press, 1966.

34. Prince, H. E., and Morrow, M. B.: Mold fungi in the etiology of respiratory allergic diseases. XV. Selection of molds for therapy. Ann. Allerg., *12:*253, 1954.

35. Prince, H. E., Selle, W. A., and Morrow, M. B.: Molds in the etiology of asthma and hayfever. Texas State Med. J., *30:*340, 1934.

36. Prince, H. E., *et al.:* Molds and bacteria in the etiology of respiratory allergic diseases. XXI. Studies with mold extracts produced from cultures grown in modified synthetic media. Ann. Allerg., *19:*259, 1961.

37. Salvaggio, J., Seabury, J., and Schoenhardt, E. A.: New Orleans asthma. V. J. Allerg. and Clin. Immunol., *48:*96, 1971.

38. Shulman, S.: Insect allergy: biochemical and immunological analysis of allergens. *In* Kallós, P., and Waksman, B. H., (eds.): Progress in Allerg. vol. 12. Basel, S. Karger, 1968.

39. Solomon, W. R.: Aeroallergens. I. Techniques of air sampling. *In* Sheldon, J. M., Lovell, R. G., and Mathews, K. P.: A Manual of Clinical Allergy. ed 2. Philadelphia, W. B. Saunders, 1967.

40. ———: A simplified application of the Anderson sampler to the study of airborne fungus particles. J. Allerg., *45:*1, 1970.

41. Storm van Leeuwen, W., Bien, Z., and Varekamp, H.: Experimentable allergische Krankheiten. Z. Immunitot., *40:*552, 1924.

42. Storm van Leeuwen, W., and Brutel de la Riviere, J. J.: Hausstaub als Asthmaursache. Munchen Med. Wschr., *24:*990, 1929.

43. Stull, A., and Sherman, W. B.: Further studies on the allergenic activity of protein and nonprotein nitrogen fractions of ragweed pollen extract. J. Allerg., *10:*130, 1939.

44. Van der Werff, P. J.: Mould Fungi and Bronchial Asthma. Springfield, Charles C Thomas, 1958.

45. Voorhorst, R., Spieksma, F. Th. M., and Varekamp, H.: House-Dust Atopy and the House-Dust Mite (*Dermatophagoides pteronyssinus* Trouessart 1897). Leiden, Scientific Publishing Co., 1969.

46. Voorhorst, R., Spieksman-Boezeman, M. I. A., and Spieksma, F. Th. M.: Is a mite (*Dermatophagoides sp.*) the producer of the house-dust allergen? Allergie u. Asthma, *6:*329, 1964.

47. Wodehouse, R. P.: Hayfever Plants. Waltham, Mass., Chronica Botanica Co., 1945.

5

Pollen Survey

Walter W. Y. Chang, M.D.

"The physician should know his pollens"; this statement by the late Owen C. Durham,[1] a noted pioneer in the fields of aerobiology and pollen surveys, emphasizes an important aspect of clinical allergy. The allergist must know the identity of common aeroallergen-producing plants in general and those specific and peculiar to his area. By knowing the different types and the quantity of pollen produced by these plants, the physician can significantly increase his clinical knowledge and diagnostic skills. Patients with pollinosis have symptoms in relationship to their seasonal pollen exposure. The diagnosis of pollinosis in a patient is dependent on the correlation of the time of onset of symptoms with the time of pollenation of the plant. Variations in symptoms during a season or during different seasons will depend, in part, on the abundance of pollen in the air. Daily variations in pollen production and distribution will affect the patient's management. The physician should be aware of the short- and long-term factors affecting pollen concentration.

Yearly pollen surveys correlating closely with botanical field studies should be done wherever possible in an effort to document and to further clarify these factors. The equipment and methodology may be obtained from the Secretary of the Pollen and Mold Committee of the American Academy of Allergy.[8] Briefly, one needs an aeroallergen sampling device; a microscope to scan and record the aeroallergens caught on the sampler slide; reference books on botany, pollen grain characteristics and identification, and on regional flora; and lastly, reference pollen slides obtained personally or commercially. The following general pollen calendar and pollen survey is intended as a short synopsis for the physician. It is arranged by states into geographical sections of the United States including the Northeast, Southeast and the South, the Midwest and the West. The survey is not all-inclusive, although efforts have been made to bring it up to date. Various factors do affect this survey data. These include (1) wind, rain and other meteorological conditions during a particular season and year; (2) geographical and topographical considerations; (3) population growth and virgin land usage; (4) industrialization and population pollution problems and (5) lack of adequate surveys of aeroallergens in local and statewide areas. Other references of interest are included at the end of this chapter [2,3,5-11] and in the chapter on aeroallergens.

NORTHEASTERN UNITED STATES

CONNECTICUT	NEW YORK
DELAWARE	OHIO
DISTRICT OF COLUMBIA AND MARYLAND	PENNSYLVANIA
MAINE	RHODE ISLAND
MASSACHUSETTS	VERMONT
NEW HAMPSHIRE	VIRGINIA
NEW JERSEY	WEST VIRGINIA

COMMON NAME	BOTANICAL NAME	IMPORTANCE	SEASON
CONNECTICUT			
Trees			
Ash, white	Fraxinus americana	Secondary	Early May
Elm, American	Ulmus americana	High	April
Oak, white	Quercus alba	High	May
Hickory, shagbark	Hicoria ovata	Secondary	April–May
Birch, red	Betula nigra	Secondary	April
Cottonwood	Populus deltoides	Secondary	April
Grasses			
June/Kentucky blue	Poa pratensis	High	Late May–Mid July
Orchard	Dactylis glomerata	High	Same
Red top	Agrostis alba	High	Same
Timothy	Phleum pratense	High	Same
Sweet vernal	Anthoxanthum spp.	High	Same
Weeds			
Ragweeds—giant	Ambrosia trifida	High	Mid August–Mid
short	Ambrosia elatior	High	September
Cocklebur	Xanthium canadense	Secondary	Same
Lambs quarters	Chenopodium alba	Secondary	August–September
Pigweed, rough	Amaranthus retroflexus	Secondary	August–September
Plantain, English	Plantago lanceolata	Secondary	May–July

Common Name	Botanical Name	Importance	Season
	DELAWARE		

Trees

Elm, American	Ulmus americana	High	April
Oak, white	Quercus alba	High	May
Cottonwood	Populus deltoides	Secondary	April–May
Ash, white	Fraxinus americana	Secondary	May
Maple, red	Acer rubrum	Secondary	April
Sycamore	Platanus occidentalis	Secondary	April–May
Walnut, black	Juglans nigra	Secondary	Same
Birch, red	Betula nigra	Secondary	Same

Grasses

June/Kentucky blue	Poa pratensis	High	Mid May–July
Orchard	Dactylis glomerata	High	Same
Red top	Agrostis alba	High	Same
Sweet vernal	Anthoxanthum spp.	High	Same
Timothy	Lolium perenne	Secondary	Same
Rey, perennial	Phleum pratense	High	June–July
Bermuda	Cynodon dactylon	Secondary	Late spring to early frost
Fescue meadow	Festuca elatior	Secondary	Summer
Johnson	Holcus halepensis	Secondary	Summer
Velvet	Holcus lanatus	Secondary	Summer

Weeds

Ragweed, giant	Ambrosia trifida	High	Mid August–October
short	Ambrosia elatior	High	Same
Cocklebur	Xanthium canadense	Secondary	Summer
Dock, yellow	Rumex crispus	Secondary	Summer
Lambs quarters	Chenopodium alba	Secondary	Summer
Pigweed, rough	Amaranthus retroflexus	Secondary	Summer
Plantain, English	Plantago lanceolata	Secondary	Summer

	MAINE		

Trees

Elm, American	Ulmus americana	High	April
Oak, white	Quercus alba	High	May
Ash, white	Fraxinus americana	Secondary	Early May
Beech	Fagus grandifolia	Secondary	May
Birch, paper	Betula papyrifera	Secondary	April–May
Cottonwood	Populus deltoides	Secondary	April–May
Hickory, shagbark	Hicoria ovata	Secondary	May
Maple, hard	Acer saccharum	Secondary	April

COMMON NAME	BOTANICAL NAME	IMPORTANCE	SEASON

MAINE (Continued)

Grasses

June/Kentucky blue	Poa pratensis	High	May–June
Orchard	Dactylis glomerata	High	Same
Red top	Agrostis alba	High	Same
Sweet vernal	Anthoxanthum spp.	High	Same
Rye, perennial	Lolium perenne	High	Same
Timothy	Phleum pratense	High	May–July

Weeds

Same as Delaware above

MARYLAND AND DISTRICT OF COLUMBIA

Trees

Elm, American	Ulmus americana	High	March–April
Oak, white,	Quercus alba	High	April–May
Ash, white	Fraxinus americana	Secondary	Late April
Birch, red	Betula nigra	Secondary	April–May
Cottonwood	Populus deltoides	Secondary	March–April
Hickory, white	Hicoria alba	Secondary	April–May
Sycamore	Pla tanus occidentalis	Secondary	April–May
Walnut, black	Juglans nigra	Secondary	April–May

Grasses

June/Kentucky blue	Poa pratensis	High	May–July
Orchard	Dactylis glomerata	High	Same
Red top	Agrostis alba	High	Same
Sweet vernal	Anthoxanthum spp.	High	May–June
Rye, perennial	Lolium perenne	High	May–July
Timothy	Phleum pratense	High	June–July
Bermuda	Cynodon dactylon	Secondary	May–October
Fescue, meadow	Festuca elatior	Secondary	May–July
Johnson	Holcus halepensis	Secondary	May–July

Weeds

Ragweeds, giant	Ambrosia trifida	High	Mid August to
short	Ambrosia elatior	High	Mid September
Cocklebur	Xanthium canadense	Secondary	August–September
Dock, yellow	Rumex crispus	Secondary	May–July
Lambs quarters	Chenopodium alba	Secondary	August–September
Pigweed, rough	Amaranthus retroflexus	Secondary	June–August
Plantain, English	Plantago lanceolata	Secondary	May–August

Common Name	Botanical Name	Importance	Season

MASSACHUSETTS

Trees

Common Name	Botanical Name	Importance	Season
Ash, white	Fraxinus americana	High	April
Elm, American	Ulmus americana	High	April
Hickory, shagbark	Hicoria ovata	High	April
Oak, white	Quercus alba	High	May—June
Birch, red	Betula nigra	Secondary	April—May
Cottonwood	Populus deltoides	Secondary	April
Willow, black	Salix nigra	Secondary	April—May

Grasses

Common Name	Botanical Name	Importance	Season
June/Kentucky blue	Poa pratensis	High	May—July
Fescue, meadow	Festuca elatior	High	Same
Orchard	Dactylis glomerata	High	Same
Red top	Agrostis alba	High	Same
Sweet vernal	Anthoxathum spp.	High	May—July
Timothy	Phleum pratense	High	Same
Rye, perennial	Lolium perenne	Secondary	Same

Weeds

Common Name	Botanical Name	Importance	Season
Ragweeds, giant	Ambrosia trifida	High	Mid August—Late
short	Ambrosia elatior	High	September
Cocklebur	Xanthium canadense	Secondary	August—September
Dock, yellow	Rumex crispus	Secondary	Same
Lambs quarters	Chenopodium alba	Secondary	Same
Pigweed, rough	Amaranthus retroflexus	Secondary	Same
Plantain, English	Plantago lanceolata	Secondary	May—August
Marsh elder, burweed	Iva xanthifolia	Secondary	August—September

NEW HAMPSHIRE

Trees

Common Name	Botanical Name	Importance	Season
Elm, American	Ulmus americana	High	April
Oak, white	Quercus alba	High	May
Birch, paper	Betula papyrifera	Secondary	April
Cottonwood	Populus deltoides	Secondary	April
Hickory, shagbark	Hicoria ovata	Secondary	April
Maple, hard	Acer saccharum	Secondary	Spring

Grasses

Common Name	Botanical Name	Importance	Season
June/Kentucky	Poa pratensis	High	May—July
Orchard	Dactylis glomerata	High	Same
Red top	Agrostis alba	High	Same
Rye, perennial	Loluim perenne	High	Same

COMMON NAME	BOTANICAL NAME	IMPORTANCE	SEASON
	NEW HAMPSHIRE (Continued)		
Vernal, sweet	Anthoxanthum spp.	High	Same
Timothy	Phleum pratense	High	Same

Weeds

Similar to Massachusetts above including cocklebur, yellow dock, lambs quarters, rough pigweed, English plantain, giant and short ragweeds. Pollinating seasons may vary locally.

	NEW JERSEY		
Trees			
Ash, white	Fraxinus americana	High	April
Elm, American	Ulmus americana	High	March–April
Hickory, shagbark	Hicoria ovata	High	April–May
Oak, white	Quercus alba	High	May
Birch, red	Betula nigra	Secondary	April
Cottonwood	Populus deltoides	Secondary	April
Maple, hard	Acer saccharum	Secondary	March
Sycamore, eastern	Platanus occidentalis	Secondary	April–May
Walnut, black	Juglans nigra	Secondary	April–May
Grasses			
June/Kentucky blue	Poa pratensis	High	May–July
Orchard	Dactylis glomerata	High	Same
Red top	Agrostis alba	High	Same
Fescue, meadow	Festuca elatior	High	Same
Timothy	Phleum pratense	High	Same
Brome, smooth	Bromus inermis	Secondary	Same
Rye, perennial	Lolium perenne	Secondary	Same
Vernal, sweet	Anthoxanthum spp.	Secondary	Same
Velvet	Holcus lanatus	Secondary	Same
Weeds			
Ragweeds, giant	Ambrosia trifida	High	Mid August–
short	Ambrosia elatior	High	October First
Cocklebur	Xanthium spp.	Secondary	July–August
Dock, yellow	Rumex crispus	Secondary	Same
Lambs quarters	Chenopodium alba	Secondary	Same
Pigweed, rough	Amaranthus retroflexus	Secondary	Same
Plantain, English	Plantago lanceolata	Secondary	May–August
Kochia	Kochia scoparia	Secondary	July–August

Common Name	Botanical Name	Importance	Season
	NEW YORK		

Trees

Common Name	Botanical Name	Importance	Season
Elm, American	Ulmus americana	High	April
Oak, red	Quercus rubra	High	May
Birch, red	Betula nigra	High	April—May
Cottonwood	Populus deltoides	High	April—May
Maple, hard	Acer saccharum	Secondary	March—May
Ash, white	Fraxinus americana	Secondary	April—May

Grasses

Common Name	Botanical Name	Importance	Season
June/Kentucky blue	Poa pratensis	High	Mid May—July
Orchard	Dactylis glomerata	High	Same
Red top	Agrostis alba	High	Same
Timothy	Phleum pratense	High	June—July
Fescue, meadow	Festuca elatior	High	May—June

Weeds

Common Name	Botanical Name	Importance	Season
Ragweeds—giant	Ambrosia trifida	High	Mid August to
short	Ambrosia elatior	High	Mid September
Cocklebur	Xanthium canadense	Secondary	August—September
Lambs quarters	Chenopodium alba	Secondary	August—September
Pigweed, rough	Amaranthus retroflexus	Secondary	August—September
Plantain, English	Plantago lanceolata	Secondary	May-August

	OHIO		

Trees

Common Name	Botanical Name	Importance	Season
Elm, American	Ulmus americana	High	April
Oak, red	Quercus rubra	High	May
Sycamore, Eastern	Platanus occidentalis	High	April
Elder, box	Acer negundo	Secondary	April
Cottonwood	Populus deltoides	Secondary	May
Hickory, shagbark	Hicoria ovata	Secondary	April
Birch, red	Betula nigra	Secondary	April—May
Maple, sugar	Acer saccharum	Secondary	April—May

Grasses

Common Name	Botanical Name	Importance	Season
June/Kentucky	Poa pratensis	High	Mid May—Mid July
Fescue, meadow	Festuca elatior	High	Same
Orchard	Dactylis glomerata	High	Same
Red top	Agrostis alba	High	Same
Timothy	Phleum pratense	High	Same
Sweet vernal	Anthoxanthum spp.	Secondary	Same

Common Name	Botanical Name	Importance	Season
		OHIO (Continued)	

Weeds

Common Name	Botanical Name	Importance	Season
Ragweeds—giant	Ambrosia trifida	High	Early August—Mid
short	Ambrosia elatior	High	September
Kochia	Kochia scoparia	High	August
Cocklebur	Xanthium commune	Secondary	August
Lambs quarters	Chenopodium alba	Secondary	July—August
Pigweed, rough	Amaranthus retroflexus	Secondary	August
Plantain, English	Plantago lanceolata	Secondary	June—August
Thistle, Russian	Salsola pestifer	Local	July—August

PENNSYLVANIA

Trees

Common Name	Botanical Name	Importance	Season
Elm, American	Ulmus americana	High	March—April
Oak, red	Quercus rubra	High	April—May
Sycamore, eastern	Platanus occidentalis	High	April—May
Birch, red	Betula nigra	High	April—May
Maple, hard	Acer saccharum	Secondary	March—April
Cottonwood	Populus deltoides	Secondary	April—May
Ash, white	Fraxinus americana	Secondary	April—May

Grasses

Common Name	Botanical Name	Importance	Season
June/Kentucky blue	Poa pratensis	High	Mid May—Mid July
Orchard	Dactylis glomerata	High	Same
Canadian blue	Poa compressa	High	Same
Red top	Agrostis spp.	High	Same
Vernal, sweet	Anthoxanthum spp.	High	Same
Timothy	Phleum pratense	High	Same

Weeds

Common Name	Botanical Name	Importance	Season
Ragweeds, giant	Ambrosia trifida	High	Mid August—October
short	Ambrosia elatior	High	First
Cocklebur	Xanthium commune	Secondary	August—September
Lambs quarters	Chenopodium alba	Secondary	July—September
Pigweed, rough	Amaranthus retroflexus	Secondary	Same
Plantain, English	Plantago lanceolata	Secondary	June—September

RHODE ISLAND

Trees

Common Name	Botanical Name	Importance	Season
Elm, American	Ulmus americana	High	April
Oak, white	Quercus alba	High	May
Walnut, black	Juglans nigra	Secondary	May

Common Name	Botanical Name	Importance	Season

RHODE ISLAND (Continued)

Common Name	Botanical Name	Importance	Season
Cottonwood	Populus deltoides	Secondary	April
Maple, hard	Acer saccharum	Secondary	April
Birch, red	Betula nigra	Secondary	April–May

Grasses

June/Kentucky blue	Poa pratensis	High	Mid May–Mid July
Orchard	Dactylis glomerata	High	Same
Red top	Agrostis alba	High	Same
Vernal, sweet	Anthoxanthum spp.	High	Same
Timothy	Phleum pratense	High	Same

Weeds

Ragweeds—giant	Ambrosia trifida	High	Mid August–Mid
short	Ambrosia elatior	High	September
Cocklebur	Xanthium commune	High	July–September
Dock, yellow	Rumex crispus	High	May–July
Lambs quarters	Chenopodium alba	High	June–September
Pigweed, rough	Ameranthus retroflexus	Secondary	July–August
Plantain, English	Plantago lanceolata	Secondary	May–June

VERMONT

Trees

Elm, American	Ulmus americana	High	April
Oak, white	Quercus alba	High	May
Walnut, black	Juglans nigra	Local	April–May
Maple, hard	Acer saccharum	Secondary	April

Grasses

June/Kentucky blue	Poa pratensis	High	May–July
Orchard	Dactylis glomerata	High	Same
Red top	Agrostis alba	High	Same
Rye, perennial	Lolium perenne	High	Same
Vernal, sweet	Anthoxanthum spp.	High	Same
Timothy	Phleum pratense	High	Same

Weeds

Ragweeds—giant	Ambrosia trifida	High	Mid August to
short	Ambrosia elatior	High	Mid September
Cocklebur	Xanthium commune	Secondary	July–August
Lambs quarters	Chenopodium alba	Secondary	Same
Pigweed, rough	Amaranthus retroflexus	Secondary	Same
Plantain, English	Plantago lanceolata	Secondary	June–August

Common Name	Botanical Name	Importance	Season

VIRGINIA

Trees

Elm, American	Ulmus americana	High	February–April
Oak, Virginia live	Quercus virginiana	High	April–May
Hickory, white	Hicoria alba	High	April–May
Maple, red	Acer rubrum	High	February–April
Ash, white	Fraxinus americana	Secondary	Same
Sycamore, eastern	Platanus occidentalis	Secondary	April–May

Grasses

Bermuda	Cynodon dactylon	High	May–July
June/Kentucky blue	Poa pratensis	High	Same
Johnson	Holcus halepensis	High	Same
Orchard	Dactylis glomerata	High	May–July
Red top	Agrostis alba	High	Same
Rye, Italian	Lolium multiflorum	High	Same
Vernal, sweet	Anthoxanthum spp.	High	Same
Timothy	Phleum pratense	High	Same
Velvet	Holcus lanatus	Secondary	Same

Weeds

Ragweeds—giant	Ambrosia trifida	High	Early August–
short	Ambrosia elatior	High	Early October
Cocklebur	Xanthium commune	Secondary	August–October
Lambs quarters	Chenopodium alba	Secondary	August–October
Pigweed, rough	Amaranthus retroflexus	Secondary	August–October
Plantain, English	Plantago lanceolata	Secondary	June–August

WEST VIRGINIA

Trees

Elm, American	Ulmus americana	High	April
Oak, red	Quercus rubra	High	May
Sycamore, eastern	Platanus occidentalis	High	April
Walnut, black	Juglans nigra	High	April–May
Ash, white	Fraxinus americana	Secondary	April
Birch, red	Betula nigra	Secondary	April
Cottonwood	Populus deltoides	Secondary	April

Grasses

Bermuda	Cynodon dactylon	Secondary	May–July
June/Kentucky blue	Poa pratensis	High	Same
Johnson	Holcus halepensis	High	Same

Common Name	Botanical Name	Importance	Season

WEST VIRGINIA (Continued)

Common Name	Botanical Name	Importance	Season
Orchard	Dactylis glomerata	High	Same
Red top	Agrostis alba	High	Same
Timothy	Phleum pratense	High	Same

Weeds

Common Name	Botanical Name	Importance	Season
Ragweeds—giant	Ambrosia trifida	High	Mid August—October
short	Ambrosia elatior	High	First
Plantain, English	Plantago lanceolata	High	May—July
Cocklebur	Xanthium commune	Secondary	July—August
Lambs quarters	Chenopodium alba	Secondary	July—September
Pigweed, rough	Amaranthus retroflexus	Secondary	Same

SOUTHEASTERN AND SOUTHERN UNITED STATES

Alabama	**North Carolina**
Arkansas	**Oklahoma**
Florida	**South Carolina**
Georgia	**Tennessee**
Louisiana	**Texas**
Mississippi	

ALABAMA

Trees

Common Name	Botanical Name	Importance	Season
Pecan	Hicoria pecan	High	April—May
Elm, American	Ulmus americana	High	February—March
Oak, white	Quercus alba	High	April
Walnut, black	Juglans nigra	High	April
Ash, white	Fraxinus americana	Secondary	March
Birch, red	Betula nigra	Secondary	April
Cedar, red	Juniperus virginiana	Secondary	January—February

Grasses

Common Name	Botanical Name	Importance	Season
Bermuda	Cynodon dactylon	High	March—November
June/Kentucky blue	Poa pratensis	High	Same
Blue, annual	Poa annua	High	April—Frost
Johnson	Holcus halepensis	High	April—September
Orchard	Dactylis glomerata	High	April—September
Red top	Agrostis alba	High	Same
Timothy	Phleum pratense	High	May—September

Weeds

Common Name	Botanical Name	Importance	Season
Ragweeds—short	Ambrosia elatior	High	Mid August—Late
giant	Ambrosia trifida	High	October

Common Name	Botanical Name	Importance	Season
ALABAMA (Continued)			
Dock, yellow	Rumex crispus	Secondary	April–July
Lambs quarters	Chenopodium alba	Secondary	June–August
Pigweed, rough	Amaranthus retroflexus	Secondary	June–August
Plantain, English	Plantago lanceolata	Secondary	May–July
ARKANSAS			
Trees			
Elm, American	Ulmus americana	High	February–March
Oak, red	Quercus rubra	High	March–May
Pecan	Hicoria pecan	High	April–May
Cottonwood	Populus deltoides	Secondary	March–April
Hickory, white	Hicoria alba	Secondary	April–May
Walnut, black	Quercus nigra	Secondary	April–May
Grasses			
Bermuda	Cynodon dactylon	High	May–November
June/Kentucky blue	Poa pratensis	High	March–June
Johnson	Holcus halepensis	High	May–November
Orchard	Dactylis glomerata	High	March–June
Red top	Agrostis alba	High	Same
Timothy	Phleum pratence	High	Same
Weeds			
Ragweeds–giant	Ambrosia trifida	High	Mid August–Mid
short	Ambrosia elatior	High	October
southern	Ambrosia bidentata	Secondary	Same
western	Ambrosia psilostachya	Secondary	Same
Marshelder, burweed	Iva xanthifolia	Secondary	Same
Kochia	Kochia scoparia	Secondary	Summer
Lambs quarters	Cheopodium alba	Secondary	June–September
Pigweed, rough	Amaranthus retroflexus	Secondary	Same
Thistle, Russian	Salsola pestifer	Secondary	Same
Western Water Hemp	Acnida tamarascina	Secondary	Same
FLORIDA			
Trees			
Oak, white live	Quercus alba, virginiana	High	February–April

COMMON NAME	BOTANICAL NAME	IMPORTANCE	SEASON
	FLORIDA (Continued)		
Pecan (Northern Fla)	Hicoria pecan	High	December–April
Pine, Australian (South)	Casuarina spp.	Local	February–April
Grasses			
Bermuda	Cynodon dactylon	High	April–October
Johnson	Holcus halepensis	High	Same
June/Kentucky blue	Poa pratensis	Secondary	Same
Timothy	Phleum pratense	Secondary	Same
St. Augustine	?	Local	Same
Natal	?	Local	Same
Weeds			
Ragweeds–short	Ambrosia elatior	High	July–October
giant North)	Ambrosia trifida	High	Same
Pigweed, spiny	Amaranthus spinosa	Secondary	May–August
Dock, yellow	Rumex crispus	Secondary	May–September
Lambs quarters	Chenopodium alba	Secondary	Same
	GEORGIA		
Trees			
Elm, American	Ulmus americana	High	February–March
Oak, Virginia Live	Quercus virginiana	High	March–May
Birch, red	Betula nigra	Secondary	March–April
Pine	Pinus spp.	Local	March–May
Pecan	Hicoria pecan	Local	April–May
Grasses			
Bermuda	Cynodon dactylon	High	May–October
Johnson	Holcus halepensis	High	Same
June/Kentucky blue	Poa pratensis	High	March–July
Orchard	Dactylis glomerata	Secondary	Same
Red top	Agrostis alba	Secondary	Same
Rye, Italian	Lolium multiflorum	Secondary	Same
Weeds			
Ragweeds–giant	Ambrosia trifida	High	August–October
short	Ambrosia elatior	High	Same
Cocklebur	Xanthium canadense	Secondary	Same
Pigweed, spiny	Amaranthus spinosa	Secondary	March–September
Dock, yellow	Rumex crispus	Secondary	April–July
Kochia	Kochia scoparia	Local	Summer
Plantain, English	Plantago lanceolata	Local	May–October

COMMON NAME	BOTANICAL NAME	IMPORTANCE	SEASON

LOUISIANA

Trees

Elm, American	Ulmus americana	High	February—April
Oak, Virginia Live	Quercus virginiana	High	Same
Pecan	Hicoria pecan	High	March—May
Sycamore	Platanus occidentalis	Secondary	February—May

Grasses

Bermuda	Cynodon dactylon	High	April—December
Johnson	Holcus halepensis	High	Same
June/Kentucky	Poa pratensis	Secondary	Same
Rye, Italian	Lolium mutiflorum	Secondary	Same
Orchard	Dactylis glomerata	Secondary	Same

Weeds

Ragweeds—giant	Ambrosia trifida	High	August—November
short	Ambrosia elatior	High	Same
Marsh elder	Iva ciliata	High	Same
Lambs quarters	Chenopodium alba	Secondary	Summer
Pigweed rough	Amaranthus spinosa	Secondary	Summer
Kochia	Kochia scoparia	Secondary	Summer
Thistle, Russian	Salsola pestifer	Secondary	Summer

MISSISSIPPI

Trees

Elm, American	Ulmus americana	High	March—April
Oak, Virginia Live	Quercus virginiana	High	April—May
Pecan	Hicoria pecan	High	March—April
Ash, white	Fraxinus americana	Secondary	March
Hickory, white	Hicoria alba	Secondary	April—May

Grasses

Bermuda	Cynodon dactylon	High	April—October
Johnson	Holcus halepensis	High	Same
June/Kentucky blue	Poa pratensis	Secondary	Same
Orchard	Dactylis glomerata	Secondary	Same
Rye, Italian	Lolium multiflorum	Secondary	Same

Weeds

Ragweeds—giant	Ambrosia trifida	High	August—October
short	Ambrosia elatior	High	Same
Marsh elder	Iva ciliata	High	Same
Lambs quarters	Chenopodium alba	Local	Summer
Pigweed, rough	Amaranthus retroflexus	Local	Summer

COMMON NAME	BOTANICAL NAME	IMPORTANCE	SEASON

NORTH CAROLINA

Trees

Elm, American	Ulmus americana	High	February–April
Oak, Virginia Live	Quercus virginiana	High	March–May
Pecan	Hicoria pecan	Secondary	April–May
Hickory, white	Hicoria alba	Secondary	April
Ash, white	Fraxinus americana	Secondary	April
Maple, red	Acer rubtum	Secondary	February–May
Sycamore, Eastern	Platanus occidentalis	Secondary	April

Grasses

June/Kentucky blue	Poa pratensis	High	March–September
Timothy	Phleum pratense	High	Same
Orchard	Dactylis glomerata	High	Same
Red top	Agrostis alba	High	Same
Bermuda	Cynodon dactylon	High	Same
Johnson	Holcus halepensis	High	Same

Weeds

Ragweeds–giant	Ambrosia trifida	High	Mid July–
short	Ambrosia elatior	High	Early October
Cocklebur	Xanthium canadense	Secondary	July–August
Lambs quarters	Chenopodium alba	Secondary	Same
Pigweed, rough	Amaranthus retroflexus	Secondary	Same
Plantain, English	Plantago lanceolata	Secondary	Same

OKLAHOMA

Trees

Elm, American	Ulmus americana	High	March–April
Oak, post	Quercus stellata	High	May
Walnut, black	Juglans nigra	High	April
Cottonwood	Populus deltoides	Secondary	April
Hickory, shagbark	Hicoria ovata	Secondary	April
Ash, green	Fraxinus pennsylvanica	Secondary	March–April
Sycamore, eastern	Platanus occidentalis	Secondary	April

Grasses

Bermuda	Cynodon dactylon	High	May–August
Johnson	Holcus halepensis	High	Same
June/Kentucky blue	Poa pratensis	High	Same
Orchard	Dactylis glomerata	Secondary	Same
Red top	Agrostis alba	Secondary	Same

Common Name	Botanical Name	Importance	Season

OKLAHOMA (Continued)

Common Name	Botanical Name	Importance	Season
Rye, Italian	Lolium multiflorum	Secondary	Same
Timothy	Phleum pratense	Secondary	Same

Weeds

Ragweeds—giant	Ambrosia trifida	High	Late August—
short	Ambrosia elatior	High	October
western	Ambrosia psilostachya	High	Same
southern	Ambrosia bidentata	High	Same
Marsh elder	Iva ciliata	High	August—September
Pigweed, rough	Amaranthus retroflexus	Secondary	June—September
Plantain, English	Plantago lanceolata	Secondary	May—August
Dock, yellow	Rumex crispus	Secondary	Same
Lambs quarters	Chenopodium alba	Secondary	June—September
Kochia	Kochia scoparia	Secondary	Same
Thistle, Russian	Salsola pestifer	Secondary	Same
Cocklebur	Xanthium canadense	Secondary	Same

SOUTH CAROLINA

Trees

Elm, American	Ulmus americana	High	April
Oak, Virginia, live	Quercus virginiana	High	May
Pecan	Hicoria pecan	High	April—May
Hickory, white	Hicoria alba	Secondary	April
Maple, red	Acer rubrum	Secondary	April
Ash, white	Fraxinus americana	Secondary	March—April
Sycamore, eastern	Platanus occidentalis	Secondary	Same

Grasses

Bermuda	Cynadon dactylon	High	May—September
Johnson	Holcus halepensis	High	Same
June/Kentucky blue	Poa pratensis	High	Same
Orchard	Dactylis glomerata	Secondary	Same
Rye, Italian	Lolium multiflorum	Secondary	Same

Weeds

Ragweeds—giant	Ambrosia trifida	High	July—October
short	Ambrosia elatior	High	Same
Cocklebur	Xanthium canadense	Secondary	Same
Marsh elder, seaside	Iva fructescens	Secondary	July—September
Lambs quarters	Chenopodium alba	Secondary	Same
Pigweed, rough	Amaranthus retroflexus	Secondary	Same
Plantain, English	Plantago, lanceolata	Secondary	Same

COMMON NAME	BOTANICAL NAME	IMPORTANCE	SEASON
		TENNESSEE	

Trees

Elm, American	Ulmus americana	High	February–April
Oak, red	Quercus rubra	High	April–May
Pecan	Hicoria pecan	High	April
Walnut, black	Juglans nigra	Secondary	April–May
Ash, white	Fraxinus americana	Secondary	March
Maple, red	Acer rubrum	Secondary	March
Sycamore, eastern	Platanus occidentalis	Secondary	April–May

Grasses

June/Kentucky blue	Poa pratensis	High	March–November
Bermuda	Cynodon dactylon	High	Same
Johnson	Holcus halepensis	High	Same
Orchard	Dactylis glomerata	Secondary	Same
Red top	Agrostis alba	Secondary	Same
Timothy	Phleum pratense	Secondary	Same

Weeds

Ragweeds–giant	Ambrosia trifida	High	Mid August–
short	Ambrosia elatior	High	Late October
Cocklebur	Xanthium canadense	Secondary	June–September
Dock, yellow	Rumex crispus	Secondary	April–July
Plantain, English	Plantago lanceolata	Secondary	May–August
Kochia	Kochia scoparia	Secondary	June–August
Lambs quarters	Chenopodium alba	Secondary	Same
Pigweed, rough	Amaranthus retroflexus	Secondary	Same

		TEXAS	

Trees

Elm, American	Ulmus americana	High	February–April
Cedar, mountain	Juniperus sabinoides	Local	December–February
Oak, live	Quercus virginiana	Secondary	March–April
Pecan	Hicoria pecan	Secondary	April
Ash, white	Fraxinus americana	Secondary	February–April
Cottonwood	Populus deltoides	Secondary	March
Elder, box	Acer negundo	Secondary	March
Willow, black	Salix nigra	Secondary	March
Mesquite	Prosopsis spp.	Local	February–April

Grasses

Bermuda	Cynodon dactylon	High	February–August
Johnson	Holcus halepensis	High	Same
June/Kentucky	Poa pratensis	High	Same

Common Name	Botanical Name	Importance	Season

TEXAS (Continued)

Weeds

Ragweeds—giant	Ambrosia trifida	High	End August—
short	Ambrosia elatior	High	Early October
southern	Ambrosia bidentata	High	Same
western	Ambrosia psilostachya	Secondary	Same
March elder	Iva ciliata	Secondary	July—October
Careless weeds	Amaranthus paleri	Secondary	June—October
Kochia	Kochia scoparia	Secondary	Same
Pigweed, rough	Amaranthus retroflexus	Secondary	Same
Thistle, Russian	Salsola pestifer	Secondary	Same
Lambs quarters	Chenopodium alba	Secondary	Same
Western Water Hemp	Acnida tamarascina	Secondary	Same
Sagebrush, prairie	Artemesia ludoviciana	Secondary	Same

MIDWESTERN UNITED STATES

Illinois   Minnesota
Indiana   Missouri
Iowa   Nebraska
Kansas   North Dakota
Kentucky   South Dakota
Michigan   Wisconsin

ILLINOIS

Trees

Elm, American	Ulmus americana	High	February—April
Oak, white	Quercus alba	High	May
Ash, white	Fraxinus americana	Secondary	April—May
Maple, hard	Acer saccharum	Secondary	March—April
Walnut, black	Juglans nigra	Secondary	March—April
Cottonwood	Populus deltoides	Secondary	April—May

Grasses

June/Kentucky blue	Poa pratensis	High	Mid May—Mid July
Orchard	Dactylis glomerata	High	Same
Red top	Agrostis alba	High	Same
Timothy	Phleum pratense	High	Same

Common Name	Botanical Name	Importance	Season

ILLINOIS (Continued)

Weeds

Common Name	Botanical Name	Importance	Season
Ragweeds—giant	Ambrosia trifida	High	Early August—
short	Ambrosia elatior	High	Late September
Marsh elder, burweed	Iva xanthifolia	Local	Same
Ragweed, southern	Ambrosia bidentata	Local	Same
Ragweed, western	Ambrosia psilostachya	Local	Same
Cocklebur	Xanthium canadense	Local	Same
Kochia	Kochia scoparia	Secondary	July—October
Thistle, Russian	Salsola pestifer	Secondary	Same
Lambs quarters	Chenopodium alba	Secondary	Same
Pigweed, rough	Amaranthus retroflexus	Secondary	Same
Plantain, English	Plantago lanceolata	Secondary	June—August

INDIANA

Trees

Common Name	Botanical Name	Importance	Season
Elm, American	Ulmus americana	High	February—March
Oak, red	Quercus rubra	High	April—May
Sycamore, eastern	Platanus occidentalis	Secondary	April
Ash, white	Fraxinus americana	Secondary	April—May
Cottonwood	Populus deltoides	Secondary	April—May
Walnut, black	Juglans nigra	Secondary	March—April
Hickory, shagbark	Hicoria ovata	Secondary	May—June

Grasses

Common Name	Botanical Name	Importance	Season
June/Kentucky blue	Poa pratensis	High	May—June
Orchard	Dactylis glomerata	High	Same
Red top	Agrostis alba	High	Same
Timothy	Phleum pratense	High	Same

Weeds

Common Name	Botanical Name	Importance	Season
Ragweeds, short	Ambrosia elatior	High	August—September
giant	Ambrosia trifida	High	Same
Marsh elder, burweed	Iva xanthifolia	Local	Same
Cocklebur	Xanthium canadense	Secondary	Same
Thistle, Russian	Salsola pestifer	Local	Same
Kochia	Kochia scoparia	Local	Same
Sagebrush, annual	Artemisia annua	Local	Same
Lambs quarters	Chenopodium alba	Secondary	Same
Pigweed, rough	Amaranthus retroflexus	Secondary	Same

Common Name	Botanical Name	Importance	Season

IOWA

Trees

Elm, American	Ulmus americana	High	March–April
Oak, red	Quercus rubra	High	April–May
Walnut, black	Juglans nigra	High	March–April
Box elder	Acer negundo	Secondary	March–April
Cottonwood	Populus deltoides	Secondary	Same
Sycamore, eastern	Platanus occidentalis	Secondary	April–May

Grasses

June/Kentucky blue	Poa pratensis	High	May–June
Orchard	Dactylis glomerata	High	Same
Red top	Agrostis alba	High	Same
Timothy	Phleum pratense	High	Same
Brome, smooth	Bromus inermis	Secondary	Same

Weeds

Ragweeds—short	Ambrosia elatior	High	Mid August–Late
giant	Ambrosia trifida	High	September
Marsh elder, burweed	Iva xanthifolia	High	Same
Ragweed, western	Ambrosia psilostochya	Local	Same
Kochia	Kochia scoparia	Secondary	July–August
Thistle, Russian	Salsola pestifer	Secondary	Same
Hemp, wesetrn water	Acnida tamarascina	Secondary	Same
Hemp	Cannabis sativa	Local	July–September
Plantain, English	Plantago lanceolata	Secondary	June–July
Cocklebur	Xanthium commune	Secondary	July–August
Lambs quarters	Chenopodium alba	Local	Same
Pigweed, rough	Amaranthus retroflexus	Local	Same

KANSAS

Trees

Elm, American	Ulmus americana	High	March
Oak, post	Quercus stellata	High	May
Cottonwood	Populus deltoides	Secondary	March–April
Elder, box	Acer segundo	Secondary	Same
Ash, white	Fraximus americana	Secondary	April–May
Walnut, black	Juglans nigra	Secondary	Same
Hickory, shagbark	Hicoria ovata	Secondary	Same

Grasses

June/Kentucky blue	Poa pratensis	High	May–July
Orchard	Dactylis glomerata	High	Same
Red top	Agrostis alba	High	Same

Common Name	Botanical Name	Importance	Season
KANSAS (Continued)			

Timothy	Phleum pratense	High	Same
Bermuda	Cynodon dactylon	Secondary	Same
Johnson	Holcus halepensis	Secondary	Same
Fescue meadow	Festuca elatior	Secondary	Same

Weeds

Ragweeds—giant	Ambrosia trifida	High	Mid August—
short	Ambrosia elatior	High	Mid October
western	Ambrosia psiloatachya	High	Same
southern	Ambrosia bidentata	Secondary	Same
Thistle, Russian	Salsola pestifer	High	July—October
Kochia	Kochia scoparia	High	Same
Marsh elder, burweed	Iva xanthifolia	Secondary	August—October
Lambs quarters	Chenopodium alba	Secondary	July—September
	Amaranthus	Secondary	Same
Pigweed, rough	retroflexus		
Western water hemp	Acnida tamarascina	Secondary	Same

| KENTUCKY | | | |

Trees

Elm, American	Ulmus americana	High	February—March
Oak, red	Quercus rubra	High	April—May
Sycamore, eastern	Platanus occidentalis	Secondary	April—May
Walnut, black	Juglans nigra	Secondary	April—May
Hickory, white	Hicoria alba	Secondary	April—May
Maple, hard	Acer sacchaum	Secondary	March—April

Grasses

June/Kentucky	Poa pratensis	High	May—July
Timothy	Phleum pratense	High	Same
Bermuda	Cynodon dactylon	Secondary	May—August
Red top	Agrostis alba	Secondary	Same
Orchard	Holcus halepensis	Secondary	Same
Fescue, meadow	Festuca elatior	Secondary	Same

Weeds

Ragweeds, short	Ambrosia elatior	High	Mid August—Early
giant	Ambrosia trifida	High	October
Cocklebur	Xanthium canadense	Secondary	Same
Marsh elder, burweed	Iva xanthifolia	Secondary	Same
Lambs quarters	Ambrosia bidentata	Local	Mid August—Early October
Amaranth, spiny	Rumex crispus	Local	July—September
Plantain, English	Chenopodium alba	Secondary	July—September

Common Name	Botanical Name	Importance	Season
	KENTUCKY (Continued)		
Kochia	Amaranthus spinosus	Secondary	Same
Ragweed, southern	Plantago lanceolata	Secondary	June–July
Dock, yellow	Kochia scoparia	Local	July–September

MICHIGAN

Trees

Elm, American	Ulmus americana	High	April
Oak, red	Quercus rubra	High	May
Walnut, black	Juglans nigra	Secondary	May–June
Hickory, shagbark	Hicoria ovata	Secondary	Same
Maple, red	Acer saccharum	Secondary	April
Cottonwood	Populus deltoides	Secondary	Same
Sycamore, eastern	Platanus occidentalis	Secondary	Same

Grasses

June/Kentucky blue	Poa pratensis	High	May–July
Timothy	Phleum pratense	High	Same
Orchard	Dactylis glomerata	High	Same
Red top	Agrostis alba	High	Same

Weeds

Ragweeds—short	Ambrosia elatior	High	Mid August–
giant	Ambrosia trifida	High	Mid September
Dock, yellow	Rumex spp.	Secondary	May–July
Lambs quarters	Chenopodium alba	Secondary	July–September
Pigweed, rough	Amaranthus retroflexus	Secondary	Same
Plantain, English	Plantago lanceolata	Secondary	June–August
Cocklebur	Xanthium canadense	Secondary	July–August

MINNESOTA

Trees

Elm, American	Ulmus americana	High	April–May
Oak, red	Quercus rubra	High	May
Birch, paper	Betula papyrifera	Secondary	April–May
Ash, white	Fraxinus americana	Secondary	Same
Hickory, shagbark	Hicoria ovata	Secondary	May
Maple, hard	Acer saccharum	Secondary	March–April
Walnut, black	Juglans nigra	Secondary	May

Grasses

June/Kentucky blue	Poa pratensis	High	May–August
Orchard	Dactylis glomerata	High	Same

Common Name	Botanical Name	Importance	Season

MINNESOTA (Continued)

Red top	Agrostis alba	High	Same
Timothy	Phleum pratense	High	Same

Weeds

Ragweeds—short	Ambrosia elatior	High	August—September
giant	Ambrosia trifida	High	Same
Marsh elder, burweed	Iva xanthifolia	High	Same
Cocklebur	Xanthium canadense	Secondary	Same
Lambs quarters	Chenopodium alba	Secondary	July—September
Pigweed, rough	Amaranthus retroflexus	Secondary	Same
Plantain, English	Plantago lanceolata	Secondary	June—July
Hemp, western water	Acnida tamarascina	Secondary	July—August
Sagebrush	Artemisia spp.	Secondary	July—September

MISSOURI

Trees

Elm, American	Ulmus americana	High	March
Oak, red	Quercus rubra	High	May
Sycamore, eastern	Platanus occidentalis	Secondary	April—May
Ash, white	Frraxinus americana	Secondary	April
Cottonwood	Populus deltoides	Secondary	March—April
Walnut, black	Juglans nigra	Secondary	April—May
Hickory, shagbark	Hicoria ovata	Secondary	May

Grasses

June/Kentucky blue	Poa pratensis	High	May—August
Orchard	Dactylis glomerata	High	Same
Red top	Agrostis alba	High	Same
Timothy	Phleum pratense	High	Same
Blue, Canada	Poa compressa	Secondary	Same

Weeds

Ragweeds—short	Ambrosia elatior	High	August—First of
giant	Ambrosia trifida	High	October
southern	Ambrosia bidentata	Local	Same
Hemp, western water	Acnida tamarascina	Secondary	July—August
Lambs quarters	Chenopodium alba	Secondary	July—September
Kochia	Kochia scoparia	Secondary	Same
Thistle, Russian	Salsola pestifer	Secondary	July—August
Amaranth, pigweed	Amaranthus retroflexus	Secondary	Same
Plantain, English	Plantago lanceolata	Secondary	June—July

Common Name	Botanical Name	Importance	Season

NEBRASKA

Trees

Elm, American	Ulmus americana	High	March
Oak, burr	Quercus macrocarpa	High	May
Hickory, shagbark	Hicoria spp.	Secondary	April–May
Cottonwood	Populus deltoides	Secondary	April
Walnut, black	Juglans nigra	Secondary	April–May
Ash, white	Fraxinus americana	Secondary	Same
Box elder	Acer segundo	Secondary	Same

Grasses

June/Kentucky blue	Poa pratensis	High	May–July
Orchard	Dactylis glomerata	High	Same
Red top	Agrostis alba	High	Same
Timothy	Phleum pratense	High	Same
Western wheat	Agropyron smithii	Secondary	Same

Weeds

Ragweeds—short	Ambrosia elatior	High	Mid August–
giant	Ambrosia trifida	High	October
western	Ambrosia psilostachya	Secondary	Same
Marsh elder, burweed	Iva xanthifolia	High	Same
Kochia	Kochia scoparia	Secondary	July–August
Thistle, Russian	Salsola pestifer	High	Same
Lambs quarters	Chenopodium alba	Secondary	Same
Pigweed, rough	Amaranthus retroflexus	Secondary	Same
Hemp, western water	Acnida tamarscina	Secondary	Same
Plantain, English	Plantago lanceolate	Secondary	June–July
Sagebrush	Artemesia spp.	Secondary	July–September

NORTH AND SOUTH DAKOTA

Trees

Elm, American	Ulmus americana	Secondary	April
Box elder	Acer negundo	Secondary	April–May
Willow, pussy	Salix discolor	Secondary	Same
Aspen	Populus tremuloides	Secondary	Same
Birch, paper	Betula papyrifera	Secondary	Same

Grasses

June/Kentucky blue	Poa pratensis	High	May–July
Timothy	Phleum pratense	Secondary	Same
Western wheat	Agropyron smithii	Secondary	Same
Brome, smooth	Bromus inermis	Secondary	Same
Crested wheat	Agropyron cristatum	Secondary	Same

COMMON NAME	BOTANICAL NAME	IMPORTANCE	SEASON

NORTH AND SOUTH DAKOTA (Continued)

Weeds

Ragweeds—short	Ambrosia elatior	High	July—September
giant	Ambrosia trifida	High	Same
Marsh elder, burweed	Iva xanthifolia	High	Same
Kochia	Kochia scoparia	High	July—August
Thistle, Russian	Salsola pestifer	High	Same
Sagebrush	Artemisia spp.	Secondary	September
Hemp, western water	Acnida tamarascina	Secondary	July—August
Lambs quarters	Chenopodium alba	Secondary	Same
Pigweed, rough	Amaranthus retroflexus	Secondary	Same
Plantain, English	Plantago lanceolata	Secondary	June—July

WISCONSIN

Trees

Oak, red	Quercus rubra	High	May
Elm, American	Ulmus americana	High	April
Birch, red	Betula nigra	Secondary	April—May
Maple, hard	Acer saccharum	Secondary	April
Cottonwood	Populus deltoides	Secondary	Same
Ash, white	Fraxinus americanus	Secondary	Same

Grasses

June/Kentucky blue	Poa pratensis	High	June—July
Orchard	Dactylis glomerata	High	Same
Red top	Agrostis alba	High	Same
Timothy	Phleum pratense	High	Same

Weeds

Ragweeds, short	Ambrosia elatior	High	Early August—
giant	Ambrosia trifida	High	Late September
Marsh elder, burweed	Iva xanthifolia	Secondary	Same
Cocklebur	Xanthium canadense	Secondary	Same
Lambs quarters	Chenopodium alba	Secondary	July—August
Pigweed, rough	Amaranthus retroflexus	Secondary	Same
Plantain, English	Plantago lanceolata	Secondary	June—July
Kochia	Kochia scoparia	Local	July—August
Thistle, Russian	Salsola pestifer	Local	July—August

WESTERN UNITED STATES

ARIZONA	UTAH
CALIFORNIA	WASHINGTON
COLORADO	WYOMING
IDAHO	ALASKA
MONTANA	HAWAII
NEVADA	PUERTO RICO
NEW MEXICO	VIRGIN ISLANDS
OREGON	

COMMON NAME	BOTANICAL NAME	IMPORTANCE	SEASON
ARIZONA			
Trees			
Cottonwood	Populus deltoides	Secondary	January–April
Olive	Olea europaea	Secondary	March–May
Juniper	Juniperus spp.	Secondary	December–April
Mesquite	Prosopis spp.	Secondary	April–June
Ash, Arizona	Fraxinus velutina	Secondary	February–April
Mulberry	Morus spp.	Local	March–April
Grasses			
Bermuda	Cynodon dactylon	High	February–November
Johnson	Holcus halepensis	Secondary	Same
Rye, perennial	Lolium perenne	Secondary	Same
June/Kentucky blue	Poa pratensis	Local	Same
Weeds			
Careless weed	Amaranthus palmeri	High	May–September
Thistle, Russian	Salsola pestifer	Secondary	May–October
Ragweeds, false	Franseria spp.	Secondary	March–May
Ragweed, slender false	Franseria tenuifolia	Secondary	August–October
western	Ambrosia psilostachya	Secondary	August–October
Sagebrush	Artemisia spp.	Secondary	April–October
Atriplex-scale	Atriplex spp.	Secondary	Same
Plantain, English	Plantago lanceolata	Secondary	Same
Pigweed, rough	Amaranthus retroflexus	Secondary	May–November
Sugarbeet	Beta vulgaris	Local	April–June
CALIFORNIA, NORTHERN			
Trees			
Elm, American	Ulmus americana	High	February–March
Oak	Quercus spp.	High	February–May
Olive	Olea europaea	High	April–June

Common Name	Botanical Name	Importance	Season
CALIFORNIA, NORTHERN (Continued)			
Walnut, black	Juglans nigra	High	Same
Cottonwood	Populus spp.	High	March–April
Birch	Betula spp.	High	February–May
Box elder	Acer negundo	Secondary	February–April
Alder	Alnus spp.	Secondary	March–June
Acacia	Acacia spp.	Secondary	January–December
Sycamore	Platanus spp.	Secondary	March–April
Grasses			
Red top	Agrostis alba	High	April–September
Oat, wild	Avena fatua	High	Same
Bermuda	Cynodon dactylon	High	Same
Bromes	Bromus spp.	High	Same
Ryes	Lolium spp.	High	Same
Fescue, meadow	Festuca elatior	Secondary	Same
Orchard	Dactylis glomerata	Secondary	Same
Timothy	Phleum pratense	Secondary	Same
Weeds			
Ragweed, false western	Franseria acanthicarpa	Secondary	June–October
Sheep sorrel	Rumex acetosella	Secondary	March–September
Pigweed, rough	Amaranthus retroflexus	High	May–October
Plantain, English	Plantago lanceolata	Secondary	April–August
Sagebrush	Artemisia spp.	High	July–October
Atriplex-scales	Atriplex spp.	Secondary	June–September
Lambs quarters	Ambrosia psilostachya	Local	July–November
Cocklebur	Chenopodium alba	Secondary	April–September
Ragweed, western	Xanthium canadense	Secondary	July–November
CALIFORNIA, SOUTHERN			
Trees			
Oaks	Quercus spp.	High	March–May
Walnut, black	Juglans nigra	High	Same
Cottonwood, fremont	Populus fremontii	High	February–March
Sycamore, western	Platanus racemosa	High	March–May
Maple, big leaf	Acer macrophyllum	Secondary	March–April
Cypress, Arizona	Cupressus arizonica	Secondary	February–March
Olive	Olea europaea	Secondary	April–June
Mesquite	Prosopis spp.	Local	Spring–summer
Grasses			
Bermuda	Cynodon dactylon	High	April–October

Common Name	Botanical Name	Importance	Season
CALIFORNIA, SOUTHERN (Continued)			
Oats, wild	Avena fatua	High	April—June
Brome	Bromus spp.	Secondary	Same
June/Kentucky	Poa pratensis	Secondary	Same
Ryes	Lolium spp.	Secondary	April—October
Johnson	Holcus halepensis	Secondary	Same
Salt	Distichlis spicata	Secondary	April—September
Weeds			
Ragweeds—western	Ambrosia psilostachya	Secondary	July—September
false	Franseria acanthicarpa	High	Same
Sagebrushes	Artemesia spp.	High	July—October
Atriplex-scales	Atriplex spp.	Secondary	June—September
Lambs quarters	Chenopodium alba	Secondary	June—October
Thistle, Russian	Salsola pestifer	Secondary	June—September
Cocklebur	Xanthium canadense	Secondary	June—October

COLORADO			
Trees			
Cottonwood	Populus deltoides	High	April—May
Elm	Ulmus americana	High	February—May
Oak, scrub	Quercus gambellii	Secondary	May—June
Maple	Acer saccharum	Secondary	March—May
Cedars	Juniperus spp.	Secondary	Same
Grasses			
June/Kentucky	Poa pratensis	High	May—September
Timothy	Phleum pratense	Secondary	Same
Red top	Agrostis alba	Secondary	Same
Orchard	Dactylis glomerata	Secondary	Same
Fescue, meadow	Festuca elatior	Secondary	Same
Weeds			
Kochia	Kochia scoparia	High	July—September
Thistle, Russian	Salsola pestifer	High	Same
Lambs quarters	Chenopodium alba	Secondary	Same
Pigweed, rough	Amaranthus retroflexus	Secondary	Same
Ragweeds—giant	Ambrosia trifida	Secondary	August—September
short	Ambrosia elatior	Secondary	Same
western	Ambrosia psilostachya	Local	Same
Marsh elder, burweed	Iva xanthifolia	Secondary	Same
Sagebrushes	Artemisia spp.	Secondary	Same
Plantain, English	Plantago lanceolata	Secondary	June—August

COMMON NAME	BOTANICAL NAME	IMPORTANCE	SEASON

IDAHO

Trees

Alder	Alnus tenuifolia	Secondary	March–April
Cottonwood, black	Populus trichocarpa	Secondary	April–May
Aspen	Populus tremuloides	Secondary	April
Birch, spring	Betula spp.	Secondary	May

Grasses

June/Kentucky blue	Poa pratensis	High	May–September
Red top	Agrostis alba	High	Same
Timothy	Phleum pratense	Secondary	Same
Brome, smooth	Bromus inermis	Secondary	Same
Orchard	Dactylis glomerata	Secondary	Same

Weeds

Thistle, Russian	Salsola pestifer	High	June–September
Marsh elder, burweed	Iva xanthifolia	Secondary	August–September
Sorrel, sheep	Rumex acetosella	Same	May–October
Sagebrush	Artemisia spp.	Same	July–August
Ragweed, false western	Franseria acanthicarpa	Same	August–September
Plantain, English	Plantago lanceolata	Same	June–September
Atriplex-scale	Atriplex spp.	Same	August–September
Pigweed, rough	Amaranthus retroflexus	Same	July–September
Lambs quarters	Chenopodium alba	Same	Same

MONTANA

Trees

Cottonwood	Populus trichocarpa	Secondary	April–May
Aspen	Populus tremuloides	Secondary	May
Box elder	Acer negundo	Local	April
Willow	Salix lasiandracaudata	Secondary	March–April
Pines	Pinus	Local	June

Grasses

June/Kentucky blue	Poa pratensis	High	May–June
Red top	Agrostis alba	High	Same
Brome, smooth	Bromus inernis	Secondary	Same
Timothy	Phleum pratense	Secondary	Same
Orchard	Dactylis glomerata	Secondary	Same

Weeds

Thistle, Russian	Salsola pestifer	High	July–September

Common Name	Botanical Name	Importance	Season
MONTANA (Continued)			
Ragweeds—short	Ambrosia elatior	Secondary	August—September
giant	Ambrosia trifida	Secondary	Same
western	Ambrosia psilostachya	Local	Same
Marsh elder, burweed	Iva xanthifolia	Secondary	Same
Lambs quarters	Chenopodium alba	Secondary	July—September
Atriplex-scales	Atriplex spp.	Secondary	June
Sagebrushes	Artemisia spp.	Secondary	September—October
Pigweed, rough	Amaranthus retroflexus	Secondary	July—August
Sorrel, sheep	Kochia scoparia	Local	July—September
Kochia	Rumex acetosella	Secondary	May—October

NEVADA

Trees

Elms	Ulmus spp.	Secondary	February—April
Cottonwood	Populus spp.	Secondary	Same
Willow, narrow leaf	Salix exigua	Secondary	April—May
Sycamore, maple leaf	Platanus acerifolia	Secondary	April
Juniper, Utah	Juniperus utahensis	Local	March—May
Mesquite	Prosopis spp.	Local	April—July
Box elder	Acer negundo	Local	April—May
Ashes	Fraxinus spp.	Secondary	February—May

Grasses

Bermuda	Cynodon dactylon	High	March—October
June/Kentucky	Poa pratensis	High	May—July
Salt	Distichlis stricata	High	May—July
Timothy	Phleum pratense	Secondary	Same
Ryes	Lolium spp.	Secondary	Same
Quack	Agropyron repens	Local	Same
Redtop	Agrostis alba	Local	Same
Orchard	Dactylis glomerata	Local	Same

Weeds

Thistle, Russian	Salsola pestifer	High	July—September
Sagebrushes	Artemisia spp.	High	August—September
Ragweeds—false	Franseria acanthacarpa	Secondary	Same
Atriplex—scales	Atriplex spp.	Secondary	July—September
Lambs quarters	Chenopodium alba	Secondary	Same
Pigweed, rough	Amaranthus retroflexus	Secondary	Same

Common Name	Botanical Name	Importance	Season
		NEVADA (Continued)	
Plantain, English	Plantago lanceolata	Secondary	April—August
Kochia	Kochia scoparia	Secondary	July—September
Dock	Rumex crispus	Local	May—July

NEW MEXICO

Trees

Juniper, cherrystone	Juniperus monosperma	Secondary	March
Cottonwood	Populus deltoides	Secondary	April
Elms	Ulmus spp.	Secondary	February—March
Oak, scrub	Quercus gambellii	Secondary	May
Box elder	Acer negundo	Secondary	April—May

Grasses

Bermuda	Cynodon dactylon	High	April—August
Johnson	Holcus halepensis	Secondary	Same
June/Kentucky blue	Poa pratensis	Secondary	Same
Fescue, meadow	Festuca elatior	Secondary	Same
Rye, perennial	Lolium perenne	Secondary	Same

Weeds

Thistle, Russian	Salsola pestifer	High	June—September
Kochia	Kochia scoparia	High	Same
Careless weed	Amaranthus palmeri	Secondary	Same
Pigweed, rough	Amaranthus retroflexus	Secondary	Same
Atriplex—scales	Atriplex spp.	Secondary	Same
Ragweed, false	Franseria acanthacarpa	Secondary	August—October
Plantain, English	Artemisia spp.	Local	Same
Sagebrushes	Plantago lanceolata	Secondary	June—September

OREGON

Trees

Alder	Alnus spp.	High	March—April
Birches	Betula spp.	High	Same
Walnut, English	Juglans regia	High	May—June
Willows	Salix spp.	Local	February—March
Poplars	Populus spp.	Secondary	March—April
Box elder	Acer negundo	Secondary	Same

Grasses

June/Kentucky blue	Poa pratensis	High	May—September
Timothy	Phleum pratense	High	Same

Common Name	Botanical Name	Importance	Season
OREGON (Continued)			
Orchard	Dactylis glomerata	Secondary	Same
Red top	Agrostis alba	Secondary	Same
Rye, perennial	Lolium perenne	Secondary	Same
Velvet	Holcus lanatus	Secondary	Same
Weeds			
Dock, yellow	Rumex crispus	High	May–September
Lambs quarters	Chenopodium alba	High	June–September
Plantain, English	Plantago lanceolata	High	May–September
Pigweed, rough	Amaranthus retroflexus	High	June–September
Thistle, Russian	Salsola pestifer	High	July–September
Sagebrush	Artemisia spp.	Secondary	August–September
Atriplex–scales	Atriplex spp.	Secondary	July–September
UTAH			
Trees			
Box elder	Acer negundo	High	April–May
Cottonwood	Populus deltoides	Secondary	Same
Juniper	Juniperus spp.	Secondary	March–May
Alder, mountain	Alnus tenuifolia	Secondary	April–May
Elm	Ulmus spp.	Secondary	March
Grasses			
June/Kentucky blue	Poa pratensis	High	May–July
Koelers	Koeleria cristata	Secondary	Same
Timothy	Phleum pratense	Secondary	Same
Orchard	Dactylis glomerata	Secondary	Same
Red top	Agrostis alba	Secondary	Same
Weeds			
Thistle, Russian	Salsola pestifer	High	July–September
Kochia	Kochia scoparaia	High	Same
Ragweeds–short	Ambrosia elatior	Local	August–September
western	Ambrosia psilostachya	Local	Same
Cocklebur	Xanthium canadense	Secondary	Same
Sagebrush	Artemisia spp.	Secondary	Same
Atriplex–scale	Atriplex spp.	Secondary	June–September
Lambs quarters	Chenopodium alba	Secondary	Same
Pigweed, rough	Amaranthus retroflexus	Secondary	Same
Plantain, English	Plantago lanceolata	Secondary	May–August
Ragweed, false	Franseria acanthacarpa	Secondary	August–September

COMMON NAME	BOTANICAL NAME	IMPORTANCE	SEASON
		WASHINGTON	

Trees

Aspen	Populus tremuloides	Secondary	April
Willow	Salis lasiandrocaudata	Secondary	March—April
Elm	Ulmus spp.	Local	March
Birch	Betula spp.	Secondary	April—May
Box elder	Acer negundo	Secondary	April
Cottonwood	Populus trichocarpa	Secondary	April

Grasses

June/Kentucky blue	Poa pratensis	High	May—September
Timothy	Phleum pratense	High	June—July
Rye	Lolium spp.	Secondary	Same
Orchard	Dactylis glomerata	Secondary	Same
Red top	Agrostis alba	Secondary	Same
Brome	Bromus spp.	Local	Same
June, annual	Poa annua	Secondary	April—October

Weeds

Plantain, English	Plantago lanceolata	High	June—September
Dock, yellow	Rumex crispus	Secondary	June—July
Lambs quarters	Chenopodium alba	Secondary	July—September
Ragweeds—short	Ambrosia elatior	High	August—September
false	Franseria acanthacarpa	High	Same
western	Ambrosia psilostachya	Secondary	Same
Marsh elder, burweed	Iva xanthifolia	High	Same
Pigweed, rough	Amaranthus retroflexus	Secondary	June—September
Thistle, Russian	Salsola pestifer	High	Same
Sagebrushes	Artemisia spp.	Secondary	August—September

		WYOMING	

Trees

Alder	Alnus tenuifolia	Secondary	April
Cottonwood	Populus trichocarpa	Secondary	April—May
Birch	Betula spp.	Secondary	Same
Willow	Salix lasiandrocaudata	Secondary	February—March

Grasses

June/Kentucky blue	Poa pratensis	High	May—July
Fescue, meadow	Festuca elatior	Secondary	Same
Orchard	Dactylis glomerata	Secondary	Same
Red top	Agrostis alba	Secondary	Same
Timothy	Phleum pratense	Secondary	Same

Common Name	Botanical Name	Importance	Season

WYOMING (Continued)

Weeds

Common Name	Botanical Name	Importance	Season
Thistle, Russian	Salsola pestifer	High	July–September
Kochia	Kochia scoparaia	High	Same
Ragweeds—giant	Ambrosia trifida	Secondary	August–September
short	Ambrosia elatior	Secondary	Same
western	Ambrosia psilostachya	Local	Same
false	Franseria acanthacarpa	Local	Same
Marsh elder, burweed	Iva xanthifolia	Secondary	Same
Sagebrush	Artemisia spp.	Secondary	Same
Atriplex—scale	Atriplex spp.	Secondary	May–July
Lambs quarters	Chenopodium alba	Secondary	Same
Pigweed, rough	Amaranthus retroflexus	Secondary	Same

ALASKA

Data is insufficient from this state and Durham [4] in 1939 found no ragweed pollen in Fairbanks, Nome or Juneau. Grasses in June and July may play a role in inhalant allergy in the southern Alaskan area and about Nome. The grasses would be similar to that in British Columbia as June-Kentucky blue, Timothy, red top, and orchard.

HAWAII

Roth and Shira [4] felt that frequent rains, tradewinds, mountain barriers and insect pollination partially explained the low pollen counts obtained in Hawaii. Olive, mesquite, and Australian pine—casuarina are occasional wind borne tree pollen offenders while insect pollinated trees of local importance included hibiscus, mango, eucalyptus, acacia and mimosa. Grasses pollinated most of the year long and important grasses included Bermuda, red top, Johnson, sugar cane, panicum and pennisetum. False western ragweed is found in the western Oahu area but apparently caused little difficulty. Other weeds of local importance were lambs quarters, pigweed, redroot and English plantain.

PUERTO RICO

Trees were found to be a minor inhalant allergy cause and included Australian pine—casuarina; palms, mango, acacia and the mimosa family. Bermuda grass was the chief grass offender followed by sugar cane, panicum, pennisetum and chloris grasses. False western ragweed, chenopods, amaranths and English plantain were the primary weeds noted.

VIRGIN ISLANDS

Durham and Fafalla [1] found no ragweed in the National Park area in 1961. Tree pollens noted were mango and coconut. However coconut trees were close to the sampler. Bermuda grass, elephant or pennisetum grass and chloris grass were the chief grass offenders.

REFERENCES

1. Durham, O. C., and Fafalla, H.: A Pollen Survey at the National Park and St. Johns Island, Virgin Islands. Journal of Allergy, 32:27, 1961.
2. Feinberg, S. M.: Allergy in Practice. Chicago, Ill., Yearbook Publishers, Inc., 1946.
3. Hollister-Stier Laboratories. Pollen Guide.
4. Roth, A., and Shira, J.: Allergy in Hawaii. Annals of Allergy, 24:73, 1966.
5. Samter, M., and Durham, O. C.: Regional Allergy of The United States, Canada, Mexico, and Cuba. Springfield, Ill., Charles C Thomas, 1955.
6. Sheldon, J. A., Lovell, R. G., and Matthews, K. P.: A Manual of Clinical Allergy. Philadelphia, W. B. Saunders, 1967.
7. Sherman, W. B.: Hypersensitivity Mechanics and Management. Philadelphia, W. B. Saunders, 1968.
8. Statistical Report of the Pollen and Mold Committee of The American Academy of Allergy, 1970.
9. Vaughan, W. T., and Black, J. H.: Practice of Allergy. Saint Louis, Mo., C. V. Mosby, 1954.
10. Wodehouse, R. P.: Pollen Grains. New York, McGraw-Hill, 1935.
11. Wodehouse, R. P.: Hayfever Plants. Waltham, Mass., Chronica Botanica, 1945.

6

Allergic Rhinitis

James I. Tennenbaum, M.D.

SEASONAL ALLERGIC RHINITIS

Seasonal allergic rhinitis (pollinosis, hay fever) is a specific allergic reaction of the nasal mucosa, principally to pollens, and is characterized mainly by watery rhinorrhea, nasal congestion, sneezing, and itching of the eyes, nose, and throat. The symptoms are periodic in nature, occurring during the pollinating season of the plants to which the patient is sensitive. The term "hay fever" is a misnomer. Fever is not associated with the disease and the symptoms are not caused by hay. Use of the term "hay fever" is common among lay people and among some physicians and undoubtedly will remain in common usage for many years.

Incidence

Allergic rhinitis may begin at almost any age. The incidence of onset is greatest in children and young adults and decreases with advancing age. Occasionally, symptoms may first become manifest in middle or older age. There does not appear to be any racial, ethnic or sexual variation in its incidence. Heredity seems to play an important role in the occurrence of seasonal allergic rhinitis, as it does in other atopic dieases. Most investigators feel that the mechanisms permitting the development of hay fever, asthma, and infantile eczema are governed by an autosomal dominant gene with incomplete penetrance.[46] The degree of penetrance is the factor upon which investigators differ. Specific allergic syndromes are not hereditary; what is inherited is a heightened capacity to become sensitized following exposure to adequate concentrations of an allergen.[8] Although hay fever has been reported in infants as young as six months old,[19] in most cases an individual requires two or more seasons of exposure to a new antigen before exhibiting the clinical manifestations of allergic rhinitis.[33] This fact is supported by the observations that foreign students usually give a history of having been in the United States two or three years before suffering the symptoms of ragweed pollinosis.

It has been estimated that allergic rhinitis, both seasonal and perennial forms, accounts for the loss of 1.5 million school days per year.[2] Eleven of every 10,000 medical disqualifications from the military service are due to allergic rhinitis.[2] The exact incidence of the disease in the United States is unknown. Most figures have been obtained by studying relatively small population groups. A national survey performed by the United States Public Health Service estimated that in 1963 there were 12.5 million individuals with allergic rhinitis, asthma, or both.[5] Various authors suggest that up to 20 per cent of the population has allergic rhinitis alone.[18, 29, 44] An accurate estimate of the incidence of allergic rhinitis is difficult to obtain for several reasons. The primary reason is that the various studies have been performed in different geographic locations where the concentration and types of pollen have varied greatly. Thus, some patients with definite ragweed hay fever in Chicago, where the concentration of ragweed in the air is quite high, might be relatively asymptomatic in New York State, where the daily concentration of ragweed is lower. Such patients might be missed in a survey taken in New York. Another reason for inaccurate surveys is the failure of patients to recognize that they have allergic rhinitis believing that they suffer from "summer colds" or sinusitis instead. Regardless of the exact incidence, allergic rhinitis is an important ailment. Although the disease is not fatal, the suffering and annoyance that many patients experience should not be underestimated. Vast expenditures of money are involved when considering the cost of medication, physicians' fees, and economic loss due to patients' inability to perform efficiently in their jobs.

The disease tends to persist indefinitely after clinical symptoms appear. The severity of symptoms, however, may vary from year to year, depending in part on the quantity of pollen released during the specific pollinating season. Occasionally, the disease undergoes a spontaneous remission without specific therapy, although the mechanism for such a remission is unknown.

Etiology

Pollens and mold spores are the allergens responsible for seasonal allergic rhinitis. Pollens important in the etiology of allergic rhinitis are from plants which depend on the wind for cross-pollination. Many grasses, trees, and weeds produce lightweight pollen in sufficient quantities to sensitize genetically susceptible individuals. Plants depending on insect pollination, such as goldenrod, dandelions, and most flowers, do not cause allergic rhinitis symptoms unless the patient is in close contact with the plant, as when smelling flowers or gardening.

The pollinating season varies with the individual species and its geographic location. However, for any particular plant in a given locale, the pollinating season is constant from year to year. Weather conditions, such as temperature and rainfall, influence the amount of pollen produced but not the actual onset or termination of a specific season.

Pollens and fungi are discussed in greater detail in Chapters 4 and 5. However, certain important features must be considered here in relation to the appearance of symptoms for use in diagnosis. Ragweed pollen, a significant cause of allergic rhinitis, produces the most severe and long-lived of the seasonal rhinitis problems in the Eastern and Midwestern portions of the United States. In general, ragweed pollen appears in significant amounts from the second or third week of August through September or early October. Occasionally very sensitive patients may exhibit symptoms as early as the first few days of August, when smaller quantities of pollen first appear. Western ragweed and marsh elder in the Western States, sagebrush and franseria in the Southwestern United States, are important allergens in the late summer and early fall. In the Northern and Eastern parts of the United States the earliest pollens to appear are tree pollens, which usually occur in April, May, and June. Late spring- and early summer allergic rhinitis in this locale are due to grass pollens which appear from May to late June or very early July. It is during this season that patients complain of "rose fever"; like "hay fever," this term is a misnomer. It is coincidental that roses are in full bloom during the grass pollinating season; thus, the misconception. Approximately 75 percent of "hay fever" patients in the United States suffer from ragweed allergic rhinitis, 40 percent from grass allergic rhinitis, and 9 percent with allergic rhinitis from tree pollen sensitivity.[39] Approximately 25 percent suffer from both grass- and ragweed allergic rhinitis and about 5 percent suffer from all three allergies.[39] In other geographic locations these generalizations are not correct because of the particular climatic area and because some less common plants may predominate. For example, grass pollinates from early spring through late fall in the Southwestern regions and accounts for allergic rhinitis which is almost perennial.

Airborne mold spores, the most important of which throughout the United States are *Alternaria* and *Hormodendrum*, may also be the cause of seasonal allergic rhinitis. Warm, damp weather favors the growth of molds and thereby influences the severity of the season. Although there is no definite seasonal pattern, they generally first appear in the air in early spring, become most significant during the warmer months, and usually disappear with the first severe frost. Thus patients with a marked hypersensitivity to molds may exhibit symptoms from early spring through the first frost, while those patients with a lesser degree of hypersensitivity may have symptoms from early summer through late fall only. A more detailed discussion of the regional allergens in the United States is found in Chapter 5.

Pathophysiology

The nose has five major functions. It is (1) an olfactory organ, (2) a resonator for phonation, (3) a passageway for airflow in and out of the lungs, (4) a means of humidifying and warming inspired air, and (5) a filter of noxious particles from inspired air.

Heating and humidifying inspired air are important functions of the nasal mucosa. The highly vascularized mucosa of the turbinates and septum provide an effective structure to heat and humidify air as it passes over them. The blood vessels are under control of the autonomic nervous system, which controls reflex adjustments for efficient performance of this function.

Protecting and cleansing are also very important functions of the nasal mucosae. Relatively large particles are filtered out of inspired air by the hairs within the nostrils. The cilio-mucus transport system of the nasal mucosa helps to keep the nose clean thus supplying relatively pure air to the lungs. A thin, tenacious, and adhesive mucous blanket covering the nasal mucosa is produced by mucous- and serous glands and epithelial goblet cells in the mucosa. Nasal secretions contain an enzyme, lysozyme, which is bacteriostatic. The pH of the nasal secretions remain relatively constant at pH 7. Lysozyme activity and ciliary action are optimal at this pH. The major portions of the nose, septum, and paranasal sinuses are lined by ciliated cells. The cilia beat at a frequency of 10 to 15 beats per minute producing a streaming movement of the mucous blanket at an approximate rate of 2.5 to 7.5 mm. per minute. This blanket containing the filtered materials is moved toward the pharynx to be expectorated or swallowed.

Allergic reactions occurring in the nasal mucous membranes markedly affect the major functions of the nose. The immunologic nature of an allergic reaction has been discussed in detail in preceding chapters. The nasal mucosa is particularly vulnerable to the effects of an allergic reaction of the immediate type for several reasons. In performing its functions of cleansing and air passage, the nasal mucosa is exposed to allergens which are deposited directly on it. This enables the reaction to occur immediately in the local area. Plasma cells in the submucosal areas of the nose and respiratory tree have been shown to contain Immunoglobulin E,[45] suggesting local production of allergic antibody. The mediators of immediate allergic reactions, such as histamine, are very active in the nasal mucosa because of the huge vascular bed. The activity of histamine, which results in dilatation of small vessels and increased capillary permeability with edema formation, is more pronounced in a highly vascularized area.

Histologic changes due to an allergic reaction involving the nasal mucosa consist of dilatation of the vascular bed with edema formation, enlarged active mucous glands and goblet cells, and infiltration of the submucosa and mucosa with large numbers of eosinophiles. Plasma cells and lymphocytes may also be seen. These changes are completely reversible for when the specific pollinating season is over the mucosa returns to normal. If the patient's symptomatology remains limited to a seasonal pattern, no permanent alterations in the nasal mucosa and nasal function may occur.

Clinical Features

Symptoms. The major symptoms of allergic rhinitis are sneezing, rhinorrhea, nasal pruritus and nasal congestion. Some patients may not have the complete symptom complex. Sneezing is the most characteristic symptom, occasionally occurring in paroxysms of ten to twenty sneezes in rapid succession. Such episodes may leave a patient exhausted. Sneezing episodes may occur without warning or they may be preceded by an uncomfortable itching or irritated feeling in the nose. During the pollinating season, nonspecific factors, such as dust exposure, sudden drafts, or noxious irritants, may also trigger violent sneezing episodes.

The rhinorrhea is typically a watery, thin discharge which may be quite profuse and continuous. Because of the copious nature of the rhinorrhea, the skin covering the external nares and the upper lip may become irritated and tender. Purulent discharge is never present in uncomplicated allergic rhinitis; its presence indicates secondary infection. Nasal congestion, due to swollen turbinates, is a prominent complaint. Early in a season, the nasal obstruction may be intermittent or more troublesome in the evening and at night only to become almost continuous as the season progresses. If the nasal obstruction is severe, interference with aeration and drainage of the paranasal sinuses or Eustachian tube may occur, resulting in the complaints of headache or earache. The headache is of the so-called vacuum type presumed to be caused by the development of negative pressure as air is absorbed from the obstructed sinus or middle ear. Patients may also complain that their hearing is decreased and that sounds seem muffled. Nasal congestion alone, particularly in children, may occasionally be the major or sole complaint. With continuous severe nasal congestion the loss of smell and taste might occur. Itching of the nose may also be a prominent feature, inducing frequent rubbing of the nose, particularly in children.

Eye symptoms are itching and lacrimation. These often accompany the nasal symptoms. Patients with severe eye symptoms often complain of photophobia and sore, "tired" eyes. Occasionally, marked itching of the ears, palate, throat, or face may occur and may be extremely annoying. Because of irritating sensations in the throat and the posterior drainage of the nasal secretions, a hacking, nonproductive cough may be present. A constricted feeling in the chest, sometimes severe enough to cause the patient to complain of shortness of breath, may accompany the cough. The sensation of tightness in the chest is particularly bothersome to patients with severe nighttime cough. Some clinicians interpret this symptom as a warning signal of the possible development of asthma.

Some patients have systemic symptoms with seasonal allergic rhinitis. Such complaints include weakness, malaise, mental depression and irritability, fatigue, and anorexia.

A characteristic feature of the symptom complex is the periodicity of its appearance. Symptoms usually recur each year for many years in relation to the time and duration of the pollinating season of the causative plant. The most sensitive patients exhibit symptoms early in the season almost as soon as the pollen appears in the air. The intensity of the symptoms tends to vary with the concentration of pollen in the air, becoming more severe when the pollen concentration is highest and waning as the season comes to an end and the amount of pollen in the air decreases. Some patients find that their symptoms disappear suddenly when the pollinating season is over. In others, the symptoms may gradually disappear over a period of 2 or 3 weeks after the pollinating season is completed. Recent studies suggest that there is an increased reactivity of the nasal mucosa following repeated exposure to pollen.[7] This local and nonspecific increased reactivity has been termed a priming effect. The nonspecificity of this effect was suggested by demonstration under experimental conditions that a patient would respond to an allergen not otherwise considered clinically significant if he had been exposed or "primed" to a clinically significant allergen. This effect may account for the presence of symptoms in some patients beyond the termination of the pollinating season, because an allergen not important clinically by itself may induce symptoms in the "primed nose." For example, a patient with positive skin tests to mold antigens and ragweed and no symptoms until August may have symptoms until late October, after the ragweed pollinating season is over. The symptoms persist because of the presence of molds in the air which affect a primed mucous membrane. The presence of a secondary infection or the effects of nonspecific irritant factors on inflamed nasal mucous membranes may also prolong rhinitis symptoms beyond a specific pollinating season.

To a lesser degree the symptoms of allergic rhinitis may exhibit periodicity within the season. Many patients tend to exhibit more intense symptoms in the morning hours because most wind borne pollens are released in greatest numbers between sunrise and 9:00 a.m. Other specific factors modify the intensity of rhinitis symptoms. While it is raining, symptoms may diminish due to the clearing of pollen from the air. Windy days aggravate the patient's symptoms because a high concentration of pollen may be distributed over large areas. Automobile rides in the country, where an abundance of plants may result in higher pollen concentration, often are accompanied by a marked exacerbation of symptoms.

In addition to specific factors, nonspecific factors may also influence the intensity of rhinitis symptoms. Rapid atmospheric changes may aggravate symptoms in predisposed patients. In addition, nonspecific air pollutants may also potentiate the symptoms of allergic rhinitis.

In general, the disease tends to increase in severity for two or three years until a stabilized condition is reached. Symptoms then recur annually. Occasionally patients spontaneously lose their hypersensitivity for reasons which are not well understood.

Physical Examination. The most abnormal physical findings are present during the acute stages of the patient's seasonal complaints. The physical findings aid in the diagnosis. Rubbing of the nose and mouth breathing are common findings in children. Some children will rub the nose in an upward and outward fashion which has been termed the "allergic salute." The eyes may exhibit excessive lacrimation and the sclera and conjunctiva may be reddened. The conjunctiva may be swollen and appear granular in nature. In addition, the eyelids are often swollen. The skin about the nose may be reddened and irritated due to the continuous rubbing and blowing of the nose. Examination of the nasal cavity reveals a pale, wet, edematous mucosa, frequently bluish in color. A clear, thin nasal secretion may also be seen. Swollen turbinates may completely occlude the nasal passageway in severely affected patients. The pharynx is usually normal. The nose and eyes will appear normal during asymptomatic intervals.

Laboratory Aids

The only characteristic laboratory finding in allergic rhinitis is the presence of large numbers of eosinophils in a Wright, Giemsa, or Hansel stained smear of the nasal secretions obtained during a period of symptoms. In classic seasonal allergic rhinitis, this test is usually not necessary to make the diagnosis. Its use is limited to questionable cases and, more often, to defining chronic allergic rhinitis. Peripheral blood eosinophilia of 4 to 8 percent may or may not be present in active seasonal allergic rhinitis, and presence or absence of eosinophilia should not be relied upon to make this diagnosis.

Diagnosis

The diagnosis of seasonal allergic rhinitis usually presents no difficulty by the time the patient has symptoms severe enough to make him seek medical attention. The seasonal nature of the condition, the characteristic symptom complex, and the physical findings should establish a diagnosis in almost all cases. A physician, seeing a patient during the initial or second season or one whose major symptom is conjunctivitis might cause delay in making the diagnosis from history alone. Additional supporting evidence is the presence of a positive history of allergic disorders in the immediate family and a collateral history of other allergic disorders in the patient. After the history is taken and the physical examination is performed, skin tests should be performed to determine the reactivity of the patient against the suspected allergens. For proper interpretation of the meaning of a positive skin test, it is important to remember that patients with allergic rhinitis may exhibit positive skin tests to allergens other than those which are clinically important. (The methodology, interpretation, and the value of skin testing are discussed in Chapter 3.) Only in rare cases are direct skin tests negative in a classic case of allergic rhinitis. A diagnosis of allergic rhinitis when properly conducted skin tests have produced a negative result is always open to question. In such cases direct nasal and conjunctival mucosal testing may be useful.

The major clinical entity that enters into the differential diagnosis of allergic rhinitis is that of infectious rhinitis. Fever, sore throat, thick, purulent rhinorrhea, erythematous nasal mucosa, and the presence of cervical lymphadenopathy are helpful differential findings in infectious rhinitis. Stained smears of the nasal secretions usually show a predominance of polymorphonuclear neutrophiles. In addition, the short duration of symptoms, 4 to 10 days, is another helpful sign because pollinating seasons are usually much longer.

PERENNIAL (NONSEASONAL) ALLERGIC RHINITIS

Perennial allergic rhinitis is a condition characterized by intermittent or continuous nasal symptoms due to an allergic reaction without seasonal variation. The symptoms are generally persistent throughout the year. Some clinicians have used the term perennial allergic rhinitis to include both allergic and nonallergic forms of nonseasonal rhinitis. The term should be applied only to those cases in which an allergic etiology is shown to exist. The use of the term allergic in this book is used to designate only those responses mediated by or presumed to be mediated by an immunologic reaction. Although many aspects related to the etiology, pathophysiology, symptomatology, and diagnosis have been discussed in the preceding section, separate consideration of perennial allergic rhinitis is warranted because of certain complexities of the disease, particularly regarding diagnosis, management, and complications.

Etiology

The disease has the same basis as seasonal allergic rhinitis. The difference is only that chronic antigen challenge results in recurring symptoms throughout the year. Inhalant allergens are the most important cause of perennial allergic rhinitis. The major perennial allergens are house dust, feather pillows, mold antigens, furniture upholstery, and animal danders. Pollen allergy may contribute to seasonal exacerbations of rhinitis in patients with perennial symptoms. Occasionally perennial allergic rhinitis may be the result of exposure to an occupational allergen. Occupational chronic allergic rhinitis has been described in flour industry workers,[38] detergent workers,[31] and wood workers,[43] among others.

Although some clinicians believe that food allergens may be significant factors in the etiology of perennial allergic rhinitis, a direct immunologic relationship between ingested foods and persistent rhinitis symptoms has been difficult to establish. Most patients with proven food allergies exhibit other symptoms, including gastrointestinal disturbances, urticaria, asthma or anaphylaxis, in addition to rhinitis, following ingestion of the specific food.

Nonspecific irritants and infection may influence the course of perennial allergic rhinitis. Children with this condition appear to have a higher incidence of respiratory infections, which tend to aggravate the condition and often lead to the development of complications.[18,40] Irritants such as tobacco smoke, air pollutants, and chemical fumes can aggravate the symptoms of perennial allergic rhinitis. Drafts, chilling, and sudden changes in temperature also have a tendency to aggravate the symptoms. The latter symptoms may also indicate that the patient has nonallergic vasomotor rhinitis.

Pathophysiology

The alterations of normal physiology that have been described under seasonal allergic rhinitis are present to a lesser degree in the perennial form of the disease but are more persistent. These alterations are more chronic and permanent in nature and are significant factors in the development of many of the complications associated with nonseasonal allergic rhinitis. The histopathologic changes that occur are initially identical to those found in seasonal allergic rhinitis. With persistent disease, more chronic and irreversible changes, such as thickening and hyperplasia of the mucosal epithelium, more intense mononuclear cellular infiltration, connective tissue proliferation, and hyperplasia of adjacent periosteum may be noted.

Clinical Features

Symptoms. The symptoms of nonseasonal perennial allergic rhinitis are those of seasonal allergic rhinitis, although they are frequently less severe. This is due to the almost constant exposure to low concentrations of an allergen such as house dust. The less severe symptoms may lead the patients to attribute their symptoms to "sinus trouble" or "frequent colds." Nasal obstruction may be the major or sole complaint, particularly in children, whose nasal passageways are relatively small. Sneezing, clear rhinorrhea, itching of the nose, eyes, and throat and lacrimation may also occur. The presence of itching in the nasopharyngeal and eye areas is an indication of an allergic etiology of the chronic rhinitis. The chronic nasal obstruction may cause mouth breathing, snoring, almost constant sniffing, and a nasal twang to speech. Because of the constant mouth breathing, patients may complain of a dry, irritated or sore throat. Loss of smell and taste may occur in patients with marked chronic nasal obstruction. In some patients, the nasal obstruction is worse at night and may interfere with sleep. Sneezing episodes on awakening or in the early morning hours is a common complaint. Because the chronic edema involves the openings of the Eustachian tube and the paranasal sinuses, dull frontal headaches and ear complaints such as decreased hearing, fullness in the ears, or popping of the ears are common. In children, recurrent episodes of serous otitis media may occur. Persistent low grade nasal pruritus leads to almost constant rubbing of the nose and nasal twitching. In children, recurrent epistaxis may occur because of the friability of the mucous membranes, sneezing episodes, forceful nose blowing or nose picking. After sudden marked exposure to an allergen—by close contact with a pet or by dusting the house—the symptoms may be as severe as in the acute stages of seasonal allergic rhinitis. Constant excessive postnasal drainage of secretions may be associated with a chronic cough or a continual clearing of the throat.

Physical Examination. Physical examination of the patient with perennial allergic rhinitis will aid in the diagnosis, particularly in children. A child may constantly rub his nose or eyes. He may have certain facial characteristics which have been identified with chronic allergic nasal disease.[26] These include a gaping appearance due to the constant mouth breathing and a broadening of the midsection of the nose. In addition, there may a transverse nasal crease across the lower third of the nose where the soft cartilaginous portion meets the rigid bony bridge. This is a result of the continual rubbing and pushing of the nose to relieve itching.

The mucous membranes are pale, moist, and boggy and may have a bluish tinge. Polyps may be present in cases of chronic perennial allergic rhinitis of long duration. Their characteristic appearance is smooth, glistening, and white. They may appear as grapelike masses. The nasal secretions are usually clear and watery (but may be more mucoid in nature) and show large numbers of eosinophils when examined microscopically.

Dark circles under the eyes, known as allergic shiners, appear in some children. These are presumed to be due to venous stasis secondary to the constant nasal congestion. The conjunctiva may be infected or appear granular. In children affected with perennial allergic rhinitis early in life, narrowing of the arch of the palate may occur, leading to the "Gothic arch." In addition, these children may develop facial deformities such as a dental malocclusion. Examination of the throat is usually normal; although the posterior pharyngeal wall may exhibit prominent lymphoid follicles.

Laboratory Aids

A nasal smear examined for eosinophils may be of value in diagnosing perennial allergic rhinitis. It is particularly useful in cases in which there is no clear clinical relationship of symptoms to positive skin tests. The presence of large numbers of eosinophils suggests an allergic etiology for the chronic rhinitis. The absence of eosinophils does not exclude an allergic etiology, especially if the smear is taken during a relatively quiescent period of the disease or in the presence of bacterial infection when large numbers of polymorphonuclear neutrophils obscure the eosinophils. There is no particular diagnostic relationship between the presence or absence of a low grade peripheral blood eosinophilia and the presence of the disease although eosinophilia is suggestive evidence.

Diagnosis

Following the principles, discussed in Chapter 3, positive skin tests to aero-allergens are an important confirmatory finding in the patients whose history and physical examination suggest chronic allergic rhinitis. In rare patients in whom food allergy might play a significant role, skin tests to the specific food may fail to react. Only when avoidance of suspected foods reduces or completely abates the symptoms, which then recur with the reintroduction of the food, can one be assured of a specific food allergy. It should be emphasized that food allergy is rarely an important factor in perennial allergic rhinitis, particularly in adults.

Therefore good medical judgement must be used to avoid misdiagnosis of food allergy.

Differential Diagnosis. Incorrect diagnosis may result in expensive treatments and alteration of the patient's environment. Therefore, the diagnosis must be established carefully. The major disease entities that may be confused with perennial allergic rhinitis are chronic sinusitis, recurrent infectious rhinitis, abnormalities of nasal structures, and non-seasonal, nonallergic, noninfectious rhinitis of unknown etiology (vaso-motor rhinitis). The history and physical examination are usually helpful in differentiating these conditions from perennial allergic rhinitis. In addition, skin tests in these conditions are usually negative or do not correlate clinically with the symptomatology. In infectious rhinitis and chronic rhinitis, eosinophils are not common in the nasal secretions. The predominant cell found in the nasal secretions in these conditions is the neutrophil, unless there is a coexisting allergic rhinitis. These entities are discussed in greater detail in the last section of this chapter. Other causes of chronic nasal congestion and discharge are rhinitis medicamen-tosa, therapy with reserpine, nasal foreign bodies, and cerebrospinal rhinorrhea.

Rhinitis Medicamentosa. A condition that may enter into the differential diagnosis is that of rhinitis medicamentosa, which results from the overuse of vasoconstricting nose drops. Every patient who presents with the complaint of chronic nasal congestion should be questioned carefully as to the amount and frequency of use of nose drops. This condition will be discussed in more detail under the section on symptomatic therapy of allergic rhinitis.

Reserpine Rhinitis. Occasionally a patient who is taking reserpine will complain of marked nasal congestion, which is a common side effect of this drug. The medical history of current drug therapy will suggest this diagnosis. Discontinuation of this drug for a few days will result in marked symptomatic improvement.

Foreign Bodies. On rare occasions, a patient with a foreign body in the nose may be thought to have chronic allergic rhinitis. A foreign body usually presents as a unilateral nasal obstruction accompanied by a foul purulent nasal discharge. Children often put foreign bodies into the nose, most commonly peas, beans, buttons and erasers. Sinusitis is often diagnosed if the nose is not examined properly. Examination is best done after secretions are removed so that the foreign body may be visualized.

Cerebrospinal Rhinorrhea. Cerebrospinal rhinorrhea may follow a head injury. Cerebrospinal fluid is clear and watery in appearance simulating that seen in allergic rhinitis. In the majority of cases, the cerebrospinal rhinorrhea is unilateral. Because spinal fluid contains sugar and mucous does not, testing for the presence of glucose should be done to make the diagnosis. Cerebrospinal rhinorrhea results from a defect in the cribriform plate which usually requires surgical repair.

Complications

Allergic rhinitis accounts for the largest number of patients with respiratory allergy. The possibility of developing asthma as a sequel to allergic rhinitis may worry the patient (or his parents if the patient is a child). It has been generally stated that approximately 30 percent of patients with allergic rhinitis not treated with specific hyposensitization, eventually develop allergic asthma. However, a recent study of the population of an entire city indicated that only 7 percent of patients with allergic rhinitis develop asthma as a late sequela.[3] If asthma develops, the patient's concern for these symptoms overshadows the symptoms of allergic rhinitis. It is frequently stated that the patient with more severe allergic rhinitis has a greater risk of developing asthma.

Patients with allergic rhinitis may develop complications due to chronic nasal inflammation including recurrent otitis media with hearing loss, sinusitis and nasal or sinus polyps. These complications are discussed in detail in the last section of this chapter. It is apparent therefore that allergic rhinitis is not an insignificant problem. For these reasons, early diagnosis and treatment of chronic or seasonal allergic rhinitis is recommended.

TREATMENT

There are three types of management of seasonal or perennial allergic rhinitis. These methods are avoidance therapy, symptomatic therapy, and specific therapy, also termed hyposensitization or immunotherapy.

AVOIDANCE THERAPY

Complete avoidance of an allergen results in a cure when there is only a single allergen. For this reason, attempts to minimize contact with any important allergen should be made, regardless of what other mode of treatment is instituted. Allergic rhinitis due to the dander of a household pet can be completely controlled by having the pet removed from the home. If the patient is allergic to feathers, changing his feather pillow to a Dacron pillow should be advised. Although foods are very rarely the cause of allergic rhinitis, a patient may easily eliminate from his diet any food known to induce rhinitis symptoms. Mold sensitive patients occasionally note the precipitation or aggravation of symptoms following ingestion of certain foods having a high mold content. Avoidance of such foods as beer, wine, cantaloupe, melons, mushrooms, and various cheeses may help.

In most cases of allergic rhinitis complete avoidance therapy is difficult, if not impossible, because aero-allergens are so widely distributed. Attempts to eradicate sources of pollen or molds have not proven to be significantly effective. However, there are measures which the patient may take to decrease his exposure to certain aero-allergens. In cases of pollen or mold allergy, the amount of inhaled allergen can be decreased by such measures as sleeping with the bedroom windows closed and avoiding the countryside during pollination seasons. Ragweed-sensitive children should avoid fields where ragweed is abundant. Mold sensitive patients should avoid damp, musty basements, barns and moldy hay and straw. They should not rake or burn leaves and they must disinfect or destroy moldy articles. An effective means of avoiding pollens and molds is to stay in a controlled environment. Air conditioners are often beneficial: most units contain filters which reduce the aero-allergen concentration by filtration. A central air conditioning unit with an electrostatic precipitating filter is the most efficient air filtration system. A limitation of this form of therapy is that most patients can not remain continuously at home. On might travel to an area where the offending aero-allergen is not present. This approach is inconvenient, expensive and not always completely effective because most areas contain some aero-allergens.

In the case of house dust allergy, complete avoidance is not possible. Certain measures can be practiced which will decrease the exposure to household dust. An electrostatic precipitator in conjunction with a central heating and air conditioning unit is effective in reducing house dust. Other instructions for a dust control program should also be given to the patient with house dust sensitivity. The patient should have at least one room in his house which is relatively dust free. The most practical program is to make the bedroom as dust free as possible so that the patient may have the sleeping area as a controlled environment.

Certain measures to decrease house dust exposure are relatively easy to perform. The patient should wear a mask when cleaning house if such activity precipitates significant symptoms. Exposure to dust from feather pillows, mattresses and box springs can be effectively controlled. Both the mattress and box springs should be encased in plastic covers. Upholstered furniture, wall to wall carpeting, chenille spreads, bed pads, and stuffed toys can be eliminated from the bedroom for more complete control. Old foam rubber may harbor mold spores; therefore, it is best for the patient to obtain a Dacron pillow or a plastic pillow cover. These simple measures are often enough to render the patient's symptoms fewer and milder. For more detailed instructions on house dust control, see Appendix D.

Antihistamines

The ideal agent would be a compound which prevents all the effects of histamine without side effects. No such agent has been found, but antihistaminic drugs are still the foundation of symptomatic therapy for allergic rhinitis. They are most useful in controlling sneezing, rhinorrhea, and pruritus of seasonal allergic rhinitis but are less effective against the nasal obstruction and eye symptoms.

Antihistamines are compounds of varied chemical structures which have the property of antagonizing *some* of the actions of histamine.[17] The exact mode of action of these compounds is unknown. Many of them bear a slight structural resemblance to the histamine molecule, a fact which has led to the speculation that they act by competitive inhibition of histamine at reactive sites on cell surfaces. There are certain facts that do not support this idea. Some compounds without this structural resemblance are potent antihistamines, and other compounds with the same structural features as histamine may be inactive as antihistamines. The antihistaminic agents do not block the release of histamine nor do they interfere with antigen-antibody reactions. The do not block all actions of histamine; for example, histamine induced release of gastric juice is particularly resistant to blockade. They are most effective in preventing histamine induced capillary permeability. In clinical use, these drugs are most effective when given early—at the first appearance of symptoms—since they do not abolish existing effects of histamine but rather prevent the development of new symptoms due to further histamine release. The antihistamines may also exhibit sedative, antiemetic and local anesthetic effects depending upon the particular antihistamine, route of administration and dosage used. Many of them also exhibit atropinelike effects; this accounts for such side effects as blurred vision or dry mouth.

Chemistry. The basic structure of the antihistamines is a substituted ethylamine which has the following structural formula:

$$R-X-CH_2-CH_2-N\begin{smallmatrix} \nearrow R' \\ \searrow R'' \end{smallmatrix} \quad .$$

The ethylamine radical (CH_2-CH_2-N=) is also present in histamine. It is presumed that it is this common structural portion of the antihistamines that competes with histamine for the cell receptors. In most cases the R′ and R″ groups are CH_3 radicals. The R group represents a large basic radical which generally accounts for the majority of the molecular weight of the particular antihistamine. These large groups are linked to the basic ethylamine structure by a nitrogen-, oxygen-, or carbon atom, represented by X. If the X is a nitrogen, then the compound is an ethylenediamine derivative; if oxygen, an aminoalkyl ether derivative; and if carbon, an alkylamine derivative. There are a number of compounds having cyclic structures which are not related to the other classes, that also exhibit antihistaminic properties. Each individual class of antihistamines has certain properties that can be generalized as follows:

Ethanolamines (oxygen linkage) are potent and effective histamine antagonists with a marked tendency for sedative and atropinelike activity. They exhibit a low incidence of gastrointestinal side effects. An example of this group is diphenhydramine (Benadryl).

Ethylenediamines (nitrogen linkage) are highly effective antihistamines. They tend to cause less central nervous system depression but gastrointestinal disturbances are quite common with their use. An example of this group is tripelennamine (Pyribenzamine).

Alkylamines (carbon linkage) are extremely active as antihistamine antagonists and are very effective in relatively low doses. Representative of this group is chlopheniramine (Chlor-Trimeton). These compounds tend to have milder side effects and therefore are advantageous for use in individuals whose occupations make drowsiness a distinct hazard.

Miscellaneous Antihistaminic Agents. These compounds of various chemical structures are difficult to group together, but in general they are cyclic compounds. Only a limited number of drugs in this miscellaneous group have use in the treatment of allergic rhinitis. Most of these compounds exhibit prominent sedative effects which has led to their primary use as central nervous system depressants. The phenothiazines fall into this general category.

Clinical Use. All of the antihistamines are readily absorbed after oral administration. They vary in speed, intensity and duration of effect. Since there are so many antihistamines available, it is best to become familiar with selected ones for use. In practice, clinical choice should be based on effectiveness of antihistaminic activity and the limitation of side effects. Dryness of the mouth, vertigo, gastrointestinal upset, irritability in children and drowsiness account for over 90 percent of the side effects seen with these drugs. The depressant effect on the central nervous system is the major limiting side effect. Drowsiness may be mild and temporary, and it may disappear after a few doses of the drug. Since patients exhibit marked variability in the response to various antihistamines, individualization of dosage is important. Table 6-1 summarizes data for representative antihistamines from each group.

Sympathomimetic Agents

Sympathomimetic drugs mimic certain effects of epinephrine and norepinephrine and are used as vasoconstrictors for the nasal mucous membranes. The current concept regarding the mechanism of action of these drugs postulates two types of adrenergic receptors called alpha and beta receptors.[1] Activation of the alpha receptors produces constriction of smooth muscles of the vessels of the skin, viscera, and mucous membranes, whereas activation of beta receptors induces dilatation of vascular smooth muscle, relaxation of bronchial smooth muscle (bronchodilatation) and cardiac stimulation. The edema of the nasal mucous membranes in allergic rhinitis can be reduced by topical or systemic administration of drugs which stimulate alpha receptors.[17] In large doses these drugs induce nervousness and insomnia. They should be used with caution in patients who have hypertension, organic heart disease, angina pectoris, and hyperthyroidism. In addition to their use as decongestants, the sympathomimetic drugs are also combined with antihistamines in many oral preparations to decrease the drowsiness that often accompanies antihistamine therapy.

Nose drops or nasal sprays containing sympathomimetic agents may be overused. The topical application of these drugs is often followed by a "rebound" phenomenon in which the nasal mucous membranes become even more congested and edematous as a result of the use of the drug. This leads the patient to use the drops or spray more frequently and in higher doses to obtain relief from the nasal obstruction. This condition resulting from the overuse of topical sympathomimetic agents is called rhinitis medicamentosa. The patient must abruptly discontinue their use to alleviate the condition. Other symptomatic measures are needed to decrease the nasal congestion until this distressing side effect of topical vasoconstrictors disappears. Because of the duration of seasonal or perennial allergic rhinitis, it is best not to use the topical vasoconstrictors in the allergic patient except temporarily during periods of infectious rhinitis. The systemic use of the sympathomimetic drugs has not been associated with rhinitis medicamentosa.

Phenylephrine, ephedrine, iso-ephedrine, phenylpropanolamine and cyclopentamine are some of the more common vasoconstricting agents used in association with various antihistamines in oral preparations. Representative useful combinations are outlined in Table 6-2.

TABLE 6-1

Representative Antihistamines Useful in the Treatment of Allergic Rhinitis

GENERIC NAME	TRADE NAME	HOURS DURATION OF ACTION	SEDATION	AVERAGE DOSE (Mgm.)	
				ADULT	CHILD (60 lbs.)
Ethanolamines					
Diphenhydramine	Benadryl	4-6	Marked	50	20
Carbinoxamine	Clistin	3-4	Moderate	4	2
Doxylamine	Decapryn	4-6	Moderate	12.5 to 25	6.25
Ethylenediamines					
Tripelennamine	Pyribenzamine	4-6	Moderate	50	25
Thenylpyramine	Histadyl	4-6	Moderate	50	30
Alkylamines					
Chlorpheniramine	Chlor-Trimeton	4-6	Mild	4	2
Dexchlorpheniramine	Polaramine	4-6	Mild	2	1
Brompheniramine	Dimetane	4-6	Mild	4	2
Triprolidine	Actidil	8-12	Mild	2.5	1.25

TABLE 6-2 **Representative Antihistamine–Sympathomimetic Combinations**

TRADE NAME	INGREDIENTS	MGM. PER TABLET OR CAPSULE	DOSAGE FORMS	RECOMMENDED ADULT DOSAGE
Pyribenzamine with Ephedrine	Tripelennamine Ephedrine	25 12	Tablet	1 or 2 tablets q.i.d.
Co-Pyronil	Thenylpyramine Pyrrobutamine Cyclopentamine	25 15 12.5	Capsule Suspension	1 capsule t.i.d. 1 tsp. t.i.d. (child)
Ornade	Chlorpheniramine Phenylpropanolamine Isopropamide iodide	8 50 2.5	Timed released Spansule	1 Spansule b.i.d.
Naldecon	Chlorpheniramine Phenyltoloxamine Phenylpropanolamine Phenylephrine	5 15 40 10	Sustained action tablet Syrup	1 tablet t.i.d. 1 tsp. q.i.d. (child)
Extendryl	Chlorpheniramine Phenylephrine Methscopolamine	8 20 2.5	Timed action capsule Syrup	1 capsule b.i.d. 1 tsp. q.i.d. (child)
Algic	Chlorpheniramine Phenyltoloxamine Racephedrine	3 50 30	Tablets Sustained action tablet	1 tablet q.i.d.
Isochlor	Chlorpheniramine d-Isoephedrine	4 25	Tablets Syrup Sustained release capsule	1 tablet q.i.d. 1 tsp. q.i.d. (child)
Dimetapp	Brompheniramine Phenylpropanolamine Phenylephrine	12 15 15	Extended release tablet Elixir	1 Extentab b.i.d. 1 tsp. q.i.d. (child)
Actifed	Triprolidine d-Isoephedrine	2.5 60	Tablet Syrup	1 tablet t.i.d. 1 tsp. q.i.d. (child)
Disophrol Drixoral	Dexbrompheniramine d-Isoephedrine	6 120	Chronotab Extended release sustained action tablet	1 tablet b.i.d.

Corticosteroid Hormones

Cortisone and its derivatives have marked beneficial effects in the management of various allergic processes.[17] The mechanism of their therapeutic effect is not completely understood. In doses commonly used for reaginic allergic disease in man, antibody production and anti-gen-antibody reactions have not been shown to be altered. It has been suggested that the anti-inflammatory activity of these drugs is responsible for their effectiveness in allergic states. Adrenocorticosteroids inhibit several aspects of the inflammatory process, including edema formation, capillary permeability and migration of leukocytes into the inflamed area. Local edema and capillary permeability are prominent features of reaginic mediated reactions which respond to steroid therapy.

The indications for the use of steroid therapy in the management of allergic rhinitis are relatively few. The side effects of long term use of these drugs are well known and have been discussed extensively in textbooks of internal medicine. Therefore, these drugs should be used only for very short periods of time to treat allergic rhinitis. An example of a possible indicated use is during the height of a pollen season, when an individual is markedly symptomatic and when other measures for symptomatic control have been ineffective. In these cases, a few days to 1 or 2 weeks of corticosteroids may be justified. Fifteen to 20 milligrams of prednisone per day for 3 or 4 days followed by decreasing doses over the next few days will usually afford the patient marked relief and may enable antihistamine therapy to become effective. Some clinicians have found that injectable steroid drugs in a depot form also are effective for a week or two following a single injection. Since perennial rhinitis does not produce serious disabilities, steroids should be used only during periods of marked increase of unmanageable symptoms. They are particularly useful in the management of rhinitis medicamentosa during the period of withdrawal of topical vasoconstricting drugs. In an effort to decrease their systemic effects, the use of corticosteroids topically may also be effective. Dexamethasone phosphate in a freon propelled spray (Turbinaire) is an easy-to-use, dose-regulated topical steroid preparation. The usual adult dosage is two sprays in each nostril three or four times a day. Dexamethasone is more effective in topical administration than oral administration and side effects are less. Because the steroid is absorbed through the mucous membranes, the possibility exists that if the patient uses the spray in excess of the recommended dose or over a prolonged period of time, absorption of sufficient quantities may induce such undesirable effects as those associated with oral corticosteroid therapy.

Another indication for the use of topical steroids is in the treatment of nasal polyposis. Use of the dexamethasone spray for several weeks is effective in reducing the size of the polyps. In some cases, reduction is so remarkable that the effect has been termed a medical polypectomy. The relief may only be temporary, and surgical removal may be required later. However, in many cases the relief may last for extended periods.

IMMUNOTHERAPY

Immunotherapy or hyposensitization is treatment which attempts to raise the threshold level for symptom appearance following exposure to the aero-allergen. This altered degree of sensitivity may be the result of (1) the induction of a new antibody, the so-called blocking antibody [24]; (2) a decrease in reaginic (allergic) antibody [6]; (3) a change in the cellular histamine release phenomena [35]; or (4) an interplay of all three possibilities.[30] The therapeutic and practical aspects of immunotherapy are discussed in detail in Chapter 9.

Principles of Immunotherapy

Indications for Treatment. The severity of allergic rhinitis and its complications ranges from minimal to marked symptoms and from short to prolonged durations. The indications for the type and intensity of therapy varies depending on the clinical situation. Therefore, the indications for immunotherapy, a relatively long term treatment modality, are relative rather than absolute. For example, a patient who has mild grass pollinosis for only a few weeks in June may be well managed by symptomatic therapy alone. In such cases, immunotherapy can be instituted if the symptoms become more severe over a longer period of time or if asthma appears. Some patients are quite sensitive to the sedative effect of antihistamines and may be uncomfortable either because of the allergic rhinitis symptoms or the side effects of drug therapy. Immunotherapy may be offered to such an individual. Patients with perennial allergic rhinitis or allergic rhinitis in multiple pollen seasons who require almost daily symptomatic treatment for long periods of time may also be considered as candidates for specific immunotherapy. The advantages of long term relief by such therapy, which is relatively expensive, should be considered in relationship to the expense of taking daily medication. In addition, specific therapy may help to deter the development of some of the complications of chronic rhinitis. Antigens used for immunotherapy should be those allergens which can not be avoided; for example, pollens, molds, and house dust. Animal dander injection therapy should be restricted to veterinarians and laboratory personnel whose occupation makes avoidance impossible.

Choice of Antigen. Following the principles of diagnosis discussed in

Chapter 3, immunotherapy should be given for only those antigens which are clinically important and which cannot be completely avoided to permit control of symptoms. The allergic individual may form skin sensitizing antibodies to many allergens some of which may have no clinical significance. For example, a patient with ragweed hay fever may show a positive skin test to grass pollen extract without symptoms during the grass pollinating season. Such a patient should receive ragweed antigen alone. In some cases, because of overlapping seasons, such as grass pollen and mold spores or mold spores and ragweed pollen, the choice would be to treat with both antigens because neither can be excluded. If in the patient's future course, new allergens become clinically important, they can be added to the program with only temporary inconvenience. There is no substantial evidence that inclusion of allergens not shown to be clinically significant will prevent the future development of symptoms. Inclusion of them may tend to increase local reactions. *A very important principle is that the clinician should treat the patient and not the skin test.*

Efficacy of Treatment. Only in the past few years have properly controlled double blind studies of immunotherapy been carried out to determine the clinical value of such therapy. Most studies [10, 15, 25, 32] have indicated that in pollen allergy, 70 to 80 per cent of treated patients will experience beneficial results from immunotherapy. It should be emphasized that such patients are not necessarily cured of their disease; rather, they have fewer symptoms which are more easily controlled by symptomatic medication. Some patients, however, are fortunate enough to have a clinical remission following treatment with immunotherapy; this is the exception rather than the rule. Although improvement of symptoms may occur during the first year of immunotherapy in some patients, more definite evidence of improvement appears in the second and third years of treatment. Studies involving house dust immunotherapy indicate that the therapeutic effects appear to be less than those produced by pollen extract therapy.[27] There are no adequately controlled double blind studies for mold immunotherapy, although some allergists have the clinical impression that the results are not as good as those obtained for pollen allergic rhinitis. It is important for the clinician to discuss with the patient in great detail what may be expected from immunotherapy. A frequent cause of treatment failure is that a patient will expect too much, too soon and thus prematurely discontinue the injection program because of dissatisfaction. Another important cause of treatment failure occurs in patients with vasomotor rhinitis who have positive but clinically insignificant skin tests and have received immunotherapy based upon the skin tests. Immunotherapy based upon positive skin tests alone should not be expected to be beneficial.

Duration of Treatment. There is no adequate clinical or laboratory method of indicating to the patient how long immunotherapy must be continued. There are no long term clinical studies comparing therapies of varying durations. Therefore, the clinical response to therapy dictates the decision concerning the duration of specific treatment. It is recommended that a minimum of three years of immunotherapy be given in an effort to avoid the rapid recurrence of symptoms in uncomplicated allergic rhinitis. In patients who have persisting complications such as polyps, sinusitis, or otitis media, it may be advisable to continue therapy somewhat longer since clinical improvement may take longer in such patients. A decision to discontinue therapy may be made after the patient has experienced relatively few symptoms for two successive pollen seasons. If signficant symptoms should recur later, immunotherapy can be reinstituted. Some patients do not experience improvement from correctly chosen and properly administered immunotherapy. If no improvement is noted after a reasonable trial of therapy—usually through two seasons—immunotherapy should be discontinued.

MISCELLANEOUS FORMS OF RHINITIS

Vasomotor Rhinitis

Vasomotor rhinitis is a disease of unknown etiology. It is associated with an altered vasomotor control of the nose resulting in the development of chronic nasal congestion. Many physicians use the term vasomotor rhinitis as a descriptive term to include both nonseasonal, perennial allergic rhinitis and the nonallergic forms of rhinitis. In this discussion, the use of the term vasomotor rhinitis is restricted to the nonimmunologic, noninfectious, chronic type of rhinitis.

Pathophysiology. The nasal mucous membrane has a rich blood supply which is under the control of the autonomic nervous system. The vasculature derived from branches of the ophthalmic, maxillary, and facial arteries forms an extensive subepithelial plexus of arterioles. Blood drains from the internal nose via a very rich superficial venous plexus forming cavernous spaces which resemble those found in erectile tissue. Autonomic nerves controlling this vascular bed travel with the sensory nerves in the area, the maxillary division of the fifth cranial nerve. Parasympathetic function originates in the superior salivatory nucleus and reaches the nose via the vidian nerve and sphenopalatine ganglion. Cervical sympathetic branches from the carotid nerves join the vidian nerve to distribute to the nose.

Many nonspecific stimuli act upon the autonomic nerves resulting in reflex changes in the nasal mucosa, in particular that covering the turbinates, where the venous plexus is especially abundant. Emotional stimuli have been shown to trigger nasal obstruction and rhinorrhea.[20] In addition, rapid changes in body temperature and changes in humidity may induce similar nasal changes in susceptible patients.[42] Horner's syndrome, in which the cervical sympathetic nerves are ablated, is associated with unilateral nasal obstruction and overactivity of the mucous glands. By altering laminar air flow, a deviated nasal septum may induce reflex changes in the nasal mucosa leading to the development or aggravation of vasomotor rhinitis. Although the exact mechanism is not known, endocrine factors may be important causes in some patients with vasomotor rhinitis. Pregnancy, menstruation, menopause, and marked hypothyroidism may be accompanied by the symptoms of a nonallergic chronic rhinitis.

Clinical Features. Patients with vasomotor rhinitis complain of chronic nasal congestion, rhinorrhea and sneezing. Frequently the patients state that the nasal blockage alternates from side to side. No seasonal absence of symptoms is noted, although during the summer, when temperatures are more constant, the symptoms may be milder than in the winter. The symptoms do not change significantly in relation to any geographic changes. In patients with vasomotor rhinitis, no definite allergic or infectious factors can be shown to be clinically important. Physical factors and psychological stresses may trigger nasal symptoms. The symptoms may be worse upon awakening in the morning. Sudden changes in body temperature, exposure to drafts, high humidity, chemical fumes, tobacco smoke and emotional upsets are common nonspecific stimuli which precipitate or aggravate the nasal symptoms in susceptible patients. In vasomotor rhinitis of pregnancy, symptoms appear late in the first or second trimester, and disappear shortly after parturition. Occasionally, the use of birth control pills, which essentially induces a pseudo-pregnancy, may cause vasomotor rhinitis.

Examination of the nose will usually reveal marked edema resulting in nasal obstruction. The nasal mucosa usually appears erythematous, but occasionally it may appear pale. The nasal secretions are usually mucoid, and only on rare occasion does the stained nasal smear reveal the presence of significant numbers of eosinophils. Most patients with vasomotor rhinitis show no reactions to skin tests. In a small proportion of patients, skin tests may be positive but do not correlate with the clinical history and are coincidental. Nasal polyps frequently complicate long-standing vasomotor rhinitis and add to the nasal obstruction. The important features of allergic rhinitis and vasomotor rhinitis are compared in Table 6-3.

TABLE 6-3

Comparison of Characteristics of Allergic and Vasomotor (Nonallergic) Rhinitis

	ALLERGIC	VASOMOTOR
Seasonal variation	Yes	No
Nasal, ocular, or palatal itching	Yes	Rarely
Rhinorrhea	Watery	Mucoid
Pale nasal mucosa	Almost always	Not uncommon
Nasal polyps	Occasionally	Occasionally
Collateral allergy	Common	Unusual (coincidental)
Family history of allergy	Usual	Coincidental
Nasal secretion eosinophil smear	Usually positive	Rarely positive
Skin test reactivity	Almost always positive	Coincidental

Treatment. Therapy consists of symptomatic treatment with anti-histamines and oral nasal decongestants and avoidance of precipitating factors. Thyroid replacement therapy will diminish the nasal symptoms associated with hypothyroidism. Discontinuing the use of oral con-traceptive pills will alleviate the nasal symptoms in the occasional pa-tient in whom they induce vasomotor rhinitis. Surgical correction of a deviated nasal septum is indicated in patients with an associated marked nasal obstruction. The patient with vasomotor rhinitis of preg-nancy should be reassured of the limited nature of the nasal symptoms. The chronic use of nose drops should not be prescribed for chronic nonallergic, noninfectious rhinitis, because these patients may easily develop rhinitis medicamentosa. Because of the chronicity of symptoms, corticosteroid therapy should not be used for fear of inducing dangerous side effects.

Infectious Rhinitis

Acute infectious rhinitis is characterized by the systemic manifesta-tions of fever and malaise associated with local symptoms consisting of sneezing, nasal congestion, a purulent nasal discharge, and, occasionally, headache. The disorder typically lasts from 5 to 14 days.

Etiology. It is generally believed that any one of a variety of filterable viruses are responsible for acute infectious rhinitis although rarely a bacterial infection may be the cause. It is not unusual, however, for bacteria to act as secondary invaders and thereby be responsible for the occurrence of complications.

Clinical Manifestations. A viral rhinitis usually begins in the nose or throat and may progress to involve other parts of the respiratory tract. Initially changes of hyperemia, exudation, and serum extravasation occur. Inflammatory cells invade the mucous membranes and surface mucosal cells are shed. Within several days, the nasal secretions which are watery at the onset, become thick and tenacious and appear grossly purulent. The nasal mucosa appears markedly erythematous at examination, and often purulent secretions may be visable. Microscopic examination of the secretions reveal large numbers of polymorphonuclear leucocytes and epithelial cells. No eosinophils are seen unless the infection occurs in a patient with active allergic rhinitis. In this situation eosinophils may be seen along with the characteristic inflammatory cells.

The majority of episodes of acute infectious rhinitis run a course of around 10 days. In approximately 10 percent of cases the infection may extend to other respiratory structures such as the bronchi, trachea, or middle ear and may cause complications such as bronchitis or otitis media. If a secondary bacterial infection occurs, there is a greater chance of complications, particularly acute infectious sinusitis. It appears that recurrent episodes of acute infectious rhinitis occur more frequently in children with chronic allergic rhinitis.[18, 40] One explanation for this fact may be that the chronically inflamed nose exhibits less natural resistance to viral infections.

Treatment. Bed rest, increased oral intake of fluid, and aspirin (300 to 600 mg. every 4 hours) should be prescribed for febrile patients. An oral antihistamine-nasal decongestant tablet or syrup may afford some relief of the local symptoms. In the case of acute infectious rhinitis, topical nasal decongestants may be used for a few days to relieve the nasal congestion. Such therapy may also help maintain a patent Eustachian tube and sinus cavity orifices and diminish the chances of the complications of sinusitis or otitis media. If a secondary bacterial infection occurs, such as acute senusitis, otitis media, or bacterial bronchitis, or if the rhinitis is bacterial in origin, the use of anti-microbial agents may be indicated. Prophylactic use of anti-microbial agents in the treatment of viral rhinitis is not indicated.

Differential Diagnosis. Patients with infectious rhinitis rarely present a problem in differential diagnosis from allergic rhinitis. However, patients with chronic allergic rhinitis, children in particular, are prone to develop secondary infections and an increased incidence of upper respiratory infections. Helpful diagnostic findings in infectious rhinitis are the presence of fever, sore throat, erythematous nasal mucous membranes and cervical lymphadenopathy. The nasal secretions are thick and purulent with an absence of eosinophils. Throat cultures and white blood counts are generally not helpful in establishing a diagnosis of viral infection.

Sinusitis

Acute Sinusitis. The symptoms of acute paranasal sinusitis are localized pain and tenderness over the involved sinus, nasal obstruction, purulent nasal discharge, fever and malaise. The pain may radiate into the upper teeth causing the patient to see a dentist. The nasal mucosa appears hyperemic and edematous and the turbinates are enlarged and may be covered with purulent discharge. Tenderness over the sinus area is almost always present. If the maxillary or frontal sinus is involved, they may not transmit light on transillumination. The involved sinus will appear cloudy on roentgenographic examination. Occasionally, a fluid level may be visible on the roentgenograph.

Immediate treatment is aimed at eradicating the infection, promotion of drainage of the sinuses, and control of fever and other systemic symptoms. This is accomplished by bed rest, analgesics, antibiotics, topical and systemic nasal decongestants and local application of hot or cold compresses to the sinus areas. Local irrigation of the maxillary sinuses may be performed by the patient using a modification of the Proetz technique,[12] which consists of irrigation with a tepid saline solution several times per day. If these measures to not afford relief, consultation with an otolaryngologist for more intensive treatment should be considered.

Allergic nasal disease may contribute to the incidence of acute paranasal sinusitis. Acute sinusitis is a rare complication of acute seasonal allergic rhinitis, occurring only if a secondary bacterial infection occurs in a sinus the drainage of which is occluded by an obstructed meatus. Acute sinusitis may occur more frequently in the patient with chronic nasal obstruction due to allergic factors. The therapy of the sinusitis in this situation follows the same program as outlined above. Immunotherapy and control of the basic allergic process are useful measures in preventing the occurrence of this complication.

Chronic Sinusitis. If recurrent episodes of acute sinusitis occur, subacute and chronic sinusitis may follow with irreversible changes in the sinal mucosa. Chronic nasal obstruction, nasal discharge, and postnasal discharge are common symptoms. Mouth breathing is common in children. Patients may have a chronic cough due to irritation by the postnasal drainage. In some cases, associated infection of the bronchial mucosa results in the development of sino-bronchitis. To make the diagnosis, the physician should prove that the purulent discharge is due to pus in an involved sinus. Roentgenograph, transillumination, and irrigation procedures are necessary to establish a diagnosis. The sinus may appear clouded on x-ray or have a thickened lining.

Uncontrolled chronic allergic rhinitis, vasomotor rhinitis, and the presence of nasal polyps are factors which lead to the development of chronic sinusitis. Treatment of these disorders, including symptomatic measures and immunotherapy when indicated, often result in good control of the sinusitis. Evidence has been presented which suggests that chronic sinusitis may be one etiologic factor in the development of nasal and sinal polyps.[36] Intensive efforts directed toward the control of chronic sinusitis should be instituted in an effort to prevent the development of polyps. The principles of the treatment of chronic sinusitis are similar to those used in the treatment of acute sinusitis. The most important are long term appropriate antibiotic therapy as determined by a culture and sensitivity of the nasal discharge. Should medical measures fail, surgical intervention is usually necessary for long term management.

Hyperplastic Rhinitis. Purulent sinusitis superimposed upon allergic rhinitis and associated with marked mucosal edema has been termed hyperplastic rhinitis. Chronic hyperplasia of the mucosa occurs associated with a tendency to polyp formation. Hyperplastic sinusitis is most often treated by surgical procedures. However, anti-allergic therapy is also necessary if recurrence of infection is to be controlled successfully.

Nasal Polyps

Patients with nasal polyps are seen frequently by the allergist. Polyps may form in paranasal sinuses as well as in the nasal cavity. They occasionally occur as a complication of uncontrolled allergic rhinitis. Polyps may also develop as a result of chronic inflammation, as in chronic sinusitis, chronic vasomotor rhinitis, and cystic fibrosis. They may also occur without explanation.

Pathogenesis. The mechanism for the development of polyps is uncertain. Two possible pathways have been suggested. Kern and Schenck [22] first presented evidence to suggest that allergic factors are important in the development of polyps. The continuous nasal edema found in a chronic nasal allergic condition is associated with epithelial hypertrophy which may then develop into papillary formation. If this process persists, hypertrophy and increased activity of the mucous glands may result in polyp formation. A second pathway for polyps to form follows chronic infection. Chronic infection may result in hyperplasia of the nasal mucosa associated with inflammatory changes, mucous gland dilatation, and fibrosis with the final result being the formation of polyps. Over 50 percent of patients with polyps do not have allergic rhinitis. Chronic infection may be significant in such patients. In patients with a chronic allergic process, both mechanisms may be implicated, as secondary chronic infection is not infrequent. Rappaport [36] believes that infection is the major factor in the development of polyps in patients with severe chronic allergic rhinitis.

The typical allergic nasal mucous polyp appears grossly as a smooth, soft, glistening mass usually bluish white in color. It is attached to the nasal or sinal mucosa by a narrow stalk. It may look gelatinous and often appear as a grapelike mass. Microscopic examination reveals the polyp to consist mainly of edema fluid. The nasal mucosa covering the polyp may be squamous in nature rather than columnar with an absence of cilia. Perivascular infiltration by leukocytes and eosinophils is usually found. In addition, thickening of the basement membrane may be seen along with hypertrophy and dilatation of the mucous glands. The mucopolysaccharides in the ground substance lose their ability to take up a PAS stain, suggesting the presence of hydrophilic colloid.

Polyps associated with chronic infection appear more granular, firm, and reddened than those primarily associated with allergic disease. Morphologically, there is an increase in fibrous tissue in the submucosa associated with marked polymorphonuclear cellular infiltration. Few eosinophils are found. In polyps associated with both allergic and infectious elements, varying degrees of both types of pathologic findings may be present, depending upon the severity and duration of the various factors.

Symptoms. The patient with chronic allergic rhinitis or chronic sinusitis may not be aware of the presence of relatively large nasal polyps. Symptoms of perennial rhinitis or sinusitis usually cause these patients to seek medical care. The most distressing symptom is that of continual nasal congestion which is resistant to local and systemic decongestant therapy. Rarely, the patient may note large polyps appearing at the external nasal orifice. An additional common complaint is the loss of smell or taste. Since nasal polyps have a marked tendency to recur, some patients may give a history of having had multiple polypectomies.

Diagnosis. Most nasal polyps can be seen on physical examination particularly with the use of a nasal speculum. Those associated with allergy, usually appear as gray or white gelatinous, glistening masses and those associated with chronic infection appear more erythematous, granular, and firm. Purulent secretions may be observed around those polyps associated with chronic infection. Radiographic films are necessary to diagnose paranasal sinus polyps. These will appear as rounded shadows within the sinus cavity or completely fill the sinus making it opaque.

Treatment. Surgical removal of nasal polyps is usually indicated if they produce marked nasal obstruction. Usual symptomatic therapy will not afford the patient with this degree of involvement much relief. Because of the high rate of recurrence of nasal polyps, surgery should be reserved for those cases with marked nasal obstruction or obstruction which causes recurrent infections. In some patients with a history of multiple surgical polypectomies, the periodic use of the dexamethasone nasal spray may be useful in controlling polyp size.

In patients, with allergic rhinitis, intensive allergic management, including immunotherapy, is thought to result in a diminution of the size

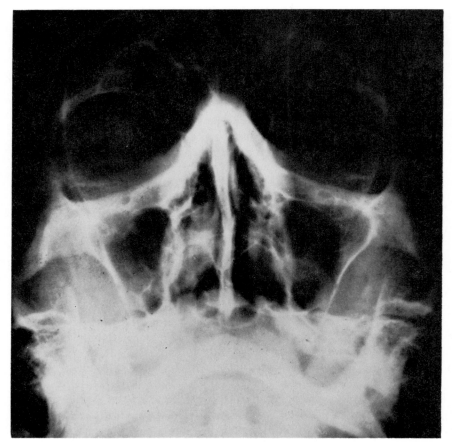

Fig. 6-1. Sinus film, with polyp in left antrum.

or actual disappearance of the nasal polyps. A good program of intensive immunotherapy should be given before surgery is performed for two major reasons. First, this may enable better control of the allergic problem so that the chances for recurrence of the polyps are diminished. Second, it has been suggested that surgical removal of polyps may provoke asthma or even worsen it in some patients. Allergy injection therapy may lessen this complication, although no studies are available to support this opinion.

Triad of Nasal Polyps, Asthma, and Aspirin Sensitivity

Certain patients exhibit a marked tendency to have recurrent nasal polyps. Some of these patients have severe asthma of unknown etiology and a marked sensitivity to aspirin. Several studies have been reported of patients with nasal polyps, asthma, and aspirin sensitivity.[16, 34, 37, 41] The polyps in these patients may antedate the asthma which generally first appears around middle age. Nasal polypectomy has appeared to precede the onset of asthma in some patients. Asthma is the major manifestation of the aspirin sensitivity. Urticaria or angioedema are uncommon expressions of the aspirin sensitivity in patients with this triad. The asthma precipitated by aspirin is severe and occurs within minutes after ingestion. It is often less responsive to usual bronchodilator therapy than ordinary asthma and it may be fatal.

The asthma in patients with this triad may be easily managed by standard bronchodilator therapy in its early stages. The asthma may become more refractory and intractable after several years. Samter and Beers [37] recently reported that the overall prognosis was better in a group of 182 patients that they studied than that suggested in the older literature. Aspirin intolerance is not considered to be the cause of the nasal polyps or asthma because the respiratory symptoms usually precede the appearance of aspirin sensitivity and continue even if aspirin ingestion is completely avoided.

The mechanism of aspirin intolerance is not understood. Circulating antibodies against aspirin which mediate the reaction have not been conclusively demonstrated in such patients. Because local positive reactions do not occur in these patients skin tests to aspirin are not helpful and are contraindicated, since severe systemic reactions may occur.[9] Few patients with this triad have unequivocal evidence of an atopic state, suggesting that aspirin sensitivity is not due to a classic IgE-mediated allergy.

Three nonimmunologic mechanisms have been suggested as possible causes of the adverse aspirin reactions. Samter and Beers [37] postulate that aspirin acts directly upon respiratory mucous membranes and skin chemoreceptors which have been altered by a preexisting disease. This increased activity of the chemorecptors to chemical mediators then results in smooth muscle contraction, capillary permeability, and mucous secretion: the characteristics of allergic reactions. Yurchak et al [47] suggest that aspirin might activate certain complement components directly releasing "anaphylatoxins" which then release histamine. They also suggest that aspirin may inactivate a hypothetical enzyme system, which, because of a deficiency of the enzyme's inhibitor in the aspirin sensitive patient, could lead to tissue damage and release of various chemical mediators.

The diagnosis of aspirin sensitivity is made by history. Occasionally patients may not recognize that aspirin is the inciting agent since it occurs in many combination "cold" tablets and analgesics. Therefore the history must be detailed carefully. An oral challenge dose of aspirin is contraindicated, because it can precipitate a violent, even fatal, reaction. Patients known to be sensitive to aspirin should be warned of its presence in most over-the-counter cold and headache remedies. Because of the possibility of sudden unexpected development of aspirin sensitivity, it is suggested that patients who exhibit nasal polyps and asthma should avoid medications containing aspirin whether or not a history of aspirin sensitivity has been obtained.

Serous Otitis Media

Serous otitis media is characterized by the accumulation of fluid in the middle ear associated with a conductive hearing loss. It is a frequent complication in children with chronic allergic rhinitis.[28] Factors other than allergy, such as bacterial and viral infections, chronic adenoiditis, congenital abnormalities of the eustachian tube, hypertrophied adenoidal tissue, and sinusitis, have also been implicated as causes of this condition.[11, 14, 21] Obstruction of the eustachian tube is followed by the absorption of air creating negative pressure in the middle ear. A transudation of serum then appears in the middle ear. The fluid varies in consistency from a thin watery material to a thick viscous mucoid material. The peak age of incidence of this disease is between 5 and 7 years. A history of recurrent earaches and a loss of hearing in a child with perennial or seasonal allergic rhinitis should alert the physician to serous otitis media. A fluctuating or constant hearing loss is characteristic of this condition in addition to the characteristic symptoms of allergic rhinitis. Allergic factors have been implicated in from 14 to 80 percent of children with serous otitis media.[4, 13, 23] If the child exhibits symptoms of allergic rhinitis, an allergic evaluation is indicated. Presumptive evidence for allergy is the finding of significant numbers of eosinophils in the middle ear effusion or in a nasal smear. Inhalant allergens are the major offenders in cases of allergic serous otitis media. Allergy may also be a contributing factor in children with infection or adenoidal hyperplasia and should not be overlooked.

Management of serous otitis media associated with allergic rhinitis consists of antihistamines, oral decongestants, hyposensitization, and environmental control measures. Until adequate control of the accumulation of fluid occurs following initiation of these measures, it may be necessary to surgically remove the fluid and prevent its reaccumulation. Treatment of other contributing factors such as infection and enlarged adenoids is also indicated. Failure to recognize allergic factors in this complication will result in treatment failures and, often, serious, permanent hearing loss.

REFERENCES

1. Abboud, F. M.: Clinical importance of the adrenergic receptors. Arch. Intern. Med., *118:*418, 1966.
2. Barkin, G. D., and McGovern, J. P.: Allergy statistics. Ann. Allerg., *24:*602, 1966.
3. Broder, I., Barlow, P. P., and Horton, R. J. M.: The epidemiology of asthma and hay fever in a total community, Tecumseh, Michigan. 2. The relationship between asthma and hay fever. J. Allerg., *33:*524, 1962.
4. Chan, J. C. M., Logan, G. B., and McBean, J. B.: Serous otitis media and allergy. Relation to allergy and other causes. Amer. J. Dis. Child., *114:*684, 1967.
5. Chronic Condition and Activity Limitation. Public Health Service Publication No. 1000, Series 10, No. 17. U. S. Government Printing Office, Washington, 1965.
6. Connell, J. T., and Sherman, W. B.: Hay fever symptoms related to immunological findings. Ann. Allerg., *25:*239, 1967.
7. Connell, J. T.: Quantitative intranasal pollen challenges. III. The priming effect in allergic rhinitis. J. Allerg., *43:*33, 1969.
8. Cooke, R. A., and Vander Veer, A.: Human sensitization. J. Immunol., *1:*201, 1916.
9. Cooke, R. A.: Allergy in drug idiosyncrasy. JAMA, *73:*759, 1919.
10. Criep, L. H.: The march of allergy. Therapeutic results. JAMA, *116:* 572, 1958.
11. Davison, F. W.: Middle ear effusion: the systemic factors. Laryngoscope, *68:*1228, 1958.
12. Di Weese, D. D., and Saunders, W. H.: Textbook of Otolaryngology. ed. 3. pp. 228-231. St. Louis, C. V. Mosby, 1968.
13. Fernandez, A. A., and McGovern, J. P.: Secretary otitis media in allergic infants and children. Southern Med. J., *58:*581, 1965.
14. Fitz-Hugh, G. S., and Stone, R. T.: Serous otitis media in children. A new treatment. Virginia Medical Monthly, *93:*61, 1966.
15. Frankland, A. W.: Seasonal hay fever and asthma treated with pollen extracts. Internat. Arch. Allerg., *6:*45, 1955.
16. Geraldo, B., Blumenthal, M. N., and Spink, W. W.: Aspirin intolerance and asthma. A clinical and immunological study. Ann. Intern. Med., *71:*479, 1969.
17. Goodman, L. S., and Gilman, A.: The Pharmacological Basis of Therapeutics. ed. 4. New York, MacMillan, 1970.
18. Hagy, G. W., and Settipane, G. A.: Bronchial asthma, allergic rhinitis, and allergy skin tests among college students. J. Allerg., *44:*323, 1969.
19. Hill, L. W.: Certain aspects of allergy in children. New Eng. J. Med., *265:*1194, 1961.

20. Holmes, T. H., Goodell, H., Wolf, S., and Wolff, H. G.: Evidence of the genesis of certain common nasal disorders. Am. J. Med. Sc., *218:*16, 1949.

21. Kapun, Y. P.: Serous otitis media in children. Arch. Otolaryng., *79:*38, 1964.

22. Kern, R. A., and Schenck, H. P.: Allergy, a constant factor in the etiology of so-called mucous nasal polyps. J. Allerg., *4:*485, 1933.

23. Lecks, R. I.: Allergic aspects of serous otitis media in childhood. New York J. Med., *61:*2737, 1961.

24. Loveless, M. H.: Immunological studies of pollenosis. IV: The relationship between thermostabile antibody in the circulation and clinical immunity. J. Immunol., *47:*165, 1943.

25. Lowell, F. C., and Franklin, W.: A double-blind study of the effectiveness and specificity of injection therapy in ragweed hay fever. New Engl. J. Med., *273:*675, 1965.

26. Marks, M. B.: Physical signs of allergy of the respiratory tract in children. Ann. Allerg., *25:*310, 1967.

27. May, C. D., Lyman, M., Alberto, R., and Cheng, J.: Immunochemical evaluation of antigenicity of house dust extract. Specificity of dermal wheal reactions and responses to injections for immunotherapy. J. Allerg., *46:*73, 1970.

28. McGovern, J. P., Haywood, T. J., and Fernandez, A. A.: Allergy and secretory otitis media. An analysis of 512 cases. JAMA, *200:*124, 1967.

29. McKee, W. D.: The incidence and familial occurrence of allergy. J. Allerg., *38:*226, 1966.

30. Melam, H. L., Pruzansky, J. J., and Patterson, R.: Correlations between clinical symptoms, leukocyte sensitivity, antigen-binding capacity, and Prausnitz-Kustner activity in a longitudinal study of ragweed pollinosis. J. Allerg., *46:*292, 1970.

31. Newhouse, M., Tagg, B., Polock, S., and McEwan, A.: An epidemiological study of workers producing enzyme washing powders. Lancet, *1:*689, 1970.

32. Pedvio, S., Fox, Z. R., and Bacal, H. L.: Long term follow-up of ragweed hay fever in children. Ann. Allerg., *20:*569, 1962.

33. Phillips, E. W.: Time required for production of hay fever by a newly encountered pollen. J. Allerg., *11:*28, 1939.

34. Prickman, L. E., and Buchstein, H. F.: Hypersensitivity to acetylsalicylic acid (aspirin). JAMA, *108:*445, 1937.

35. Pruzansky, J. J., and Patterson, R.: Immunologic changes during hyposensitization therapy. JAMA, *203:*805, 1968.

36. Rappaport, B. Z.: Physiology of the nose and pathophysiology of allergic rhinitis. *In* Samter, M., *et al.:* Immunological Diseases. Boston, Little, Brown and Co., 1965.

37. Samter, M., and Beers, R. F., Jr.: Intolerance to aspirin. Clinical studies and considerations of its pathogenesis. Ann. Int. Med., *68:*975, 1968.

38. Schwartz, M.: Heredity in Bronchial Asthma. Copenhagen, Munksgaard, 1952.
39. Sherman, W. B.: Hypersensitivity Mechanisms and Management. Philadelphia, W. B. Saunders, 1968.
40. Siegel, S. C., Goldstein, J. D., Sawyer, W. A., and Glaser, J.: Incidence of allergy in persons who have many common colds. Ann. Allerg., *10:*24, 1952.
41. Snyder, R. D., and Siegel, G. L.: An asthma triad. Ann. Allerg., *25:*377, 1967.
42. Soloman, W. R.: Comparative effects of transient body surface cooling, recumbency, and induced obstruction in allergic rhinitis and control subjects. J. Allerg., *37:*216, 1966.
43. Sosman, A. J., Schleuter, D. P., Fink, J. N., and Barborak, J. J.: Hypersensitivity to wood dust. New Engl. J. Med., *281:*977, 1969.
44. Spain, W. C., and Cooke, R. A.: Studies in specific hypersensitiveness. XI. The familial occurrence of hay fever and bronchial asthma. J. Immunol., *9:*521, 1924.
45. Tada, T., and Ishizaka, K.: Distribution of γ E-forming cells in lymphoid tissues of the human and monkey. J. Immunol., *104:*377, 1970.
46. Tennenbaum, J. I.: Immunology and Allergy. *In* Goodman, R. M.: Genetic Disorders of Man. Boston, Little, Brown and Co., 1970.
47. Yurchak, A. M., Wicher, K., and Arbesman, C. E.: Immunologic studies on aspirin. Clinical studies with aspiryl-protein conjugates. J. Allerg., *46:*245, 1970.

7

Asthma: General Concepts

Donald W. Aaronson, M.D.

Bronchial asthma is a disease characterized by an increased responsiveness of the trachea and bronchi to various stimuli. As proposed by the Committee on Diagnostic Standards for Nontuberculous Respiratory Diseases it is an illness which appears to manifest clinically by intermittent episodes of wheezing and dyspnea,[28] it is generally associated with a hyperresponsive state of the bronchi which may be antigen-mediated (allergic). The main characteristic of asthma which differentiates it from other obstructive airway diseases is its reversibility. The great majority of patients with asthma have symptom-free intervals between attacks. In some cases chronic wheezing is present but even in these patients alterations in severity occur.

Although in many instances the allergic state can be demonstrated, this is not always the case. Intrinsic or infectious bronchial asthma has been thought of as having an etiologic relationship with infection, while the acute asthma occurring after the ingestion of aspirin is due to the aspirin. In neither of these instances has an antigen-antibody reaction been demonstrated. The symptoms of wheezing, coughing and shortness of breath may be stimulated by such nonspecific factors as cold air, air pollutants, changes in barometric pressure, psychic factors and varying degrees of exertion. These precipitating factors are not considered to have any etiologic relationships other than nonspecific stimulation. Whatever the etiology, or the precipitating factors, the basic pathology is contraction of bronchial smooth muscle, edema of the bronchial mucosa and hypersecretion of mucus in the bronchial tree. In asthma resulting from an immunologic reaction, the antigen-antibody reaction is thought to result in the release of chemical mediators which produce the pathologic changes. This is incompletely understood. In asthma in which no antigen-antibody reaction is involved, the mechanism is even more uncertain.

INCIDENCE AND SIGNIFICANCE

Asthma is a common condition and, although considered a benign disorder by some, is responsible for a significant number of deaths annually. It is also a disease responsible for a great many days of absence from school or work and is an important disease from the socioeconomic point of view.

Among the diseases which may result from allergy, bronchial asthma is the most important source of morbidity and mortality. The incidence of fatalities has increased through the decade of the 60's although it may now be declining. In England and Wales the annual number of deaths from asthma in patients between the ages of 5 and 64 increased from 720 in 1959 to 1,401 in 1966, with almost doubling of the death rate from 2.0 to 3.7 per 100,000 population.[49] Comparative figures for the United States were not available. Lawrence showed that in the United States in 1964 there were 4,441 deaths from asthma, representing a rate of 2.3 deaths from asthma per 100,000 population.[24] Perhaps even more significant is the fact that an additional 13,000 death certificates listed asthma as an underlying cause; a figure which may signify that this disease is an even greater cause of death than is suspected. In 1964, a further breakdown of the statistics of asthma mortality in the United States revealed that significantly more males died than did females, except during the childbearing years, when more females did. The death rate for nonwhites was from two to five times higher at every age than for whites, except for the oldest age groups, when the rates for the two groups were about the same. If we consider the amount of morbidity caused by asthma, this disease assumes an even greater importance. In 1964 asthma was responsible for 1.3 hospitalizations per 1000 population. As a secondary or contributory diagnosis it assumes even greater importance, since hospital surveys show that the first listed cause of hospitalization constitutes less than half of the total allergic diseases entered in the records. Asthma is the major cause of hospitalization among the allergic diseases. In 1964 in an interview series on chronic disease in the United States, almost 19 million people reported an allergic disease of sufficient importance to be reported to an interviewer. Of these 19 million people, there were about 5.5 million with asthma (53 percent male and 47 percent female). These figures demonstrate that allergic diseases occur in about 10 percent of the population and that about 2.5 percent of the population appear to have significant asthma. This figure may be below the true incidence because of inaccurate reporting. During 1964, about 78 million days of disability caused by asthma were reported and of these there were 30 million days during which the entire day was spent in bed. This represents about 14 days of restricted activity for each asthmatic, and of these, five and one half days were spent completely in bed.

In considering the economics and educational importance of bronchial asthma as a cause of disability in this same reporting period, almost two million out of the total working population of 70 million had asthma. Each of these lost an average of four days of work that year because of asthma. An average of 29,000 persons were absent from work each day because of asthma. Excessive school absence may be important as a cause of economic retardation in later life. Of the 1.2 million school children with asthma there were 6.5 million days of school absence. This represents about 25 percent of all school days lost for all of the chronic diseases combined, and would, therefore, rank asthma as number one in a list of chronic diseases responsible for school absences. These figures demonstrate that bronchial asthma is a national problem of extreme importance.

THE CLINICAL PICTURE

Hereditary Aspects

It has been shown that asthma seems to occur with increased frequency in certain families. Reports of this familial incidence date back to 1650. In 1916 Cooke and Vander Veer showed that 48 percent of a group of patients suffering from bronchial asthma had a family history of this or other allergic diseases, compared to 7 percent in a group of control patients.[14] In 1920, the same figure of 48 percent was reported by Adkinson in a study of 400 asthmatic patients.[1] In 1924, Spain and Cooke studied a group of patients with hay fever and asthma for the occurrence of these same diseases in their families.[48] They found that these occurred in 58.4 percent while the same diseases occurred in only 7 percent of the relatives of controls. The major study of heredity in bronchial asthma was reported in 1952 by Schwartz.[44] He studied the families of 191 patients with asthma, 200 control families and 50 families of patients suffering from Baker's asthma. After establishing a diagnosis of bronchial asthma in the study group as carefully as possible he then divided this group into an allergic category, in which definite precipitating factors could be demonstrated, and a nonallergic group, where no definite precipitating factors could be determined. Although he disclaims a relationship of these groups to the extrinsic and intrinsic categories, to be discussed later, it seems that this may well be the correct relationship. He concluded that "bronchial asthma is a hereditary disease regardless of whether or not it is of definite allergic origin." A study done in 1967 showed that significantly more first degree relatives of patients with asthma suffered from the disease than did first degree relatives of controls and that the mode of inheritance appeared to be a single autosomal dominant gene with incomplete penetrance.[25]

Characteristics

The clinical picture of asthma is the same no matter what the cause or the precipitating factor. It is generally noted to be sporadic in its appearance.

During the symptom-free intervals, results of physical examination may not be abnormal (although, as we shall see later, pulmonary function studies may show reversible airflow obstruction during this stage). In some patients, the diagnosis may have to be made entirely from historical accounts until the patient is seen with clinical symptoms. Not uncommonly, a few short wheezes may be heard during a forced expiratory effort in the asymptomatic patient. In some patients expiratory wheezing at examination is present at all times, regardless of the degree of symptoms described by the patient.

During an attack of asthma, the amount of airway obstruction determines the degree of symptoms and physical findings. In the early or mild episodes, the complaints may only be those of mild chest tightness or cough, and the only physical findings a prolongation of the expiratory phase of respiration. Wheezing may not be heard in the milder episodes. As the episodes of asthma become more severe, we note increasing cough with sputum production, expiratory wheezing along with prolongation of the expiratory phase of respiration, and rhonchi which are progressively more audible. At this stage dyspnea may become apparent. As airway resistance increases we may now note inspiratory wheezing, use of the accessory muscles of respiration in association with hyperinflation and distention of the chest. If this stage occurs somewhat persistently in early childhood, we may find a barrel chest in a teenager or adult.

As the asthma becomes more severe, the patient is noted to be progressively more anxious, restless and apprehensive. He may be found sitting erect or leaning forward and becoming more fatigued and exhausted. At this point serious and possibly fatal diagnostic errors may occur. The fatigued state may result in the appearance of respirations which are less labored and associated with less audible wheezing. This is also associated with a decrease in the inspiratory breath sound, as there is now a decreased amount of air being moved by the greatly fatigued patient. The patient may now progress to respiratory failure with hypercapnia, respiratory acidosis and hypoxemia.

There are no diagnostic radiographic features of asthma. The most frequent picture is that of hyperinflation as a sign of obstructive airway disease with an increased anteroposterior diameter of the chest and an increase in the retrosternal air space along with flattened and depressed diaphragms. Not uncommonly atelectasis may be noted as a result of mucus plugging of bronchi. Patchy pneumonic areas may also be present. There may be noted an increase in the number of eosinophils on examination of the peripheral blood. A moderate leukocytosis may also be noted during the acute episode, which most often is associated with a respiratory infection. There are no specific or diagnostic laboratory findings except for pulmonary function studies. As will be described later these will usually demonstrate the presence of reversible obstructive pulmonary disease.

Examination of the sputum reveals a variable finding at times related to the severity of the asthma. In the mildest stages there may be no sputum produced. The sputum in mild asthma is generally foamy and is clear or white. As the asthma becomes more severe the sputum becomes thicker, more tenacious and mucoid tending to form bronchial casts of mucus. If infection is present the sputum becomes purulent, changing in color to greenish or yellowish. If there has been excessive coughing the sputum may be blood tinged, but the presence of gross blood is uncommon in asthma. Microscopic examination of the sputum in uncomplicated asthma reveals the presence of many eosinophils. These may be entirely replaced by polymorphonuclear cells when infection is present.

Classification

Extrinsic Bronchial Asthma. Extrinsic or atopic bronchial asthma is that form of asthma caused by an immediate type hypersensitivity reaction to allergens. It is considered to be mediated by Immunoglobulin E which is the major carrier of reaginic antibody activity. It has been reported that Immunoglobulin E levels may be elevated in extrinsic asthma and are only uncommonly elevated in intrinsic asthma: [20] This is discussed elsewhere in this volume. This type of asthma begins most frequently between the ages of 3 and 45 years, although it may have its onset at any age. It is most commonly caused by inhalant allergens. Foods as a cause of significant extrinsic asthma are distinctly uncommon.

The diagnosis of extrinsic asthma depends upon a correlation of symptoms with exposure to aeroallergens and confirmation with positive skin tests. The prognosis in extrinsic asthma appears to be significantly better than in intrinsic asthma. The response to bronchodilators as well as to specific therapy is more favorable. Occasionally patients may be seen who at first seem to have extrinsic asthma but whose disease seems to change over the course of several years, the extrinsic factors apparently completely replaced by intrinsic factors. There is no ready explanation for this occurrence.

The major inhalant allergens responsible for reagin-mediated asthma are house dust, mold spores, the various pollens, feathers and animal danders. If foods play much of a role they generally do so in the first year or two of life only and are decidedly unimportant as a cause of asthma after this.

Intrinsic Bronchial Asthma. Intrinsic asthma is that form of the disease in which there is no definite inciting cause. Immediate type hypersensitivity due to inhalant allergens mediated by Immunoglobulin E is not a factor. It generally has its primary onset before age 5 or after age 35. There are no adequate studies of the familial incidence of intrinsic asthma although Schwartz's study suggested the same mode of inheritance and the same familial incidence as in extrinsic asthma. Skin tests to the common inhalant antigens and to foods are usually negative. Even when there are positive skin tests, they are not correlated with the precipitating factors of the disease. It is possible that our testing methods or the allergens used in testing are not sophisticated enough to determine the actual causative factors in intrinsic asthma. It is possible that as we refine our testing we will be able to show extrinsic agents in this category and thereby combine the extrinsic and intrinsic into one group. It is even more likely that this is a noninhalant disease.

Many physicians consider the most important factor in intrinsic asthma to be infection. The manner in which infection affects the asthmatic is obscure. Whether intrinsic asthma is due to an allergic reaction to bacterial or viral antigens or whether these infectious agents are merely nonspecific inflammatory factors is not apparent. Infection may mechanically exacerbate asthma by increasing obstruction of the bronchi and bronchioles because of edema and infiltration of the bronchi, together with increased mucus production. In any event, infection of the bronchial tree is an important factor in intrinsic asthma and not infrequently is the only factor besides the bronchospasm with which we can deal specifically. Skin testing to bacterial antigens is of no value.

The prognosis for remission of intrinsic asthma is not favorable. Chronic asthma which may be difficult to control with the usual modalities of therapy and which may be lifelong is not uncommon. Although some irreversible changes in pulmonary tissue may result from the recurrent infectious processes, they are not thought to be significant, and it is not felt that chronic asthma leads to the development of emphysema.

Mixed Asthma. The term mixed asthma has been applied to patients in whom immediate type reactivity appears to be combined with infectious factors in the production of asthma. Either the allergic or infectious factor will usually predominate, but this may vary in the same patient at different times. The separation of asthma into purely extrinsic or intrinsic is usually difficult.

Aspirin-Induced Asthma. A special category of intrinsic asthma is that induced by the ingestion of aspirin. This may occur as the triad of bronchial asthma, nasal polyposis and severe, potentially fatal, reactions to aspirin. This clinical subject has been reviewed by Samter and Beers.[42] In these patients, symptoms may begin with vasomotor rhinitis manifested initially by rhinorrhea and then followed by severe chronic nasal congestion. The onset of the asthma usually occurs in middle age. The onset of the asthma has seemed to follow nasal polypectomy in some patients. Nasal polypectomy did not seem to be permanently helpful, the polyps generally tended to reappear in a significant number of patients, and multiple polypectomies were required. In these cases of recurrent polyposis no specific therapy seems consistently effective, although topical steroids may reduce polyp size temporarily. The asthma in this syndrome has been described as varying from moderate and fairly responsive to bronchodilators and small doses of corticosteroids, to severe and intractable. These patients have a lower incidence of atopy than expected in a random population. Skin sensitivity tests to aspirin are always negative and provocative oral challenge has been accompanied by fatal reactions and should never be tried. The order of appearance of the triad varies, and the respiratory symptoms may precede the first reaction to aspirin by years.

According to Samter, the time of onset of symptoms after ingestion of aspirin, may vary from 20 minutes to two hours. The reaction usually begins with severe watery rhinorrhea followed by marked flushing of the upper body. Occasionally this may be followed by gastrointestinal symptoms of nausea and vomiting. Wheezing, dyspnea and cyanosis usually occur within minutes of the nasal symptoms. Certain other chemically dissimilar compounds such as indomethacin, hydrazine yellow and mefenamic acid cause a similar reaction. No other salicylate (e.g., sodium salicylate) causes similar reactions in these patients. The pathogenesis of the entity has not been explained.

Non-Antigen Precipitating or Inciting Stimuli in Asthma

A group of triggering factors, which by an irritant type effect may be responsible for a single episode of bronchospasm in the asthmatic individual should be considered. Asthmatic patients have a hyperreactive bronchial tree when compared with normals. Inhalation of aerosols of histamine, acetylcholine or methacholine causes a much greater bronchoconstriction in asthmatics than in normals.[36] The asthmatic bronchial tree appears to be uncommonly sensitive and is susceptible to nonspecific or irritating factors.

Among these nonspecific factors, emotional components have always been stressed. There is no established evidence which proves that the emotions are a primary cause of asthma. Psychic factors are recognized as having a triggering or precipitating effect of varying importance in different patients.

Reversible airway obstruction has been shown to result from exposure to dust or other noxious particles (air pollutants),[30] the inhalation of cold air,[29] chemical irritants, the fumes of fresh paint, gasoline or turpentine or by damp weather or changes in barometric pressure.

Bronchoconstriction after inhalation of sulfur dioxide has been demonstrated.[31] The level of sulfur dioxide used in the study, however, was probably higher than even the levels measured on days of high pollution in many cities in the United States. Increases in respiratory disease are associated with days of high pollution, and asthma is included in the diseases thereby demonstrating a relationship between asthma and air pollutants.[9, 10] The mechanism of action of these factors has not yet been demonstrated adequately, but many of the physiologic changes occurring are the same as those caused by exertion. They will be described below. Although exertion seems to fit the category of nonspecific stimuli, its importance indicates a separate discussion.

Exercise-Induced Asthma

Exercise may cause bronchoconstriction in asthmatic individuals.[21, 23, 26] In all probability wheezing on exertion merely represents the initial stages of developing asthma. There is at this time no indication that exertional asthma has any other relationship to reagin-mediated asthma than do any of the other nonspecific irritating or precipitating factors. In all of these instances the physiologic changes are the same as those occurring in other types of asthma, but no immunologic hypersensitivity has been demonstrated.

Measurements of airflow during exercise reveal that after 1 to 2 minutes there may be bronchodilation which is followed by a progressive fall in the forced expiratory volume to levels denoting mild to severe bronchospasm.[19] The bronchoconstriction is readily prevented by isoproterenol or by disodium chromoglycate inhalation prior to the exercise period,[18] but reports vary as to reversibility by drugs once it is fully established. It should be considered as at least partially reversible following isoproterenol inhalation. McNeill et al. showed, in a few patients, a lessening of the effect of exercise by repeated exercise on the same day.[26] Although the mechanism of exercise asthma is not known, this could suggest mediation via release of a humoral substance, as will subsequently be discussed. Acidosis has also been suggested as the underlying cause.[45] Both of these causes may prove important when this condition is finally explained.

Differential Diagnosis of Wheezing

There are many conditions in which wheezing, coughing and dyspnea are important. A differential diagnosis of some of the more important causes follows:

I. Commonly Encountered Diseases

    A. Bronchial Asthma

    B. Respiratory Infections

        1. Croup (laryngotracheobronchitis) ⎫

        2. Bronchiolitis ⎬ Children

        3. Acute and Chronic Bronchitis ⎫

        4. Pneumonia ⎬ Any Age

    C. Chronic Obstructive Lung Disease

    D. Heart Disease

        1. Left Ventricular Failure

        2. Mitral Stenosis

    E. Hyperventilation Syndrome

    F. Pulmonary Embolism

II. Less Common Problems

    A. Obstructions of the Respiratory Tract

        1. Larynx

            a. Stenosis (lye and burns)

            b. Angioedema

        2. Larynx, Trachea and Bronchi

            a. Neoplasms (benign and malignant)

            b. Foreign Bodies

    B. Mucoviscidosis

    C. Tuberculosis

    D. Pneumonoconiosis

    E. Hypersensitivity Pneumonitis

III. Unusual Disorders

    A. Restrictive Pulmonary Disease

    B. Polyarteritis Nodosa

    C. Pressure from Mediastinal Structures

    D. Diphtheria

    E. Carcinoid Syndrome

    F. Paralysis of the Recurrent Laryngeal Nerve

    G. Immunologic deficiency diseases and recurrent respiratory infections with coughing and wheezing

EVALUATION OF THE PATIENT WITH ASTHMA

The patient may be evaluated in the hospital or in the office. The objectives are the establishment of the diagnosis and establishment of long range therapeutic and rehabilitation programs. An outline of the approach is as follows:

I. Diagnosis
    A. History
    B. Physical Examination
    C. Chest X-Ray
    D. Complete Blood Count
    E. Sputum Examination
    F. Pulmonary Function Studies
    G. Sweat Test (usually only in children)

II. Differential Diagnosis (See the preceding section; each of these should be considered and appropriate diagnostic procedure instituted.)

III. Classification (This is necessary to facilitate an orderly approach to therapy.)
    A. Extrinsic—IgE-mediated hypersensitivity reaction generally to inhaled allergen; may be seasonal or perennial; has a strong family history of atopy; has positive skin tests; eosinophilia up to 10%; generally responds well to therapy
    B. Intrinsic—non-IgE-mediated; probably related to infection; during acute infection may have 10 to 20% eosinophilia; generally negative or noncorrelating skin tests; less responsive to therapy
    C. Mixed—mixture of extrinsic and intrinsic forms with one form generally predominating
    D. ASA Sensitive—usually consists of aspirin sensitivity (severe); bronchial asthma and nasal polyposis; preceded in onset by vasomotor rhinitis; asthma onset usually in middle age; negative skin test to ASA; provocative test with aspirin may cause a fatal reaction
    E. Exercise—may be a special case; rarely is the only cause of wheezing but usually only precedes a full blown case of asthma. May be prevented by isoproterenol, disodium chromoglycate or ephedrine administered prior to exercise

IV. Precipitating factors—any of these may trigger a single asthma attack in the asthmatic patient
    A. Strong odors and fumes: paints, turpentine, perfumes, flowers, chemicals, tobacco smoke

B. Cold air and other weather changes with increase in barometric pressure and humidity

C. Air pollutants

D. Emotions

V. Evaluation of the severity of the asthma—once the diagnosis is established (usually not a difficult problem) and the prognosis considered (more difficult to predict), therapy must be guided by severity of disease and degree of disability. This is done by considering the following:

1. Amount of school or work missed

2. In the case of the mother, ability to maintain the home in normal fashion

3. Frequency of hospitalizations and visits to emergency rooms

4. Response to previous therapy, including previous use of steroids and indications for its use

5. Emotional problems resulting from asthma disrupting normal family life; the effect of the emotional response to the disease must be evaluated and the ability of the patient and his family to deal with the disease must be considered.

6. Complications and associated diseases. These may be the final arbiter of the degree of disability and the ability to cope with the total problem.

FUNCTIONAL ANATOMY OF THE LUNGS

The function of the lungs is for the exchange of gases with the passage into the body of oxygen and the removal of carbon dioxide. The lung is a vast network of capillaries passing through the walls of the alveoli and separated from the air by a thin moist membrane. Air is transported to the alveoli via the trachea and the bronchi with their branching subdivisions. The structure of the bronchi is the same as that of the trachea until they enter the lung (Fig. 7-1) at which time the cartilage rings are replaced by irregularly shaped cartilage plates which completely surround the bronchus. They disappear when the diameter of the bronchiole becomes 1 mm. A smooth muscular layer completely surrounds the bronchus. The lining mucous membrane layer is continuous from the trachea. Mucous and mucoserous glands extend from the tissue surrounding the trachea as far out as the cartilage goes and lie under the muscles. As the bronchi and bronchioles progressively decrease in size on the passage to the distal sections of the lung, their walls become progressively thinner. The smooth muscle remains to the end of the respiratory bronchi and into alveolar ducts. The respiratory unit of the lungs

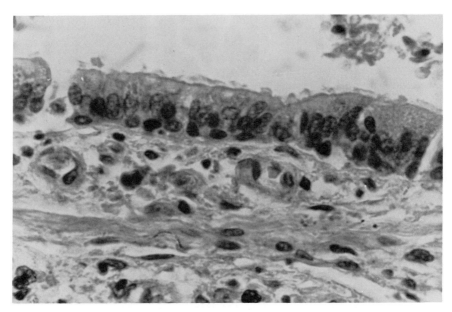

Fig. 7-1. Section of normal bronchial wall showing the normal pseudo-stratified ciliated columnar epithelium with occasional goblet cells and their basement membrane. (× 450)

is that portion beginning with the respiratory bronchioles and extending to and including the alveoli with all of the nerves, lymphatics, blood vessels and connective tissue. The alveoli are thin-walled polyhedral units which are always lacking one side, so that air may freely pass into the alveolar cavity.

The larger bronchi and bronchioles are surrounded by a connective tissue sheath which separates them from the adjacent lung and allows them to change in width and length without affecting this adjacent lung tissue. It becomes a part of the interlacing connective tissue at the area where the cartilage disappears. Since the respiratory unit contains no cartilage, its patency depends upon this network of collagenous, elastic and reticular fibers.[27]

Innervation of the Airways

The autonomic nervous system is responsible for the innervation of the airway.[57] Efferent parasympathetic (vagal) and sympathetic nerves pass through the cardiac and pulmonary plexuses, then spread through the lung to form many plexuses innervating the major components of the respiratory tree. There is also a nerve plexus around the large pulmonary vessels. The parasympathetic postganglionic nerve fibers are derived from all of these plexuses. Two of the three main types of afferent end organs in the bronchial wall appear to be important in terms of reflexly affecting the smooth muscle of the airway. The subepithelial receptors, which lie in the trachea and bronchi and at points of bronchial branching up to the respiratory bronchioles, send many branches between the epithelial cells to terminate just below the ciliary layer. These appear to be responsible for the cough reflex.

The smooth muscle endings which occur throughout the smooth muscle of the respiratory tract and less frequently in the narrower airways, appear to be responsible for the Hering-Breuer inflation reflex which results in bronchodilatation on inflation of the lungs. Although this reflex is probably weak in man as compared to other mammals its importance lies in the fact that with bronchoconstriction and secondary hyperinflation of the lungs this reflex bronchodilatation may help to correct the bronchoconstriction physiologically. It must be noted that this effect is partially countered by the normal muscular contraction which occurs when airway or other smooth muscle is stretched. The smooth muscle of the air passage is in tonic contraction during normal quiet respiration.

The most effective bronchodilating drug is isoproterenol, which can also decrease this tonicity as can vagotomy and epinephrine injections. This effect can be shown by the increase in anatomic dead space, dilation of the air passages and decrease in airway resistance. Acetylcholine and vagal nerve stimulation cause marked bronchoconstriction, as do methylcholine and histamine aerosols. The increased airway resistance resulting from histamine aerosol can be blocked by isoproterenol or atropine. It has been proposed, but not definitely established, that part of the histamine constriction is mediated by nervous pathways.

The Lining Mucous Membrane

The lining epithelium of the trachea and bronchi is a pseudostratified ciliated columnar epithelium which rests on a distinct basement membrane.[27] The ciliated epithelial cells are tall cells with about 270 cilia per cell. Goblet cells, found interspersed among the ciliated cells, are tall, nonciliated cells which secrete mucus. This mucus combines with that secreted by the submucosal mucous glands to overlie the cilia. The cilia themselves are bathed by a watery fluid and covered by the mucus layer. Underlying the basement membrane is a lamina propria consisting of elastic fibers, connective tissue, nerves, blood vessels and lymphatics, together with lymphocytes and mast cells. Beneath this lamina propria are the smooth muscles followed by the bronchial mucous glands and then the cartilaginous layer. The relative volume of the goblet cells to the mucus secreting cells is approximately 1 to 40. In the early phases of an irritative pulmonary state (nonbacterial) the lining respiratory epithelium may change into sheets of goblet cells, however, in the more advanced stages of pulmonary disease they disappear completely with atrophy of the respiratory mucosa. At the same time, the mucous glands undergo hypertrophy and hyperplasia. It has long been recognized that acetylcholine is active as a chemical mediator in stimulating these cells. Since the mechanism for removal of particulate matter from air prior to its passage into the lungs is not completely effective, this is one of the functions of the overlying mucus blanket. This blanket is constantly being moved towards the trachea and larynx by the continuous beating of the cilia. Nervous control of ciliary action has not yet been established.

Pathologic Changes in Bronchial Asthma

The major physiologic lesion in asthma is the obstruction to air flow which occurs because of three major pathologic changes: smooth muscle contraction, mucosal edema, and production and secretion of a thick tenacious sputum. The pathology of asthma may be studied by consideration of the cytology of the sputum, bronchial biopsy and by evaluation of the entire lung obtained at autopsy from patients dying in status asthmaticus. Several excellent studies of the pathology have been reported.[7, 17]

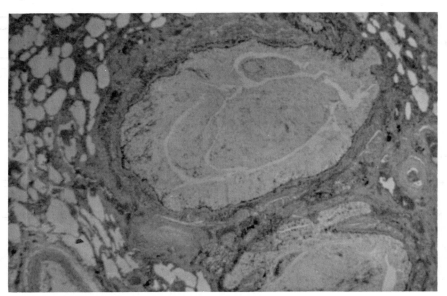

Fig. 7-2. Low power photograph of whole mount of bronchus from lung of patient who succumbed in status asthmaticus. The lumen is filled with a mucoid plug. (See Fig. 7-3 for details.)

On opening the chest of patients who have died in status asthmaticus, it is observed that the grossly overdistended lungs fail to collapse.[7] Occasionally, atelectasis may be noted. The cut surface of the lungs allows observation of the bronchi, many of which demonstrate obstruction with gray, glistening, thick, tenacious, plugs of mucus. Areas of cystic bronchiectasis have been found distal to areas of complete occlusion of a bronchus.[17] There is no evidence that destructive emphysema of the centrilobular, panacinar or bullous varieties occurs more frequently in patients with asthma than in the general population. Subpleural pneumonic lesions which progress to fibrosis have been noted in the superior and anterior margins of the lungs. These have been considered to be due to an allergic pneumonitis which eventually causes scarring.

The most striking aspect in examination of histologic sections from the lung of an asthmatic dying in status asthmaticus is the mucous exudate completely occluding the bronchi (Fig. 7-2, 7-3). The mucus contains

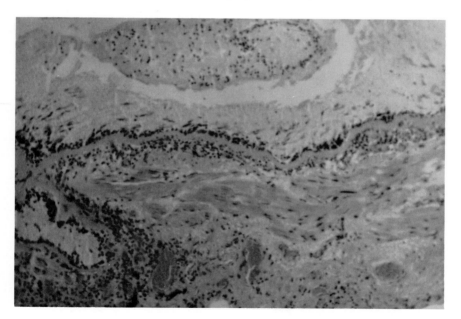

Fig. 7-3. High power field from Figure 7-2. The hypersecreting goblet cells have dissolved into a sea of mucus. The basement membrane is prominently thickened. The underlying muscularis is hypertrophied. The subepithelial tissue is edematous, congested, and contains inflammatory cells which can be identified as eosinophils and lymphocytes in the original sections. The bronchial mucous glands in the lower left corner are not especially hyperplastic in this field.

large numbers of eosinophils and variable numbers of clusters of columnar epithelial cells. These cells are considered to be fragments of mucosa
which had become detached from the lower respiratory tract. They are
found almost exclusively in the sputum of asthmatics, and in even greater
quantity in the sputum of asthmatics during attacks of asthma. It has
been suggested that they contribute even more to the difficulty in
clearance of mucus from the lower respiratory tract and thereby to a
worsening prognosis. It has been shown that increased numbers of clusters of epithelial cells correlated generally with duration of hospitalization
for asthma.[32] The mucus itself is not homogeneous. It consists of a mixture of mucous and serous components. In examination of the mucosa
of the bronchi of patients dying in status asthmaticus normal areas are
difficult to find. Mucosal edema as well as separation of mucosal cells is
evident. There are areas of metaplastic regenerating epithelium at many
points. No cilia are seen.

There is also marked thickening of the basement membrane which
was thought to be characteristic but is also seen in other conditions.[16]
Histologic evaluation of lung parenchymal tissue reveals no characteristic
lesions. The changes herein described are those associated with death
from status asthmaticus. It must be remembered that the less severe
episodes must be associated with less marked pathology. It is logical
that the prominent mucus plugging of the bronchioles in fatal status
asthmaticus is not as important in the clinically less severe cases. In
these instances smooth muscle contraction is a more important factor. It
is not felt that bronchospasm results in the shedding of the mucosal
cells.[32]

PHYSIOLOGY OF ASTHMA

The reaction which we clinically refer to as extrinsic bronchial asthma,
occurs as the result of release of certain chemicals into tissues or into the
bloodstream, following a reaction between antigen and antibody.
Whether this same mechanism exists in intrinsic asthma has not yet
been established. The specific antibody responsible for the reaction of
extrinsic asthma is skin-sensitizing antibody or reaginic antibody, classified as belonging to Immunoglobulin E. The IgE antibodies have been
discussed in more detail elsewhere in this book. They are found in serum
and nasal washings and in sputum obtained from some asthmatic patients. Apparently they are more common in patients with extrinsic or
mixed asthma than in those with intrinsic asthma but are found in both
groups of patients. The major mediators which have been considered
are histamine, slow reacting substance of anaphylaxis (SRS-A), acetylcholine, serotonin, bradykinin, prostaglandins, rabbit aorta contracting

substance (RCS) and permeability factors. Other mediators have also been described, including those of the autonomic nervous system. It has been shown that IgE will sensitize monkey tissues for antigen-induced release of histamine and SRS-A.

Chemical Mediators of the Allergic Reaction

Histamine. In the past it had been thought that the most important of the mediators was histamine. Research, however, into the other mediators noted above, has raised questions concerning its role. Histamine is formed from C-Histidine by decarboxylation.[6] It is present in many tissues in minute amounts, and is found in the granules of tissue and free mast cells of many species. It is probably stored as a complex with a protein from which it is readily displaceable. That it is also present in other cells such as basophils and also in rabbit platelets in much smaller quantity is also agreed. It was shown by Schild et al. to be specifically present in lungs.[43] They demonstrated its release from isolated portions of lungs, removed at surgery from asthmatic patients, when the tissue was exposed to antigens to which the patient was sensitive. Its major pharmacologic actions involve primarily smooth muscles, the vascular system and exocrine glands. Of primary importance is the observation that histamine causes contraction of smooth muscle, including human bronchioles. Many studies have shown that patients with asthma are much more susceptible to histamine than are persons without asthma. Histamine also stimulates many of the exocrine glands, particularly the gastric glands but also the nasal, lacrimal and probably the bronchial glands.[6] After intradermal injection there is a reaction of capillary dilatation, a diffuse flare because of dilatation of surrounding arterioles caused by local axon reflexes and localized vascular edema. It is this response which probably occurs when there is histamine release due to tissue injury. It has also been shown that histamine has a role in stimulating phagocyte mobilization and in facilitating tissue repair, by the indirect mechanism of releasing ground substance material from mast cells.[6] Histamine given intravenously causes headache, flushing of the face and a drop in carotid pressure. For all of these described actions of histamine, its specific role in body function is yet to be established. It has been suggested that the antigen-antibody induced release of histamine does not disrupt cell membranes but is rather a specific reaction of degranulation of mast cells and basophils.

SRS-A. Slow reacting substance released by anaphylaxis was first described in 1940 by Kelloway and Trethewice,[22] but its significance has not yet been established and its structure is unknown. Several different preparations have been called SRS-A. It has been suggested that in guinea pigs, conditions which cause SRS-A formation also lead to histamine release. Both of these substances usually appear together. A number of liberators of SRS-A have been demonstrated, including snake and bee venoms, phospholipase A,[55] antigen acting on sensitized tissue. Vogt has defined SRS-A as "all those substances which slowly contract the guinea pig ileum and are released from tissues or cells as opposed to body fluids like plasma—by any injury or potentially injurious stimulation." [55] It has been shown by Brocklehurst that "human bronchioles in vitro, and the bronchial tree in vivo, show a long lasting bronchoconstriction in the presence of amounts of SRS-A no greater than those obtained from asthmatic lung challenged by allergen in vitro." [6] This action is not blocked by antihistamines. The prolonged bronchospasm in asthma may be primarily caused by SRS-A and the development of specific therapy against this substance may improve therapy of bronchial asthma.

Miscellaneous Mediators. No role has been established linking serotonin with human anaphylaxis.[6] It is important in immediate type reactions in rats and mice.

Bradykinin is the best known of a group of plasma substances called kinins.[6] It causes contraction of many types of smooth muscle, including bronchial smooth muscle; causes increased vascular permeability; and possibly stimulates bronchial mucous gland secretion. It has been shown that kinins are formed during anaphylactic shock in animals. Bradykinin inhalation has been shown to cause significant bronchoconstriction in a group of asthmatics, whereas there was no effect in a group of controls. The production of symptoms by bradykinin depends upon the duration of its presence prior to its destruction. This rate of destruction is unknown.

Acetycholine was once thought to be a mediator of importance in asthma because atropine had been shown to be useful in relieving bronchospasm, especially that induced by mecholyl, a derivative of acetylcholine. No evidence exists suggesting a direct relationship for acetylcholine, and its release in anaphylaxis has not been demonstrated.

Prostaglandins are a group of hydroxyaliphatic acids found in many tissues and released in a number of conditions. Piper and Vane recently showed that prostaglandins F2a and E2 were present after anaphylaxis in guinea pigs.[37] They suggest that large quantities may be released in the lungs in anaphylaxis. Some of the prostaglandins have been shown to increase airway resistance in the cat and guinea pig. One of the prostaglandins reduces histamine-induced bronchoconstriction in guinea pigs. Other reports are equally confusing. They do not appear to be important mediators and the last noted may even be a therapeutic agent. The role of prostaglandins is under intensive investigation.

A substance released following anaphylaxis in the lungs strongly contracts the rabbit aorta. It has been called rabbit aorta constricting substance (RCS). It is released within a few seconds of anaphylactic shock. Its activity disappears after standing at room temperature for 20 minutes. This short life probably explains the long delay in discovery of this compound. Its role as a mediator has not yet been determined.[37]

Some other substances which may play a role in mediating allergic responses should be mentioned. Several permeability factors have been described. G2 alphaglobulin may be important in increasing vascular permeability, particularly in vessels already altered by histamine or bradykinin. In addition to increasing vascular permeability, another factor, lymph node permeability factor also may play a role in leukotaxis into areas of allergic reactions. Another mediator may be anaphylatoxin the generation of which is intimately related to c'3, the fifth component of complement. It is generated by immune precipitates among others. Its presence may have some role in histamine release.

Autonomic Mediators. A number of autonomic nervous system mediators must be considered in relation to allergic reactions. It has been proposed by some workers, that the underlying defect in asthma is a deficit in or abnormal function of the enzyme, adenyl cyclase. Several recent reviews summarize this system well and point out the early state of the development of our knowledge.[33, 51, 52] In brief review, it is postulated that cyclic 3'5' adenosine monophosphate (cyclic AMP) mediates the actions of a great many hormones upon cells. This is accomplished via the action of the hormone on adenyl cyclase, which catalyzes the formation of cyclic AMP from ATP. Cyclic AMP then goes on to effect the end result of the hormone stimulation within the cell. Adenyl cyclase has been found in the cell membranes of all animal tissues studied to date. Most hormones act by increasing cyclic AMP, probably by stimulating adenyl cyclase. The only enzyme known to inactivate cyclic AMP is phosphodiesterase, which converts it to 5' AMP. This enzyme has been shown to be inhibited by a number of drugs. Levels of cyclic AMP, therefore, may be increased by blocking its degradation by phosophodiesterase or by increasing its production by stimulating adenyl cyclase. Among hormones which have been shown to stimulate adenyl cyclase, some of the most prominent are the catecholamines. Although not fully studied, it appears that the results of this stimulation of adenyl cyclase are those clinical effects which have been described as being mediated by alpha and beta adrenergic receptors.

Some explanation of alpha and beta adrenergic receptors is appropriate. Effector or target cells are those which, when activated by contact with certain chemicals, give certain predictable responses. These effector cells are further described as having a receptor site with a steric configuration complementary to that of the effector chemical. Because of natural affinity, the released chemical combines with the complementary receptor site which initiates a series of biochemical reactions resulting in a clinically definable response. It is this clinical response of the receptor to which the name alpha and beta has been given. Unfortunately, as pointed out by Robinson and Associates,[40] "what should be apparent . . . from data of long standing, is that seldom, if ever, has it been possible to define an alpha or beta receptor in one tissue and find that its properties coincide exactly with a similar receptor in another tissue, or even in the same type of tissue in another part of the body, no matter whether the event under consideration is mechanical or metabolic in nature."

With this in mind, a working definition of alpha and beta adrenergic receptors can be advanced. Both are defined by their response to catecholamines. This group of responses varies in various tissues, and other sources should be consulted for a complete review. For practical purposes, a working classification would describe an alpha effect as that causing contraction of smooth muscles as manifested by bronchial contraction, contraction of the iris dilator of the eye, of the trigone and sphincter of the bladder, of the myometrium, of the splenic capsule and of vasoconstriction. A beta receptor effect would be described as that resulting in vasodilation and smooth muscle relaxation, as manifested by bronchial relaxation, relaxation of the ciliary muscle, of the detrusor muscle of the bladder and the myometrium. The beta receptor has been postulated as adenyl cyclase. Stimulation of the production of this enzyme would, in mechanisms already described, result in effects referred to as beta responses. The alpha receptor is even more poorly established. It has been suggested that adenyl cyclase is both the beta and the alpha receptor.[41] A reaction with an alpha agent would then result in a decrease in adenyl cyclase activity while reaction with a beta agent would stimulate the same activity.

As Ahlquist pointed out, "Although a receptor is a very useful concept to describe drug actions, tissue responses and structure-activity relationships, it should be kept in mind that invoking a receptor mechanism does not explain the real nature of the interaction between a tissue and a drug. When better knowledge of a receptor is obtained, for example, the exact identification of the enzyme or enzyme system involved, the need for the receptor vanishes."[2] We know that antigen-antibody reactions result in the release of a number of chemical mediators described above. These mediators may result in a group of clinical responses which we describe as alpha or beta in nature. Similar responses may also be caused by a group of other nonspecific factors such as infection, air pollutants of various kinds, aspirin, exertion and cold. Because of this, it has been proposed that asthma is a deficiency in or a partial blockade of beta receptors in the lung. This merely means that we are still unable to characterize the mechanisms of the bronchoconstrictive response for every stimulus at the cellular level. In the light of our current thinking, however, certain drug actions can or should be expected, based upon the above considerations.

NORMAL PULMONARY PHYSIOLOGY

The lungs play a major role in assuring that adequately oxygenated blood is distributed to the tissues of the body, and that sufficient carbon dioxide is removed. Both of these functions are altered in asthma. In order to understand the effects of asthma on pulmonary ventilation, a knowledge of normal ventilatory physiology is necessary. For greater detail, reference can be made to one of the standard texts.[3, 13, 15, 47]

The role of the lungs in oxygenating venous blood and removing carbon dioxide is achieved by a process of pulmonary gas exchange involving three primary functions. The first is ventilation which involves provision of an adequate volume of inspired air evenly distributed to all of the alveoli and then traveling the reverse route. The second function is diffusion, which involves the passage of these gases across the alveolar membrane from and to the pulmonary capillary blood. The third function is that which involves the circulation, both in assuring that all the venous blood is presented evenly to all of the ventilated capillaries and that it then adequately reaches all the other tissues of the body. Each of these processes will be considered, because they may be altered by the abnormalities that occur in the physical state known as asthma.

Lung Volumes and Capacities

In order to understand many of the studies of ventilation, lung volumes and capacities within which this ventilation takes place must be defined. Lung volumes (the four primary volumes do not overlap): (1) *Tidal volume* (Vt) is the volume of gas inspired or expired during each respiratory cycle. (2) *Inspiratory reserve volume* (IRV) is the maximal amount of gas that can be inspired from the end-inspiratory position. (3) *Expiratory reserve volume* (ERV) is the maximal volume of gas that can be expired from the end-expiratory level. (4) *Residual volume* (RV) is the volume of gas remaining in the lungs at the end of a maximal expiration. Lung capacities (each of the four capacities includes two or more of the lung volumes); (1) *Total lung capacity* (TLC) is the volume of gas contained in the lung at the end of a maximal inspiration. (2) *Vital capacity* (VC) is the maximal volume of gas that can be expelled from the lungs by a forceful effort following a maximal inspiration. (3) *Inspiratory capacity* (IC) is the maximal volume of gas that can be inspired from the resting expiratory level. (4)

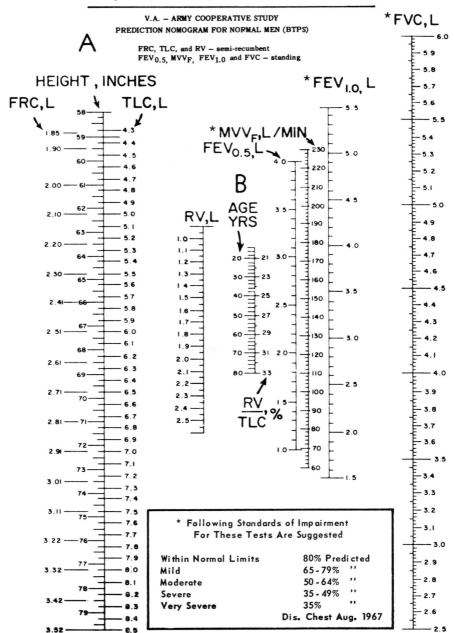

V.A. – ARMY COOPERATIVE STUDY
PREDICTION NOMOGRAM FOR NORMAL MEN (BTPS)

A

FRC, TLC, and RV – semi-recumbent
$FEV_{0.5}$, MVV_F, $FEV_{1.0}$ and FVC – standing

HEIGHT , INCHES

FRC,L   TLC,L

*FEV$_{1.0}$, L

*MVV$_F$,L /MIN
FEV$_{0.5}$,L

B

RV,L   AGE
          YRS

RV
——,%
TLC

*FVC,L

* Following Standards of Impairment
  For These Tests Are Suggested

Within Normal Limits	80% Predicted
Mild	65-79% ''
Moderate	50-64% ''
Severe	35-49% ''
Very Severe	35% ''

Dis. Chest Aug. 1967

Figure 7-4

Functional residual capacity (FRC) is the volume of gas remaining in the lung at the resting expiratory level. Many of these measurements can be made in the office.

The vital capacity and its subdivisions can be measured by having the patient breathe into a recording spirometer, bellows or meter. Standard nomograms for this and all other measurements of ventilation are readily available; a useful one is in Figure 7-4. The functional residual capacity and total lung capacity measurements usually cannot be done in the physicians' office,[8] since these measurements require gas analyses which are usually available only in pulmonary function testing laboratories.

The FRC may be determined by several methods. In the nitrogen washout method, the patient inspires pure oxygen while expiring into a spirometer in an open circuit for seven minutes. During this time, almost all of the nitrogen originally present is washed out of the lung and into the spirometer. At the end of the test, the amount of nitrogen is calculated from the concentration of nitrogen and the volume of gas in the spirometer. The nitrogen concentration in the lungs at the end of the test is also determined. Since we know that the patient breathing room air is breathing 80 percent nitrogen and since we know how many milliliters of N_2 were in his lungs at the start of the study (it was washed into the spirometer and then measured), the FRC can now be calculated as the milliliters of N_2 washed out of the lung $\times$ 100/80. Other methods can also be employed for which standard texts should be consulted. The residual volume equals the functional residual capacity minus the expiratory reserve volume. Total lung capacity is usually calculated by measuring FRC and adding the inspiratory capacity. It may be estimated from the calculated normal vital capacity by dividing vital capacity by 0.8 for ages 15 to 34 years, 0.75 for 35 to 49 years and 0.65 for 50 years of age and over.[13]

METHODS OF TESTING LUNG FUNCTIONS

Spirographic recordings of normal breathing patterns together with those of forced inspiration, forced expiration, and maximum voluntary ventilation, allow us to analyze breathing patterns. Although these tests are not completely objective, since they require the cooperation of the patient, they usually are the initial tests carried out and point the way to further testing. Since the major respiratory disorders involve disturbances in airflow and since these measurements of airflow in and out of the lungs can readily be done in the office, they have become an important part of the diagnostic evaluation.

Many available varieties of spirometers with rapidly moving kymographs have recently been reviewed.[8] The devices which provide a graphic recording of both flow and volume are the most practical. The

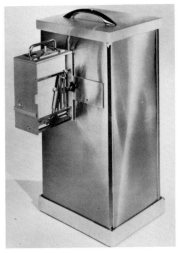

Fig. 7-5. The Jones Pulmonor—A useful spirometer for office evaluation of breathing patterns, flow rates, and volumes. (Jones Medical Instruments, Oak Brook, Ill.)

Jones Pulmonor (Fig. 7-5) is a very useful recording instrument which can be used with both children and adults and gives fairly accurate and reproducible results. As you can see (Fig. 7-6) the spirographic recording of the pulmonor allows for a number of calculations. Since abnormalities in airflow are most apparent when maximal amounts of airflow are measured, the forced expiratory volume (FEV) in which the patient is asked to inspire maximally then blow out as fast and as hard as he can, is a very useful measurement. If a machine with a rapid paper speed is used, a fairly quantitative measurement can be obtained. The normal patient will be able to expel 75 percent of the FEV in the first second (FEV_1 75%), 85 percent by the end of the second second and 95 percent by the end of three seconds. Another very useful measurement, the maximal midexpiratory flow rate (MMFR) can also be calculated from the FEV curve. This measurement is of the mid-50 percent of the FEV curve and can easily be calculated. In routine work, there is value in calculating both FEV_1 and MMFR to make it easier to detect errors in the calculation of either of these procedures.

Another measurement which can be simply made in the office is the maximum breathing capacity (MBC) or maximum voluntary ventilation (MVV). This is the maximal volume of air that an individual can breathe per minute. It is measured by having a subject breathe maximally for 15 seconds. It should be remembered that the duration of the test period requires a greater than normal amount of cooperation from the patient and a physical ability to breathe maximally for this length of time. In addition, it may be greatly influenced by the use of instruments with high resistance. With these limitations in mind, the MBC is still highly useful as an indication of overall ventilatory capacity.

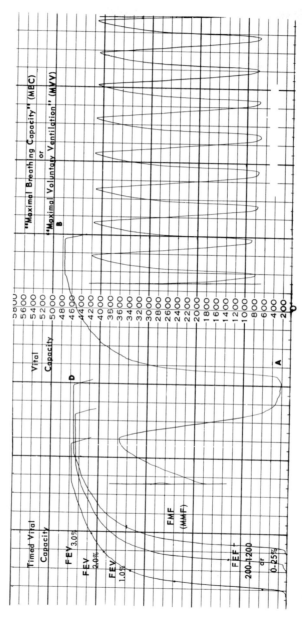

Fig. 7-6. Spirographic recording of Jones Pulmonor demonstrating that vital capacity, timed vital capacity and maximum breathing capacity can be measured on a single graph. (Jones Medical Instruments, Oak Brook, Ill.)

INTERPRETATION OF SPIROGRAPHIC CURVES

Evaluation of the spirographic data just discussed should begin with an overall inspection of the graph. Certain inferences can be drawn from this concerning patient cooperation and a gross estimate of the normality or abnormality of the vital capacity or the ventilatory capacity. The emotionally distressed patient can be recognized by a pattern of hyperventilation with increased rate and depth of respiration, irregularity of the breathing pattern and frequent deep inspirations. The elevation of the spirographic recording of the MBC which may occur with the first few breaths or persist throughout, is a sign of increased airway resistance and outflow obstruction.[47] If one notes notching (2 or occasionally 3 notches) of the initial portion of the expiratory recording of the MBC or FVC, this indicates airway collapse due to loss of normal airway support.[47] This is a common finding in moderately severe emphysema. A pattern of rapid and regular respirations of low tidal volume is seen in patients with very low vital capacities and diffuse bronchopulmonary fibrosis.

All of the capacities and volumes of the lung which have been described vary with the age, sex, height and posture of the patient. There is, therefore, a broad range of normal values. The proportion of the total lung capacity taken up by each of these volumes is quite stable over the range of varying physical characteristics. Vital capacity represents about 75 percent of the total lung capacity while the residual volume represents the other 25 percent. Functional residual capacity represents about 40 percent of the total lung capacity. Vital capacity depends upon patient cooperation. Malingering, or lack of understanding of instructions therefore may be responsible for abnormalities. The vital capacity may vary as much as 20 percent from the average and still be normal. It may also vary as much as 200 ml. from the mean in a single patient with multiple repeat studies. Changes of 250 ml. or more in the same patient are considered significant if daily or weekly measurements are made in the same patient and in the same way.[11] In a patient whose predicted normal vital capacity was 4000 ml. a reading of 3400 ml. therefore could be considered normal, as it is only 15 percent below the predicted. If repeat studies after specific therapy for bronchial obstructive disease revealed an improvement in vital capacity to 3800 ml., then the originally determined value of 3400 ml. would not have been normal. Serial measurements of vital capacity are useful, therefore, in following the effectiveness of drug therapy in the treatment of asthma. Serial determinations of MVV are probably of more value, however, in following the effectiveness of drug therapy.[13] There may be a narrowing of the bronchioles great enough to cause increased resistance to airflow but not enough to completely block the airway and thereby decrease the vital capacity. Other causes of decreased vital capacity include (1) an absolute decrease in the amount of distensible lung tissue due to causes such as large neoplasms or pneumonia; (2) a decrease in expansion of the thorax or the lungs by causes such as pneumothorax, pain from rib fracture, scleroderma or myasthenia gravis; and (3) a limitation of diaphragm descent due to pregnancy or phrenic nerve lesions. Since a decreased vital capacity may occur in so many conditions, it has no diagnostic significance by itself. A normal vital capacity is not uncommon in pulmonary emphysema, so that normal values do not assure normal lungs. It cannot, therefore, be relied upon as an isolated test. In conjunction with other tests and for repeated testing over a period of time it is very useful.

Changes in the expiratory reserve volume are not generally useful in diagnosis of abnormal pulmonary function. An increased functional residual capacity shows hyperinflated lungs during quiet breathing, while an increase in residual volume denotes that the lung has remained hyperinflated after a maximal expiratory effort. These two capacities may return to normal in patients with bronchial asthma but may remain abnormally elevated in patients with emphysema, or those with persistent bronchial obstruction caused by such things as secretions or edema. In elderly patients an elevated functional residual capacity may not signify an abnormality of lung function. It has been noted that alveolar ventilation is more important to good function than is alveolar volume, as the major requirement is to maintain alveolar Po_2 at about 100 mg. Hg to insure adequate oxygenation of the blood. This is primarily a ventilatory requirement, as it only requires the replacement of the volume of O_2 removed per minute by the blood. An increased FRC is undesirable when rapid changes in alveolar gas composition are desired, as the equilibration time is longer. It is also a disadvantage because of muscular inefficiency and the increased mechanical work requirements to move this volume of air. If both FRC and RV are increased, then, barring an increase in total lung capacity, there must be a decrease in both vital capacity and inspiratory capacity, which results in a lessened capacity to increase ventilatory volume. A very small FRC leads to a disadvantage because of wide fluctuations of alveolar Po_2 throughout the respiratory cycle, ultimately leading to uneven ventilation and slight hypoxemia.

A somewhat useful ratio is that of the residual volume to total lung capacity. This represents the proportional amount of lung tissue which cannot be used to increase ventilation. The normal value is 20 to 35 percent. An increased value may represent an increase in absolute volume, as in emphysema or asthma, or a decreased total lung capacity as in pulmonary restrictive diseases or with pulmonary congestion. The value of the ratio over 35 percent does not in itself mean pulmonary insufficiency, since the aged may have a value up to 50 percent with little or no disability.

PULMONARY VENTILATION

Concern with alveolar ventilation and assurance that the volume of ventilation and its distribution are adequate to maintain, at optimal levels, the partial pressures of O_2 and CO_2 within the alveoli, thereby assuring adequate oxygenation of arterial blood, along with removal of CO_2 is of obvious importance. It is, therefore, recognized that the supply of O_2 each minute must be equal to the O_2 requirements each minute. The minute ventilation volume is an important measure of respiration. This minute ventilatory volume, however, contains two parts. The first is a volume of air which has not participated in gas exchange, the dead space, and the second volume which does participate in gas exchange, the alveolar ventilation volume. Since these are not anatomic but rather functional spaces, they cannot be measured directly. The dead space consists of two portions. The first is that referred to as the anatomic dead space and consists of the volume of the conducting air passages, i.e., the trachea and bronchial air passages, where no gas exchange occurs. This anatomic dead space may be reduced in asthma because of bronchial obstruction or increased in diseases such as bronchiectasis. The alveolar dead space is more important in consideration of the altered pulmonary physiology of asthma. This space represents that portion of the inspired air which enters the alveoli but does not take part in gas exchange. (Standard texts should be consulted for a discussion of the measurement of alveolar ventilation).[3, 13, 15, 47]

For clinical purposes, alveolar hypoventilation refers to inadequate supply of air into the alveoli to maintain adequate oxygenation or to adequately remove CO_2. Alveolar hypoventilation may be defined by an arterial Pco_2 greater than 44 mg. Hg. The more common causes of alveolar hypoventilation are respiratory center depression (by anesthetics, narcotics, barbiturates or elevated arterial CO_2 concentrations), limited thoracic or lung movement (by diseases of respiratory muscles, scleroderma, or pneumothorax) or, most commonly, by obstructive lung disease (asthma, emphysema or chronic bronchitis). The result of the inadequate movement of air in and out of the alveoli is arterial hypoxemia, carbon dioxide retention and respiratory acidosis. When the patient is breathing high concentrations of O_2, hypoventilation will not result in hypoxemia but only in CO_2 retention and respiratory acidosis. Hypoxemic patients, therefore, given O_2 to breathe, may further complicate their hypoventilation disturbance because of removal of the hypoxic respiratory drive. This may be an important therapeutic consideration, primarily in the older patient with a combination of bronchial asthma and pulmonary emphysema.

Alveolar hyperventilation is defined as ventilatory effort greater than that required for maintenance of normal arterial oxygen and carbon dioxide pressures. It may also be defined by an arterial Pco_2 less than 38 mm. Hg. The most common cause, one which plays a role in the differential diagnosis of asthma, is the hyperventilation syndrome, acute or chronic. Other causes include hypoxia, hypothyroidism, fever, drugs such as epinephrine, and pain responses. Hyperventilation results in decreased aleveolar partial pressure of CO_2 and increased partial pressure of O_2. The decrease in alveolar Pco_2 results in a decreased arterial Pco_2 and CO_2 content with resultant respiratory alkalosis, whereas the increased alveolar Pco_2 has rather less effect on arterial O_2 saturation owing to the shape of the O_2 dissociation curve of hemoglobin. In the normal lung inspired air is uniformly delivered to and removed uniformly from all alveoli. In a number of pulmonary disorders, including asthma, this gas distribution may not be uniform, so that even with normal alveolar ventilation arterial hypoxemia may occur. Carbon dioxide retention and respiratory acidosis may result only if there is not compensatory hyperventilation of another lung area.

DIFFUSION

In order for oxygen and carbon dioxide to enter or leave the blood they must diffuse across the alveolar-capillary membrane. Diffusion refers to the process by which O_2 molecules move from an area of higher partial pressure (the alveoli) to an area of lower pressure (the pulmonary capillary blood). The diffusing capacity of the lung for a gas—O_2—may be defined as the rate of oxygen transfer per unit of pressure difference across the alveolar capillary membrane (ml. O_2/min./mm. Hg). The diffusion distance normally is about 1.0 micron but may be greatly increased in disease. The alveolar or capillary wall may be thickened, the membranes may be further separated by exudate or edema fluid, and the interstitial space may be fibrotic. The capillary may be dilated, allowing several red blood cells to travel alongside each other. All of these factors which widen the path that gases must travel, cause a decrease in diffusing capacity. Since the diffusing capacity of CO_2 is about 20 times greater than that of O_2, practically speaking, CO_2 retention does not result from diffusion defects. Diffusion defects because of membrane disorders do not generally occur in asthma. For reasons of convenience CO_2 is used for measuring airway diffusing capacity rather than O_2.

PULMONARY CIRCULATION

The final consideration is that of the circulation, which is responsible for assuring that all the venous blood is presented evenly to all the ventilated capillaries and that it then adequately reaches all the other tissues of the body. Any consideration of blood flow beyond the confines of the lung are beyond the scope of this text. As important as the volume and the distribution of alveolar ventilation are to gas exchange in the lungs so are the volume and the distribution of the pulmonary capillary blood flow. Since the pulmonary capillaries at any moment contain only 75 to 100 ml. of blood and since about 98 percent of the cardiac output is pumped through, the amount of time available for gas exchange for each erythrocyte is less than one second. The normal pulmonary blood flow is 5 liters per minute. In asthma, as well as in a number of disorders, the distribution of gases to the alveoli is not equal. Indeed there is some unevenness of ventilation in normal people. This is also the situation when we consider the pulmonary capillary blood flow. Recent studies have shown that a combination of abnormalities in ventilation and in pulmonary capillary blood flow result in many of the abnormalities of blood gases seen in asthma.[34, 58] The control of vascular tone and, thereby, of perfusion within the lung is not completely understood. We know that inhalation of air with reduced oxygen tension causes an increase in pulmonary artery pressure. This hypoxic response is not affected by denervation of the lung or by drugs which block the effects of acetylcholine or histamine. Pulmonary vasomotor tone is also increased by histamine, norepinephrine and serotonin. Pulmonary vascular mechanisms must be more adequately explained for us to fully comprehend the disturbances we note in asthma.

PULMONARY PHYSIOLOGY IN ASTHMA

The major feature of an asthma attack is obstruction of the airway. Much of the testing and most of the abnormalities, therefore, are those of ventilation. Since asthma is a dynamic disease, the levels of abnormality may vary widely in the same patient over very short periods of time. Therefore consideration of the asymptomatic asthmatic, the patient who has significant symptomatic asthma but is not in status asthmaticus, and the patient in status asthmaticus is appropriate.

The Asymptomatic Asthmatic

Studies of pulmonary function in patients with bronchial asthma during their symptom-free intervals may be normal or markedly abnormal.[4, 56] Measurements of vital capacity and inspiratory capacity may be decreased. The MBC may also be decreased, usually proportionately more than the vital capacity. The residual volume is increased as is the RV/TLC ratio. As previously noted, the Po_2 may also be decreased while the Pco_2 and pH remain normal. This change is caused by abnormalities in ventilation and perfusion. The measurements of forced expiratory volume along with the percentage of air expired each second may also be decreased. In some of these patients, values may be obtained which appear to be within the range of normal. For this reason, all ventilatory testing of asthmatic patients should include studies after inhalation of isoproterenol or injection of Adrenalin. Apparently normal studies may show significant improvement after this treatment. Thus, it is highly reasonable, and well advised, to obtain routine tests of lung function in all patients with asthma, in order to make therapy more accurate. This type of testing is done most easily and economically with one of the portable office machines, such as the Pulmonor, and does not generally require all the studies available through more sophisticated hospital laboratories. As will be noted in the chapter on treatment of asthma, it is probably advisable to obtain serial studies up to every 15 minutes for four determinations after isoproterenol inhalation in every patient whose illness may be exacerbated by overuse of a Freon-propelled isoproterenol inhaler. Lack of significant improvement or a drop of FEV 60 minutes after inhalation may indicate the patient who should completely discontinue the use of these inhalers.[39]

The Moderately Symptomatic Asthmatic

In the patient who is not asymptomatic but is also not in status asthmaticus, the changes we note are similar to, but more severe than, those just described. The primary feature of an asthma attack is airway obstruction. The major findings, therefore, relate to studies of ventilatory function. Vital capacity is reduced in almost all patients with bronchospasm and tends to improve to near normal levels with adequate treatment. Most commonly the reduction in vital capacity is accompanied by equivalent reductions in the inspiratory capacity and expiratory reserve volumes. Functional residual capacity is usually increased in the acute stages of asthma and generally, but not always, decreases with treatment. In a series of 30 patients [56] studied throughout the course of an asthma attack, it was found that the FRC remained elevated even after the VC, ERV, IC and FEV had returned to normal. The residual volume showed changes similar to that of the FRC. The total lung capacity varies from normal to being significantly increased. In general the RV/TLC ratio is increased because of the greater abnormality in RV. Unfortunately, there is much variation in the findings in the patients with asthma and any or all of these parameters and no constant pattern of change can be described. The changes described above, however, are the ones generally present.

As previously noted, the airway obstruction of asthma is usually accompanied by an increase in airflow resistance, even in asymptomatic patients. The one-second forced expiratory volume is always decreased as is the maximal mid-expiratory flow rate. The maximal breathing capacity is usually reduced by an even greater percentage than the other studies observed. The marked increase in resistance to airflow during an asthma attack is accompanied by a marked increase of from six to ten times in the work of breathing.

In recent years, more sophisticated techniques have led to a greater understanding of some of the abnormalities noted in blood gases during asthma. Several groups have now reported studies in which there were simultaneous measurement of blood gases and ventilation-perfusion in the same patients.[34, 58] These studies have shown that, despite the observation that most patients with asthma hyperventilate, there remain areas of decreased ventilation. These areas have a relative decrease in perfusion which is physiologically useful, as less blood is exposed to underventilated areas, thereby decreasing the arterial unsaturation which is present. Hypoxia is the result of incomplete shutting off of the perfusion of the poorly ventilated alveoli. This hypoxia becomes worse as the asthma becomes more severe. Since we know that blood coming from hyperventilated areas will not have an elevated Po_2 while blood coming from poorly ventilated alveoli is less than normally saturated, the end result is arterial oxygen unsaturation. Conversely, the ready transfer of CO_2 requires that a great amount of hypoventilation occurs before we find an increase of CO_2. Indeed, the somewhat paradoxic finding of low CO_2 levels in the early stage of an asthma attack reflects the alveolar hyperventilation which predominates at this stage. It becomes reasonable therefore, to place emphasis on CO_2 levels in describing the severity of the disease at any given stage and thus in determining the intensity of therapy required. It has been shown that these ventilation-perfusion abnormalities will disappear with complete relief of bronchospasm but that they may be present in asymptomatic patients, giving further reason for continuous drug therapy even during symptom-free periods.[34] It has also been shown that these ventilation-perfusion abnormalities may be produced by pollen inhalation, by methacholine injection and by exercise.

The severity of the ventilation-perfusion abnormality seemed to parallel closely the clinical severity of symptoms in all of these situations, thereby suggesting that induced asthma is an entity which is closely related to the natural disease and that ventilation-perfusion abnormalities occur as an early part of the abnormal pathophysiology of asthma.

Status Asthmaticus

As an asthma attack becomes more severe we now begin to note that the Pco_2 returns to normal and then becomes elevated. When hypercapnia is demonstrated we must acknowledge the failure of conventional therapy. It is this state which we refer to as status asthmaticus. Status asthmaticus may, therefore, be defined as that state of severe bronchial asthma in which there has been no response to conventional therapy (epinephrine and theophylline) and in which alveolar hypoventilation has progressed to ventilatory failure with arterial Pco_2 greater than 44 mm. Hg. This constitutes a medical emergency and requires extraordinary therapeutic measures.

Although some authors would place more stringent requirements upon the diagnosis of status asthmaticus, application of this definition will result in the institution of a more aggressive therapeutic approach at an earlier time, thereby decreasing the frequency of occurrence of the most severe episodes. The etiology of status asthmaticus is not fully understood. Why does a refractory state develop in which there is no response to epinephrine? Possibly it is due to the acidosis which has developed secondary to CO_2 retention. Other important factors in the development of status asthmaticus appear to be infection and dehydration. The adverse effect of both nebulized isoproterenol and the Freon vehicle used in some of the hand nebulizers has been blamed for some of the very refractory asthmatic states.

Another complicating cause in some cases is overuse of sedation. The adverse effects of narcotics, barbiturates, sedatives and tranquilizers should be recognized and their use in patients who are wheezing is contraindicated. Once the patient in status asthmaticus has responded to treatment there will be no need for any type of sedative. Many patients who progress into status asthmaticus are those requiring corticosteroids for control of their disease. Perhaps early increase of their steroid dosage during acute exacerbations of asthma would prevent progression into the unresponsive phase. These patients may establish a clinical pattern of repeated progression into status asthmaticus. This may be prevented by administration of large doses of corticosteroids at the first indication of an exacerbation of symptoms. Occasionally some patients become acutely worse when exposed to the humidified oxygen conveyances (tents or masks) in general use. Although they represent a small group, their recognition is important, since in these people progression into status asthmaticus can be prevented by not using humidified air.

Treatment of status asthmaticus is generally directed by the degree of derangement of blood gas tensions. The rapidity of change in the pH and in the blood gases requires their rapid and frequent measurement. Since repeated arterial punctures are not desired in any patients and since it is an even less desirable procedure in infants and children, other methods are necessary. In the past few years reliable equipment has been introduced with which electrometric analyses of pH, Po_2 and Pco_2 on microliter samples of blood can be obtained.[46] This, coupled with the demonstration that properly obtained samples of capillary blood gave results either identical with or differing insignificantly from arterial blood samples obtained from patients with a variety of pulmonary diseases, has made possible a more rational management of patients with status asthmaticus. The capillary measurements are not accurate in patients with major circulatory disturbances. In recent years, studies of the changes in arterial blood gas tensions during an attack of asthma, including episodes of status asthmaticus, have given a clearer picture of the problem.[35, 38, 54] Studies of ventilatory function during status asthmaticus are not commonly available because of the inability of the patient to cooperate in the study. In a group of 20 patients[38] described as having severe airway obstruction, the mean FEV_1 was 0.46 liters (range 0.20 to 0.80 liters), which is one fifth the predicted normal value. The mean FVC in this same group was one liter (range 0.70 to 1.85 liters); one fourth the predicted normal value. In this group of patients, daily measurement of these two parameters revealed a very slow increase to near normal levels about 14 days after the start of the acute attack.

The characteristic blood gas pattern found in patients during an acute asthma attack is that of hypoxemia with a respiratory alkalosis.

	Blood Gas Changes in Asthma		
	Early	Moderately Severe	Status
pH	↑	Normal	↓↓
Pco_2	↓	Normal Range	↑
Po_2	↓	↓	↓↓

In a study of 64 patients with moderately severe asthma it was found that only two had a Po_2 of 90 or above and only nine had a Pco_2 of 45 mm. Hg or above, while 31 had a Pco_2 under 50 mm. Hg.[53] These data demonstrate that most asthma attacks are associated with hypoxemia but that alveolar hyperventilation results in hypocarbia with a resultant respiratory alkalosis. As the acute asthma worsens, there is a progressive increase in the ventilation-perfusion abnormality. With severe airway obstruction, the number of hypoventilated but relatively overperfused alveoli increases enough to result in alveolar hypoventilation, and the Pco_2 begins to rise. At this time a blood sample may show hypoxemia with a normal pH and Pco_2. During therapy the patient in this stage must be followed with frequently repeated blood samples, because the direction of the pH and the Pco_2 must be determined. As the alveolar hypoventilation progresses, the pH begins to fall with concomitant rise in the Pco_2. Levels of Pco_2 as high as 150 mm. Hg with pH of 6.92 have been described. The need for frequent determination of pH, Pco_2 and Po_2 cannot be overemphasized.

As the attack of acute asthma progresses into status asthmaticus, we note a number of clinical changes which are the result of the alterations in blood gases. The gray matter of the central nervous system is most affected by hypoxia, since these CNS cells have no recourse to anaerobic metabolism, with resultant mental disturbances including fatigue, headache, irritability, dizziness and impaired cerebration. These symptoms are insidious in onset and may not be recognized initially. As the condition worsens and CO_2 retention occurs, muscle twitching, somnolence, asterixis and diaphoresis occur. Together with the cerebral changes caused by hypoxemia and hypercarbia, a tachycardia with an increased cardiac output and elevation in systolic and diastolic blood pressures occurs. Irregularities in cardiac rhythm may also occur. At very low O_2 levels and high CO_2 levels, sudden hypotension may occur. These changes may also lead to pulmonary vasoconstriction with right heart strain and acute heart failure. All of these alterations may then lead to death from suffocation. A group of patients in status asthmaticus was reported in whom there was a sudden onset of hypotension following the relief of airway obstruction, accompanied by an increase in pulse rate.[50] All of these patients were found to be significantly hemoconcentrated. When the hemoconcentration was relieved by infusion of plasma, all parameters returned to normal. It was postulated that this was related to some of the unexpected deaths from status asthmaticus. If patients are adequately treated, this condition should not occur. The management of status asthmaticus with ventilatory failure has become a team effort, requiring an allergist, a chest physician and an anesthesiologist.

PSYCHIC FACTORS IN ASTHMA

Consideration of psychic factors in asthma must encompass two separate but closely related areas. The first is consideration of the effect of the emotional environment on the patient with bronchial asthma. The second is consideration of the emotional effect of the patient with bronchial asthma upon his environment. In consideration of the first area, the best approach was summarized by Leigh and Marley who noted, "The evidence either for a specific personality, or for a specific psychopathology is poor; such concepts are already falling into disrepute." [25] It is well known that emotional disturbances as triggering mechanism are related to attacks of asthma in some patients. Beyond this statement there is little scientific information. There are no controlled studies which tend to clarify psychic mechanisms and asthma. It has been suggested, but not confirmed, that depression is more common in asthma. Although there is a need for further studies, it can be concluded that psychic factors do play an important role as triggering mechanisms in a number of patients.

In considering the effect that the asthmatic has upon his environment, several factors must be considered. The wheezing child imparts a great deal of stress to his environment. Asthma causes more school absence than any other chronic illness. Because of the increasing importance of education in our society, the asthmatic is at a disadvantage and may be prevented from achieving his socioeconomic goals. The cost of his illness, and the extra attentions usually directed at the asthmatic child may focus the attention of the family toward the asthma to a much greater degree than necessary or normal. This abnormal focus, coupled with necessary environmental changes, such as removal of a pet or inability of the mother to work outside the home, either may result in a hostile environment for the child or conversely may result in guilt feelings, with the end result of an equally unhealthy atmosphere of overprotection. Should either of these situations occur, a family counseling program may be beneficial.

COMPLICATIONS OF ASTHMA

Specific complications attributable to the disease are not common. A number of complications related to drug therapy will be discussed in the chapter on treatment of asthma. Infection is not uncommon with asthma and is very common in status asthmaticus. Whether this can be considered a complication or a concomitant occurrence is not important as long as the importance of infection is recognized.

The relationship of asthma to chronic obstructive pulmonary disease has not been answered. The old opinion that asthma caused irreversible structural changes in the lungs is probably incorrect. No structural changes occur in patients with extrinsic asthma, even in chronic cases. Severe intrinsic asthma with repeated infection possibly does lead to irreversible structural changes. Further investigation of this area is necessary. Long standing severe chronic asthma that has caused irreversible structural lung changes may also result in right heart failure or cor pulmonale. This complication is rare.

Complications that appear to be much more common that their reported incidence are those of pneumomediastinum and pneumothorax.[5] These complications occur most often in children. It has been suggested that severe asthma with obstruction leads to overdistention of the alveoli and alveolar ducts. This is well tolerated by the alveoli but the supporting structures, such as the pulmonary arteries, alveolar septi and pulmonary veins having only a limited elasticity, do not withstand this well. As the overdistention increases, rupture at the alveolar bases results in either pneumomediastinum or pneumothorax depending upon the location of the ruptured alveolus. It may result in no symptoms if there is only a small pneumothorax. In more serious cases the symptoms are those of severe air hunger, anxiety and restlessness, hard, brassy cough and either neck or chest pain or both. On examination there may be absence of cardiac dullness, subcutaneous emphysema and cyanosis. The diagnosis is made by roentgenogram.

Treatment is generally conservative usually calling for control of asthma and careful observation. Occasionally tracheotomy or insertion of a water sealed intercostal tube for drainage of a pneumothorax is necessary. Another common and frequently unrecognized complication is atelectasis. This is usually mild and results from mucus plugging a bronchiole. Large areas of lung tissue are rarely involved. Specific therapy is usually not indicated.

REFERENCES

1. Adkinson, J.: Behavior of bronchial asthma as an inherited character. J. Genetics, 5:363, 1920.
2. Ahlquist, R. T.: Development of the concept of alpha and beta adrenotropic receptors. Ann. N.Y. Acad. Sci., 139:552, 1967.
3. Bates, D. V., Macklem, P. T., and Christie, R. V.: Respiratory function in disease. ed. 2. Philadelphia, W. B. Saunders, 1971.
4. Beale, H. D., Fowler, W. F., and Comroe, J. H., Jr.: Pulmonary function studies in 20 asthmatic patients in the symptom free interval. J. Allerg., 23:1, 1952.
5. Bierman, C. W.: Pneumomediastinum and pneumothorax complicating asthma in children. Amer. J. Dis. Child., 114:32, 1967.
6. Brocklehurst, W. E.: In Gell, P. G. H., and Coombs, R. R. A.: Clinical Aspects of Immunology. Chap. 22, ed. 2. Philadelphia, F. A. Davis, 1968.
7. Bullen, Sterns S., Sr.: Correlation of clinical and autopsy findings in 176 cases of asthma. J. Allerg., 23:193, 1952.
8. Callaway, J. J., et al.: Measurement of lung function in the doctor's office. Med. Clin. N. Amer., 53:37, 1969.

9. Carnow, B. W.: Air pollution and respiratory diseases. Scientist and Citizen, May, 1966.
10. Carnow, B. W., Lepper, M. H., Shekelle, R. B., and Stamler, J.: Chicago air pollution study. Arch. Environ. Health, *18*:768, 1969.
11. Comroe, J. H., Forester, R. E., DuBois, A. B., Briscoe, W. A., and Carlsen, E.: The Lung. p. 9. Chicago, Yearbook Medical Publishers, 1962.
12. ———: The Lung. p. 11. Chicago, Yearbook Medical Publishers, 1962.
13. ———: The Lung: Clinical physiology and pulmonary function tests. ed. 2. Chicago, Yearbook Medical Publishers, 1962.
14. Cooke, R. A. and VanderVeer, A., Jr.: Human sensitization. J. Immun., *1*:201, 1916.
15. Cotes, J. E.: Lung function. ed. 2. Philadelphia, F. A. Davis, 1968.
16. Crepea, S. B., and Harman, J. W.: The pathology of bronchial asthma. The significance of membrane changes in asthmatic and nonallergic pulmonary diseases. J. Allerg., *26*:453, 1955.
17. Dunnill, M. S.: The pathology of asthma, with special reference to changes in the bronchial mucosa. J. Clin. Path., *13*:27, 1960.
18. Falliers, C. J.: Cromolyn Sodium, An Editorial. J. Allerg., *47*:298, 1971.
19. Fisher, H. K., *et al.*: Mechanism of exercise induced bronchoconstriction in asthma. Clinical Research, Vol. 16, 162, 1968.
20. Henderson, L. L., *et al.*: Value of serum IgE concentrations in the practice of allergy. Presented at the American Academy of Allergy meeting, February, 1971.
21. Jones, R. F., Buston, M. H., and Warden, M. J.: The effect of exercise on ventilatory function in the child with asthma. Brit. J. Chest Dis., *56*: 78, 1962.
22. Kellaway, C. H. and Trethewice, E. R.: The liberation of a slow reacting smooth muscle stimulating substance in anaphylaxis. Quar. J. Exp. Physiol., *30*:121, 1940.
23. Kjellman, B.: Ventilatory capacity and efficiency after exercise in healthy and asthmatic children. Scand. J. Resp. Dis., *50*:41, 1969.
24. Lawrence, P. F.: Morbidity and mortality from asthma and other allergic diseases. Conference on Research in Asthma and Other Allergic Disease, April 6-8, 1967, National Jewish Hospital and Research Center, Denver, Colorado.
25. Leigh, D., and Marley, E.: Bronchial Asthma: A Genetic Population and Psychiatric Study. p. 39. Oxford, Pergamon Press, 1967.
26. McNeill, R. S., Nairn, J. R., Millar, J. F., and Ingram, C. C.: Exercise induced asthma. Quar. J. Med., *25*:55, 1966.
27. Maximow, A. A., and Bloom, W.: A Textbook of Histology. ed. 7. pp. 435-449. Philadelphia, W. B. Saunders, 1957.
28. Meneely, G. R., *et al.*: Chronic bronchitis, asthma and pulmonary emphysema. Amer. Rev. Resp. Dis., *85*:762, 1962.
29. Millar, J. F., Narin, J. R., Unkles, R. D., and McNeill, R. S.: Cold air and the ventilatory function. Brit. J. Chest Dis., *59*:23, 1965.

30. Nadel, J. A.: Mechanism of airway response to inhaled substances. Arch. Environ. Health, *16:*171, 1968.
31. Nadel, J. A., Salem, H., Tamplin, B., and Tokiwa, Y.: Mechanism of bronchoconstriction during inhalation of sulfur dioxide. Journal of Applied Physiology, *20:*164-167, 1965.
32. Naylor, B. The shedding of the mucosa of the bronchial tree in asthma. Thorax, *17:*69, 1962.
33. Newer adrenergic blocking drugs: Their pharmacological, biochemical and clinical actions. Annals of the New York Academy of Sciences, *139:*, 541-1009, 1967. Chairman Neil C. Moran.
34. Novey, H. F., Wilson, A. F., Suprenant, E. L., and Bennett, L. R.: Early ventilation perfusion changes in asthma. J. Allerg., *46:*221, 1970.
35. Palmer, K. N. V., and Diament, M. L.: Dynamic and static lung volumes and blood gas tensions in bronchial asthma. Lancet, *1:*591, 1969.
36. Parker, C. D., Bilbo, R. E., and Reed, C. E.: Methacholine aerosol as test for bronchial asthma. Arch. Intern. Med., *115:*452, 1965.
37. Piper, P. J., and Vane, J. R.: Release of additional factors in anaphylaxis and its antagonism by anti-inflammatory drugs. Nature, *223:*29, 1969.
38. Rees, H. A., Millar, J. F., and Donald, K. W.: A study of the clinical course and arterial blood gas tensions of patients in status asthmaticus. Quar. J. Med., *148:*541, 1968.
39. Reisman, R. E.: Asthma induced by adrenergic aerosols. J. Allerg., *46:*162, 1970.
40. Robinson, G. A., Butcher, R. W., and Sutherland, E. W.: Adenyl cyclase as an adrenergic receptor in new adrenergic blocking drugs: their pharmacological, biochemical and clinical actions. Ann. N.Y. Acad. Sci., *139:*706, 1967.
41. ———: Adenyl cyclase as an adrenergic receptor. Ann. N.Y. Acad. Sci., *139:*703, 1967.
42. Samter, M., and Beers, R. F., Jr.: Intolerance to aspirin. Ann. Inter. Med., *68:*975, 1968.
43. Schild, H. O., Hawkins, D. F., Mongar, J. L., and Herxheimer, H.: Reactions of isolated human asthmatic lung and bronchial tissue to a specific antigen. Lancet, *2:*376, 1951.
44. Schwartz, M.: Heredity and bronchial asthma. Acta Allerg., [Supp. 2], *5:*1-288, 1952.
45. Seaton, A., Davies, G., Gaziano, D., and Hughes, R. O.: Exercise induced asthma. Brit. Med. J., *3:*556, 1969.
46. Sharp, J. T.: Measurement of pH and blood gases in arterialized capillary blood. Med. Clin. N. Amer., *53:*137, 1969.
47. Slonim, N. B., and Chapin, J. L.: Respiratory physiology. St. Louis, C. V. Mosby, 1967.
48. Spain, W. C., and Cooke, R. A.: Studies in specific hypersensitiveness. J. Immunol., *9:*521, 1924.
49. Speizer, F. E., Doll, R., and Heaf, P.: Observations on recent increase in mortality from asthma. Brit. Med. J., *1:*335, 1968.

50. Straub, P. W., Buhlmann, A. A., and Rossier, P. H.: Hypovolemia in status asthmaticus. Lancet, 2:923, 1969.
51. Sutherland, E. W.: The biological role of cyclic AMP. JAMA, 214:1281, 1970.
52. Szentivanyi, A.: The beta adrenergic theory of the atopic abnormality in bronchial asthma. J. Allerg., 42:203, 1968.
53. Tai, E., and Reed, J.: Blood gas tensions in bronchial asthma. Lancet, 1:644, 1967.
54. Teculescu, D. B., and Stanescu, D. C.: Blood oxygen tension during induced asthma attacks. Amer. Rev. Resp. Dis., 98:842, 1968.
55. Vogt, W.: Slow reacting substances. *In* Movat, H. Z. (ed.): Cellular and Humoral Mechanisms in Anaphylaxis and Allergy. New York, S. Karger, 1969.
56. Weng, T. R., and Levinson, H.: Pulmonary function in children with asthma at acute attack and symptom free status. Amer. Rev. Resp., 99:719, 1969.
57. Widdicombe, J. V.: Regulation of tracheobronchial smooth muscle. Physiol. Rev., 43:1, 1963.
58. Wilson, A. F., *et al.:* The significance of regional pulmonary function changes in bronchial asthma. Amer. J. Med., 48:416, 1970.

8

Asthma: Management

Angelo E. Falleroni, M.D.

Asthma afflicts approximately 6 to 8 million Americans and represents about 25 percent of the chronic diseases of childhood. Although the prevalence of asthma has remained essentially unchanged, its attendant morbidity is probably increasing. Paradoxically, with a seemingly better understanding of its pathophysiology and more effective modes of treatment, the last decade has seen an increasing mortality from asthma. In 1967 there were 4,137 deaths attributable to asthma in the United States.[41]

Except for anaphylaxis, asthma can be considered the most serious condition that the allergist treats. Factors which can cause or precipitate asthma are numerous and vary from patient to patient. Some of these can be treated directly; others are partially controllable. The central theme of proper treatment is the realization that it must be individualized according to the specific characteristics of each patient's problem.

Because of its chronicity as well as the wide scope of factors which adversely affect asthma, proper management must involve the physician in the psychologic and socioeconomic situation of each patient. Other factors, such as atmospheric pollution, may also involve the physician and the medical profession in general in a politically more dominant role in assuring control and improvement of the environment.[6]

At the present time there is no cure (in the absolute sense of the word) for asthma. Significant advances in understanding some of the underlying abnormalities in asthma have been made, but a concise, unifying mechanism remains unknown. Despite these negative remarks, however, it must be stressed that employment of the presently available treatment modalities will provide significant improvement and adequate control for most patients with asthma.

BASIC CONCEPTS

Asthma is characterized by reversible episodes of cough, sputum pro‧ duction and wheezing dyspnea with variable degrees of pulmonary insufficiency. Clinically, asthma is classified into four basic types: extrinsic, intrinsic, mixed (extrinsic and intrinsic) and aspirin-sensitive. Extrinsic asthma is also known as allergic or atopic asthma and refers to that type which results from the allergic reaction of the immediate or reaginic type. Intrinsic asthma encompasses, in general, all other nonallergic types of asthma. Infection of the respiratory tract appears to be a significant precipitating factor in the majority of this group, but in the remaining patients the cause is unknown. The mixed type includes both reaginic allergy and infection as significant precipitating factors. The aspirin-sensitive type of asthma is clinically similar to the intrinsic type but has the additional features of rhinitis, nasal polyposis and aspirin intolerance. A few of these patients may have coexistent atopic (extrinsic) factors which may contribute to symptoms.

Asthma should be considered not solely as a symptom complex or syndrome but as a definitive disease entity with specific and concise characteristics. The disease is characterized by an enhanced bronchial hyperreactivity. This hyperreactivity helps differentiate asthma from other pulmonary conditions. Clinically it is made manifest by the asthmatic's adverse reaction to stimuli which have no untoward affect on normal individuals. Cold air, changes in environmental factors (temperature, humidity and barometric pressure), exercise, odors, fumes, emotional stress and laughter are examples of such stimuli. Similarly, asthmatics require lesser amounts of atmospheric pollution to develop significant pulmonary symptoms.

Pharmacologically this hyperreactivity can be shown by the administration of mediators such as methacholine (and acetylcholine), histamine, and bradykinin. In asthmatics of all types, these substances induce significant bronchospasm in lower concentrations than are required in normals or patients with other pulmonary conditions. There have been many attempts to explain the various complexities of asthma by one common pathophysiologic mechanism. Although various theories have been propounded, none has been able to unify all the facts known about asthma. A recent theory suggests that asthma results from a partial β-adrenergic receptor blockade of the lung. Although there is indirect evidence consistent with this theory, direct proof is still wanting. This theory is discussed in detail in Chapter 7.

Proper treatment and management of asthma depends on the establishment of an accurate diagnosis. Usually a careful history and physical examination with only a few laboratory studies are sufficient to establish the diagnosis. But wheezing dyspnea, the central feature of asthma, is also a common complaint and finding of other conditions which may or may not be directly cardiopulmonary in origin. A discussion of the clinical aspects, laboratory studies and differential diagnosis of asthma is presented in Chapter 7.

TREATMENT

The treatment of an asthmatic episode varies according to its clinical severity. Similarly, long range treatment regimens depend on the type of asthma and its severity. In general the prognosis for recovery or control is good for the patient with extrinsic asthma. However, intrinsic asthma is often more severe and has a less favorable prognosis. Indeed in most patients with intractable asthma, the disease is the intrinsic type. The basic objective of treatment, as in other chronic illnesses, is to achieve significant control of symptoms in order to prevent physical as well as psychologic incapacitation. In addition to the observation of clinical improvement, the practical goals of treatment are best measured by a decreasing number of hospitalizations and lessening of school or work absenteeism.

PRINCIPLES OF TREATMENT

The treatment of asthma consists of therapeutic measures to reverse bronchial mucosal edema, bronchospasm, hypersecretion of mucus and ventilation-perfusion imbalance. Depending on the severity of the attack, various degrees of hypo- or hypercarbia with its resultant acid-base changes may also require specific therapy. Finally, other emergency measures may be necessary to prevent or reverse acute respiratory failure when it occurs.

Preventive measures are important in the proper management of asthma. In allergic asthma, of primary importance is the removal of the offending allergen. If this is impossible, immunotherapy should be considered when applicable. Protective measures must also be included to lessen the deleterious effects of certain aggravating factors. In addition, drugs the pharmacologic effects of which may aggravate asthma must be avoided when possible.

The treatment of asthma can be considered as a threefold approach consisting of drug therapy, nonspecific measures applicable to all patients, and specific management depending on the clinical classification.

DRUG THERAPY

Sympathomimetic Amines

The peripheral effects of an adrenergic drug are dependent on its specific receptor stimulating capacity as well as the type of receptor present in the organ or tissue stimulated. The bronchi contain predominantly β receptors which promote bronchodilatation, and only those sympathomimetics possessing β-stimulating activity are effective in the

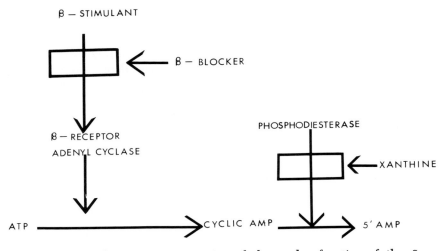

Fig. 8-1. A schematic representation of the mode of action of the β-stimulating drugs and xanthines on the adenyl cyclase-ATP system.

treatment of asthma. Beta receptors themselves may differ from organ to organ; those in the bronchi have been termed β_2 and those in the heart β_1.

The biochemical mechanisms of action (Fig. 8-1) of the β-stimulating adrenergic drugs have not been completely elucidated, but they are known to increase the rate of formation of 3'5'-cyclic adenosine monophosophate (cyclic AMP) from adenosine triphosphate (ATP) in the presence of adenyl cyclase. The increased cyclic AMP in turn triggers other intermediate reactions which ultimately results in bronchodilatation.

Epinephrine

Epinephrine (Adrenalin), because of its potent bronchodilating effect and rapid onset of action, is the drug of choice in acute asthma. It possesses both α- and β-stimulating properties. The recommended adult dose is 0.30 to 0.50 ml. of the 1:1000 solution administered subcutaneously. In infants and children the dose is 0.01 ml./kg. with a maximum of 0.25 ml. The dose may be repeated in 15 to 30 minutes if necessary. Nebulized epinephrine is also effective but is less commonly used today. Sus-Phrine,* a 1:200 aqueous suspension of epinephrine, may be used when a longer duration (6 to 8 hours) of action is desirable. Its dose is 0.20 to 0.30 ml. subcutaneously for adults and 0.005

* Trademark, Cooper Laboratories.

ml./kg. (maximum 0.15 ml.) for infants and children. A portion of the epinephrine (20 per cent) in this preparation is in solution and thus available for an immediate effect, while the remainder in crystalline form, provides more sustained relief.

The common side effects of epinephrine include pallor, agitation, hypertension, tremulousness, tachycardia, palpitation, arrhythmias, headache, nausea and vomiting. Subarachnoid hemorrhage and hemiplegia have been reported to result from 0.50 ml. of 1:1000 aqueous epinephrine subcutaneously. Epinephrine must be administered with caution in patients with cardiovascular disease and hypertension.

Ethylnorepinephrine Hydrochloride (Bronkephrine) *

This sympathomimetic acts on β-adrenergic receptors predominantly, but it also possesses minimal α-adrenergic properties. Its α-stimulating potential is less than that of epinephrine and thus represents a good substitute when the vasopressor and other α-adrenergic effects of epinephrine are not desired. It is most effective by parentral administration, but may also be given orally or by aerosol. The dose for adults is 0.5 to 1.0 ml. given subcutaneously or intramuscularly. If necessary, it may be repeated in 20 minutes. For infants and children the dose is 0.01 to 0.02 ml./kg. (maximum 0.5 ml).

Isoproterenol

Isoproterenol (Isuprel, Aludrine, Norisodrine) † stimulates predominantely β-receptors (both bronchial and cardiac). When administered by aerosol it has a rapid onset of action and it is most commonly used by this route. Its duration of action is comparatively short, since it is rapidly metabolized to 3-methoxyisoproterenol by the enzyme catechol-o-methyl transferase. For aerosol treatment it is available in pressurized aerosol cartridges and as a 1:200 solution, which when diluted in warm saline can be used in hand propelled nebulizers, motor driven nebulizers and by intermittent positive pressure.

The recommended dose from the pressurized aerosols is 1 to 2 inhalations 4 to 6 times daily. Aerosol treatments with the isoproterenol solution should also be limited to 4 to 6 treatments per day unless they are being used in the treatment of status asthmaticus. In this situation they may be used more frequently (every 2 to 4 hours) provided the patient is watched closely for adverse effects. The nebulized mixture in children should range from 0.15 to 0.50 ml. of isoproterenol (1:200) diluted in 1 to 2 ml. of warm saline. In adults the ratio may be 0.25 to 0.50 ml. of isoproterenol in 1 ml. of saline.

* Trademark, Breon Laboratories.
† Trademarks, respectively, of Winthrop, Lilly, and Abbott.

Isoproterenol is also effective by the sublingual route. The suggested dose for adults is 10 to 15 mg., and it may be repeated every 4 to 6 hours if necessary. The dose for children ranges from 5 to 10 mg. For patients who tend to overuse their nebulizers, sublingual administration may be an effective substitute. Isoproterenol is least effective when administered orally. This probably results from gastrointestinal inactivation of the drug.

Side effects of isoproterenol are similar to those of epinephrine, but because of its vasodilating properties hypertension is less apt to occur. An immediate hypersensitivity reaction to isoproterenol was recently reported in one patient.[43] The prevalence of this presumably rare reaction and its importance as a possible cause of paradoxical bronchospasm seen in an occasional patient may deserve further study.

Overuse of aerosolized isoproterenol (see below) may result in serious side effects, but to completely ban its use is not indicated. When properly and judiciously used it remains a beneficial form of treatment.

Bronkosol *

Bronkosol is another adrenergic preparation commonly used for aerosol therapy. It is a solution consisting of isoetharine HCl (β-adrenergic stimulator), phenylephrine HCl (an α-adrenergic stimulator) and thenyldiamine HCl (an antihistamine). Unlike isoproterenol, isoetharine stimulates predominantly bronchial β-receptors (beta$_2$) and therefore results in less cardiac stimulation. This solution may be used undiluted (0.50 ml) in the hand nebulizer. For motor driven or IPPB aerosolization the recommended dose is from 0.25 ml. to 0.50 ml. diluted in 3 volumes of saline. This preparation is also available in a pressurized hand aerosol cartridge (Bronkometer *).

Overuse of Adrenergic Aerosols

Aerosols containing adrenergic drugs have been used in the treatment of asthma for many years. The immediate and effective relief offered by this form of therapy has made it popular and widely accepted by both patients and physicians. Unfortunately, many patients become practically addicted to this therapy. With exacerbation of symptoms both adults and children tend to overuse the nebulizer. Adverse effects from aerosolized adrenergic drugs were reported as early as 1939, but only within the last few years has the full extent of their deleterious effect been realized.

The overuse of these aerosols has been shown to increase and perpetuate the severity of symptoms in certain chronic asthmatics. Many

* Trademark, Breon Laboratories.

Some Pressurized Aerosols Available for the Treatment of Asthma

Trade Name	Contents
Aerolone Compound	Isoproterenol Cyclopentamine Hydrochloride
Asthma Meter Mist	Epinephrine
Bronkometer	Isoetharine Phenylephrine Thenyldiamine
Duo-Medihaler	Isoproterenol Phenylephrine
Isuprel Mistometer	Isoproterenol
Medihaler–Epi	Epinephrine
Medihaler–Iso	Isoproterenol
Norisodrine Aerotrol	Isoproterenol
Vaponefrin	Racemic Epinephrine
Vapo-N-Iso	Racemic Epinephrine Isoproterenol
Alupent *	Metaproterenol

* Not available in the U.S.A.

of these patients improve remarkably when the aerosol therapy is discontinued. Retrospective studies have also suggested the overuse of aerosols often antedated and possibly contributed to the development of status asthmaticus. Certain English investigators have suggested that the recent increase in mortality from asthma may be related to the increased use of pressurized nebulizers.[20] Although not definitely proven, there is some evidence lending credence to this contention.

A method to detect those patients who are adversely affected by the overuse of aerosolized isoproterenol has recently been described.[33] A group of patients who chronically overused isoproterenol aerosol were studied. The baseline FEV_1 and the FEV_1 60 minutes after inhaling 0.5% isoproterenol for 1 minute were compared. A 60-minute FEV_1 similar to or less than the baseline FEV_1 was noted in those patients in whom discontinuing aerosol therapy provided dramatic improvement in symptoms. Other patients who overused aerosols but in whom the 60-minute FEV_1 was 10 percent or greater than the baseline did not improve with cessation of aerosol treatment. These studies indicate that the deleterious effect of these aerosols may also depend on individual susceptibility.

How these aerosolized drugs aggravate asthma is not known. They probably are irritating to the bronchial mucosa, but this may not be the only reason for their untoward effects. The metabolic end product of isoproterenol, 3-methoxyisoproterenol, has been shown to block beta adrenergic receptors. The possible accumulation of this substance may account for the aggravation of asthma. Chronic users of isoproterenol have been shown to be more resistant to the adverse cardiac effects of isoproterenol.[29] This resistance is also thought to possibly result from the blocking effects of accumulated 3-methoxyisoproterenol.

Although subjective and objective improvement of airway obstruction results from aerosolized isoproterenol, the associated hypoxemia of asthma is not improved and is often worsened. This probably results from enhancing the already existing ventilation-perfusion imbalance by either increasing aeration of those alveoli already over-ventilating in relation to their perfusion, or by reestablishing ventilation to nonperfused alveoli. Other alterations of diffusion, pulmonary blood flow and pulmonary capillary volume resulting from isoproterenol may also contribute in enhancing hypoxemia.[14]

The cardiotoxic effects of isoproterenol, probably heightened by the hypoxemia commonly present with asthma, has been suggested as a possible mechanism for some of the sudden deaths seen in asthma. Fatal arrythmias and tachycardias may occur, but it must be remembered that sudden deaths in asthma have been reported before the common usage of aerosols.

Fluorinated hydrocarbons (Freons), the propellants used in pressurized aerosols, have also been implicated as possible aggravating factors. Sudden deaths in young people after sniffing solvents and aerosols have been reported.[4] It is speculated that these deaths may result from cardiac arrhythmias caused by the sensitizing effect of the halogenated hydrocarbons to circulating endogenously released catecholamines. Studies in mice have revealed that these substances may sensitize the heart to asphyxia-induced bradyarrhythmias.[39] It is possible that these hydrocarbons may induce cardiotoxic effects in the asthmatic, who not only may be hypoxemic, but also may have an abundance of circulating catecholamines from both endogenous and exogenous sources. Recent studies [12, 30] have shown that some of these hydrocarbons can be measured in the venous and arterial blood of normal volunteers and asthmatics when inhaled in normal or large amounts. For example, blood levels of trichlorofluoromethane (Freon 11) after inhaling two puffs of commercially available aerosols containing this hydrocarbon were similar in asthmatics (including those overusing aerosols) and normal controls. Peak blood levels ranged from 0.13 to 2.60 μg./ml. and the blood half life was 0.3 to 1.5 minutes. The clinical significance of the possible adverse effect of these hydrocarbons must await further studies.

Ephedrine

Ephedrine, although less potent than isoproterenol and epinephrine, has the advantages of being effective by oral administration and possessing a longer duration of action (3 to 6 hours). It is an integral component of the many oral preparations commonly used for treatment. The adult dose is 25 mg. every 4 to 6 hours. For infants and children the recommended dose is 0.5 to 1 mg./kg. every 4 to 6 hours. Its side effects are similar to those of the other sympathomimetics discussed above.

Alpha Adrenergic Drugs

As expected, specific alpha adrenergic stimulating drugs alone are not efficacious in the treatment of asthma. There is a rationale for combining them with isoproterenol or isoetharine for aerosolization. Theoretically, by promoting vascular constriction their net effect would result in decreasing bronchial obstruction by decreasing bronchial mucosal edema. Their combined use with isoproterenol has also been shown to prevent isoproterenol-induced hypoxemia.[19] Phenylephrine and cyclopentamine are the most commonly used alpha adrenergics.

Newer Sympathomimetics

Continuing pharmacologic and biochemical research not only has resulted in a better understanding of the adrenergic receptor system but also in the development of drugs with more specific stimulating or blocking action. Slight alterations in the isoproterenol molecule, for example, have resulted in new compounds possessing predominantly $beta_2$ (lung) stimulating properties. Metaproterenol (orciprenaline, Alupent *), salbutamol and terbutaline are three such drugs presently being evaluated for the treatment of asthma (Fig. 8-2). Preliminary studies have suggested their superiority to isoproterenol.[13, 25, 28, 32] The chemical changes of the benzene ring render these compounds more

* Trademark, Geigy.

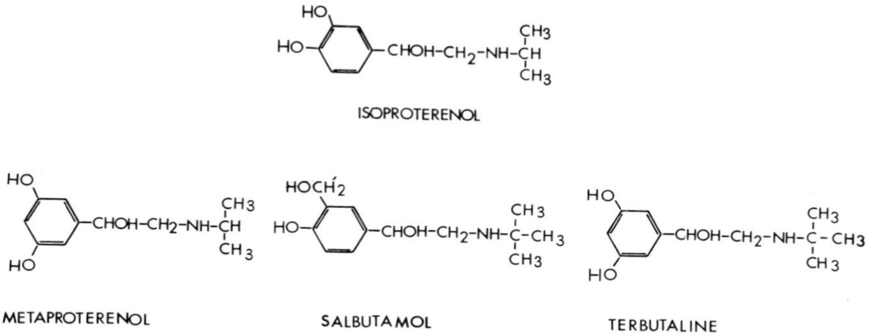

ISOPROTERENOL

METAPROTERENOL   SALBUTAMOL   TERBUTALINE

Fig. 8-2. The chemical structures of the new β-adrenergic drugs as compared to that of isoproterenol.

resistant to the action of catechol-o-methyl transferase thus prolonging their duration of action as compared to isoproterenol. Changes in the side chain have increased their specificity for beta$_2$ receptors with only minimal beta$_1$ (cardiac) receptor activity. Another advantage over isoproterenol is that these drugs are effective by aerosol, oral and subcutaneous administration.

Studies in asthmatics have shown that these compounds promote a significant bronchodilatation of 4 to 5 hours duration with a maximum response between 2 to 4 hours (oral and aerosol treatment). Little or no change in arterial oxygen levels occurs in contrast to the increased hypoxemia commonly seen with isoproterenol. An increase in pulse rate is seen with minimal changes in blood pressure. Slight increases in systolic pressure with a tendency to lower diastolic pressure commonly occur. Side effects from these drugs are minimal; tremulousness, headache and palpitations are most prominent.

The recommended adult oral dose for salbutamol is from 2 to 4 mg. t.i.d. and for terbutaline it is 5 mg. t.i.d. The dose of metaproterenol is 20 to 30 mg. t.i.d. Aerosol treatment with these drugs could probably be limited to 2 to 3 inhalations per day. Theoretically, aerosol treatment with these drugs would be safer and more effective than with isoproterenol. They all are potent bronchodilators and possess the least cardiac stimulating capacity and hypoxemic potential.

Theophylline

The most important pharmacologic action of theophylline (1-3 dimethylxanthine) is bronchodilation. It also possesses diuretic properties as well as central nervous system and respiratory stimulating capacities.

The mechanism by which the methylxanthines cause bronchodilatation may result from their effect upon the adenyl cyclase-ATP system (Fig. 8-1). These compounds inhibit phosphodiesterase, the enzyme which is required for the conversion of 3'-5' cyclic AMP to 5' AMP. The net effect of this action is an increase in 3'5'-cyclic AMP, an end result similar to that of the β-stimulating drugs but resulting from a different mechanism. This site of action also explains how a patient unresponsive to epinephrine often obtains relief with theophylline. It is also known that theophylline and epinephrine (as well as other β-stimulating drugs) result in an "additive" bronchodilator response.

Theophylline is relatively insoluble and not well absorbed from the gastrointestinal tract. Combining ethylenediamine with theophylline (aminophylline) renders it more soluble. The choline salt of theophylline (choline theophyllinate-Choledyl*) also results in a more soluble form of theophylline. The latter compound is available for oral

* Trademark, Chilcott.

administration only; it is well absorbed from the gastrointestinal tract and causes minimal gastric irritation. Dyphylline, 7-(2-3-dihydropropyl) theophylline, (Lufyllin *) is another more soluble preparation of theophylline. This form of theophylline presumably causes the least gastric irritation when taken orally. The hydro-alcoholic solutions of theophylline not only increase the solubility of theophylline but also enhance its gastrointestinal absorption. These preparations produce rapid and prolonged therapeutic blood levels of theophylline.

Rectal preparations are also available. This form of therapy causes less gastrointestinal side effects but absorption may be unpredictable and prolonged use of suppositories (aminophylline) may cause proctitis. Theophylline monoethanolamine (Fleet Theophylline) as a retention enema provides effective and rapid bronchodilatation. Table 8-1 lists some of the commonly used oral and rectal preparations of theophylline.

Toxic effects of theophylline include nausea, vomiting, epigastric pain, palpitation, agitation and convulsions. When given intravenously (aminophylline) or intramuscularly (dyphylline) it must be administered slowly over a 10- to 15-minute period in order to avoid hypotension or cardiac arrest. Urticaria and pruritis resulting from intravenous aminophylline was recently reported in one patient.[42] A positive wheal and flare reaction to aminophylline, which was passively transferred by the Prausnitz-Küstner technique, was found. This type of reaction to aminophylline is considered quite rare.

Aminophylline

Aminophylline (theophylline ethylenediamine) is a potent bronchodilator. Although it is available for intravenous, oral and rectal administration, it is most effective by the intravenous route. When given intravenously its onset of action is within minutes. The adult dose is from 250 to 500 mg. administered slowly as mentioned above. This dose may be repeated every 6 to 8 hours.

Children are unusually sensitive to the toxic effects of aminophylline and the dosage should not exceed 3 to 5 mg./kg. (intravenously) every 8 hours. Aminophylline overdose has been cited as a cause of death in childhood asthma. To prevent overdosage, when aminophylline is administered in severe asthma it is important to ascertain the amount of theophylline taken orally or rectally within the previous 12 hours.

Dyphylline (Lufyllin)

Dyphylline is available in both intramuscular and oral preparations. When this drug is used, other theophylline derivatives should be dis-

---

* Trademark, Mallinckrodt.

continued to avoid toxicity. The usual intramuscular dose for adults is 250 to 500 mg. given slowly over a period of 5 to 10 minutes. The recommended dose of the tablets and elixir is 200 mg. three to four times daily. For children, the dosage is 5 to 10 mg./kg./day in divided doses, but it is not recommended for children below the age of 6.

Expectorants and Mucolytic Agents

Bronchial mucus is formed by the bronchial glands and goblet cells in the bronchial epithelium. Both are stimulated by irritation from particulate matter, but the bronchial glands also respond to nervous (vagal) and humoral (atropine) influences. The function of bronchial mucus is twofold: it traps and removes particles, and it moistens the bronchial mucosa. Two layers of mucus are present. A thin layer bathes the cilia and a thicker, superimposed layer, is propelled cephalad by the cilia.

In asthma there is an increased production of highly viscid mucus. For this reason mucus flow and removal by ciliary action is impaired. This causes additional obstruction of the airway, atelectasis and may also enhance the colonization of bacteria. When bronchial infection is superimposed, the problem is worsened because of the production of an even more viscid mucus. It is imperative therefore to institute measures to maintain the mucus liquefied and thin so that it is continually propelled by the cilia and becomes more easily removed by coughing. For these reasons it is not wise to suppress cough in the asthmatic unless it is irritative, fatiguing and nonproductive.

Simply increasing fluid intake maintains a more liquefied mucus. All asthmatics should be instructed to make a conscious effort to increase their fluid intake.

Iodides

Iodides are the most commonly used expectorants. The underlying mechanism by which they exert their expectorant action has not been fully established. They are known to promote bronchorrhea by producing a more watery secretion. Iodides may also alter the protein substrate of mucus so that it is more readily hydrolyzed by the natural leukocytic proteases. A saturated solution of potassium iodide (SSKI) is the cheapest and probably most effective form of therapy. The adult dose is 10 to 15 drops four times daily and must be taken diluted in water, milk or juice. In children the dose is 1 drop per year of age four times daily. Iodides are also incorporated in many drug mixtures used in the treatment of asthma.

Iodinated glycerol, Organidin,* is another oral preparation which may

* Trademark, Wampole Laboratories.

Table 8-1. Some Theophylline Preparations Used in the Treatment of Asthma

Name	Content	Available Forms	Adult Dose	Child Dose
Elixophylline	Theophylline	Liquid	30-45 ml. t.i.d.	0.2-0.3 ml./lb. t.i.d.
Elixophylline-KI	Theophylline KI	Liquid	30-45 ml. t.i.d.	0.2-0.3 ml./lb. t.i.d.
Theokin	Theophylline KI	Liquid / Tablets	15 ml. every 8-12 hrs. / 1 tablet every 8-12 hrs.	5 ml./30 lb. every 12 hrs. / ½ tablet/45 lb. every 12 hrs.
Quibron	Theophylline Glyceryl Guaiacolate	Liquid / Capsules	15 or 30 ml. b.i.d. or t.i.d. / 1 or 2 capsules b.i.d. or t.i.d.	2⅔ ml./10 lb. b.i.d. or t.i.d. / 1 capsule b.i.d. or t.i.d. (age 6-12)
Choledyl	Oxtriphylline	Liquid (100 mg./5 ml.) / Tablets (100 and 200 mg.)	100-200 mg. q.i.d.	5 ml./60 lb. q.i.d.
Brondecon	Oxtriphylline Glyceryl Guaiacolate	Liquid / Tablets	10 ml. q.i.d. / 1 tablet q.i.d.	5 ml./60 lb. q.i.d.
Asbron	Theophylline Glyceryl Guaiacolate / Phenylpropanolamine	Liquid / Tablet	15 or 30 cc. b.i.d. or t.i.d. / 1 or 2 tablets b.i.d. or t.i.d.	age 1-3: 2½-5 ml. b.i.d. or t.i.d. / age 3-6: 5-7½ ml. b.i.d. or t.i.d. / age 6-12: 10-15 ml. b.i.d. or t.i.d.
Lufyllin	Dyphylline	Liquid (100 mg./15 ml.) / Tablet (100 and 200 mg.)	100-200 mg. t.i.d. or q.i.d.	5-10 mg./kg./day in divided doses
Aminodur Dura Tabs	Aminophylline (0.3 g)	Tablet	1-2 tablets every 8-12 hrs.	Not recommended for children under 6
Aerolate Sr. & Jr.	Theophylline (Sr.—4 grains; Jr.—2 grains)	Capsules	1 capsule every 12 hrs.	
Aminets Children ¼ strength	Aminophylline 125 mg. Pentobarbital sodium 25 mg.	Suppositories		35 lbs. or over 1 every 12 hrs.
Children ½ strength	Aminophylline 250 mg. Pentobarbital sodium 50 mg.			80 lbs. or over 1 every 8 to 12 hrs.
Adults full strength	Aminophylline 500 mg. Pentobarbital sodium 100 mg.		1 every 8-12 hrs.	
Fleet Theophylline	Theophylline monoethanolamine 250 or 500 mg.	Enema	250 to 500 mg. every 8 to 12 hrs.	

be used. This product presumably causes fewer gastrointestinal side effects than iodides, but it is probably less effective as an expectorant. It is available as a solution, tablet and elixir. The dose for adults is either 20 drops of the solution four times daily taken with a liquid or two of the tablets four times daily with a liquid. The adult dose of the elixir is one teaspoon four times daily. One third to one half of the adult dose is recommended for children.

Intravenous sodium iodide, 0.5 to 1.0 g., added to a bottle of intravenous fluids may also be used in severe status asthmaticus when the patient is unable to take oral medication. In adults the dose should not exceed 1 g. per 24 hours and in children it should not exceed 0.3 to 0.5 g. per 24 hours.

The most frequent side effects of iodides include metallic taste, nausea, vomiting, pyrosis, acniform skin eruption, parotitis and nasal congestion. Rarer more serious side effects include erythema nodosum, urticaria, bullous eruptions, fever and hypersensitivity angiitis. In children receiving prolonged iodide therapy goiter may develop; this finding warrants its discontinuation. Although rare, hypothyroidism from prolonged use of iodides may occur.

Glyceryl Guaiacolate

Glyceryl guaiacolate (Robitussin *), 100 to 200 mg. four times daily, may be used in patients with iodide intolerance, but its expectorant action is less than that of iodides. It is present in many of the commonly used drug mixtures (see list below). No serious side effects have been reported from the use of glyceryl guaiacolate, but recently it has been shown to decrease platelet adhesiveness. Because of the latter property it should probably be avoided in patients with an active peptic ulcer or in patients with a bleeding diathesis. Ingestion of glyceryl guaiacolate gives rise to a colored metabolic end product which may result in a false positive elevation of urinary 5-HIAA (5-hydroxyindoleacetic acid).[31] Patients in whom this study is contemplated should avoid glyceryl guaiacolate for at least 24 to 48 hours. This laboratory study is important in establishing the diagnosis of carcinoid, a condition which itself may be associated with wheezing.

Bromhexine

Bromhexine, a new oral expectorant currently undergoing clinical trials in England and the United States, is a synthetic derivative of vasicine, an alkaloid derived from the plant *Abhatoda vasica*. Its expectorant action is thought to result from depolymerization of the high molecular weight mucopolysaccharide protein fibers. Although the first clinical trials yielded conflicting results, a recent study utilizing a higher

* Trademark, A. H. Robins, Inc.

dose revealed objective evidence of its expectorant action.[18] The dose given in the latter study was 16 mg. three times daily. The drug appears to be well tolerated. Mild epigastric distress and nausea are the only untoward effects thus far reported.

N-acetylcysteine

N-acetylcysteine (Mucomyst *) enjoys common clinical use and is effective on both purulent and nonpurulent sputum. A 10 or 20 percent solution is sufficient to exert its mucolytic activity. To insure efficient contact with respiratory secretions it is best administered by positive pressure aerosolization. When a lot of thick sputum is present, 1 to 2 ml. may be poured directly into the tracheobronchial tree (at bronchoscopy, through tracheostomy or endobronchial tube) followed by immediate suction. The mucolytic action of N-acetylcysteine results from the activity of its free sulfhydryl group acting upon the disulfide bonds of mucoprotein.

One disadvantage of its use is the propensity to induce bronchospasm, especially in asthmatics. When used in an asthmatic it is important to observe the patient closely; and it is advisable to use it with isoproterenol. A suggested aerosol mixture is 3 ml. of the 10 per cent N-acetylcysteine combined with 0.25 ml. of 1:200 isoproterenol.

Pancreatic Dornase

Pancreatic dornase (Dornavac †) is another effective mucolytic. Its use is limited since it promotes liquefaction of purulent sputum only. The mucolytic activity of this enzyme is mediated by its ability to depolymerize DNA, which is present only in purulent sputum. Bronchospasm may also occur with its use but to a lesser extent as is seen with N-acetylcysteine. Pancreatic dornase can be effectively administered by ultrasonic nebulization or by jet nebulizer. The dose is 1000 units dissolved in 10 ml. of diluent (10 percent propylene glycol or saline) for ultrasonic nebulization or 2 to 3 ml. of diluent for the jet nebulizer.

Combination Drug Preparations

Many tablet and liquid preparations containing a mixture of ephedrine, theophylline, expectorants and sedatives provide a simplified and economical approach to drug therapy. The many combinations enable adequate alternatives when one or other ingredient cannot be tolerated. Sustained action preparations, such as Tedral-SA,‡ are helpful in controlling mild nocturnal exacerbations and may offer smooth control

* Trademark, Mead, Johnson.
† Trademark, Merck Sharp & Dohme.
‡ Trademark, Warner-Chilcott.

of mild symptoms when taken every 8 to 12 hours. Enteric coated (i.e., Tedral) preparations are also available when gastric irritation may be a problem.

Some Combination Drugs Used in Management of Asthma

TRADE NAME	CONTENTS
* Tedral	Ephedrine, theophylline, phenobarbital
* Tedral Expectorant	Ephedrine, theophylline, phenobarbital, glyceryl guaiacolate
* Quadrinal	Ephedrine, theophylline, phenobarbital, KI
* Veraquard	Ephedrine, theophylline, phenobarbital, glyceryl guaiacolate
* Marax	Ephedrine, theophylline, hydroxyzine
* KIE	Ephedrine, KI, (also available with phenobarbital)
* Asbron	Phenylpropanolamine, glyceryl guaiacolate, theophylline
Amesec	Ephedrine, aminophylline, amobarbital
* Bronkotab (Bronkolixir)	Ephedrine, theophylline, phenobarbital, glyceryl guaiacolate
* Brondecon	Oxtriphylline, glyceryl guaiacolate
* Quibron	Theophylline, glyceryl guaiacolate
Ephedrine-Amytal	Ephedrine, amobarbital
* Lufyllin-GG	Dyphylline, glyceryl guaiacolate
* Lufyllin-EP	Dyphylline, ephedrine, phenobarbital
* Lufyllin-EPG	Dyphylline, ephedrine, phenobarbital, glyceryl guaiacolate
Amodrine	Theophylline, racephedrine, phenobarbital

* Available in tablet and liquid preparations.

Antibiotics

Early and judicious antibiotic treatment of respiratory infection in asthma is an important aspect of therapy. Clinical signs of fever and malaise may not be present, and often the only index of infection may be increased sputum viscosity. The change in color of sputum from white-gray to yellow or green is another indication of the presence of respiratory infection. Similarly, this change in the color of sputum may be the only clinical evidence of infection. Ideally, gram stain study and culture of the sputum should be obtained, but in the routine outpatient care of asthmatics, these studies may be impractical and antibiotics may be given without their benefit. If symptoms persist with evidence of continuing infection despite the addition of an antibiotic, it is advisable to obtain sputum culture and sensitivities before changing to another antibiotic.

The most common causative bacterial organisms encountered with respiratory infections in asthmatics are pneumococci, streptococci and *Hemophilus influenzae*. Penicillin and broad spectrum antibiotics such as tetracycline and ampicillin are the drugs of choice. Studies have shown possible benefit of prophylactic antibiotic therapy (continuous or intermittent courses) during the winter months. To prevent emergence of resistant organisms this practice should be limited and not used indiscriminately for all asthmatics.

Corticosteroids

Corticosteroids represent the most effective drugs in the treatment of asthma. Because of their potentially serious side effects, they are advised when other measures have not provided sufficient control of acute or chronic symptoms. Their indiscriminate use for every episode of asthma is to be criticized. On the other hand, failure to use them when indicated may result in unwarranted morbidity and mortality. In life-threatening asthma, corticosteroids are essential, but because of their delayed onset of action they cannot replace other necessary emergency measures including epinephrine, aminophylline, patent airway and oxygen. Balanced clinical judgment must be exercised before they are used in any given situation.

The exact mode of action of corticosteroids in asthma is not known but probably results from their anti-inflammatory effects. Reduction of bronchial mucosal edema, suppression of the inflammatory response, stabilization of membrane (vascular and lysozomal) permeability are but a few of their known effects which may benefit asthma. In addition, studies in vitro have shown that large amounts of corticosteroids induce relaxation of bronchial muscle preparations. It has also been suggested that corticosteroids might restore responsiveness to bronchodilator (β stimulator) drugs by enhancing their activation of adenyl cyclase. Reaccumulation of histamine granules in mast cells is inhibited by corticosteroids. This latter property could also be helpful in controlling asthmatic symptoms; but it must be emphasized that the fate of the mast cell after it has released histamine is not definitely known.

Not only are these compounds of therapeutic importance, but they may be useful as a diagnostic tool. Often it is helpful to document the exact amount of reversibility of a patient's signs and symptoms in order to establish whether the basic underlying process is asthma or irreversible obstructive airway disease. Suppressive doses of corticosteroids for 3 to 7 days would significantly reverse the airway obstruction of asthma but would result in little or no reversibility in bronchitis or emphysema. The suppressive dose of prednisone in children is 2 mg./kg./day in divided doses and in adults it is from 40 to 80 mg. per day.

Numerous analogues of cortisone and hydrocortisone are now available. Varying their chemical configurations has conferred changes in duration of action, but, more specifically, it has resulted in a lessening of their mineralocorticoid effect. Unfortunately, the development of the newer synthetic analogues has not resulted in any preparation with only anti-inflammatory properties without the concomitant undesirable effects on glucose and protein metabolism. Serious side effects can therefore result from prolonged use of any of these preparations and certain preparations appear to have an increased propensity for a specific side effect (Table 8-2).

Despite the many side effects resulting from the use of corticosteroids, there are only a few absolute contraindications to their use. The presence of varicella and herpes simplex ophthalmicus constitute the commonly listed absolute contraindications. Most of the serious side effects result from prolonged chronic treatment with large doses. In most asthmatics chronic maintenance doses of corticosteroids are relatively low. The dosage range is usually 2.5 to 15 mg. of prednisone or its equivalent per day. Long term studies of steroid dependent asthmatics have accordingly shown predominately tolerable side effects.

In order to minimize side effects it is important to use these drugs for the least possible length of time necessary to achieve their clinical goal. A 3-day course of corticosteroids in suppressive doses may be sufficient to reverse an occasional acute episode which has not responded adequately to the common modes of therapy. If corticosteroids are required for longer periods abrupt discontinuation may exacerbate symptoms, and it is therefore advisable to discontinue therapy by gradual tapering over 7 to 10 days or even longer. In a small group of patients who have abruptly discontinued corticosteroids a withdrawal syndrome consisting of malaise, emotional lability, myalgia and low grade fever may occur. It is not exactly known why these symptoms arise in these individuals.

In patients requiring maintenance therapy, the lowest possible dose compatible with adequate control of symptoms should be used. In patients with a history of peptic ulcer, adjunctive measures of diet restriction and antacid therapy should be included. To protect against osteoporosis the elderly are advised to drink a quart of milk per day and maintain an adequate protein intake. Supplemental calcium and vitamin D may be indicated. In postmenopausal females estrogen therapy would be included provided there is no contraindication. Prophylactic isoniazid (INH) therapy may be prescribed in patients with a history of tuberculosis. It is also wise to check tuberculin reactivity in patients requiring chronic therapy. A positive reaction in adults need not necessarily demand chronic INH therapy provided frequent chest x-rays are obtained. In every patient requiring chronic corticosteroid therapy, follow-up surveillance is necessary for early detection and management of possible side effects. It is suggested that yearly physical

TABLE 8-2
Corticosteroids: Their Relative Dose Equivalents and Propensity for Specific Side Effects

	Equivalent Anti-inflammatory Dose	Mineralocorticoid Potency (Fluid Retention)	Increased Appetite	Growth Suppression	Myopathy	Purpura Ecchymosis	Adrenal Suppression
Short Acting							
Hydrocortisone	20 mg	+++	++	+	+	+	++
Prednisone	5 mg	++	++	++	+	++	++
Methylprednisone	4 mg	+	++	++	+	++	++
Prednisolone	5 mg	++	++	++	+	++	++
Methylprednisolone	5 mg	+	++	++	+	+++	++
Intermediate Acting							
Paramethasone	2 mg	+	+	++	+	+	++
Triamcinolone	4 mg	0	±	?	+++	++	+++
Long Acting							
Betamethasone	0.6 mg	+	++	++	+	++	++
Dexamethasone	0.75 mg	+	+++	++	+	++	+++

Possible Complications of Corticosteroids

TOLERABLE COMPLICATIONS:

Increased appetite and weight gain
Edema
Eccymosis
Striae
Hypertrichosis
Insomnia
Euphoria
Leg cramps
Leukocytosis
Cushingoid body changes

MORE SERIOUS COMPLICATIONS:

Endocrine
Adrenal suppression
Diabetes

Cardiovascular
Hypertension
Congestive heart failure
Thromboembolism
Arteritis

Gastrointestinal
Peptic ulcer
Gastritis
Esophagitis
Pancreatitis

Hematopoietic
Agranulocytosis

Musculoskeletal
Myopathy—proximal
Tendon rupture
Osteoporosis
Aseptic necrosis
Growth suppression

Ocular
Subcapsular cataracts
Glaucoma
Exophthalmos
Enhances herpes and fungal keratitis

Central nervous
Psychosis
Pseudotumor cerebri
Seizures

Serum electrolytes
Hypokalemia—weakness
alkalosis

Adverse effect on infection
Enhances virulence
Masks symptoms
Activates latent infection

Subcutaneous tissue
Panniculitis

examinations with chest x-ray, complete blood count, urine analysis and 2-hour postprandial blood sugar determination be done. Lumbosacral x-rays every 2 to 4 years are helpful in determining the presence or progression of osteoporosis. In children an accurate record of growth is indicated.

It is desirable to use those preparations with the shortest duration of action and with the least suppressive capacity on the adrenals. Prednisone best fulfills these criteria and furthermore is the least expensive of all the corticosteroids. It is not available in a liquid preparation, but for small children the tablet can be crushed and given in a teaspoon of apple sauce.

A serious side effect from corticosteroids is suppression of the hypothalamic-pituitary-adrenal (HPA) axis. This results in an impaired ability to tolerate stress and for this reason patients must receive increased doses during stressful situations such as surgery, infectious illnesses, and even exacerbations of asthma. Significant HPA suppression occurs with as little as 3 to 5 days of systemic therapy and may also result from chronic local administration (i.e., inhalation or topical). The extent of suppression, however, is variable from patient to patient. The time required for a return to normal HPA activity after discontinuation of corticosteroids also varies and is unpredictable. In some patients, inability of the HPA axis to respond to stress may persist for up to a year after the cessation of therapy, and in others normal HPA reactivity may persist despite taking corticosteroids for as long as 10 years.

In addition to direct measurements of blood cortisol and ACTH, other specific tests are available to determine the functional integrity of each part of the HPA axis. These tests involve measurements of blood and/or urinary steroid levels before and after a specific stimulus is directed to only one component of the HPA axis. The ACTH stimulation test reveals adrenal responsiveness. The oral metapyrone test indicates the pituitary's ability to secrete ACTH. Metapyrone inhibits 11-β-hydroxylase, the enzyme that converts compound S to compound F (cortisol). The resultant decrease of cortisol stimulates the pituitary to secrete ACTH (negative feedback) which in turn stimulates the adrenal; compound S increases and is measured as an increase in urinary 17-hydroxysteroids. Thus, if metapyrone does not result in a urinary rise of 17-hydroxysteroid, the pituitary release of ACTH is impaired provided the adrenal gland is itself not suppressed. The administration of arginine vasopressin, a substance which releases ACTH from the pituitary, constitutes another test of pituitary responsiveness. Insulin hypoglycemia produces an increase in cortisol levels by releasing hypothalamic CRF (corticotropin releasing factor). The response to insulin hypoglycemia correlates well with the ability of the HPA axis to mount an adequate response to stress. Studies utilizing these various testing parameters have suggested that with corticosteroid therapy the following sequence of HPA suppression occurs: the hypothalamus first, then the pituitary and finally the adrenal. In evaluating the HPA axis the ACTH stimulation test should be done first. If it is subnormal it can be assumed that there is gross HPA suppression. When the ACTH test is normal, the metapyrone test and insulin hypoglycemia response will indicate the presence or absence of pituitary or hypothalamic insufficiency. An abnormal HPA axis can therefore exist in the presence of normal cortisol levels and a normal ACTH test. For example, if the latter two parameters are normal, a patient may still be unable to withstand the stress of major surgery.

To minimize the occurrence of adverse side effects as well as HPA suppression the use of intermittent (3 to 4 days out of 7), or alternate day corticosteroid therapy has been advocated. In addition, the total daily dose should be taken in the morning. Most asthmatics obtain adequate control of symptoms by these forms of therapy. These methods of administration are applicable primarily to patients requiring corticosteroids for more than 10 days and especially those requiring chronic maintenance doses. When utilizing these forms of therapy it is important to use short-acting corticosteroids. Intermittent or alternate day therapy with dexamethasone (long-acting) is as suppressive as that resulting from its daily use.

Studies have shown that the use of alternate day or intermittent therapy has resulted in a decrease in some side effects such as moon face, growth retardation, obesity, hypertension, mental abberations and possibly osteoporosis. A study by Malone et al.,[26] however, has shown that four of five asthmatics on chronic intermittent prednisone therapy had an impaired insulin hypoglycemia response. Four of five on daily therapy similarly had an impaired insulin response. It can be assumed therefore, that despite the lowered incidence of side effects resulting from intermittent or alternate day corticosteroid therapy, these forms of therapy may still be associated with suppression of the HPA axis (especially as related to stress). Even in these patients, corticosteroids should therefore be temporarily increased during periods of stress.

Parenteral Corticosteroids. Intravenous corticosteroids are generally utilized for status asthmaticus. Hydrocortisone (Solu-Cortef *) is the most commonly used. Other intravenous preparations available are methyl prednisolone (Solu-Medrol *), prednisolone (Hydeltrasol †) and dexamethasone.

Collins et al.[8] conducted a study to determine the fate of intravenously

* Trademark, Upjohn Co.
† Trademark, Merck Sharp & Dohme.

injected hydrocortisone hemisuccinate in acutely asthmatic and non-asthmatic subjects given varying loading doses. In both groups peak plasma levels occurred at the same time, and the plasma half life was identical. Peak plasma levels occurred within 60 minutes, and the half life of a 4 mg./kg. dose was 125 minutes. These investigators felt that a plasma cortisol level of 150 μg. percent was necessary for a satisfactory clinical response, but others have suggested that a level of at least 100 μg. percent was sufficient. A dose of 4 mg./kg. given at intervals of 140 minutes would maintain a plasma cortisol level of 150 μg. percent. This dose given at intervals of 220 minutes was required to maintain a cortisol level in excess of 100 μg. percent. These findings suggest that in the treatment of status asthmaticus the appropriate dose of hydrocortisone is 4 mg./kg. every 2 to 4 hours. When using such large doses of hydrocortisone, replacement of potassium is important.

Aerosol Corticosteroids. Dexamethasone phosphate (Decadron Respihaler *) is available in pressurized hand cannister aerosols. The recommended starting dose is three inhalations (two for children) four times daily. When symptoms are controlled the dose should gradually be reduced. One presumed advantage of this type of administration is that a lesser amount of corticosteroid may be required as compared with systemic therapy. Many have found this not to be true, and as a result this form of therapy has not become generally accepted. The cautions and side effects of aerosol therapy as expressed above are also applicable to this product.

Depot Corticosteroids. Repository injectable preparations of corticosteroids have recently become available. Their superiority over oral corticosteroids has not been definitely established. Advocates claim that they bypass the local effects of corticosteroids on the gastric mucosa, have a faster onset of action, and have a lower incidence of side effects. One advantage may be better control of therapy in those patients who tend to indiscriminately abuse oral preparations. It is to be noted that some preparations have caused subcutaneous atrophy and most preparations are associated with a profound and long lasting HPA suppression.

ACTH

The use of ACTH in the treatment of asthma continues to be controversial. A critical review of the various aspects of ACTH therapy, however, suggests that it has little advantage over corticosteroids. The beneficial effect of ACTH stems from the release of endogenous corticoids; there is no evidence suggesting that ACTH, itself, has any ameliorating effect on asthma. In status asthmaticus, since the adrenal glands

* Trademark, Merck Sharp & Dohme.

are already maximally stimulated, ACTH would probably not result in further release of endogenous corticoids. In this situation ACTH is absolutely contraindicated.

Since ACTH stimulates the adrenals, its presumed major advantage would be the avoidance of adrenal suppression. Chronic ACTH therapy, however, has occasionally been noted to result in a loss of its effectiveness. This has suggested the possibility that chronic stimulation of the adrenals may eventually impair their function. Alternatively, chronic exogenous ACTH administration may suppress the hypothalamic and/or pituitary mechanisms for endogenous ACTH release. A study of 10 patients receiving daily ACTH therapy (from 2 to 17 years) for rheumatoid arthritis did reveal a suppressed cortisol response to insulin hypoglycemia [10] but most patients receiving daily ACTH for 2 years or less maintain normal HPA function.

It has been suggested that the sequential use of ACTH combined with corticosteroids may lessen the adrenal suppression resulting from corticosteroids alone. One study, however, did not document such an effect, and parenthetically, a heightened adrenal suppression resulted from the combined use.[21]

Growth retardation is a common serious side effect from chronic corticosteroid therapy. Chronic ACTH therapy in asthmatic children is significantly less growth-retarding. On the other hand, it has also been shown that intermittent or alternate day prednisone therapy lessens the incidence of this side effect, and if these forms of therapy are unable to control symptoms, ACTH therapy may be preferred.

The cited allergic reactions to ACTH derived from animal sources will probably lessen by the use of newly synthetic preparations now available. It must be cautioned, however, that allergic reactions have already been reported from the new synthetic preparations.

New Drugs for the Treatment of Asthma

Disodium Cromoglycate, Cromolyn sodium, was first shown to be effective in preventing the bronchospasm from inhaled antigens by Altounyan in 1965.[3] Since then there have been numerous reports documenting its effectiveness in from 40 to 60 percent of subjects tested. In 1968 it was made available for general clinical use in England and Europe. In the United States, clinical trials and studies have also documented its usefulness and it is expected to become available for general use.

Disodium cromoglycate is a derivative of khellin, an active principle obtained from crude extracts of seeds from an Eastern Mediterranean plant, *Ammni visnaga*. The drug is not absorbed by the gastrointestinal tract, but when inhaled, approximately 10 percent is absorbed systemically. The unchanged drug is excreted in the urine and bile. It is available as a fine micronized powder usually diluted in lactose and provided in a capsule for inhalation through a Spinhaler (Fisons Ltd.). The dose is 20 mg. four times daily.

This drug possesses no intrinsic bronchodilating or antihistaminic properties. Studies in vitro have shown that disodium cromoglycate inhibits IgE-mediated histamine and SRS-A release and does not inhibit the antigen-antibody reaction per se. Its suspected mode of action is specific inhibition, probably enzymatic, of an intermediate reaction in the mediator-releasing pathway triggered by the antigen-antibody interaction. This mechanism of action would suggest primary benefit for extrinsic asthma only, but some intrinsic asthmatics have also benefited from its use. Of interest is the recent finding that disodium cromoglycate inhibits exercise bronchospasm also.[11, 37]

Antigen inhalation challenges in patients with allergic pulmonary aspergillosis characteristically result in immediate (Type I, IgE-mediated) decreases in FEV_1 followed by another late reaction (Type III, precipitin-mediated), usually beginning from 4 to 12 hours after initial challenge. Pre-challenge treatment with disodium cromoglycate inhibited both reactions. Antigen challenge in some patients with bird fancier's disease results primarily in the precipitin-mediated bronchopulmonary type of reaction. Pretreatment with disodium cromoglycate in these patients likewise inhibited the response despite the antecedent absence of the IgE-mediated reaction. Further pharmacologic and immunologic studies of disodium cromoglycate may be helpful in clarifying the basic mechanisms of Type I and Type III reactions and how they may be interrelated.

Therapeutically, disodium cromoglycate will probably have its greatest impact in the corticosteroid-dependent asthmatic. The additional benefit it provides may allow a reduction in the maintenance dose of corticosteroid or, possibly, discontinuation. Whether disodium cromoglycate will supplant the other commonly used methods of treatment in less severe asthma remains to be seen.

No significant side effects have been reported from the use of disodium cromoglycate. Mild irritation of the tracheobronchial tree with slight bronchospasm may occur. The addition of isoproterenol in the capsule is helpful in relieving this minor side effect.

Diethylcarbamazine (Hetrazan *) is an antihelminth, which when used in the treatment of tropical eosinophilia was noted to relieve the associated bronchospasm. Although an original uncontrolled study showed promising results with its use in asthmatics, a more recent controlled study revealed it to be of no significant benefit.[5] Further studies

* Trademark, Lederle Laboratories.

are necessary, but at present its usefulness in the treatment of asthma is questionable. Diethylcarbamazine has been shown to inhibit the release of SRS-A without inhibiting the antigen-antibody reaction. It is not an antagonist of SRS-A nor does it possess bronchodilating or antihistaminic properties.

Fenspiride, developed in France, is a new nonsteroidal bronchodilator. Clinical trials have reportedly shown it to be effective in the treatment of acute and chronic asthma.[7] Its mechanism of action is not known, but it has been shown to inhibit histamine and serotonin bronchospasm in the guinea pig. Studies in vitro have also suggested an immunosuppressive potential. Further clinical trials are planned in the United States.

Leaf of Tylophora Indica. In India, the leaf of the Tylophora indica plant has been found to benefit asthmatic symptoms. Clinical trials have shown significant long lasting improvement with merely chewing one leaf daily for 6 days.[36] Studies are under way to determine the active principle of the leaf. Why the juice of this leaf should improve asthma is not known.

Prostaglandins are a group of naturally occurring long chain fatty acids. They are present in many organs and tissues and possess potent vasoactive properties. Since 1962, after the chemical structure of the first member of the group was determined, these compounds have been intensively studied. Depending on their particular ring structure they have been divided into four major groups: E, F, A and B.

Human bronchial muscle preparations in vitro have been shown to relax in the presence of prostaglandin E_1 (PGE_1) and PGE_2. PGF_2, however, contracts human bronchial muscle. A study comparing the bronchodilating effects of 55 μg. of aerosolized PGE_1 (triethanolamine salt) and 550 μg. of isoproterenol was recently reported in asthmatics.[9] It was found that PGE_1, in this dosage, produced a similar increase in FEV_1 as did isoproterenol. In one of the six asthmatics tested, PGE_1 was irritating to the respiratory tract and was associated with increase cough and bronchospasm. In this patient only 5.5 μg. was sufficient to cause irritation; other asthmatics tolerated 55 μg. with no irritation. The use of PGE_1 in these asthmatics was not associated with any significant changes in blood pressure, pulse rate, and electrocardiogram.

PGE_2 and PGF_{2a} have both been identified in the human lung. Their functions in the lung are unknown. It has been suggested that asthma may represent a condition in which there is an increase of PGF_{2a} (bronchoconstrictor). No definitive evidence of the latter has been established thus far. Whether the prostaglandins have any therapeutic advantage over the presently available bronchodilators remains to be seen. The exact mechanism by which PGE_1 promotes bronchodilatation is not known but probably results from stimulating adenyl cyclase to form cyclic AMP. This action of PGE_1 has been shown to occur with leukocyte adenyl cyclase.

DRUGS AND TREATMENTS OF LITTLE OR NO VALUE

Immunosuppressant Drugs

These drugs, because of their immunosuppressive qualities as well as their anti-inflammatory effects, may theoretically be helpful in the treatment of asthma. Their serious side effects far outweigh their presumed usefulness in a condition such as asthma. Furthermore, a study reporting the effects of aziathioprine in five asthmatics revealed no significant improvement with 3 to 4 weeks of therapy.[24]

Chloroquine

Chloroquine, a well known anti-inflammatory agent, was noted to offer possible relief in asthmatics. Because of its serious retinal toxicity, further clinical trials were not warranted, and its benefit was not confirmed.

Heparin

The various properties of heparin suggesting its possible benefit in asthma and other allergic conditions include: histamine and serotonin binding properties, liberator of histaminase, inhibitor of histamine release from platelets, anticomplementary action and mucolytic activity. Controlled studies have shown it to be ineffective in asthma and to possess virtually no mulcolytic abilities.

Gay's Solution

The use of Gay's solution is not an accepted form of treatment. Its ingredients are numerous: Fowler's solution, digitalis, phenobarbital, potassium iodide, saccharin, methylparaben, propylparaben and amaranth solution. Studies have shown it to be of some possible benefit and the ingredient which might produce an ameliorating effect is arsenic (in Fowler's solution). Significant arsenic toxicity may occur, and, for this reason, as well as the availability of superior drugs, its use is not warranted.

Macrolide Antibiotics

The macrolide antibodies include triacetyloleandomycin (TAO), oleandomycin and erythromycin. It was observed clinically that when these antibiotics were used in the treatment of respiratory infections, some asthmatics appeared to obtain more relief than expected from their antibacterial activity alone. In some asthmatics their use also appeared to result in a lowering of the maintenance dose of corticosteroids. These findings suggested that these antibiotics may promote a beneficial effect unrelated to their antibacterial properties. Animal studies subsequently showed that they indeed have a glucocorticoid sparing effect, but the inherent liver toxicity associated with these drugs precludes their clinical usefulness in achieving this purpose.

Glomectomy

Resection of the carotid body (glomectomy) was once advocated as a surgical treatment for asthma. Although immediate results appeared promising, further follow-up study has shown no objective evidence of improvement. Moreover, the rationale for such a procedure in asthmatics is obscure; the chief function of these chemoreceptors is to protect against acute hypoxia or chronic hypercapnia. This treatment is not recommended.

NONSPECIFIC MEASURES

Protection from Meterologic Factors

Increasing air pollution is a known world wide health hazard. It is considered to be a major etiologic factor in certain conditions such as bronchitis, emphysema and lung cancer. Urban surveys have adequately shown the deleterious effect of pollution on patients with chronic cardiopulmonary disease. The alarming morbidity and mortality resulting from thermal inversions in cities in the United States and elsewhere have dramatized the seriousness of stagnating pollution. The asthmatic, because of his inherent bronchial hyperreactivity, is one of the most vulnerable of the high risk group of patients. The aggravating effect of pollution probably results from local irritation on the bronchial mucosa.

The measurement of certain atmospheric substances such as SO_2, particulate matter and CO provides an estimation of pollution content. Proper evaluation of meteorologic parameters can also predict in advance the occurrence of high pollution days thus enabling the high-risk population to take protective measures. On high pollution days the chronic severe asthmatic should be instructed to stay indoors with windows closed, increase bronchodilator therapy, maintain adequate hydration, rest and avoid exertion. Those on corticosteroids may be advised to increase their dosage temporarily. Patients with a propensity to develop bronchial infections may also be advised to take a broad spectrum antibiotic prophylactically.

Other meterologic factors such as sudden changes in temperature, increases in relative humidity and increasing barometric pressure may also aggravate asthmatic symptoms. It is impossible to completely protect patients from these changes. Why these weather changes should aggravate asthma is not completely known. The associated positive air ionization which may occur with these changes has been an incriminated cause for the exacerbation of symptoms. Artificially controlled negative air ionization environments have provided some relief to patients with pollenosis, but adequate confirmation is still lacking. The combination of meteorologic factors may also be important in triggering symptoms. For example, a recent study [15] comparing the peak incidence of asthma seen in a general hospital (in Philadelphia) with comcomitant meteorologic factors revealed a threefold increase of asthma during days of high pollution and a fourfold increase on days of high barometric pressure. Of interest was when both these conditions coincided there was a ninefold increase in the incidence of asthma. In prospective studies of "New Orleans asthma" [34] epidemic days did not necessarily occur when pollen or mold spore counts alone were increased, but usually when associated with meteorologic factors such as rising barometric pressure or decreases in temperature, relative humidity and wind velocity. Although these climatic influences may increase atmospheric allergen and particulate concentrations a direct additive or synergistic effect on bronchial hyperreactivity can also be involved. Research studies utilizing artificially controlled environment units will hopefully provide a clearer understanding of the influences and mechanisms of these metereologic variables.

The breathing of cold air is a potent stimulus which precipitates symptoms in many asthmatics. This is thought to occur via vagal reflex action. The use of face masks is to be encouraged in these patients. Masks with attachable heating units are also available.

A change of climate is generally unnecessary and often economically impractical for many patients. This type of therapy must be guided by a rational and deliberate consideration of the severity of the patient's condition, and the psychologic implications of such a move and, above all, the social and economic well-being of the family unit itself. It should only be considered after appropriate medical and allergy management have proved ineffective in significantly curbing symptoms. No area of the United States is completely devoid of inhalant allergens, and the possibility of allergic patients becoming sensitized and symptomatic to the newly confronted allergens exists.

Although European physicians have notably stressed the beneficial effects of high altitude, there has really been no good objective evidence substantiating this claim. Mites are probably the most important allergen constituent of house dust. The house dust of high altitude appears to have less mites than that of lower levels, and it has been suggested that this may be one reason why some asthmatics may improve after moving to higher altitudes.[38]

In those patients (usually intrinsic or mixed asthmatics) in whom meteorologic factors and air pollution appear to be important potentiating factors, moving to a warm, less humid and less industrialized area may be helpful. Patients who live in an urban area of relatively high atmospheric pollution may note significant improvement by merely moving to a nearby area or suburb with less pollution. If it is deemed necessary to attempt a trial of climate change, a 2 to 4-week stay is not sufficient to conclude whether the change will be effective. A more realistic approach is to allow a 6 to 12-month trial period.

Home Environment

Certain controls of the internal environment of the home (especially the bedroom) are beneficial. Extremes of humidity can adversely affect the asthmatic; the optimal humidity should range from 40 to 50 percent. Low humidity dries the mucous membranes and becomes an irritative factor. It must be cautioned, however, that hypersensitivity pneumonitis resulting from mold (thermophilic actinomycetes and micropolyspora faeni) contaminated humidifiers has been reported. A detailed discussion of this type of pneumonitis can be found in Chapter 18.

The proper temperature range should be 68 to 72° F. Care should be taken to avoid rapid changes in temperature. Most asthmatics are benefited by air conditioning, but in a few, the cold air may increase symptoms.

Mechanical devices which purify circulating air may be helpful. Air filters vary in their effectiveness, but in general remove only particles greater than 5μ (pollens) in size. Many inhalant particles, such as dust, fumes, smoke, mold spores, bacteria and viruses are less than 5μ. The most efficient air cleaning device is the electrostatic precipitator, which attracts particles of all sizes by high voltage plates. Air cleaners that utilize a refined filtering system have recently become available. They are presumed to be equally efficient with the advantage of not emitting ozone, a toxic and irritative substance which may be emitted from the electrostatic precipitator.

Smoking

Cigarette smoking must be discouraged in all asthmatics. Its deleterious effects probably result from bronchial irritation and impairment of antibacterial defense mechanisms. Cigarette smoke has been shown to impair the mucociliary mechanism and to inhibit alveolar macrophage phagocytosis. The possibility that tobacco smoke may evoke symptoms on an allergic basis also exists.

Exercise

Exercise programs have been advised in the total treatment of the chronic perennial asthmatic. The two types of exercises utilized are breathing exercises and general conditioning or physical fitness exercises.

Breathing exercises to improve ventilation are so designed as to enhance the expiratory effort of breathing. This is accomplished by training the patient to voluntarily use his abdominal muscles which increases intra-abdominal pressure and results in passively displacing the diaphragm higher into the thorax. The time of expiration must also be consciously prolonged. It is assumed that the passive elevation of the diaphragm is helpful in promoting a more efficient expiratory phase, since the thoracic component of respiration is already compromised by the hyperexpanded state. It is recommended that these exercises be performed upon arising, before retiring, and at the onset of an acute episode of asthma. Studies to determine the long term effects of these exercises have consistently shown little or no objective improvement. In some patients they may be helpful in preventing or allaying the severity of an acute attack of wheezing. The latter amelioration may be due to inhibiting the hyperventilation associated with an acute attack. The exercise may also provide a psychological benefit to these patients.

Exercises to correct the musculoskeletal deformity of the chest commonly seen in the young asthmatic have also been advised. Because of the flexibility of the chest cage these thoracic changes are not permanent and usually reverse when asthma improves. The characteristic changes are increase in anteroposterior and transverse diameters of the chest, a prominent sternum, drawing in of the lower ribs and rib cartilages ("asthmatic pseudo-richets"), elevation of the shoulders and exaggeration of the kyphosis of the spine. The abnormal configuration of the chest is thought to result from an increased tonus of the muscles of inspiration to accomodate the hyperinflated lungs. These exercises are thus designed to produce muscular relaxation and increased mobility of thorax and shoulder girdle.

Publications of the above exercises have been made available for patient distribution by Breon Laboratories, Inc., and Riker Laboratories. A similar publication is also being prepared by the section of Allergy of the American Academy of Pediatrics.

Physical fitness exercises consisting of modified calisthenics, walk-jog and swimming have been encouraged in adults as well as children with asthma. Again, objective evidence of improvement of their disease is minimal.

The subjective and psychologic assets of physical conditioning, especially in asthmatic children, may be a helpful adjunct in treatment. A unique feature of asthma is the occurrence of bronchospasm with exertion; many children may thus be discouraged by their inability to partake in sports or withstand other normal exerting activities. These feelings of inferiority promote additional physical and psychologic incapacitation. An exercise program, especially in a peer group with similar disability, will result in a noticeable increase in their physical capacities. This in turn instills a sense of accomplishment and competition, attributes so desperately needed to uplift their self image. Oral bronchodilators or nebulized isoproterenol taken 15 to 30 minutes before exercise will decrease postexercise bronchospasm. Although it is generally advisable to encourage patients to exercise and participate in sports, during periods of exacerbation it is wise to temporarily suspend these activities.

A propensity for nocturnal episodes of wheezing is another common feature of asthma. Sleep studies in asthmatics have shown that the nocturnal attacks occur in both REM (rapid eye movement) as well as non-REM periods of sleep.[23] It was also found that asthmatic episodes were less prone to occur in stage 4 sleep. As compared to normals the amount of stage 4 sleep is reduced in asthmatics. It is known that exercise induces an increase in stage 4 sleep, and thus it has been suggested that exercise before going to sleep, by increasing stage 4 sleep, may reduce the frequency of nocturnal attacks. Further studies are needed to test this hypothesis.

Drugs Which May Adversely Affect Asthma

Antihistamines and anticholinergics should generally be avoided during exacerbations of asthma because of their tendency to dry bronchial secretions. Atropine, although a known bronchodilator, should also be avoided for similar reasons.

Antidepressants of the monoamine oxidase inhibitor class are not recommended since these substances may induce a hypertensive crisis when taken with sympathomimetic drugs which are commonly used in the medical treatment of asthma. The tricyclic group of antidepressants are less apt to produce this complication.

Narcotics such as morphine and meperidine, because of their respiratory depressive properties, are contraindicated during exacerbations of asthma. Moreover, morphine is a known histamine releaser. Even mild sedatives and tranquilizers should be used with caution since they also induce varying amounts of respiratory depression. Small doses of these drugs (i.e., meprobamate, chlordiazepoxide, phenobarbital, chloral hydrate, hydroxyzine and phenothiazines) may be used cautiously in the outpatient treatment of asthmatics in whom anxiety symptoms are present. Asthma should not be considered primarily as an expression of an underlying emotional disturbance, and its diagnosis alone is not an indication for the use of these drugs.

Excessive use of hypnotics for sleep must also be discouraged. A study [2] comparing the respiratory function during chloral hydrate-induced sleep (20 mg./kg.) in asthmatics and nonasthmatics has shown a significantly more prolonged hypoxemia in the asthmatics. Although the level was not dangerously low, it is conceivable that during periods of exacerbation, especially if the dose is repeated, dangerous levels of pO_2 may result.

Status asthmaticus is an absolute contraindication for the use of all sedatives or tranquilizers. In this situation, even small doses of these drugs may cause respiratory depression. Phenothiazines, in this context, deserve further comment. These drugs are not only tranquilizers but also possess alpha adrenergic blocking properties and thus may potentiate the vasodilator effects of isoproterenol, a β-stimulating drug commonly used in status asthmaticus. The combined effect of these two drugs may therefore induce severe hypotension; moreover, the associative dehydration (decrease in blood volume) present in status asthmaticus may further potentiate this problem.

Drugs possessing anticholinesterase properties may potentiate wheezing in asthmatics. This results from their net parasympathomimetic enhancing effect due to the inhibition of acetylcholine catabolism. These drugs represent the primary drug treatment of myasthenia gravis; if asthma coexists, a therapeutic problem arises. When anticholinesterases are necessary, maximal doses of ephedrine, aminophylline and expectorants must be used. The addition of corticosteroids may be indicated for more adequate control of asthma, but it must be remembered that in some patients myasthemic symptoms may initially worsen with addition of corticosteroids.

Reserpine may also trigger bronchospasm in asthmatics. With the common oral dosage used in the treatment of hypertension, the aggravating effect on asthma, although noted by some investigators in the past, has not been widely publicized. When used parenterally in higher dosage (1.0 to 2.5 mg.) as in severe hypertension, it has reportedly caused clinically significant bronchospasm. The mechanism by which reserpine induces bronchospasm is not known but presumably may result either from its catecholamine-depleting potential or its known cholingergic effects.

Propranolol (Inderal *), a β-adrenergic blocking drug, has recently gained wide clinical use in the treatment of cardiac arrhythmias, angina,

* Trademark, Ayerst Laboratories.

hypertension, hypertrophic subaortic stenosis and thyrotoxicosis. This drug exerts its blocking properties on both cardiac and pulmonary β-receptors. As a result of the latter it enhances and triggers wheezing in overt and latent asthmatics. The adrenergic receptors of the lung are predominately beta in type and they subserve bronchodilatation. When these receptors are blocked, bronchoconstriction may result. The aggravating effect of this drug is in keeping with the theory that asthma represents an inherent partial beta receptor blockade of the lung. Practalol, a new β-blocking drug, the blocking property of which is directed predominantly to the β-receptors of the heart alone, should theoretically be safer in asthmatics. Preliminary clinical studies thus far appear to substantiate this claim.[17]

SPECIFIC THERAPY

Allergic Asthma

Specific allergy management must be included in the treatment regimen of extrinsic and mixed asthmatics. When one allergen is the primary cause (e.g., animal dander), and it can be removed from the environment, symptomatic relief is achieved. Most allergic patients, however, are sensitive to more than one antigen and many cannot be completely removed. In adults, inhalant allergens are the most frequent causative agents. Foods are rarely the cause of asthma except in occasional children and infants. Since food skin tests are often not accurate indicators of clinical sensitivity, food evaluation is best accomplished by observation after diet manipulation. Continuation of symptoms despite avoidance of a suspect food for at least 5 to 7 days usually suffices to rule out allergic reactivity to that food.

Certain basic environmental controls in the house are generally advisable. These efforts are of paramount importance in those patients with dust, dander, and mold hypersensitivities. Frequent dusting with a moistened cloth is advisable. Furnishings in the bedroom are best kept simple and should include only the basic necessities. Upholstered materials, rugs or carpeting, and draperies should be avoided in the bedroom. Dacron or foam rubber pillows are preferred and should be enclosed in plastic zip covers. Mattresses should similarly be enclosed. Wool blankets, because of their ability to trap dust and other particles should be replaced with cotton or synthetic fabric quilts. Closets should be kept neat and orderly, and loose clothing and other objects should be stored in plastic bags.

Other aspects may be considered in regard to the environmental control of the home. Basement apartments, because of increased moisture, are most apt to have higher levels of airborne mold and mite antigens. Radiant heating systems are preferred to the blowing hot air types. Indoor plants should be limited in number since they may also contribute to an increased amount of dust and mold spores. In patients with perennial symptoms it is generally advisable that pets (cats, dogs and birds) be removed from the house if there are symptoms from contact or a positive skin test to the respective antigen. Mechanical aids for the removal of allergens and other airborne irritants have been discussed on page 266.

When environmental control is either impossible or insufficient to control symptoms, specific hyposensitization (inhalants) therapy must be included. The details of hyposensitization therapy are discussed in Chapter 9. It is the clinical impression of many practicing allergists that allergic asthma appears more responsive to hyposensitization than is allergic rhinitis and that pollen-sensitive asthmatics respond better to hyposensitization than those with dust and mold sensitivity. These impressions unfortunately have not been subjected to clinical study.

Johnstone and Dutton [22] in a 14-year prospective study of allergic asthmatic children have shown that 72 percent of the hyposensitized group were symptom free at age 16 as compared to only 22 percent of the placebo treated group. Of greater importance was a significantly increased improvement rate in those receiving the highest tolerable dose of antigen. Others have also shown the necessity of administering the highest possible antigen doses to assure the best results with hyposensitization.

Intrinsic Asthma

Treatment of intrinsic asthma primarily involves the judicious use of drug therapy. General and nonspecific measures of treatment (as described above) are included according to their importance in a given patient.

Bacterial hyposensitization is a controversial mode of therapy. Although not conclusive, some controlled studies have shown that it may be beneficial, especially if large doses are employed. The use of bacterial hyposensitization presupposes that infection-induced asthma and asthma of unknown cause may be mediated by an immunologic reaction to bacteria. Factors which have suggested such a mechanism have been: the immediate occurrence of wheezing with bronchopulmonary infection; the occurrence of wheezing with infection of the upper respiratory tract, suggesting an allergic reaction to an absorbed bacterial antigen; the induction of symptoms with injection of bacterial antigens given in treatment; the reproduction of symptoms with inhalation challenges of bacterial antigens; the onset of asthma occuring after an overt respiratory infection in occasional patients and the positive immediate and delayed skin reactions to bacterial antigens observed in some patients.

Despite these observations, there is no data documenting unequivocally (by our present day knowledge of immunologic mechanisms) that intrinsic asthma results from either immediate or delayed hypersensitivity to bacteria. Quantitative measurements of IgE in intrinsic asthma are much lower than those found in allergic asthma. The clinical significance of the skin test reactions to bacterial antigens is questionable. These may be either irritative phenomena or possibly immunologically mediated (i.e., immediate, Arthus or delayed). Even if the positive skin tests were immunologically significant, their presence need not necessarily reflect the cause but might also be the result of the disease. Finally, the associated wheezing with natural infection or inhalation of bacterial antigen can be possibly explained by the β-adrenergic blockade theory of asthma. Bacterial infection and the injection of bacterial products in animals have been shown to result in pharmacologic and physiologic changes suggesting a blockade of β-receptors. Although not definitely proven, there is some evidence of a similar response in man. Thus in an asthmatic who would already have a partial blockade of his pulmonary β-receptors, the addition of natural infection (and injected or inhaled bacterial antigens) could conceivably precipitate symptoms by increasing the already existent beta blockade.

The use of bacterial vaccine is based on empiricism alone. When other modes have not been helpful, a trial of bacterial hyposensitization may be attempted. Endogenous vaccines show no apparent superiority to the available stock vaccines.

Aspirin-Sensitive Asthma

In aspirin-sensitive asthma treatment is generally similar to that of the intrinsic type with exception to those patients in whom there is clinical and skin test evidence of contributing allergy. Of additional importance is the avoidance of aspirin and other drugs which may also produce adverse reactions. Patients must be informed of the numerous proprietary mixtures which contain aspirin (See list below). Acetominophen may be used as a safe substitute for aspirin, and other salicylates such as sodium salicylate can be taken safely. It is advisable that these patients wear or carry Medic-Alert materials (cards, bracelets, necklaces, etc.) stating their hypersensitivity. The ingestion of aspirin by these patients commonly causes urticaria, angioedema, or increased asthma, but it can also result in an explosively severe reaction resembling anaphylaxis.

Other drugs which may cause similar reactions include the pyrazones (antipyrine and aminopyrine), indomethacin (Indocin*) and mefanamic acid (Ponstel †). Approximately 25 percent of the patients may also experience similar adverse reactions with the ingestion of the coal tar dye tartrazine (Food, Drug and Cosmetic yellow No. 5). This dye is commonly found in yellow colored candies and drinks (Tang and probably others). Vitamin tablets as well as other medicines (Decadron, Paracort, Premarin and Deronil ‡) containing this dye have been reported to cause symptoms. Pyrvinium pamoate (Povan §) tablets contain tartrazine in their coating and should be avoided by aspirin-sensitive patients. This drug is an effective antihelminth used for the treatment of pinworms. It has been suggested that sodium benzoate, a common food additive, may also trigger symptoms in some of these patients.

The exact mechanism by which these patients become intolerant to aspirin and the other substances mentioned is not known. What relationship this intolerance has to the rhinitis, nasal polyposis and asthma is also unknown. Skin testing with aspirin is not advisable and, furthermore, may be dangerous. Extensive immunologic studies utilizing aspirin and aspirin-protein conjugates have usually resulted in negative findings. The differing chemical structures of these substances also suggest that an immunologic mechanism is unlikely. A property common to all these substances is their analgesic effect. The analgesic property of aspirin is thought to result from its bradykinin antagonism. It has been theorized that aspirin-sensitive disease may result from altered chemoreceptor reactivity (in the skin and respiratory tract). In some unknown fashion, it is felt that aspirin and the other incriminated drugs, instead of antagonizing bradykinin, now become agonists and it is this property that accounts for the drug intolerance and the typical signs and symptoms seen in this condition.[35] Recently, two other speculations have been offered as possible mechanisms by which these drugs may produce their adverse effects: (1) complement may be activated with resultant chemotaxis of leukocytes, anaphylatoxin formation and histamine release or (2) these patients may lack a substance which normally would inhibit an enzyme (or enzymes) activated by these drugs and thus would allow this enzyme to result in release of mediators such as histamine, SRS-A, and possibly others.[44]

* Trademark, Merck Sharp & Dohme.
† Trademark, Parke, Davis.
‡ Trademarks, respectively, of Merck Sharp & Dohme, Parke Davis, Ayerst, and Schering.
§ Trademark, Parke, Davis.

Some Proprietary Drugs Containing Aspirin

Acetidine	Empirin Compound
Alka-Seltzer	Excedrin
Anacin	Inhiston
Anahist	Liquiprin
APC	Measurin
Aspergum	Midol
BC	Pepto-Bismol
Bromo-quinine	Persistin
Bromo-Seltzer	Say-Sayne
Bufferin	Stanback
Charger	Theracin
Coricidin	Triaminicin
Dristan	Trigesic
Ecotrin	Vanquish

CLINICAL MANAGEMENT

Treatment of the Acute Asthmatic Attack

In mild attacks the use of oral bronchodilators and expectorants every 4 to 6 hours may suffice. Nebulized isoproterenol may also be used, but when nebulized medications are used, patients must be advised how to use them properly and not to overuse them (see above). For more severe attacks, aqueous epinephrine, 1:1000, may be given subcutaneously and the dose may be repeated every 15 to 20 minutes if necessary. More than 3 to 4 doses is not recommended. Sus-phrine,* an aqueous epinephrine suspension, may be given subcutaneously when a more prolonged effect is desired. Once the acute attack has subsided, regular and continuous use of oral bronchodilators should follow for at least 3 to 5 days. Supplemental theophylline (oral or rectal preparations) may be used for smoother control.

If epinephrine has not proved effective, intravenous aminophylline is indicated. It is cautioned again that aminophylline must be injected over a period of 10 to 15 minutes. In most cases these measures are effective in providing relief. When symptoms are refractory to these treatment modalities, status asthmaticus exists. The treatment of status asthmaticus is presented below.

Equally important as the medical treatment of an acute episode of asthma is the attempt to delineate its possible precipitating factor. Inquiry as to activity, time and place of occurrence, ingestion of foods, presence of emotional stresses and evidence of respiratory tract infec-

* Trademark, Cooper Laboratories.

tion must be made. Accordingly, additional measures to prevent recurrence or continuation of symptoms can then be instituted.

Treatment of Chronic Asthma

The management of chronic asthma entails a continuous broad scope control which must be tailored to each individual patient. Features of general management as discussed above must be included in the treatment regimen. Significant allergic factors are treated by environmental control combined with an adequate hyposensitization program. In each patient secondary contributing factors must be evaluated and controlled when possible.

All patients will require some form of chronic bronchodilator and expectorant therapy. In those with mild intermittent symptoms oral preparations taken only when symptoms occur may suffice. Patients with persistent symptoms may require chronic daily medication. It is advisable to rely primarily on oral drugs. Aerosol adrenergics are to be discouraged but in some patients their use 4 to 6 times daily may be a helpful adjunct to oral therapy. For the routine outpatient care there is no evidence that IPBB-delivered aerosols are more effective than the hand nebulizers. In patients with copious secretions, adrenergic nebulization followed by postural drainage might be tried.

Nocturnal wheezing may respond to the use of a sustained release bronchodilator at bedtime. Another alternative would include a theophylline preparation before retiring. Aerosolized adrenergics should be used nocturnally only if the above measure are ineffective.

During periods of exacerbations oral bronchodilator therapy is increased with inclusion of theophylline derivatives on an every 6 to 8 hour basis. If the exacerbation is related to a respiratory infection, an antibiotic is required. If symptoms persist despite these measures, a short course of corticosteroids may be necessary.

When these usual conservative measures are insufficient to control symptoms, chronic corticosteroid therapy may be required. This form of treatment should always be the last resort. The lowest possible maintenance dose is desired, and alternate day or intermittent therapy should be atempted.

Bronchopulmonary infection requires early antibiotic therapy. Six- to 14-day courses are usually adequate for each acute episode. Adequate care and treatment of naso-sinal infection is also important. In many patients, with or without nasal polyps, recurrent naso-sinal infection with concomitant aggravation of asthma is common. Antibiotic therapy alone may be insufficient if local measures to relieve obstruction or loculated areas of suppuration are not included.

Because of their frequent recurrence, it is generally advisable that surgical removal of nasal polyps be done only after local dexamethasone (Decadron Turbinaire*) aerosol or cortisone injection, coupled with good medical and allergy management have not been effective in decreasing obstruction and infection. Sinus surgery also should be considered only when more conservative treatment (medical and allergic) has resulted in little or no improvement in preventing recurrent infection.

Anxiety and or depression may aggravate asthma. When present, drug therapy (sedatives, tranquilizers and antidepressants) may be used. Although helpful, these drugs may have adverse effects on asthma as described above. They should be used with caution. If safe drug therapy fails to control these symptoms, psychiatric evaluation should be obtained. It has been assumed by the lay public as well as the medical profession that asthma is primarily an expression of an underlying psychologic disturbance. This attitude unfortunately has often prevented proper medical and allergy management for many patients. In most asthmatics psychiatric factors are of little or no significance in the etiology of the disease. However, there is no doubt that psychic factors may well contribute as an initiating or aggravating factor in asthma. But this should not be construed as evidence that asthma is predominantly, or only, a disorder of the psyche. Asthma is a chronic disease which may also be associated with significant impairment of physical and social activity. These factors in themselves may lend to the development of psychoneurotic signs and symptoms. It is often seen that as asthmatic symptoms are brought under control concomitant improvement of the psyche occurs.

Intractable Asthma

Intractable asthma refers to persistent, incapacitating symptoms, which have become unresponsive to the usual therapy including corticosteroids. These patients fortunately are few in number, and most are patients with the intrinsic or mixed type of asthma. Their constant medical and nonmedical requirements are heavy social and financial burdens on their family. For these reasons institutions that care for the intractable asthmatic have been founded. Originally it was felt that mere removal of the patient from his home would be beneficial. With the accumulated years of experience, it has become quite evident that the problem is not this simple. Many patients, despite their long term residence in these institutions, with optimal medical and psychologic management, persist with equally disabling symptoms and corticosteroid dependence. Some investigators have suggested that intractable asthma, because of its unique resistance to the commonly employed asthma therapy, may represent a variant of asthma with superimposed and

* Trademark, Schering.

unknown pathophysiologic mechanisms. An example of the latter would be alpha$_1$ antitrypsin deficiency, which, it has now been shown, may present early in its course as asthma.[40] Newer drugs and further research are required to improve control of the intractable asthmatic.

STATUS ASTHMATICUS

Status asthmaticus is defined as severe asthma unresponsive to epinephrine and aminophylline. It is a medical emergency and proper and immediate treatment is necessary to avoid a fatal outcome.

A number of factors have been shown to be important in inducing status and contributing to its mortality. Approximately 50 percent of these patients have an associated respiratory tract infection. Many have overused nebulized isoproterenol before developing refractoriness. Withdrawal or too sudden reduction of corticosteroids may contribute to the development of status. In many situations both the patient and physician were unaware of the severity of symptoms and probably an earlier and more aggressive medical management would have prevented status. The unwise use of sedatives and tranquilizers in the treatment of status asthmaticus has often contributed to the development of respiratory failure. Overdose of aminophylline has been cited as a cause of death in some children with status.

Status asthmaticus is undoubtedly a stressful situation. Patients who have been on maintenance corticosteroids must receive increased doses. This would also apply to patients who have received corticosteroids within the recent past (at least 1 year). In these patients corticosteroids are necessary not only as a therapeutic measure but also to prevent a fatal outcome from adrenal crisis.

Why therapeutic hyporesponsiveness occurs is not known. Respiratory acidosis was once thought to be a cause for the epinephrine fastness. It is now known that status asthmaticus may exist with a normal or alkalotic blood pH. Proponents of the partial beta blockade theory of asthma suggest that status results from an overwhelming blockade of all the pulmonary β-receptors. Exogenous β-adrenergic stimulating drugs thus become ineffective. A study in vitro using human tracheobronchial muscle preparations has shown that the relaxing effect of epinephrine was abolished when propranolol (a beta blocker) was placed in the bath.[1] With complete beta blockade, epinephrine paradoxically caused contraction of the muscle preparation. This suggests that when beta blockade is present, a-receptor activity is enhanced. Further epinephrine administration would not only be ineffective in status but could also contribute to the existent pathophysiologic mechanisms.

Patients with status asthmaticus must be hospitalized, preferably in pulmonary intensive care units where close observation and ancillary treatment by experienced personnel are available. Optimum treatment often involves the combined efforts of the allergist, pulmonary disease specialist and anesthesiologist.

Initial laboratory studies should include a complete blood count, gram stain with culture and sensitivity study of the sputum, chest x-ray, serum electrolytes, blood pH and blood gas (arterial or arterialized capillary) studies. A bedside spirometer is also helpful in determining and following ventilatory parameters. Of these laboratory aids blood gas and pH determinations are probably the most valuable. They not only are important in guiding therapy but also provide a true assessment of severity. These determinations allow the classification of asthma into 4 stages of severity (Figure 8-3).

Stage I signifies the presence of airway obstruction only. Because of the associated hyperventilation the pCO_2 is low and the pH is therefore slightly alkalotic (respiratory alkalosis). The pO_2 in Stage I is normal. Spirometric study only reveals a decrease in FEV_1 with a normal vital capacity. As symptoms progress, obstruction of the airway increases, compliance decreases and air trapping and hyperinflation develop. As a result of the latter changes the functional residual capacity increases and the vital capacity of necessity is decreased. It is at this time, Stage II, that ventilation-perfusion imbalance with hypoxemia result. These changes, however, are not enough to impair net alveolar ventilation and thus although pO_2 is lowered, pCO_2 remains low and an alkalotic pH persists. With continuing progression, net alveolar ventilation decreases and a transitional period exists, (Stage III) where the pCO_2 increases and the pH decreases so that now both values are normal. When the blood gas study reveals hypoxemia in the presence of a normal pCO_2 and pH, close supervision with frequent determinations of pH, pCO_2 and pO_2 are important to evaluate the adequacy of treatment and the presence or absence of a trend toward respiratory failure (Stage IV). Clinical observation alone is notoriously inaccurate in reflecting the seriousness of the situation.

	FEV₁ (OBSTRUCTION OF AIRWAY)	VITAL CAPACITY (RESTRICTION OF AIRWAY)	PO₂ NORMAL 90-100 mmHg	PCO₂ NORMAL 35-40 mmHg	pH NORMAL 7.35-7.43 mmHg
STAGE I	↓	NORMAL	NORMAL	↓	> 7.43 (RESP. ALKALOSIS)
STAGE II	↓↓	↓	↓	↓↓	> 7.43 (RESP. ALKALOSIS)
STAGE III	↓↓↓	↓↓	↓↓	NORMAL	7.35-7.43 NORMAL
STAGE IV	↓↓↓↓	↓↓↓	↓↓↓	↑↑↑	< 7.35 (RESP. ACIDOSIS)

Fig. 8-3. Spirometry, blood gas and blood pH in asthma as related to the stage of severity.

Treatment of Status Asthmaticus

It is again stressed that although many of these patients manifest signs of fright, restlessness and anxiety, the use of sedatives and tranquilizers is absolutely contraindicated. Treatment directed in alleviating wheezing, hypoxemia and dyspnea will ameliorate these signs and symptoms. Even small doses of sedatives and tranquilizers in this situation will suppress respirations sufficient to induce respiratory failure.

Many patients in status asthmaticus are significantly dehydrated. This is especially true in children. The accompanying hyperventilation causes water loss via the lungs. Also because of their distress, many patients have not maintained an adequate fluid intake. Dehydration promotes continuing thickening and inspissation of bronchial secretions.

Hydration is best accomplished by intravenous fluid therapy. In adults, 1000 ml. may be given within the first 2 hours of treatment and thereafter the rate may be decreased, but a total of 3000 to 4000 ml. per 24 hours is advisable. In children, fluid therapy is dictated by the clinical state of dehydration, but generally 300 to 400 ml./M^2 of body surface can be given during the first hour and then 2.0 to 3.0 L./M^2 for the following 24 hours. Urinary output must also be closely monitored.

Solutions of 5 percent dextrose alternating with 5 percent dextrose in ½ Normal saline given intravenously will constitute basic caloric, sodium and chloride requirements. In patients with a compromised cardiovascular system, sodium and water overload must be avoided. Since a high dose of corticosteroids is used in these patients, adequate potassium supplementation must be included in the intravenous therapy. In the adult 80 to 120 milliequivalents of KCl per 24 hours (not to exceed 20 mEq./hour) is indicated. Frequent serum electrolyte determinations provide the best guide for continued electrolyte therapy.

Aminophylline should be given intravenously at a rate of 250 to 500 mg. every 6 hours for adults and 3 to 5 mg./kg. every 8 hours for children. Studies have shown that if given intermittently in individual doses, more efficient therapeutic levels are obtained as compared to that given in a continuous intravenous drip delivering the same dose over 6 to 8 hours.[27] The intermittent doses may be given in "piggy back" fashion after being dissolved in 100 to 250 ml. of fluid and infused within 10 to 15 minutes.

Since all patients will be hypoxemic, oxygen therapy is required. The oxygen must be humidified to prevent irritation of the bronchial mucous membrane. Ideally, blood gas determinations should guide proper therapy. Therapeutically, a pO_2 of 60 mm. Hg or slightly above is sufficient. This can often be accomplished with low flow rates of 2 to 3 L./minute by nasal cannula or nasal catheter. Ventimasks calibrated to deliver 24-,

28- and 35 percent oxygen may also be used. The necessity for higher concentrations of O_2 to maintain a pO_2 of 60 mm. Hg usually signifies the presence of thick tracheobronchial secretions. It is cautioned that in patients whose asthma is complicated by irreversible pulmonary damage chronic hypercapnia may be present, and hypoxemia remains as the only respiratory stimulus. Oxygen therapy during an acute respiratory insult in these patients may enhance respiratory failure. Close clinical observation and frequent blood gas monitoring are important in preventing this complication. In infants and young children, fine mist tents in an oxygen enriched atmosphere are usually used. Not only do these provide oxygen, but they also provide hydration to aid in liquefying secretions.

With clear evidence of infection (i.e., purulent sputum, fever, or x-ray evidence of pneumonitis), antibiotics must be administered after stains and culture of the sputum are obtained. In many instances, infection may be present in the absence of these suggestive findings. Furthermore, many patients with status asthmaticus may have low grade fever and leukocytosis without infection. Corticosteroids and epinephrine, alone or in combination, can result in leukocytosis. For these reasons, especially in view of the seriousness of the problem, it is the author's opinion that the early use of antibiotics in every case of status asthmaticus is advised. When culture and sensitivity studies of the sputum are done first, the adverse effects of the empiric use of antibiotics is minimal as compared to the possible deleterious effects resulting from delaying their use. Drugs of choice include ampicillin, cephalothin and tetracycline. Results of sputum culture should dictate further changes in antibiotic therapy.

The expectorant action of adequate intravenous fluid therapy usually suffices, but if the patient is able to take fluids by mouth, oral iodides (SSKI) may be given. In patients unable to take fluids orally, sodium iodide, 0.5 g. to 1.0 g. may be given in the intravenous fluids.

Intermittent positive pressure nebulization of isoproterenol is usually effective in promoting bronchodilatation and liquefaction of secretions. When it is used the patient should be watched closely, since bronchospasm may be increased in some patients. Because isoproterenol may result in increased hypoxia, positive pressure nebulization should be propelled with 50 percent oxygen rather than compressed air. These treatments, if effective, may be repeated every 2 to 4 hours. Depending on the condition of the patient, minimal postural drainage after percussion and vibration of the chest may be helpful following each treatment.

It is not advisable to use N-acetylcysteine in status asthmaticus because it may induce more bronchospasm. When there is evidence that the presence of tenacious secretions is preventing proper oxygenation and is a major factor contributing to respiratory failure, N-acetylcysteine may be combined with isoproterenol in positive pressure nebulization.

Ultrasonic nebulization may also be utilized to liquefy secretions. This method of nebulization delivers small sized droplets to the small bronchioles. Whether or not it is more effective than IPPB is not clearly established. It has been described to be quite effective especially if used in conjunction with nebulized isoproterenol. For example, if the ultrasonic aerosol mist is delivered by mask, nebulized isoproterenol can be included through an inlet in the side of the mask.

Large doses of corticosteroids are essential in status asthmaticus. Hydrocortisone (Solu-Cortef *), 4 mg./kg., may be given intravenously and repeated every 2 to 4 hours. Patients who have been receiving corticosteroids must certainly be given hydrocortisone immediately. With

* Trademark, Upjohn Co.

Treatment of Status Asthmaticus

Hospitalize
    Laboratory Studies:
      WBC and differential
      Chest x-ray
      Sputum-gram stain, culture and sensitivities
      Blood gas and electrolyte determinations
      Bedside spirometer
Avoid use of all sedatives, tranquilizers and antihistamines

Hydration—(To include adequate potassium and chloride supplementation)
    Adults—1000 ml. in first 2 hours with 24-hour total of 3000 to 4000 ml.
    Children—300 to 400 ml./M² body surface in first hour with 24-hr. total of 2.0 to 3.0 L./M²

Aminophylline (Intravenous)
    Adults—250 to 500 mg. every 6 hours
    Children—3 to 5 mg./kg. every 8 hours

Oxygen Therapy—2 to 3 L./min. (Best guided by blood gas determination)

Antibiotic Therapy—cephalothin, ampicillin, tetracycline

Corticosteroid Therapy—Children and adults: 4 mg./kg. hydrocortisone (Solu-Cortef) intravenously every 2 to 4 hours.

Expectorants—
    Oral—SSKI
    Intravenous—Sodium iodide 0.5 to 1.0 g./24 hours (diluted in a bottle of fluids)

Aerosol Therapy
    IPBB with isoproterenol or ultrasonic nebulization coupled with isoproterenol nebulization

Impending or Acute Respiratory Failure
    Sodium Bicarbonate:
Children—2 mEq./kg.   } May repeat in 30 to 45
Adults—44 to 88 mEq. intravenously } minutes if necessary

    Consider bronchial lavage or bronchoscopy

    Endotracheal intubation with assisted or controlled ventilation improvement, as evidenced by spirometry and blood gas studies, suppressive doses of prednisone can be substituted. Thereafter, gradual reduction of dosage with discontinuation (or to maintenance level) is advised over a 7- to 10-day period.

Although indiscriminate use of corticosteroids is to be avoided, the severity of status asthmaticus dictates their immediate use in all patients. It is felt that their beneficial effect, especially when given early in the course of treatment, far outweighs their risks when compared to the morbidity and mortality of status asthmaticus.

RESPIRATORY FAILURE

Most patients with status asthmaticus respond favorably with the institution of the above modes of treatment. In those who continue to deteriorate, other aggressive measures must be included in order to prevent death from respiratory failure. The important features of treatment at this stage include measures to maintain adequate ventilation and to protect from the severe acid-base disturbances which may arise. It is suggested at this point that the coordinated efforts of the anesthesiologist, chest physician and allergist are important in providing proper and effective treatment.

Signs of impending respiratory failure result from the combined effects of hypercapnia, hypoxia and acidosis. Clinically, because of fatigue and exhaustion, thoracic mobility is decreased and auscultation of the chest may reveal decreased respiratory sounds, since there is a decrease in aeration. Because of accompanying stupor the patient may appear to be struggling less to breathe. These two features may give a false impression of improvement. Other signs and symptoms of imminent respiratory failure include cyanosis, papilledema, pulsus paradoxus, marked inspiratory retraction, asterixis, muscular weakness and hypotension. Arrhythmias and cardiac arrest may also occur. Acidosis and hypoxemia also contribute to pulmonary vasoconstriction with resultant pulmonary hypertension, right heart strain and eventually cardiac failure. The acidosis is primarily respiratory in etiology, but with severe hypoxemia aerobic metabolism is impaired and there is an accumulation of pyruvic and lactic acid (end products of aneorobic metabolism). These result in a superimposed metabolic acidosis.

The presence of any of these signs and symptoms associated with a pCO_2 of 65 mm. Hg or higher demand the institution of artificial ventilation. The use of tracheal intubation is preferred to tracheostomy because of its ease and also because the potential complications of tracheostomy are prevented. Electrocardiographic monitoring with oscilloscope visualization is advised. This facilitates the early detection and treatment of arrythmias which may occur during or immediately after intubation. Electrocardiographic monitoring should continue throughout the entire time of mechanical ventilation. Before intubation, mild sedation or light halothane anesthesia is suggested. Preoxygenation with humidified 100 percent oxygen is administered with the use of mask and bag. A muscle paralyzing drug (succinylcholine, d-tubocurarine, or gallamine) is then administered to further facilitate intubation and ventilation. A cuffed nasotracheal or orotracheal tube is then inserted and attached to the ventilator. The orotracheal tube, because of its large diameter, allows for more efficient suctioning of secretions.

The volume regulated ventilator has been shown to be superior to the pressure regulated type. In status asthmaticus high pulmonary pressures are present; the volume regulated ventilators are more efficient in overcoming these pressures and provide more efficient and smoother ventilation.

After institution of artificial ventilation many patients, with only minimal sedation, will be able to trigger the machine themselves (assisted ventilation). In those patients who fight the machine and despite mild sedation are unable to accomodate to the machine, it is necessary to provide continuous muscle relaxation and have the machine completely take over their breathing (controlled ventilation). While on the ventilator it is important to obtain frequent blood gas determinations to assure proper reversal of acid-base and ventilatory abnormalities. Frequent gentle suctioning of tracheobronchial secretions is necessary.

If these measures are inadequate to correct the hypoxia and hypercarbia, especially when high concentrations of oxygen are used, other measures to remove bronchial secretions must be considered. Bronchial lavage with sterile saline, (or 1 percent sodium bicarbonate) may be used. This is done by instilling 15 to 20 ml. amounts of fluid into the endotracheal tube followed by immediate suction. A total of 300 to 500 ml. may be used in one treatment. When lavage is done by those experienced with the technique it is probably preferred to bronchoscopy and suction. Adequate steps to insure proper ventilation and oxygenation are mandatory during lavage or bronchoscopic therapy. Better removal of secretions may be accomplished by additional intermittent lavages with a mixture of 1.5 ml. of 1:10,000 epinephrine and 1 to 2 ml. of 5 percent N-acetylcysteine.

Although respiratory failure requires primarily ventilatory correction, the severe acidosis which is present (especially if the pH is 7.25 or lower) requires immediate administration of alkalinizing agents to protect from the deleterious effects of the extreme blood acidity. In adults 44 to 88 mEq. of sodium bicarbonate can be given intravenously and in children 2 mEq./kg. may be given intravenously within 5 minutes. These doses may be repeated in 30 to 40 minutes if acidosis persists. It is recommended that immediately after artificial ventilation blood gas and pH studies be obtained every 15 to 20 minutes for at least 1 hour.

Sodium lactate and THAM (tris(hydroxymethyl)aminomethane) are other alkalinizing agents which may be used. Sodium lactate may contribute to lactic acidosis, and for this reason sodium bicarbonate is preferred. THAM is a strong base and theoretically may yield a faster rise of pH than bicarbonate or lactate; but since it may cause respiratory depression it should be used only with artificial ventilation.

Overtreatment with sodium bicarbonate must be avoided. With efficient mechanical ventilation a sudden removal of CO_2 may result in acute alkalosis, since the elevated levels of bicarbonate remain uncompensated. Hyperexcitability and convulsions may then occur. This complication is best treated by temporarily decreasing ventilation. Other factors such as depletion of potassium (secondary to corticosteroids or diuretics) and chloride may occur in status asthmaticus and may also contribute to alkalosis. Adequate replacement of these ions must be included in therapy.

The only contraindication to the use of mechanical ventilation is the presense of pneumothorax or pneumomediastinum. In view of the potential lethality of acute respiratory failure these conditions are to be considered relative contraindications. Mechanical ventilation may be cautiously undertaken provided all other measures have been unsuccessful. Pneumothorax must be treated with a chest tube under water seal before ventilation is attempted. In the presence of pneumomediastinum, tracheostomy is preferred, since this would also allow for escape of air from the mediastinum.

COMPLICATIONS OF MECHANICAL VENTILATION

Mechanical ventilation, although life saving in acute respiratory failure may be associated with specific complications. Sudden occurrence of tachypnea, hypotension, tachycardia and cyanosis usually indicates a serious complication such as kinking of the endotracheal tube with obstruction of a major bronchus, a large pneumothorax or pneumomediastinum, or obstruction of the endotracheal tube by secretions.

Oxygen toxicity from the chronic use of a high concentration of oxygen (50 to 100 percent for 48 hours or longer), is another complication seen with the use of mechanical ventilation. Frequent checks of the oxygen concentration can prevent this complication. The pressure ventilators are more apt to result in delivering a higher oxygen concentration than is designated by the machine controls. The pulmonary changes found with oxygen toxicity are capillary congestion, interstitial edema, alveolar edema, fibrin deposition, hemorrhage and atelectasis. These changes themselves may impair oxygen diffusion and contribute to hypoxemia. Later and irreversible changes of oxygen toxicity include capillary proliferation and fibrosis.

Abnormal fluid retention and weight gain may also occur with prolonged mechanical ventilation. The chest x-ray may assume the appearance of pulmonary edema. As expected, a decrease in vital capacity and compliance with a tendency to hypoxemia result. The cause of the water overload is not known, but subclinical heart failure or antidiuretic hormone release have been suggested mechanisms. Water restriction and diuretic therapy constitute treatment for this complication.

Tracheal stenosis is a complication of cuffed endotracheal or tracheostomy tubes. This occurs as a result of the mucosal injury arising from cuff-induced pressure necrosis. Other factors such as local infection and hypotension may be contributory. The occurrence of stridor or loud wheezing heard best at the mouth suggest the possibility of this complication in a patient recently intubated. Modifications in tube design may lower the incidence of this complication. The most recent is a tube whose cuff is only inflated during inspiration.

A potentially fatal complication of mechanical ventilation is *Pseudomonas aeruginosa* pneumonitis. The ventilators are often the source of infection, but the concomitant use of antibiotics and corticosteroids along with an impaired bronchopulmonary defense mechanism are also important predisposing factors. The radiologic picture of this type of pneumonia is variable and may consist of bilateral or unilateral consolidation, nodular lesions or abscess formation. The diagnosis is established by repeated cultures from tracheal and bronchial secretions, and specific antibiotic therapy is best determined by sensitivity studies.

PREGNANCY AND ASTHMA

Pregnancy often results in reduction of asthmatic symptoms, but in some patients symptoms are unchanged or markedly increased. The exact reasons for this variability are not known. General principles of treatment are the same as in the nonpregnant asthmatic, but certain drugs should be avoided. Iodides are not to be used because they may produce fetal goiter and other thyroid abnormalities. Hydroxyzine (present in Marax *) should be avoided because of its possible teratogenic potential. Tetracycline may be injurious to the fetal osseous structures and dental anlage. The latter drug is also hepatotoxic, especially in the last trimester and when given in large intravenous doses.

* Trademark, Roerig.

There are no added risks for the woman who may require cortico-steroids during pregnancy. Pregnancy per se should not alter the de-cision to use corticosteroids if these appear essential for control of asthma. As yet there has been no case report of fetal adrenal insuffi-ciency occurring as a result of exogenously administered corticosteroids passing the placenta. Pregnancy is not a contraindication for beginning or maintaining hyposensitization therapy. Many allergists empirically decrease the maintainence dose of antigens, or increase treatment doses more slowly, since systemic reactions may result in uterine contractions and possible abortion.

It has generally been assumed that asthma had little or no deleterious effect on fetal morbidity. However, in a recent study of 277 pregnant asthmatics [16] from a total of 30,861 collaborative research project de-liveries, the perinatal death rate (5.9) was almost twice that of the project in general (3.2). The accuracy of this rate as a pure reflection of asthma alone is questionable. In a significant number of the perinatal deaths other complicating coexisting cardiovascular diseases were also present in the mothers.

There is no question that severe asthma can be a serious threat to mother and fetus. Sixteen of the 277 asthmatics were classified as having severe asthma. Four of these patients died during the study period and represented two thirds of all the maternal deaths in the study. Approxi-mately 28 percent of these sixteen pregnancies resulted in perinatal deaths.

PREPARATION OF THE ASTHMATIC FOR SURGERY

For elective surgery the asthmatic should be admitted a few days in advance so that adequate treatment can be instituted to insure an op-timal bronchopulmonary status. Bronchodilators, expectorants and judi-cious use of aerosol therapy are advisable. Respiratory exercises and postural drainage maneuvers may be helpful. If there is evidence of a respiratory infection, surgery must be postponed.

Patients on maintenance corticosteroids require an increased amount to prevent stress-induced hypoadrenalism. Those patients who have re-ceived corticosteroids at any time during the previous year should like-wise receive corticosteroids for surgery unless appropriate testing of the HPA axis (see above) reveals normal adrenal responsiveness. Cortisone acetate, 50 mg. intramuscularly, may be given on the night before sur-gery with a repeat dose on the morning of surgery. Hydrocortisone, 100 to 200 mg. intravenously, is then given immediately before surgery. Repeat doses of cortisone acetate or hydrocortisone are given after surgery so that at least a total of 300 to 400 mg. of cortisone is received on the day of surgery. If no postoperative complications arise the cortisone dose can then be tapered to maintenance levels or discontinued in 3 to 5 days.

Preanesthetic sedation is best achieved with hydroxyzine, since it causes minimal respiratory depression. Regional anesthesia should be used when feasible; but if general anesthesia is required, halothane is now considered superior to ether and is the anesthetic of choice for the asthmatic. It produces less salivation and less bronchial secretions than with ether. Other desirable properties of halothane are smooth and rapid induction of anesthesia and relaxation of bronchial smooth muscle with a resultant increase in bronchial caliber and pulmonary compliance. It has also been shown that halothane possesses beta adrenergic stimulating activity.

In asthmatics, inhalation induction and maintenance of anesthesia is preferred. Manipulation of the upper airway (e.g., suction, pharyngeal airways) may cause bronchospasm during light stages of anesthesia. Tracheal intubation is to be avoided when possible, but if deemed necessary should be performed during deep levels of anesthesia.

Postoperatively, the patient must be followed closely. Maintenance bronchodilators should be continued. Aerosol bronchodilators, deep breathing exercises, adequate hydration, postural drainage and gentle coughing should be instituted to avoid accumulation of secretions and atelectasis.

General anesthesia (ether and halothane) has been used as a treatment of status asthmaticus. At present these methods of treatment are considered potentially dangerous and are less effective than the method outlined above.

COMPLICATIONS OF ASTHMA

Although rare, pneumothorax, pneumomediastinum and subcutaneous emphysema can occur during an attack of severe asthma. The cause of these complications is thought to be the rupture of overdistended peripheral alveoli. The escaping air then follows and dissects through vascular sheaths of the lung parenchyma. Usually the amount of air is minimal and no specific intervention is required, but severe tension symptoms may occur, and insertion of a chest tube under a water seal for pneumothorax may be needed. Incisions of the neck tissues or tracheostomy may be needed for severe tension complications of pneumomediastinum. A common feature of these conditions is severe chest pain. Chest pain itself is unusual with uncomplicated asthma and when present should suggest the possibility of the extravasation of air. Upon auscultation of the heart, a crunching sound synchronous with the heartbeat may be present with pneumomediastinum (Hamman's sign).

Minimal areas of atelectasis may occur in asthma, but in children a not uncommon complication of asthma has been atelectasis of the right middle lobe. It is often reversible with bronchodilators, expectorants and aerosol therapy and probably results from mucus plugging and edema of the right middle lobe bronchus. When the atelectasis does not respond to the above treatment within a few days, bronchoscopy is indicated for both therapeutic and diagnostic reasons. Occasionally, children may develop atelectasis of other lobes or an entire lung.

Rib fracture and costochondral strain may occur as a result of coughing with attacks of asthma. In a few patients severe coughing from asthma may result in cough syncope.

Chronic bronchitis and emphysema are not to be considered complications of asthma. These conditions result with irreversible obstruction of the airway, whereas asthma is a reversible bronchospastic condition. In a few patients chronic asthma and bronchitis may coexist. This is especially true of those patients with asthma of the infectious (intrinsic) type.

MORTALITY

Death from asthma commonly occurs either as a result of irreversible status asthmaticus or suddenly and unexpectedly from severe bronchospasm and anoxia. Recently an unusual increase in the mortality rate of asthma has been reported in England, Wales and Australia. The age group primarily affected is 7 to 14. The exact cause of this change in mortality rate has not been definitely established. Some investigators have suggested that the use of pressurized aerosols of isoproterenol is an important causative factor. A recent report [20] has shown that since March, 1967, concomitant with a diminished use and sale of hand nebulizers in England, the mortality rate there has decreased. It is not absolutely certain that this factor alone resulted in the decreased mortality. In the United States, statistics suggest a decrease of asthma mortality in the decade from 1958 to 1967, despite a significant increase in the sale of pressurized nebulizers.

THE FUTURE

Only with continued research will the riddles of asthma be solved. Specific curative therapy can only be realized when basic pathologic mechanisms are delineated. Only then can treatment modalities be rationally devised to completely reverse the underlying pathogenetic process. The advances already made provide an optimistic speculation for the future treatment of asthma.

REFERENCES

1. Adolphson, R. L., Abern, S. B., Townley, R. G.: Demonstration of alpha-adrenergic receptors in human respiratory smooth muscle. Clin. Research, *18*:629, 1970.
2. Aldrete, J. A., Itkin, I.: Effects of chloral hydrate on the respiration of non-asthmatic and asthmatic patients. J. Allerg., 43:342, 1969.
3. Altounyan, R. E. C.: Inhibition of experimental asthma by a new compound, disodium cromoglycate. Acta Allerg., 22:487, 1967.
4. Bass, M.: Sudden sniffing death. JAMA, *212*:2075, 1970.
5. Brenner, M., Lowell, F. C.: Failure of diethylcarbamazine citrate (Hetrazan) in the treatment of asthma. J. Allerg., 46:29, 1970.
6. Carnow, B. W.: Air pollution and physician responsibility. Arch. Intern. Med., *127*:91, 1971.
7. Clinical trial of new asthma drug reported. Medical News. JAMA, 209: 1615, 1969.
8. Collins, J. V., Harris, P. W. R., Clark, T. J. H., Townsend, J.: Intravenous corticosteroids in treatment of acute bronchial asthma. Lancet, 2:1047, 1970.
9. Cuthbert, M. F.: Effect on airways resistance of prostaglandin E$_1$ given by aerosol to healthy and asthmatic volunteers. Brit. Med. J., 4:723, 1969.
10. Daly, J. R., Glass, D.: Corticosteroid and growth-hormone response to hypoglycemia in patients on long-term treatment with corticotrophin. Lancet, *1*:476, 1971.
11. Davies, S. E.: Effect of disodium cromoglycate on exercise-induced asthma. Brit. Med. J., 3:593, 1968.
12. Dollery, C. T., Davies, D. S., Draffan, G. H., Williams, F. M., Conolly, M. E.: Blood concentrations in man of fluorinated hydrocarbons after inhalation of pressurized aerosols. Lancet, 2:1164, 1970.
13. Freedman, B. J.: Trial of new bronchodilator, terbutaline, in asthma. Brit. Med. J., *1*:633, 1971.
14. Gazioglu, K., Condemi, J. J., Hyde, R. W., Kaltreider, N. L.: Effect of isoproterenol on gas exchange during air and oxygen breathing in patients with asthma. Amer. J. Med., *50*:185, 1971.
15. Girsh, L. S., Shubin, E., Dick, C., Schulaner, F. A.: A study on the epidemiology of asthma in children in Philadelphia. J. Allerg., 39:347, 1967.
16. Gordon, M., Niswander, K. R., Berendes, H., Kantor, A. G.: Fetal morbidity following potentially anoxigenic obstetric conditions. VII. bronchial asthma. Amer. J. Obstet. Gynec., *106*:421, 1970.

17. Grieco, M. H., Pierson, R. N.: Mechanism of bronchoconstriction due to β-adrenergic blockade. J. Allerg. Clin. Immunol., *48*:144, 1971.

18. Hamilton, W. F. D., Palmer, K. N. V., Gent, M.: Expectorant action of bromhexine in chronic obstructive bronchitis. Brit. Med. J., 3:260, 1970.

19. Harris, L. H.: Effects of isoproterenol plus phenylephrine by pressurized aerosol on blood gases, ventilation and perfusion in chronic obstructive lung diseases. Brit. Med. J., 4:579, 1970.

20. Inman, W. H. W., and Adelstein, A. M.: Rise and fall of asthma mortality in England and Wales in relation to use of pressurized aerosols. Lancet, 2:279, 1969.

21. James, V. H. T.: The investigation of pituitary-adrenal function; effects of corticosteroids and corticotrophin therapy. Pharmacologia Clin., 2:182, 1970.

22. Johnstone, D. E., Dutton, A.: The value of hyposensitization therapy for bronchial asthma in children—a 14-year study. Pediatrics, *42*:793, 1968.

23. Kales, A., Kales, J.: Evaluation, diagnosis and treatment of clinical conditions related to sleep. JAMA, *213*:2299, 1970.

24. Kaiser, H. B., Beall, G. N.: Azathioprine (Imuran) in chronic asthma. Ann. Allerg., *24*:369, 1966.

25. Legge, J. S., Gaddie, J., Palmer, K. N. V.: Comparison of two oral selective β_2—adrenergic stimulant drugs in bronchial asthma. Brit. Med. J., *1*:637, 1971.

26. Malone, D. N. S., Grant, I. W. B., Percy-Robb, I. W.: Hypothalamo-pituitary-adrenal function in asthmatic patients receiving long-term corticosteroid therapy. Lancet, 2:733, 1970.

27. Maselli, R., Cosal, G. L., Ellis, E. F.: Pharmacologic effects of intravenously administered aminophylline in asthmatic children. J. Pediat., *76*:777, 1970.

28. Palmer, K. N. V., Legge, J. S., Hamilton, W. F. D., Diament, M. L.: Comparison on effect of salbutamol and isoprenaline on spirometry and blood-gas tensions in bronchial asthma. Brit. Med. J., 2:23, 1970.

29. Paterson, J. W., Conolly, M. E., Davies, D. S., Dollery, C. T.: Isoprenaline resistance and the use of pressurized aerosols in asthma. Lancet, 2:426, 1968.

30. Paterson, J. W., Sudlow, M. F., Walker, S. R.: Blood levels of fluorinated hydrocarbons in asthmatic patients after inhalation of pressurized aerosols. Lancet, 2:565, 1971.

31. Pedersen, A. T., Batsakis, J. G., Vanselow, N. A., McLean, J. A.: False-positive tests for urinary 5-hydroxyindoleacetic acid. JAMA, *211*:1184, 1970.

32. Pelz, H. H.: Metaproterenol, a new bronchodilator: comparison with isoproterenol. Amer. J. Med. Sci., *253*:321, 1967.

33. Reisman, R. E.: Asthma induced by adrenergic aerosols. J. Allerg., *46*:153, 1970.

34. Salvaggio, J., Seaburg, J., Schoenhardt, E. A.: New Orleans asthma V. J. Allerg. Clin. Immunol., *48*:96, 1971.

35. Samter, M., Beers, R. F.: Intolerance to aspirin. Ann. Int. Med., *68*:975, 1968.
36. Shivpuri, D. N., Menon, M. P. S., Prakash, D.: A crossover double-blind study on *Tylophora indica* in the treatment of asthma and allergic rhinitis. J. Allerg., *43*:145, 1969.
37. Sly, R. M.: Effect of cromolyn sodium on exercise-induced airway obstruction in asthmatic children. Ann. Allerg., *29*:362, 1971.
38. Spieksma, F. T. M., Zuidema, P., Leupen, M. J.: High altitude and house-dust mites. Brit. Med. J., *1*:82, 1971.
39. Taylor, G. J., Harris, W. S.: Cardiac toxicity of aerosol propellants. JAMA, *214*:81, 1970.
40. Townley, R. G., Ryning, F., Lynch, H., Brody, A. W.: Obstructive lung disease in hereditary a_1, antitrypsin deficiency. JAMA, *214*:325, 1970.
41. U. S. Bureau of the Census, Statistical Abstract of the United States, 1970 (91st Edition) Washington, D.C.
42. Wong, D., Lopapa, A. F., Haddad, Z. H.: Immediate hypersensitivity reaction to aminophylline. J. Allerg. Clin. Immunol., *48*:165, 1971.
43. Worth, J., Rappaport, A.: Atypical reaction to isoproterenol. JAMA, *209*:417, 1969.
44. Yurchak, A. M., Wicher, K., Arbesman, C. E.: Immunologic studies on aspirin. J. Allerg., *46*:345, 1970.

9

Principles of Immunologic Management of Allergic Disease Due to Extrinsic Antigens

Howard L. Melam, M.D.

As with any disease, the optimal goal in the treatment of allergic disease is a complete cure. When this cannot be achieved, the physician attempts to relieve symptoms and prevent complications.

AVOIDANCE OF ANTIGENS

Allergic diseases result from the interaction of antigen and antibody and subsequent release of mediators which affect target organs. If exposure to the antigen or allergen can be avoided, no antigen-antibody interaction takes place and there is no allergic reaction of disease manifestation. This is the first tenet of allergic management: remove the allergen where possible.

In the case of certain allergens this can be accomplished readily. If an individual is sensitive to cat or dog dander, bird feathers or other animal protein, he should not have the animal in his home if complete control of symptoms is the goal of management. If he is sensitive to certain foods or drugs, he should avoid ingestion of these agents.

House Dust. In the case of house dust allergy, although complete avoidance is not possible, the degree of exposure to this allergen can be diminished. Intensive antidust precautions would include the following recommendations: The patient's bedroom should have nonallergenic bedding, preferably of synthetic materials. Plastic zippered covers should enclose the mattress, box spring and pillows. Bed linen may then be placed over these protective coverings for more comfort. Floors should be bare wood, linoleum, or tile. Washable scatter rugs are permissible if they are laundered frequently. Venetian blinds should be removed. If draperies are used, they should be washable and of short length. Furniture in the room should be simple and without elaborate design. No upholstered furniture should be present in the bedroom. Children should not have stuffed animals. Desks, books and writing material should not be in the bedroom. Closet doors should be kept closed at all times. The room should be dusted with a damp rag and wet-mopped daily. Wall heating vents should be covered. Furnace air filters should be changed at least twice yearly. Other rooms of the house should also be kept clean with special attention given to areas where the patient spends a great deal of time, such as a den or playroom. The patient should not be present in a room when it is being cleaned.

The recommendations described above include those which would be indicated for a complete anti-dust program. Such an intensive program might not be indicated for all patients, particularly those with very mild symptoms. A minimal anti-dust program would include covering pillows and mattress with plastic covers and thorough dusting and cleaning of the bedroom three times a week. For many patients, this simple program might be sufficient for control of symptoms.

Molds. Exposure to mold spores may also be reduced by environmental precautions. The patient should avoid barns, and mowing grass or raking leaves, since high concentrations of molds may be found in barns, old leaves and grass. A summer cabin which has been closed for several months may have a high mold concentration. If the patient's home has a basement, a dehumidifier should be used to reduce dampness. Certain foods and beverages such as aged cheese, canned tomatoes and beer may produce symptoms in some mold-sensitive patients.

Other Allergens. Other allergens such as tree-, grass- and ragweed pollens cannot be avoided except by staying out of geographic areas where they pollinate. For most individuals this is impractical socially and economically. Air conditioning and electrostatic precipitators will reduce somewhat exposure to these pollens and to dust and mold spores as well. An individual who has the opportunity to select a new area in which to live should consider his allergic diseases when making this important decision.

MEDICATIONS

When environmental precautions alone are not sufficient to control an allergic disease, the second approach is medication. As discussed in Chapters 6 and 8, drugs are available to relieve the various symptoms of allergic disease. For many patients, a combination of environmental control of antigens and drug therapy may achieve adequate relief of their symptoms.

IMMUNOTHERAPY

Introduction

In spite of good environmental control and use of proper medications, some patients continue to have difficulty from their allergic disease. For this group of patients immunotherapy is often beneficial.

Immunotherapy is a treatment in which patients receive injections of antigenic material to which they are sensitive in an attempt to reduce their sensitivity. Hyposensitization and desensitization are two other names for this form of therapy. How these terms are misleading will be discussed later in this chapter.

Immunotherapy had its beginning in 1911 when Noon and Freeman [4, 10] first treated grass pollen-sensitive patients with injections of extracts of grass pollen. A beneficial effect was noted in 16 of the 18 patients treated. It was thought then that the pollen was a toxin and that the pollen immunizations resulted in the production of an antitoxin.

Although allergy injection therapy has been used since that time to treat certain forms of allergic disease, it is only in recent years that some insight has been gained into its mode of action. Many physicians have used immunotherapy empirically because they thought they observed relief of symptoms in their patients. Controlled studies by investigators have now confirmed this clinical impression. In these studies patients were divided into treated and untreated control groups. The patients who received treatment had statistically significant improvement in symptoms.[5, 7] Other studies, of patients treated with high dose of antigen, indicate that the results achieved were superior to those of patients treated with low doses.[11, 13]

Laboratory investigations have given information on the possible mechanism of benefit achieved by allergy injection therapy. Studies showed that patients treated by immunotherapy had decreased serum reaginic antibody against the specific antigen with which they had been treated.[1] Other investigators have shown a decrease in the sensitivity of mediator releasing cells as indicated by histamine release of washed leukocytes after antigenic challenge [3, 11, 12] and an increase of serum blocking antibody activity with immunotherapy.[6] The latter antibody is presumably protective.

A unifying theory has been proposed based on the above studies and observations as to the time sequence of immunologic changes which occur in injection therapy with ragweed antigen.[8] The increase in IgG binding activity could result in the initial symtomatic improvement which follows injections of antigen. This antibody is presumed to combine with environmental antigen in or on the respiratory mucosa. The IgG antibody, by combining with the ragweed determinants, prevents ragweed from reacting with the allergic (reaginic) antibody on cell surfaces which would result in the subsequent release of chemical mediators. This causes the initial clinical improvement of symptoms that occurs in ragweed immunotherapy despite persistent cellular sensitivity and unaltered levels of reaginic antibody.

Following continued high dose therapy there is a loss of cellular sensitivity and a decrease in specific reaginic antibody available to sensitize mediator releasing cells. These changes are related to the long term improvement of symptoms with injections.

Other factors that may also be important in allergy injection therapy include possible reduction in the total numbers of mast cells, receptor sites, and receptor activity. These and other factors are currently being studied.

Because of these immunological changes which can be measured subsequent to injection therapy, the term "immunotherapy" is currently used to describe this form of treatment. Desensitization or hyposensitization more accurately describes the complete or partial decrease in reactivity resulting from administration of antigen to anaphylactically sensitive animals. The latter protection, although temporary, occurs rapidly. The experimental desensitization of animals with anaphylactic sensitivity probably occurs by exhaustion of mediators or sensitizing antibodies or both. In contrast, the effect of immunotherapy on human allergic patients is usually of long duration and is generally achieved slowly only after many months of inoculations.

Antigens Used in Immunotherapy

As a result of the studies already described the effectiveness of immunotherapy in treatment of ragweed pollen allergy appears established. Results of treatment with other pollen antigens are considered analogous. The common clinical impression is that results of immunotherapy with extracts of fungi have been less successful.

Injection therapy is not recommended for treatment of food allergy. Dietary exclusion of these foods is the therapy of choice. While some individuals advocate use of oral administration of antigen, its effectiveness is questioned. Using this method an individual is given small amounts of food to which he is sensitive. The amounts are then gradually increased until the patient is able to consume normal amounts, or until his tolerance is reached.

Immunotherapy is not recommended for treatment of animal danders except under unusual circumstances. Extracts of animal danders are very potent and often cause severe reactions. If the patient is susceptible to a family pet, avoidance of the animal is the safest and most satisfactory method of treatment. If an individual is sensitive to laboratory animals with which he must work, certain environmental precautions may decrease his exposure. He should plan his work ahead so as to be with the animals as short a time as possible. He should wear a mask, gloves and laboratory coat when he works with these animals. A fan should be placed behind the patient so that animal danders are blown away from him. If possible, the animal should be wetted down to decrease air-borne spread of danders. The patient should change his coat and discard his gloves and mask after working with the animals.

Debate continues concerning the use of bacterial vaccine. Although some investigators have reported benefit to patients treated with bacterial vaccine, most have questioned the value of this form of therapy.

The bacterial vaccines most commonly used are commercial preparations containing organisms usually cultured from the respiratory tract. Some physicians treat their patients with autogenous vaccines, which are bacterial vaccines prepared from cultures of the patient's nasal and bronchial secretions. A detailed discussion of bacterial vaccines is in Chapter 18 in Therapeutic Measures of Uncertain Value.

Selection of Antigens. Selection of antigens for immunization depends upon the sensitivity to aeroallergens as determined by clinical history and confirmed by appropriate skin tests. Immunotherapy should only be initiated with the antigens meeting these criteria. It is undesirable either to treat patients empirically with a battery of antigens common to that geographic location or to treat patients with all antigens to which they show positive skin test reactivity. These approaches would result in dilution of clinically important allergens. In addition, patients would be injected with unnecessary materials.

Antigen Mixtures. *Mixture of Related Antigens* Antigenic similarity exists between some related mold spores and pollens. For this reason it is customary to treat patients with selected mixtures of antigens of grasses, trees, weeds and fungi. The varieties of plant life which would be used by a physician for skin testing and treatment would depend upon the plants found to be important causes of disease in a particular geographic area.

Mixture of Unrelated Antigens There are two approaches in the office methodology of injection therapy. In the first method the physician uses a treatment set containing all the standard dilutions of the individual extracts of aeroallergens with which he is treating. If the patient is receiving therapy to several allergens then they are drawn into a syringe, the most dilute antigen first, and administered to the patient. This method allows the physician to vary the dose of extract the patient receives each visit. Using this form of therapy it is easy to change the amount of one allergen administered relative to the others, based on clinical considerations. There are disadvantages to this form of therapy. One vial of allergen may be contaminated with another allergen if caution is not used in drawing up the material. Unless the physician is treating a large number of patients it may be too costly to keep a complete set of fresh allergenic materials.

In the second method of treatment the patient receives a premixed vial containing the allergens to which he is sensitive. Under such circumstances the percentage of each antigen contributing to the mixture would be in proportion to its apparent importance in causing the patient's clinical symptoms. As an example, an individual with major difficulty during ragweed pollen season but with only minor symptoms during the grass pollen season might receive injections from an extract containing 60 to 75 percent ragweed pollen antigen and 25 to 40 percent grass antigen. Individuals with perennial symptoms might be treated with equal parts of tree, grass, and ragweed pollen, mold spores and dust antigens.

It is preferable to use one vial of extract to avoid confusing the dosage schedules between two separate vials. While two vials may be necessary under certain circumstances, it is extremely rare that three vials need be used. Injections from two vials should be considered when an individual is especially reactive to one antigen and less sensitive to several others. If all the antigens are combined, it might be necessary to proceed more slowly with the injection of all the antigens because of the marked reactivity to the one antigen. However, if this one antigen is removed and administered separately then the rate of increase in the concentration of the other antigens would proceed more quickly.

Techniques of Immunotherapy

Three forms of immunotherapy have been used: coseasonal, preseasonal and perennial.

Coseasonal is the least satisfactory of the three forms of therapy. It is sometimes used when the patient first presents during the season in which he is having allergic symptoms. This form of treatment involves frequent injections of very low concentrations of antigen. The intradermal method of administration of allergen is preferred over the subcutaneous injections by some physicians who give coseasonal therapy.

Preseasonal treatment is begun 3 to 6 months before the season during which the patient has allergic symptoms. The patient receives injections every 4 to 7 days, before the onset of the season, until the dose of maximum tolerance is reached. During the patient's allergy season the injections are stopped and then resumed again the following year at the same time.

Perennial is the recommended form of therapy. It consists of year round injection of antigens to which the patient is sensitive. The current evidence suggests that treatment with higher doses of pollen extracts results in better long term reduction of clinical symptoms and greater immunologic changes. The use of perennial treatment results in a higher cumulative dose of antigen than that achieved with preseasonal or coseasonal therapy and appears to be responsible for a longer and more significant clinical response.

Types of Allergy Extracts Used in Immunotherapy. Aqueous extracts are the standard form of therapy. In the studies demonstrating the effectiveness of allergy injection therapy, aqueous extracts of allergen were used. Other forms of antigen such as aqueous extracts in oil emulsion, alum precipitated antigens and other preparations have been described. Although the potential usefulness of certain of these treatments is good, they have not had the same degree of clinical or experimental evaluation as aqueous extract.

Initiation and Schedule of Treatment. Pollen extracts are standardized according to several different systems: pollen units, Freeman-Noon units, pollen weight by volume, protein nitrogen units, nitrogen units, and milligrams of total nitrogen.

The most concentrated form of extract used by many allergists, based on the weight by volume system, is a 1:50 dilution. The 1:50 dilution is prepared by extracting 1 gram of the pollen with 50 ml. of extracting fluid. One milliliter is equivalent to 20,000 pollen units; 20,000 Freeman-Noon units; 10.000 protein nitrogen units (PNU); 26,000 total nitrogen units; and 0.26 mg. total nitrogen. Two ten-fold dilutions of the 1:50 extract are usually prepared to make 1:500 and 1:5000 concentrations.

Other variations of classifying extracts according to the weight by volume method are also used and should become familiar to the reader. In one, dilutions of extract are made of 1:10,000; 1:1,000; 1:100 and 1:33 (1 gram of pollen extracted with 33 ml. of extract fluid). One of the common house dust preparations (Endo House Dust *) is made in weight by volume concentrations of 1:40,000; 1:4,000 and 1:400. Certain extracts of mold spores are prepared in weight by volume dilutions of 1:1,000; 1:100 and 1:10.

When the physician is using extracts of allergens diluted 1:5,000; 1:500 and 1:50, treatment of most patients is usually started with 0.05 ml. of the 1:5,000 concentration. If the patient gives a history of marked

* Manufactured by Endo Products, Richmond Hill, New York.

clinical sensitivity to an antigen, demonstrates very marked skin re-activity by scratch test, is pregnant, or has a history of prior reactions to injection therapy, a more dilute extract of 1:50,000 would be an appropriate starting dilution. Rarely, it may be necessary to initiate treatment with a dilution of 1:500,000 or greater.

If the first injection from the starting dilute extract is tolerated without a significant local reaction, increasing doses of that extract may be administered in a schedule similar to that shown below. The rate of increase in the early stages of treatment with the more dilute solution of extract is usually greater than with the most concentrated solution of extract. This schedule is intended only as an illustration and should be modified appropriately to the individual patient. The physician must be careful to proceed very cautiously in the highly sensitive patient who develops a large local reaction or has systemic reactions to the injections.

Allergy Treatment Tentative Dosage Schedule

DATE	EXTRACT CONCENTRATION	DOSAGE	REMARKS
—	1:5000	0.05	
		0.10	
		0.15	
		0.20	
		0.30	
		0.40	
		0.50	
	1:500	0.05	
		0.10	
		0.15	
		0.20	
		0.30	
		0.40	
		0.50	
	1:50	0.05	
		0.10	
		0.15	
		0.20	
		0.25	
		0.30	
		0.35	
		0.40	
		0.45	
		0.50	

Technique of Injections. The immunotherapy injections should always be given under the close supervision of a physician in the event that the patient should have a systemic reaction. For this reason, patients should not receive vials of their extract to be administered by themselves or friends while at home, at work or on vacation.

Before a patient receives each injection he should be asked whether he had any reaction after the previous injection or if he is presently ill. Both of these factors will influence whether the patient receives an injection and the dose of extract.

The proper injection technique can minimize the pain of injection and the degree of local reaction. The needle size should be 26 or 27 gauge to reduce discomfort. Disposable needles are preferable, but if reusable needles are used they should be sterilized after each use and sharpened frequently. The syringe should be a 1.0 ml. tuberculin type with well marked graduations. It may be either of disposable plastic or glass material. The latter requires adequate washing and sterilizing to destroy all antigens and avoid contamination.

Special care must be taken to select the correct antigen vial and draw the proper dose into the syringe before administering the injection to the patient. If antigens are being withdrawn from several vials, the most dilute antigen should be withdrawn first. It is important to avoid reflux into any of the antigen vials. The correctness of the schedule, the vials of antigens and the dose should be checked several times before the injection is made in order to avoid use of the wrong antigen or an error in the concentration or dose of the antigen.

The injection site should be the outer aspect of the arm midway between the shoulder and elbow. The area should be cleaned first with alcohol. The syringe needle should be wiped with alcohol before injecting to reduce local reactions. The angle of injection should be oblique but not too shallow. The plunger of the syringe should be pulled back before the extract is injected. **If blood is withdrawn, do not inject at that site;** withdraw the needle and select another site for injection. If antigen is injected directly into the blood stream, the possibility of an anaphylactic reaction is greatly increased.

After the injection, the patient presses an alcohol sponge to the injection site and avoids scratching or rubbing to reduce systemic absorption of antigen. The patient should always wait in the physicain's office for a period of thirty minutes. It is during this time that the majority of reactions begin.

Frequency of Injections. Therapeutic injections are usually administered weekly during the period of time that the dose and concentration of allergy extract are being increased. Once the maintenance dose has been reached and the patient's symptoms are controlled, the interval between injections may be increased to every 2 weeks. If improvement continues, the interval between injections may be gradually increased to every 3 and then every 4 weeks. If no improvement of symptoms occurs within 6 months to 1 year after initiation of treatment, the patient and his course of therapy must be carefully reevaluated.

Duration of Therapy. The duration of treatment depends on the response of the patient. His progress should be evaluated periodically. Administration of injections year after year after year without sense or reason is poor medical practice.

Duration of treatment for the average patient is 3 to 5 years. The program will vary if the patient is being treated for asthma, or asthma and rhinitis instead of rhinitis alone. Therapy for asthma may require longer treatment. Some physicians will continue to treat a patient with injections every 4 weeks until they are symptom free or near symptom free for 1 year before stopping immunotherapy.

Duration of Benefit. There are differences between individuals in the duration of benefits achieved from immunotherapy once injections are stopped. In some individuals, improvement is persistent. Other patients may have minimal allergic symptoms return which can be adequately controlled by environmental controls and infrequent use of medications. However, occasional patients, after immunization therapy has been stopped, develop increasing symptoms which may require further treatment. Unfortunately, it is not possible to predict which group the individual patient will fit. Therefore, the physician should not promise a patient that immunotherapy will "cure" all symptoms.

Maintenance Dose of Extract. The maintenance dose of extract received by a patient is variable. The goal is to give the patient the largest amount of extract which he can tolerate without having reactions to the injections. For many patients this would be approximately 0.50 ml. of 1:50 extract. For others, because of the occurrence of reactions, the maintenance dose may need to be a smaller amount of 1:50 extract or it may even be necessary to use a more dilute solution.

Reactions to Injections. Most patients will develop some swelling and redness at the injection site. Swelling or redness that persists longer than 24 hours or is larger than a walnut in size should be considered a significant local reaction. Such local reactions may indicate that a systemic reaction will occur if the dose of extract is increased. They should be viewed as a warning to the physician to proceed cautiously with increases in dose. A patient who develops an uncomfortable local reaction to an injection may be treated with an antihistaminic agent.

A patient who has a systemic reaction following an injection of allergy extract may require emergency treatment (see Chap. 12). A possible error in administration of the injection, such as a wrong dose or mix-up in vials, should be considered as causes of reactions. If no error is found, the schedule of doses should be reviewed and the next dose reduced by 50 to 90 percent.

Treatment Failures. A treatment failure occurs when a significant decrease in the patient's symptoms has not been achieved with immunotherapy. The reason should be found, if possible.

Failure to properly institute environmental control is a possible contribution to failure of treatment. This would include inadequate dust and mold control measures and failure to eliminate pets from the home. Many patients become lax in their environmental control after immunotherapy has been started and may even acquire pets at that time. They may believe it is safe to have an animal in their home because the initial skin test showed no reactivity to that animal.

Some patients develop new sensitivities to allergens different from the ones to which they are being treated. When indicated these new antigens should be added to the immunotherapy program in an appropriately cautious manner.

The antigens selected to use in the treatment mixture may be incorrect. This may be the result of an inadequate history or relying too heavily on skin test results alone; the importance of adequate diagnosis prior to initiation of a long and expensive treatment is again emphasized.

A patient may be receiving treatment with improper doses of extract. If inadequate doses are given, no immunologic changes are produced and the patient does not improve.

Some patients with vasomotor rhinitis and intrinsic asthma are diagnosed as having extrinsic allergic disease. Since these two conditions are not due to extrinsic aeroallergens, injection therapy would not relieve their symptoms.

In certain patients the diagnosis of treatment failure may not be justified. The relief that is obtained with immunotherapy may take many months and may not completely control all symptoms. If the individual being treated is impatient or expects a complete cure, he will be disappointed and may consider himself a treatment failure.

REFERENCES

1. Connell, J. T., and Sherman, W. B.: Skin-sensitizing antibody titer III. Relationship of the skin-sensitizing antibody titer to the intracutaneous skin test, to the tolerance of injections of antigens, and to the effects of prolonged treatment with antigen. J. Allerg., 35:169, 1964.
2. Cooke, R. A.: Allergy in Theory and Practice. Philadelphia, W. B. Saunders, 1947.

3. Cooke, R. A., *et al.:* The antibody mechanisms of ragweed allergy. electrophoretic and chemical studies. I. The blocking antibody. J. Exp. Med., *101:*177, 1955.

4. Freeman, J.: Further observations on the treatment of hay fever by hypodermic inoculation of pollen vaccine. Lancet, 2:814, 1911.

5. Johnstone, D. E., and Dutton, A.: The value of hyposensitization therapy for bronchial asthma in children—a 14 year study. Pediatrics, *42:*793, 1968.

6. Loveless, M. H.: Immunologic studies in pollenosis, I. The presence of two antibodies related to the same pollen antigen in the serum of treated hay fever patients. J. Immunol., *38:*25, 1940.

7. Lowell, F. C., and Franklin, W.: A double-blind study of the effectiveness and specificity of injection therapy in ragweed hay fever. New Eng. J. Med., *273:*675, 1965.

8. Melam, H., *et al.:* Clinical and immunologic studies of ragweed immunotherapy. J. Allerg., [In Press].

9. Mueller, H. L., and Lanz, M.: Hyposensitization with bacterial vaccine in infectious asthma. JAMA, *208:*1379, 1969.

10. Noon, L.: Prophylactic inoculation against hay fever. Lancet, *1:*1572, 1911.

11. Pruzansky, J. J., and Patterson, R.: Histamine release from leukocytes of hypersensitive individuals. *II* Reduced sensitivity of leukocytes after injection therapy. J. Allerg., *39:*44, 1967.

12. Sadan, N., *et al.:* Immunotherapy of pollinosis in children. New Eng. J. Med., *280:*623, 1969.

13. Van Metre, T. E., Jr., *et al.:* Hay fever symptoms, blocking antibody levels, and leukocyte histamine release in patients receiving very high dosage immunotherapy with ragweed pollen extract. [Abst.]. J. Allerg., *43:*180, 1969.

10

Ocular and Otic Manifestations of Allergy

Phillip L. Lieberman, M.D.

The eye is involved in allergic reactions of both delayed and humoral types. Although allergic reactions of the eye represent a relatively small portion of the allergist's practice, their significance in any given situation may be great. Allergic disease of the eye may be conveniently classified according to the part of the eye afflicted. Thus they are divided into reactions of the eyelid, the conjunctiva, the uvea, the lens and the cornea.

THE EYELID

Contact Dermatitis

By far the most important disease of the eyelid seen in the practice of allergy is contact dermatitis. Contact dermatitis of the eyelids is a delayed hypersensitivity reaction of the same type that occurs elsewhere on the skin (see Chap. 17). It can be associated with a conjunctival reaction.

Clinical Presentation and Etiology. Vesiculation may occur in the early stages of the disease, but, by the time the patient seeks care, the lids usually appear thickened, red, and chronically inflamed.

The sensitizing substance is usually a cosmetic or therapeutic agent. Nail polish, perfumes, mascara, eye shadow, artificial lashes and lash adhesives, aerosolized agents such as hair sprays, and eye ointments and drops, all may cause this disease. When the offending substance is an eye ointment or drop there is often a severe reaction involving the conjunctivae as well as the lids which is usually referred to as dermatoconjunctivitis. Many therapeutic agents can cause this type of lesion. Any topical antibacterial agent or local anesthetic can cause the reaction. Topical antihistamines have also been reported to cause delayed hypersensitivity reactions. The incidence of delayed hypersensitivity to most of these agents appears to be relatively low when viewed in light of their common usage; nevertheless, certain drugs (penicillin and various topical analgesics, for example) are frequent offenders.

Diagnosis and Treatment. The management of contact dermatitis of the lids should attempt to eliminate the sensitizing agent. In relatively acute cases or cases associated with topical drug administration, this agent can usually be quickly identified. However, in chronic cases, which present with a slightly swollen, red, and sometimes weeping lesion, the agent may not be readily detected. In either case, all topical applications to the eye should be stopped immediately. In addition, the use of less obvious possible offenders, such as hair sprays, colognes, and nail polishes should be discontinued. In many cases this simple measure results in rapid healing.

If the lesion is particularly severe and if one is certain that the offending agent has been removed, topical corticosteroids should be used. However, if the lesion involves the conjunctiva and if the steroids must be applied directly into the eye as well as on the lids, an ophthalmologist should be consulted prior to their administration. This precaution is advised whenever intraocular corticosteroids are indicated. The hazards associated with these drugs are well known. In the presence of herpetic lesions topical corticosteroids can result in blindness. They may predispose to fungal invasion, cause posterior subcapsular cataracts, or raise intraocular pressure, thus precipitating open angle glaucoma.

Patch testing may be used to identify the sensitizing agent after all possible offenders have been discontinued. This procedure may aid in allowing the patient to resume the use of innocuous substances which previously had been suspect. It must be remembered, however, that the offending substance may be acting as a primary irritant and not as a true sensitizing agent. In this case the patch test may be negative. Therefore the history of exposure induced symptomatology may be of more value than patch tests in outlining a therapeutic regimen.

THE CONJUNCTIVA

Acute Allergic (Atopic) Conjunctivitis

Pathophysiology. Acute allergic conjunctivitis is the ocular analogue of allergic rhinitis. It is the clinical manifestation of the interaction between antigen and IgE bound to mast cells located in the conjunctiva. Histamine and perhaps other mediators are liberated by this antigen-antibody union. The consequence is a local conjunctival reaction consisting of vasodilatation and edema. The clinical reproducibility of this reaction is dependable and was once used as a diagnostic test for immediate hypersensitivity. This was accomplished by the instillation of antigens directly into the conjunctival sac.[31] The conjunctival reaction thus produced is analogous to the presently employed cutaneous tests.

Clinical Presentation. The eye, being in constant contact with the external environment, is frequently the target organ in allergic individuals. The resultant symptomatology in the acute phase is usually easily recognized. The conjunctiva is injected and edematous. Chemosis is present. Profuse tearing occurs, and, in severe cases, there is often a mucopurulent discharge. Itching is prominent, and the resultant rubbing often intensifies the symptomatology. The lesion is almost always bilateral but may be unilateral. The eyes may be swollen shut. The etiologic agent is usually an aero-allergen; however, acute allergic conjunctivitis can be caused by manual contamination of the conjunctiva with other types of antigens. The latter should be suspected if the lesion is unilateral.

Diagnosis and Treatment. The diagnosis can usually be made on the basis of the history and physical examination. There will be an atopic personal or family history; the disease will usually be seasonal; and at times the patient may be able to accurately define the offending allergen. Of great importance is the almost universal association with allergic rhinitis. If allergic rhinitis has never been present the diagnosis is highly questionable. Allergic rhinitis may be present in a subclinical form. In such cases the nasal mucosa will appear boggy and swollen, and nasal secretions will contain many eosinophils, even though the patient has no subjective complaints of rhinitis. Skin tests are confirmatory. Hansel's staining of the conjunctival secretions or scrapings should reveal numerous eosinophils. The differential diagnosis should include other forms of acute conjunctivitis, particularly those of viral etiology. Conjunctivitis due to bacterial infection and secondary to irritation from drug instillation should also be considered.

Treatment of acute allergic conjunctivitis should follow the same outline as that of any atopic illness. Avoidance, symptomatic relief, and desensitization should be proposed in that order. Usually allergic conjunctivitis is a relatively minor problem associated with allergic rhinitis or extrinsic asthma. In this case treatment will naturally follow the course dictated by the more debilitating disorder. At times the conjunctivitis is the most prominent disease, and therapy will be directed primarily toward its relief.

Avoidance of ubiquitous aero-allergens is, of course, impractical. But avoidance measures outlined elsewhere in this text can also be employed in the treatment of allergic conjunctivitis. Symptomatic therapy may be topical or oral. Oral antihistamines are the preferred method of treatment because of their comparative safety. At times they will afford sufficient relief, but topical therapy is a necessary adjunct in many cases.

Three classes of topical medication are useful: decongestants, usually containing phenylephrine; antihistamines; and corticosteroids. Several proprietary preparations are available. These will often provide excellent relief. They may sting for a brief period upon application and may be responsible for a dermatoconjunctivitis. For the most part, however, they are beneficial and safe. Topical application of corticoids can provide dramatic relief. Once again, their use is potentially hazardous, as discussed in the section on contact dermatitis of the lids.

Although no definitive double blind studies concerning the efficacy of hyposensitization in this disease have been performed to date, it is felt, based on clinical experience, to be a useful measure. The criteria for its application are highly variable, but it is worthy of trial in cases not adequately controlled by avoidance or mild symptomatic therapy.

Allergic conjunctivitis can also exist in a rarer, chronic, form. Again it is almost always associated with allergic rhinitis. The findings of chronic allergic conjunctivitis are less striking. Edema of the bulbar conjunctiva may give the eye a glassy appearance. Photophobia and itching are common complaints. Stain of the ocular secretions shows eosinophils and lymphocytes. Treatment is much the same as for acute conjunctivitis. Response to therapy is less dramatic.

Conjunctivitis of Questionable Allergic Etiology

There are two diseases of the conjuctiva which have, in the past, been attributed to immune mechanisms. These are conjunctivitis due to hypersensitivity to the staphylococcus and vernal conjunctivitis. Several features of these diseases suggest allergic etiologies, but their true pathogeneses have not been clarified. The immunopathology involved has not been adequately defined in either case. No antigen has been discovered in vernal conjunctivitis, and in neither of the diseases (with the possible exception of staphylococcal hypersensitivity) has a specific form of immune therapy proven efficacious. However, because of the traditional approach to these illnesses, they deserve to be discussed as allergies.

Staphylococcal Hypersensitivity. Delayed hypersensitivity to the staphylococcus has been incriminated as a cause of a chronic, recurrent, nonpurulent conjunctivitis. Burning eyes, usually worse in the morning, are characteristic. In this disease the lids are described as chronically inflamed. There is folliculosis and marginal blepharitis. Coagulase-positive *Staphylococcus aureus* is often, but not always, isolated from the conjunctiva. There is a delayed hypersensitivity to staphylococcal toxin as demonstrated by intradermal injection. Improvement is claimed to follow incremental injections of staphylococcal toxin or toxoid.[30]

The role of hypersensitivity in this disease is still not firmly established. The presence of cutaneous delayed hypersensitivity to the staphylococcus may be a chance association; many asymptomatic individuals exhibit this phenomenon. The improvement apparently obtained by "desensitization" to staphylococcus is puzzling. This observation does not affirm the significance of delayed hypersensitivity in this disease, since such "desensitization" procedures have yet to be shown effective in other clinical states of delayed hypersensitivity.

Vernal Conjunctivitis. *Clinical Presentation.* Vernal conjunctivitis is a chronic conjunctivitis occurring in the spring and summer. It is characterized mainly by itching, but tearing, burning and photophobia also occur. It is always bilateral and apparently more common in warmer climates. The disease is more common in children than adults, and males are affected more often than females. It may exist in a palpebral or a limbal form. In the palpebral variety the tarsal conjunctiva of the upper lid is deformed by thickened, gelatinous vegetations with a "cobblestone" appearance. In the limbal form there is inflammation of the corneoscleral limbus which causes thickening and the formation of a gelatinous covering which may also have a "cobblestone" appearance. There is a stringy, mucoid exudate which often shows numerous eosinophils. The patient may be particularly troubled by this discharge, which often strings out a distance of over an inch when it is removed from the eye.

Etiology. Because of the seasonal occurrence, the presence of eosinophils in the ocular secretions, and the frequent coexistence of vernal conjunctivitis with confirmed allergic disease,[2] hypersensitivity has been suspected as the etiology. No firm evidence exists to substantiate this hypothesis, and response to routine allergic treatment, especially immunotherapy, is inconsistent. The disease has also been associated with intestinal parasitosis, chronic seborrhea, and warm climates. At present, the etiology of this illness remains unknown.

Treatment. Therapeutic measures in vernal conjunctivitis are, for the most part, nonspecific. At the present time topical corticosteroid drops appear to be the treatment of choice. Their use is not without the risks previously mentioned, and ophthalmological supervision should always be obtained prior to their administration. Topical antihistamines with or without phenylephrine may be employed as in acute allergic conjunctivitis. Detection and elimination of intestinal parasites, if present, and treatment of associated seborrhea or allergic rhinitis has been claimed to be effective, as has moving to cooler climates.[1] Air conditioning and filtering systems have also been advocated.[23] Fortunately, spontaneous remission usually occurs after 8 to 10 years.

THE UVEAL TRACT

The uveal tract consists of the iris, the ciliary body, and the choroid. It is the "middle coat" of the eye, lying between the sclera and the retina. The choroid is a highly vascular layer supplying blood to the retinal pigmented epithelium and the outer half of the neural retina. The ciliary body forms a ring between the iris and the choroid. It secretes aqueous humor and is responsible for changing the shape of the lens during accommodation. The iris separates the anterior and posterior chambers. It lies anterior to the ciliary body and lens and acts as a diaphragm to regulate the entrance of light into the eye.

The uveal tract is subject to inflammatory changes which can result in blindness. Immune mechanisms have long been felt to be responsible for inflammation of the uveal tract, and a wealth of experimental data has been accumulated to corroborate these impressions. The animal models by which uveitis can be reproduced experimentally are ex-

TABLE 10-1
Classification of Uveitis

I. GRANULOMATOUS
  A. Viral
    H. simplex, H. zoster, cytomegalic inclusion virus, mumps, infectious mononucleosis, influenza, vaccinia
  B. Bacterial
    tuberculosis, brucellosis, leprosy, leptospirosis
  C. Fungal
    histoplasmosis, blastomycosis, coccidioidosis, mucormycosis, cryptococcosis
  D. Protozoal
    toxoplasmosis, trypanosomiasis
  E. Helminth
    A variety of both nematodes and cestodes

II. NONGRANULOMATOUS
  A. Reiter's syndrome
  B. Rheumatoid arthritis
  C. Ankylosing spondylitis
  D. Ulcerative colitis
  E. Regional enteritis
  F. Other "connective tissue diseases" (lupus erythematosus, periarteritis nodosa, dermatomyositis)
  G. Behçet's disease
  H. Vogt-Koyanagi-Harada syndrome
  I. Serum sickness
  J. Streptococcal hypersensitivity
  K. Focal infections of the respiratory and urinary tracts and of the teeth

III. MISCELLANEOUS
  A. Phacogenic uveitis
  B. Sympathetic ophthalmia

tensive in number, and it has been shown that the uveal tract is a target organ in which many immunopathologic reactions are clinically expressed. Uveitis may be experimentally reproduced by both Arthus and delayed types of hypersensitivity.[25] Several antigens and numerous species have been studied. Unfortunately, even in the face of this intensive research, the basic mechanisms involved in the clinical diseases have not been entirely clarified. In clinical practice the etiology of any individual case of uveitis may be obscure.

The clinical classifications of uveitis have all met with major criticisms. For our purposes uveitis may be divided into granulomatous and nongranulomatous forms.[32] In addition, a third category, which consists of miscellaneous forms usually due to trauma, should be considered because of its immunologic significance (Table 10-1). The most important form of uveitis as regards allergology is nongranulomatous uveitis. The other forms are mentioned for the sake of completeness and because of the immunologic mechanisms involved in their pathogenesis.

Granulomatous Uveitis

Granulomatous uveitis, as its name implies, is characterized by a chronic tissue reaction which consists of large mononuclear phagocytes and epithelioid cells which aggregate to form granulomas. It is usually the result of direct invasion of the uveal tract by a nonpyogenic organism (See Table 10-1). The etiologic agent can often be identified by the appearance of the eye on slit lamp examination. This can be a relentless, progressive disease resulting in blindness. An extensive investigation for an etiologic agent and institution of specific therapy are indicated in all cases. Usually therapy consists of anti-infectious agents, with or without corticosteroids. A "desensitization" procedure has been recommended for the treatment of granulomatous uveitis associated with histoplasmosis.[27] The benefit of this form of therapy remains controversial.

Nongranulomatous Uveitis

Nongranulomatous uveitis is the ocular manifestation of several systemic diseases (See Table 10-1). In contrast to the granulomatous form, it is a sterile inflammatory reaction with aggregations of lymphocytes and plasma cells.

Clinical Presentation. Nongranulomatous uveitis usually takes the form of a transitory, recurrent inflammation and does not result in permanent damage unless attacks are persistent or extraordinarily severe. Nevertheless, residual synechiae and cataracts may result from repeated attacks. The eye is injected. Pain, photophobia, lacrimation, and blurred vision may be present. Slit lamp examination is useful in making the diagnosis.

Theories of Etiology. Auto-immunity in the form of classical Arthus, immune complex, or delayed hypersensitivity, has been repeatedly implicated as the cause of nongranulomatous uveitis. This hypothesis is based on both clinical and serologic findings in humans and animal models. Both anti-uveal and anti-DNA antibodies have been considered as possible participants in the production of the disease in man. [3, 21] The human uveitis that can accompany serum sickness is apparently due to immune complex deposition on the uveal tract. Human uveitis occuring after intracutaneous injection of tuberculin [16] is thought to be due to delayed hypersensitivity.

Rats,[28] guinea pigs, rabbits,[4] and other animals have been used to recreate the disease experimentally. In these experimental models the animal is injected with uveal or retinal-vitreous extracts in complete Freund's adjuvant. The resultant uveitis is considered to be auto-immune in origin and due to the production of anti-uveal antibodies.

Whenever an antigen is injected into the vitreous of an animal, it escapes very slowly resulting in a situation analogous to a depot immunization. One week after the injection, an initial uveitis occurs. This inflammation recedes spontaneously. However, if the animal is challenged again with the same antigen at a distant site, even a year later, a secondary nongranulomatous uveitis can ensue. This reaction, analogous histologically to the human disease, is believed to be due to the humoral antibody response of sensitized "lymphocyte-plasma" cells which have remained in the eye since the first injection.[26]

Of note is the questionable etiologic role of hidden focal infections of the teeth, respiratory tract and genito-urinary tract [27] and of streptococcal hypersensitivity [12] in the pathogenesis of this disease (See Table 10-1). Although the actual significance of these entities has not been established, they should not be ignored in cases for which no etiology can be found.

Diagnosis and Treatment. In practice it may be impossible to document the mechanisms involved in the production of uveitis. The allergist usually approaches the problem after an anatomical diagnosis is made by the ophthalmologist. If the ophthalmologist is also able to supply the etiologic diagnosis on the basis of the appearance of the lesion, proper treatment is then instituted. However, it is usually impossible to determine the etiology on eye exam alone. A general medical workup with history, physical examination, and routine laboratory evaluation (complete blood count, urinalysis, chest x-ray, glucose, and blood urea nitrogen) is then indicated. A VDRL, stools for ova and parasites, serological studies for "collagen disorders" are employed as deemed necessary. It must also be remembered that infectious agents can cause nongranulomatous uveitis on occasion. Therefore, skin tests and serologies may be helpful.

The treatment of nongranulomatous uveitis must always be conducted in close consultation with an ophthalmologist. Local and symptomatic therapy should be under his supervision. Corticosteroids, topical and oral, have proven beneficial. Recently, various antimetabolites have been employed to treat this disease. Cyclophosphamide,[5] methotrexate,[13] azathioprine,[19] and 6-mercaptopurine[18] have been tried with encouraging results.

Other Forms of Immune Uveitis

As has been noted, the allergist rarely has the opportunity to see uveitis other than the nongranulomatous variety. However, because of the immunopathology involved, two rarer type of uveitis warrant mention. These types are phacogenic uveitis (phacoanaphylaxis) and sympathetic ophthalmia.

Phacogenic Uveitis (Phacoanaphylaxis). Phacogenic uveitis is a sterile inflammation resulting from the liberation of lens protein into the eye. The disease is manifested by an iridocyclitis that usually follows trauma, especially surgical, causing disruption of the lens capsule. It can also occur after spontaneous disruption of the capsule. The intensity of the reaction is variable and seems to have no relation to the amount of liberated lens protein or the duration of time between the trauma and the onset of uveitis. The disease does not occur in every case of injury that results in lens capsule damage. The lesion is almost always unilateral.

The hypothesis that this disease is of immune origin is based on the idea that, since the lens is isolated anatomically from the immune system at an early embryologic stage, it is recognized as foreign protein on subsequent exposure. Thus antibodies are produced to lens protein when it is liberated into the systemic circulation. This theory has support in the fact that anti-lens antibodies are found in patients who have undergone cataract surgery and later developed uveitis,[29] and also by the observation that uveitis can be produced in rabbits that have been sensitized to lens protein and afterwards have had traumatic lens disruptions.[24] However, anti-lens antibodies have also been found in normal volunteers who had no evidence of ocular disease.[10]

The treatment of choice is removal of all residual lens material. Corticosteroids seem to be of some benefit.

Sympathetic Ophthalmia. Sympathetic ophthalmia is a uveitis, histologically distinct from phacogenic uveitis, that is thought to result from traumatic liberation of uveal tissue into the systemic circulation. It occurs as the result of a perforating eye injury that disrupts the uveal tract. A unique feature of this disease is that it is always bilateral. Trauma to one eye incites a reaction in both. Antibody formation to uveal pigment has been incriminated as the mechanism responsible for the inflammation. As in phacogenic uveitis, there is both clinical and experimental data to support this hypothesis. Circulating anti-uveal antibodies have been demonstrated in patients with the disease [17] as have positive "delayed skin tests" to uveal pigment.[8] In addition, uveitis occurs in guinea pigs sensitized to homologous uveal tissue.[7] Although such evidence is suggestive, no definitive immune pathogenesis has been established.

Treatment of this disease centers around corticosteroid administration. Prophylactic enucleation of an irreparably injured eye, prior to the onset of sympathetic ophthalmia, has also been advised.

THE LENS

A number of attempts have been made to incriminate immune mechanisms in the pathogenesis of both congenital and senile cataracts. No convincing evidence exists to date to corroborate these hypotheses. On the other hand there appears to be a definite clinical association between atopic dermatitis and premature cataract formation. Some patients with atopic dermatitis will develop cataracts prior to age 30. These lesions are usually bilateral. They are structurally distinct from congenital or metabolically induced lesions. Progression of the cataract formation may be extremely rapid and is often associated with periods of exacerbation of the dermatitis.

The allergist should also be alert to the development of cataracts in patients on long term corticosteroid therapy.

THE CORNEA

The cornea has served as an excellent organ for the study of immune phenomena. Because of its easy accessibility and its unique vascular structure, consisting of an avascular center surrounded by a highly vascular corneoscleral periphery, it has been employed to demonstrate both Arthus and delayed hypersensitivity reactions. Antigen injection directly into the cornea of a passively sensitized animal will produce a visible ring coaxial with the injection site. This ring consists of antigen-antibody precipitates and is analogous to that formed in the Mancini gel diffusion system.[9]

Of more clinical importance is the ease with which the cornea participates in delayed hypersensitivity reactions. Intracorneal injection of an antigen to which an animal exhibits delayed hypersensitivity can result in a keratitis in a matter of days. This has been demonstrated experimentally with tuberculin and staphylococcus antigens as well as horse serum. The human analogue of these experimental models is believed to be phlyctenular keratoconjunctivitis. This disease is thought to be due to delayed hypersensitivity. It is most commonly associated with tuberculosis, but other organisms, such as the staphylococcus and gonococcus, in addition to fungi, yeast and helminths have been incriminated.

The disease usually involves both the cornea and the conjunctiva. A small, gray nodule, the phlyctenule, develops at the corneoscleral limbus. The nodule ulcerates, and the ulcer usually progresses toward the center of the cornea carrying with it the neovasculature of inflammation. This process can result in corneal scarring. Several such ulcerating nodules may be present simultaneously. The lesions respond to topical corticosteroids. Whenever this disease is diagnosed, a search for tuberculosis is indicated.

Several other diseases of the cornea have been thought to result from immune pathology. These are seen solely by the ophthalmologist. They are the interstitial keratitis seen as a late manifestation of congenital syphilis, the disciform keratitis associated with herpes simplex, and the corneal ulcerations occasionally seen with blepharitis and chronic conjunctivitis. In addition, there is an apparent association between atopic dermatitis and keratoconus, a disease characterized by thinning and bulging of the central cornea.

OTIC MANIFESTATIONS OF ALLERGY

The allergist's contact with ear disease is, for the most part, limited to serous otitis media. The ear, however, is subject to delayed hypersensitivity reactions which can involve both the auricle and the external canal. Earrings, glasses and perfumes are common causes of contact dermatitis of the auricle. Objects such as hair pins, which are repeatedly placed into the external canal, can cause contact sensitivity in this area. Allergic mechanisms have also been proposed as etiologies for diseases of the inner ear, but such relationships have not been thoroughly studied or documented.

Serous Otitis Media

Serous otitis media is a disorder of the middle ear characterized by the accumulation of a nonpurulent, serous secretion. Its most disabling effect is that of hearing loss. It is the most common cause of childhood deafness in the United States today.

Pathophysiology. In the normal state the middle ear is free of any significant amount of fluid and is filled with air. Air is maintained in the middle ear by the action of the eustachian tube, which connects the middle ear and nasopharynx. This tube serves to maintain ventilation of the middle ear and equalize pressure on both sides of the tympanic membrane. The eustachian tube is closed at the pharyngeal end except during swallowing when the tensor palatini contract and open it by lifting its posterior lip. When the tube is opened, air passes from the nasopharynx into the middle ear. By means of this ventilation system equal pressure is maintained on both sides of the tympanic membrane.

When the tube is blocked, air cannot enter the middle ear and the remaining air is absorbed. This results in the formation of negative pressure within the middle ear. It is this negative pressure that is thought to cause the accumulation of a serous fluid. The fluid itself is responsible for the signs and symptoms of the disease.

The fluid is considered to consist mainly of secretions from the cells lining the middle ear. The lining of the middle ear is mainly nonsecretory, cuboidal epithelium but also contains cells capable of producing secretions, such as goblet cells. It is thought that with pathological stimuli, such as the development of negative pressure, these cells undergo hyperplasia and produce excessive secretions.[22]

The characteristics of the fluid vary with the stage of the disease. In the early stages it is usually yellow and of relatively low viscosity. As the disease progresses the fluid darkens and becomes increasingly viscuous. In the late stages it is blue-gray and extremely tenacious. In this stage it prohibits any movement of the ossicles or tympanic membrane. It is usually acellular, but eosinophils may be present. In most cases pathogenic organisms are not isolated from the fluid although the respiratory syncytial virus has been found on occasion.[6]

Etiology. Serous otitis media can result from any condition which causes eustachian obstruction. Upper respiratory infections, enlarged adenoids, postnasal tumors, dental malocclusion, malfunction of the tensor veli palatini, and upper respiratory allergies have all been associated with the disease. Allergic disorders seem to play a prominent role in the pathogenesis of the illness either as an etiologic or aggravating factor. A large percent of children with serous otitis have concomitant atopic disease, especially upper respiratory allergies.[6] The role of food allergy in the production of serous otitis is entirely speculative, and no adequate documentation of this relationship exists to date. In certain instances, especially in children under age 3, it may be worthwhile to investigate foods as a causal agent. The middle ear does not appear to be the allergic target organ, but the allergic state seems to predispose to obstruction of the eustachian tube, perhaps through inflammation and edema at the nasopharyngeal orifice.

Clinical Presentation. Serous otitis media is usually a disease of childhood occurring with greatest frequency before age 10. The most common and gravest symptom is that of hearing loss. The loss may be rapid or insidious. It is often difficult to detect in young children who have few subjective complaints. The child may appear "slow," inattentive or simply disobedient. The mother or teacher may find it necessary to speak loudly and repeat herself to be heard. Often the degree of hearing loss may vary with position of the head, and fluctuations in severity of the deficit are common. There may also be a sensation of "popping" of the ears, a dull, mild earache, or a sense of "fullness of the head." A history of rhinitis or repeated upper respiratory infections is frequently encountered.

On otoscopic examination the drum may be entirely normal in appearance or may simply have lost its normal luster. At times a fluid level may be seen, and bubbles may be evident in the fluid. As the disease progresses the drum turns a blue-gray color and becomes opaque and immobile. Marked limitation of drum movement is seen with the pneumatic otoscope. Audiometry confirms a conductive hearing loss, usually ranging from 10 to 40 decibels.

Therapy. The referring physician and the allergist must cooperate closely in the management of the patient with serous otitis media. It is the allergist's responsibility to perform the allergic workup and determine if hypersensitivity is a contributing or causative factor in the disease. A standard allergic workup is indicated. Nasal smears for the presence of eosinophils may be of diagnostic importance. If allergic factors are thought to be playing a significant role, therapy should proceed along the well established lines of avoidance of antigens, symptomatic alleviation, and desensitization.

Since aero-allergens are felt to be the major inciting antigens avoidance procedures should be carried out as outlined elsewhere in the text. The foundation of symptomatic therapy is the daily administration of an antihistamine-decongestant. The efficacy of this form of treatment has been demonstrated in certain cases.[15] If chronic respiratory infection is present, prolonged antibiotic administration (especially during the winter months) may be indicated. Decongestant nose drops may help during acute upper respiratory infections. However, because of the danger of rhinitis medicamentosa their use should be limited to a three day period. Corticosteroid nasal sprays are often beneficial.[14] Short term oral corticosteroid therapy has also been advocated.[20] The use of steroids, however, must be considered in relation to their side effects.

They should therefore be reserved for difficult cases who have shown a poor response to more standard therapy. The nasal spray would appear to be the most innocuous route of steroid administration, but systemic steroid effects can also occur during this mode of therapy. Proper humidification of the home during winter months may be of benefit. In mild cases the Valsalva maneuver is useful in aiding fluid drainage.

The decision to begin hyposensitization must be individualized according to the requirements of any given situation. There are no steadfast guidelines. However, because of the possibility of permanent ear damage or retardation of intellectual and speech development,[11] the initiation of therapy in any case with definite findings of hypersensitivity appears both justified and indicated.

Refractory or severe cases often require surgical intervention. Insertion of a Silastic or Teflon tube into the ear drum is a common procedure. The tube is usually removed in 3 to 6 months. Other types of ventilation tubes for more prolonged use (1 to 2 years) are reserved for the most severe cases. In addition the otolaryngologist may employ other techniques such as myringectomy, aspirations, and eustachian tubal inflation.

Prognosis in serous otitis media is usually good, and most children undergo spontaneous, permanent remission. However, lasting damage can occur. The disease can predispose to cholesteatoma formation or chronic suppurative otitis media.

REFERENCES

1. Alimuddin, M.: Treatment of vernal conjunctivitis. Brit. J. Ophthal., *39*:540, 1955.
2. Allensmith, M., and Frick, O. L.: Antibodies to grass in vernal conjuctivitis. J. Allerg., *34*:535, 1963.
3. Aronson, S. B., Yamamoto, E., Goodner, E. K., and O'Connor, G. R.: The occurrence of an autoantiuveal antibody in human uveitis. Arch. Ophthal. [Chicago], *72*:621, 1964.
4. Aronson, S. B.: Experimental allergic uveitis. Arch. Ophthal., *80*:235, 1968.
5. Buckley, C. E. III, and Gills, J. P.: Cyclophosphamide therapy of peripheral uveitis. Arch. Intern. Med., *124*:29, 1969.
6. Chan, J. C. M., Logan, C. B., and McBean, J. B.: Serous otitis media and allergy. Amer. J. Dis. Child., *114*:684, 1967.
7. Collins, R. C.: Experimental studies on sympathetic ophthalmia. Amer. J. Ophthal., *32*:1687, 1949.
8. Friedenwald, J., S.: Notes on the allergy theory of sympathetic ophthalmia. Amer. J. Ophthal., *17*:1008, 1934.

9. Germuth, F. G., *et al.:* Observations on the site and mechanism of antigen-antibody interaction in anaphylactic hypersensitivity. Amer. J. Ophthal., 46:282, 1958.

10. Hackett, E., and Thompson, A.: Anti-lens antibodies in human sera. Lancet, 2:663, 1964.

11. Holm, V. A., and Kunze, L. H.: Effect of chronic otitis media on language and speech development. Pediatrics, 43:883, 1969.

12. Koleckarova, M., Klenka, L., and Hana, I.: Hypersensitivity to streptococci in patients with recurrent uveitis. Acta Allerg., 20:484, 1965.

13. Lazar, M., Weiner, M. J., and Leopold, I. H.: Treatment of uveitis with methotrexate. Amer. J. Ophthal., 67:383, 1969.

14. Lecks, H. I., Kravis, L. P., and Wood, D. W.: Serous otitis media: reflections on pathogenesis and treatment. Clin. Pediat. [Phila.], 6:519, 1967.

15. Miller, G. F.: Influence on an oral decongestant on eustachian tube function in children. J. Allerg., 45:187, 1970.

16. Miller, R. K., and Smerz, A.: Bilateral posterior uveitis complicating a positive tuberculin reaction. Arch. Ophthal., 56:896, 1956.

17. Mills, P. V., and Sheehan, W. I.: Serological studies in sympathetic ophthalmia. Brit. J. Ophthal., 49:29, 1965.

18. Newel, F. W., Krill, A. E., and Thompson, A.: The treatment of uveitis with six-mercaptopurine. Amer. J. Ophthal., 61:1250, 1966.

19. Newell, F. W., and Krill, A. E.: Treatment of uveitis with azathioprine. Trans. Ophthal. Soc. U. K., 87:499, 1967.

20. Oppenheimer, P.: Short term steroid therapy, treatment of serous otitis media in children. Arch. Otolaryng., 88:138, 1968.

21. Rheins, M. S., Burno, R. M., and Suie, T.: Anti-DNA serum factors in chronic microbial diseases and endogenous uveitis. Amer. J. Ophthal., 64:437, 1967.

22. Sade, J.: Pathology and pathogenesis of serous otitis media. Arch. of Otolaryng., 84:297, 1966.

23. Scheie, H. G., and Albert, D. M.: Adlers Textbook of Ophthalmology. ed. 8. p. 186. Philadelphia, W. B. Saunders, 1969.

24. Scobee, R. G., and Slaughter, H. C.: Endophthalmitis phacoanaphylactica. Amer. J. Ophthal., 27:49, 1944.

25. Silverstein, A. M., and Zimmerman, L. E.: Immunogenic endophthalmitis produced in the guinea pig by different pathogenetic mechanisms. Amer. J. Ophthal., 48:435, 1959.

26. Smith, R. E., Jensen, A. D., and Silverstein, A. M.: Antibody formation by single cells during experimental immunogenic uveitis. Invest. Ophthal., 8:373, 1969.

27. Van Metre, T. E., Jr.: Role of the allergist in diagnosis and management of patients with uveitis, JAMA, 195:167, 1966.

28. Waksman, B. H., and Bollington, S. J.: Studies of arthritis and other lesions induced in rats by injection of mycobacterial adjuvant. III. Lesions of the the eye. Arch. Ophthal., 64:751, 1960.

29. Wirostko, E., and Halbert, S. P.: Autoimmune phenomena in the eye. *In* Miescher, P. A., and Mueller-Eberhard, H. J.: Textbook of Immuno-pathology. ed. 1. vol. 1. p. 626. New York, Grune and Stratton, 1968.
30. Woods, A. C.: Allergy and conjunctivitis. Arch. Ophthal., [Chicago], *17*:1, 1937.
31. Woods, A. C.: Ocular allergy. Amer. J. Ophthal., *32*:1457, 1949.
32. Woods, A. C.: Endogenous inflammations of the uveal tract. ed. 1. p. 22. Baltimore, Williams & Wilkins, 1961.

11

Insect Sting Allergy

Alice Solar-Mills, M.D.

The stings of certain insects may produce anaphylactic reactions. Each year in the United States, there are more deaths from anaphylaxis to insect stings than from snake bites.

Most of the insects responsible for severe reactions in man are members of the phylum *Arthropoda,* class *Insecta,* order *Hymenoptera* (meaning membrane-wing). The yellow jacket sting is most likely to produce anaphylaxis, followed by bee, wasp, and hornet stings. Systemic allergic reactions to the sting of the imported fire ant and rarely to the bite of the mosquito, deer fly, and tick have been reported.

Only female hymenoptera sting, as the stinging apparatus is a modified ovipositor. Acid, alkaline, and poison secreting glands empty their contents into the stinger. Bee venom has been shown to contain histamine, a histamine releaser which produces decarboxylation of histadine, hyaluronidase, phospholipase, and mellitin. Wasp venom contains histamine, serotonin, several kinins, and hyaluronidase. Hornet venom has very large amounts of acetyl choline in addition to histamine, serotonin and kinins. When an individual has received multiple stings, toxic reactions of varying severity to these chemicals may occur.

Yellow jackets, wasps, and hornets use their stingers to paralyze or kill insects to provide food for their larvae. The bee feeds its larva honey and pollen and stings only to protect itself or its hive. Wasp, hornet and yellow jacket stings are frequently infected by bacteria, but bee stings are seldom infected. Of the hymenoptera, only the honeybee has a barbed stinger which it is unable to withdraw from its prey. As the bee attempts to withdraw her stinger, a portion of the abdomen and the venom sac are left behind and the bee dies.

CLINICAL PICTURE

Pain and swelling at the sting site are a normal response. Local, non-allergic reactions can be quite severe.

The reactions which are allergic may be either local or systemic. The latter is anaphylaxis in man. Generalized pruritus, urticaria, or both following the sting are the most common symptoms. In decreasing order of frequency are dyspnea, weakness, feelings of anxiety, nausea, abdominal cramps, and loss of consciousness.[3] These symptoms are generally present within fifteen minutes of the sting, and almost always within 1 hour. Serum sickness reactions occurring 1 to 2 weeks after a hymenoptera sting occur occasionally. The symptoms are similar to those of serum sickness due to other causes, and include fever, arthralgia, urticaria, angioedema and lymphadenopathy. Untreated, these symptoms may persist for weeks. The nephrotic syndrome and Schöenlein-Henoch purpura have also been reported.

Certain factors appear to predispose people to allergic responses to insect stings. A statistical study conducted by the Insect Allergy Committee of the American Academy of Allergy provided the information that (1) severe reactions are more likely to occur in persons over 30 years of age; (2) August is the month in which the greatest number of reactions occur; (3) a personal history of atopy was present in only 27 percent of patients reporting reactions, and in only 19 percent of patients having severe reactions. An additional 30 percent of the patients came from families with positive histories of allergy.[2]

A group of 400 patients with histories of severe insect sting reactions was reviewed by Brown.[3] Forty one percent had a history of urticaria, or food or pollen sensitivities. Forty percent of Brown's group reported large local reactions after previous stings. Some of these patients were unable to recall ever having been stung previously.

Schwartz and Kahn evaluated 44 patients after systemic reactions to insect stings, and 11 patients who had had very large local reactions.[4] The patients were studied by scratch and intradermal testing to common inhalant and food allergens. Thirty four percent of the patients who had had systemic reactions and 36 percent of those who had experienced local reactions had no positive skin tests to these allergens.

It appears from the above studies that no good correlation exists between insect sting anaphylaxis and atopy.

IMMUNOLOGY

Foubert and Stier, using ground whole bodies of bees, wasps, yellow jackets and hornets, did double diffusion gel studies with animal antisera.[5] They found that extracts of each of the insects produced 4 to 6 precipitin bands. Two of these bands appeared to be common to all of the groups. The antigens of some of the remaining fractions were shared by honeybees and wasps.

Langlois, Shulman and Arbesman used hemagglutination and passive transfer skin testing in the study of sera collected from patients who had had immediate type hypersensitivity reactions to insect stings, using as antigens venom sacs, sacless whole body extracts, and whole body extracts of bees, wasps, and yellow jackets.[6] They demonstrated antigens common to venom sacs and sacless whole bodies plus one or two antigens specific to venom sacs. They were unable to demonstrate crossreactivity between bees and yellow jackets by gel diffusion or hemagglutination but found one common antigen to whole body extracts by immunoelectrophoresis. The same was true of crossreactivity between bees and wasps. Two common antigens were demonstrated between wasps and yellow jackets: one, a whole body antigen and one, a venom sac antigen.

Passive transfer studies were also done, using sera from patients with strongly positive skin test reactions to more than one type of hymenoptera. The skin sensitizing antibodies were readily transferable. When a test site was exhausted by daily injections of small amounts of yellow jacket extract, it still responded on challenge to bee and wasp antigens; sites exhausted with bee antigens still reacted to wasp and yellow jacket extracts; sites neutralized with wasp antigens continued to react to bee and yellow jacket extracts. No differences in results were observed if the extracts used were made from whole insects, sacless insects or venom sacs alone.

In summary, present knowledge indicates that both laboratory animals and humans who are sensitive to hymenoptera have in their sera both species specific antibodies and antibodies which react with antigens from more than one hymenoptera species.

TREATMENT

For the acute reaction in the patient with dyspnea, angioedema, altered consciousness or shock, the treatment is that for anaphylactic shock. Epinephrine is given subcutaneously at once and repeated every 15 to 30 minutes until the blood pressure is stabilized and the bronchospasm is relieved. In addition parenteral antihistamines such as diphenhydramine or chlorpheniramine can be given. Ice applied to the sting will slow absorption of antigen, and if the sting is on an extremity, a tourniquet applied proximal to it will also serve to slow absorption of antigen.

If a honey bee stinger is left in the skin it should not be squeezed by fingers or forceps in an attempt to remove it, as this will force any venom remaining in the venom sac into the sting site. The stinger should be carefully flicked away with the fingernail with the least possible amount of pressure on the sac.

The patient generally responds rapidly to emergency therapy. Failure to do so may require further intensive care in a hospital. A more extensive discussion of the treatment of anaphylaxis may be found in Chapter 12.

Urticaria or angioedema which persist beyond the acute period should be treated with oral antihistamines and ephedrine in therapeutic doses as long as they are needed. Reactions of the serum sickness type are also treated with antihistamines and ephedrine. Adrenal corticosteroids are used when these drugs are not adequate for control.

PROPHYLAXIS

Immunotherapy

Hyposensitization should be initiated in patients who have had systemic reactions to insect stings. The statistical study of the American Academy of Allergy [2] revealed that 90 percent of patients restung while receiving immunotherapy had less severe reactions, while fewer than 9 percent of untreated persons reported less severe reactions after being restung.

Skin testing is a useful procedure in determining the starting treatment doses of a program of immunotherapy. Testing should not be done within 2 weeks of a sting because this is frequently a period in which the skin is nonresponsive, due to exhaustion of the skin sensitizing antibodies by the sting reaction. The degree of skin sensitivity as determined by titration with dilutions of insect antigens does not correlate well with the degree of clinical sensitivity the patient has demonstrated.

Testing is done with the aqueous extracts of whole bodies of bees, wasps, hornets, and yellow jackets. Testing may be done for each insect separately, or a mixture such as would be used in treatment can be made from all four because of their overlapping antigenicity. The arms should be used as the testing site so that if a severe reaction to a test should occur, a tourniquet can be placed proximal to it. The initial skin test should be done by the prick or scratch method with a weight per volume (w/v) extract of 1:100 million. If after 20 minutes there is no skin response, the test is repeated at a site about 1 inch away from the first test using an extract of 1:10 million w/v concentration. If this test again produces no skin response it is probably safe to proceed with intradermal testing.

For this procedure 0.02 ml. of a 1:100 million w/v extract is injected intradermally and observed for 20 minutes. If this test is negative, the test is repeated with a tenfold increase in the concentration of the testing material. *Note that extreme caution must be used in this test procedure. Very severe systemic reactions can occur from hymenoptera skin testing and great care is truly warranted.* Erythema or wheal formation at a test site is considered the end point, and treatment is started several days later using an extract of one tenth the concentration which produced the skin response. Starting with 0.05 ml. of this extract subcutaneously, doses are given at weekly intervals doubling the amount of material with each injection until erythema lasting beyond the 20 minute observation period, or whealing, is produced at the injection site, or until a dose of 0.5 ml. of 1:100 extract is reached without reaction. This maximum tolerated dose is repeated weekly through the first summer, then once every 4 to 6 weeks. At the present time it is thought that indefinite treatment is the most appropriate choice, until further study provides a more definite answer to the duration required for complete safety from anaphylaxis.

Emergency Therapy

The individual who has had a systemic sting reaction should carry during the summer (a) a readily available form of epinephrine, such as a preloaded disposable syringe, (b) a capsule combining an antihistamine and ephedrine in a rapidly absorbed form (for example, Benadryl * with ephedrine, Parke-Davis); he should wear (c) a Medic-Alert tag around his neck identifying him as allergic to insect stings. There are insect sting emergency kits available on prescription † which contain the above drugs plus a tourniquet and an alcohol swab to clean the injection site. The patient should be shown how to give the injection and should give himself an injection of physiologic saline to demonstrate his competence to himself and to the physician. If the patient is a child, or if he is an individual who in the physician's judgment would not have the composure to give himself an injection in a stress situation, a pocket-sized pressure packed nebulizer of epinephrine (for example, Medihaler-Epi ‡) may be substituted for the syringe, and instructions given for its use. After taking emergency measures, the patient should then go to the nearest medical facility for observation. The patient with a history of insect sting allergy should be instructed on how to decrease the chances of exposure to stinging insects. This advice is summarized below.

---

* Trademark of Parke-Davis.
† Both Center Laboratories and Hollister-Stier Laboratories market such kits.
‡ Trademark of Riker Laboratories.

Advice on How to Limit Exposure to Hymenoptera Stings in Summertime

A. Wear shoes out of doors at all times.

B. Wear clothing of colors not attractive to bees: white, grey, red.

C. Wear garments that fit close to the body. Insects can become trapped in loose fitting clothing.

D. Avoid using scented soaps and cosmetics.

E. Stay away from insect feeding grounds: flower beds, fields of clover, garbage, and orchards with ripe fruit.

F. Keep automobile windows closed. Aside from the possibility of a sting, stinging insects in a car can arouse such terror in a sting sensitive driver as to make him an irresponsible driver.

G. If it is necessary to dispose of garbage, spray the area first with an effective, rapid-acting insecticide.

H. Wasp or hornet nests or bee hives noted in the vicinity of the patient's home should be destroyed by a professional exterminator.

REFERENCES

1. Brown, H.: Allergy to hymenoptera. Arch. Intern. Med., *125:*665, 1970.
2. Foubert, E. L., and Stier, R. A.: Antigenic relationship between honey bees, yellow hornets, black hornets, and yellow jackets. J. Allerg., *29:* 13, 1958.
3. Insect Allergy Committee of the American Academy of Allergy: Insect Sting Allergy. Questionaire Study of 2606 Cases. JAMA, *193:*115, 1965.
4. Langlois, C., Shulman, S., and Arbesman, C.: Allergic response to stinging insects. parts II and II. J. Allerg., *36:*12,   109, 1965.
5. Schwartz, H., and Kahn, B.: Hymenoptera sensitivity II. Role of atopy in the development of clinical hypersensitivity. J. Allerg., *45:*87, 1970.
6. Van Frisch, K.: Bees: Their Vision, Chemical Senses and Language. Cornell University Press, 1950.

FURTHER DETAILED READING

1. Frazier, C.: Insect Allergy. St. Louis, Warren H. Green, 1969.

12

Allergic Emergencies

Isaac Weiszer, M.D.

Allergic emergencies refer to allergic reactions of such severity that immediate treatment is required. The clinical picture is a manifestation of an immunologic reaction, in which an antigen-antibody reaction results in release of chemical mediators. These mediators produce the subsequent signs and symptoms.

There are three clinical situations which are allergic emergencies: anaphylaxis, laryngeal edema without other systemic manifestations and status asthmaticus. This chapter will deal with anaphylaxis in man. The term anaphylaxis is used to denote a generalized allergic reaction which is immunologically mediated.

The term anaphylaxis was first used by Porter and Richet in 1902, when they described anaphylactic shock in the dog.[14] Anaphylaxis is derived from the Greek and means "against (or removal from) protection." Richet observed that a foreign substance which was relatively harmless on the first injection could become severely toxic when reinjected in the same or smaller dose. It was also noted that an interval of several days was needed between the first and subsequent injections for this phenomenon to occur.

In the literature, the terms anaphylaxis and anaphylactoid reaction have been used to describe human systemic allergic reactions. Some have felt that the term anaphylaxis should be restricted to use in induced experimental immunologic reactions in animals. Others have said that anaphylaxis should not be used for human reactions unless there is hypotension. The term anaphylactoid is confusing because of the varying definitions given by different authors. We will use the term anaphylaxis as defined earlier: to describe human systemic allergic reactions which are immunologically mediated.

The most characteristic feature of anaphylaxis is its rapid onset after the administration of antigen and its rapid progression to severe and sometimes fatal outcome. In human anaphylaxis, early signs and symptoms indicate the onset of the reaction and immediate treatment may prevent the progression of the clinical state. In some instances, however, shock occurs without the warning signs and death may result.

The advent of modern drugs and diagnostic agents has resulted in an increased incidence of these reactions. Because the responsible agents are often used by physicians in diagnosis and treatment, an awareness of the problem and preventive measures is important.

Certain factors seem to be associated with an increased incidence of human anaphylaxis: (1) The nature of the antigen. Certain of these are more frequently the cause of a systemic reaction. (2) A history of atopy in the patient or the family is associated with an increased incidence of anaphylaxis to penicillin. (3) Anaphylaxis occurs more often following parenteral administration of a drug than after oral ingestion.

ETIOLOGY

Many antigens have been reported to cause anaphylaxis in man. These can be classified as complete antigens, or haptens. The complete antigens are mainly protein, but occasionally polysaccharide in nature. Table 12-1 lists the most common causes of human anaphylaxis.

Penicillin

Allergic reactions of any sort to penicillin occur only in about 1 percent of patients so treated. The chance of an acute, explosive reaction is between 1 and 4 in 10,000. The risk of a fatal reaction is not more than 2 in 100,000 treated cases. Idsoe and colleagues analyzed 151 penicillin deaths reported in the literature from 1951 to 1965. In 38 cases there was a history of a previous reaction, and in an additional 74 the history was unknown. A high proportion of those who died after receiving penicillin had a history of other allergic problems, particularly asthma.[16]

Parenteral administration remains the mode most likely to induce anaphylaxis. Reactions have occurred after oral administration, inhalation and skin testing. Immunologic evidence indicates that there are varying degrees of cross-reactivity among the various penicillins. It is safer to presume that patients with a history of allergy to penicillin G are also allergic to other penicillins both natural and synthetic. Recent reports suggest cross-reactivity with cephalothin.

Heterologous Antiserum

Prior to the advent of penicillin, horse serum was the most common cause of anaphylaxis. In the previously sensitized patient, a clinical picture of anaphylaxis may result after administration of horse serum or other heterologous antiserum.

TABLE 12-1
Some Materials Which have Caused Anaphylaxis in Man *

Proteins	Polysaccharides	Haptens
Heterologous serum	Dextran	Salicylates

Hormones
  ACTH
  Insulin
	Iron dextran
	  preparations
		Sodium dehydrocholate
		  (decholin)
		Sulfobromophthalein (BSP)

Enzymes
  Chymopapain
  Chymotrypsin
  Penicillinase
  L-asparaginase
		Procaine
		Penicillin and synthetic peni-
		  cillin analogues
		Aminopyrine

Pollen extracts		Iodinated contrast media
Venom of stinging insects		Demethylchlortetracycline (Declomycin)

Foods (by skin test)
  Buckwheat
  Eggwhite
  Cotton seed
		Nitrofurantoin
		Streptomycin
		Sodium cephalothin (Keflin)

Foods (by ingestion)
  Egg
  Milk
  Potato
  Rice
  Legumes (soybeans, pinto
    beans, chick-peas)
  Citrus fruits (orange,
    tangerine)
  Nuts (Brazil, pistachio,
    cashew)		

* Adapted from Austen.[1]

Insect Stings

Insect sting hypersensitivity is an important and increasingly recognized cause of severe, and sometimes fatal, human anaphylaxis. The four common stinging insects (bee, wasp, hornet, yellow jacket) account for most of these reactions, and there is antigenic cross-reactivity.

Previous sting is obviously necessary for sensitization, but a severe systemic allergic reaction may occur without any previous reaction, either local or systemic. The clinical picture is usually the same here as in anaphylaxis due to other causes. Barnard has reported occasional systemic, even fatal, reactions occurring three days after an insect sting.[2] Continued vigilance is needed in the high risk patient after insect sting.

Food

Certain foods cause anaphylaxis in man and the sequence of events usually makes the diagnosis easy.[7] Occasionally, anaphylaxis follows the ingestion of a food, but neither patient nor physician suspects the ingested antigen. Eggs, nuts, beans, seafood and milk are foods reported to cause systemic allergic reactions (see Table 12-1). The degree of sensitivity may be so extreme that skin testing may result in a systemic reaction. Cooking or other processes involved in preparing a food may alter the antigenicity sufficiently to prevent a reaction.

Injection of Allergic Extracts

Allergy injection therapy consists of subcutaneous injections of gradually increasing doses of inhalant antigens to which the patient is clinically sensitive. The risk of a systemic reaction is always present, and this risk increases with high dosage, high titer of skin sensitizing antibody, simultaneous presence of the allergen in the patient's environment and inadvertent vascular introduction of the antigen.

Rupture of Hydatid Cyst

Massive release of antigen in a sensitized host causes the anaphylactic reaction seen in puncture or spontaneous rupture of a hydatid cyst, caused by the tapeworm *Echinococcus granulosus.* Symptoms may include erythema, pruritus, urticaria, fever, cyanosis, dyspnea, abdominal pain, vomiting, diarrhea and syncope.

Physical Allergy

Physical allergy, such as cold urticaria, may result in a clinical picture resembling anaphylaxis possibly due to massive histamine release. When such a cold-sensitive patient is suddenly immersed in cold water symptoms of faintness, syncope and urticaria may result.

Hereditary Angioneurotic Edema

The patient with hereditary angioneurotic edema may present with laryngeal edema as a life threatening occurrence.

Gamma Globulin Therapy

When gamma globulin is given intravenously, there are a number of individuals who will have systemic reactions, some of which resemble anaphylaxis. Similar reactions may also occur with intramuscular administration. The mechanism may be immunologic or nonimmunologic.[5]

CLINICAL MANIFESTATIONS

The manifestations of anaphylaxis vary depending upon the animal species and the route of administration. The guinea pig usually has acute respiratory obstruction; the rat exhibits circulatory collapse with increased peristalsis; the rabbit shows acute pulmonary hypertension; and the dog typically exhibits circulatory collapse.

In man the clinical manifestations of systemic anaphylaxis vary in kind and degree, resembling those seen in many of the other animals. Typically, the four organ systems involved are the skin, respiratory tract, gastrointestinal tract and the cardiovascular system. Skin manifestations include diffuse erythema, urticaria, pruritus and angiodema. Respiratory distress results from bronchospasm or edema of the upper airways. Vomiting, abdominal cramps and diarrhea are the usual gastrointestinal signs. Vascular collapse, secondary to respiratory failure, or as a primary phenomenon may occur as the reaction becomes more severe.

The severity of the reaction may vary from one that is mild to immediate collapse and death. In general, the sooner the symptoms begin after antigen administration, the more severe the symptoms. Severe reactions may occur within seconds of injection of antigen and usually they appear within 30 to 45 minutes. Reactions following ingestion of antigen may be rapid and explosive, but more commonly they are less severe and the onset may take longer. Inhaling the antigen may cause systemic reactions in highly susceptible persons. Skin testing, usually of the intradermal type, has resulted in systemic reactions with pollen, penicillin and food antigens.

Some early manifestations of anaphylaxis include a feeling of uneasiness or apprehension, weakness, sweating, sneezing or nasal pruritus, generalized pruritus, urticaria and angioedema. Dyspnea, wheezing, dysphagia, vomiting, abdominal pain, syncope or shock may follow rapidly. There may be urgency of urination, fecal and urinary incontinence, convulsions and coma.

The pulse may be rapid, weak, irregular or unobtainable. Hypotension is usually present if the reaction progresses. Cardiovascular manifestations may suggest a primary cardiac event, and, indeed, a serious arrhythmia or a myocardial infarction may occur in an anaphylactic reaction. Electrocardiographic changes during human anaphylaxis may consist of flattening and inversion of T waves, ST segment elevation or depression and arrhythmia (nodal rhythm, atrial fibrillation). In a recent series, it was felt that some of these changes were primary, occurring in healthy persons without preexisting heart disease and not due to therapy initiated for the anaphylaxis.[4]

Signs of laryngeal edema consist of dyspnea, hoarseness, stridor or dysphagia. Bronchospasm results in wheezing, a sensation of tightness in the chest, and cough. If bronchospasm is severe, there may be no breath sounds by auscultation. Respiratory failure may follow, with cyanosis, hypotension and death. Loss of consciousness or hypotension may occur without respiratory distress. It is extremely important to recognize mild and early manifestations of anaphylaxis and to institute appropriate therapy.

PATHOPHYSIOLOGY

Immunologic Mechanism

The anaphylactic reaction in man is presumed to result from a specific immunologic interaction of antigen with an antibody known as skin-sensitizing antibody or reagin which in man is almost always (perhaps always) IgE. This interaction results in the release of chemical mediators which act on secondary sites such as smooth muscle and vascular tissue.

The chemical mediators of anaphylactic tissue injury known to be specifically formed or released from mammalian tissue by antigen-antibody interaction include histamine, serotonin, bradykinin and slow reacting substance of anaphylaxis (SRS-A).[3] Each mediator can cause contraction of a particular group of smooth muscles and can increase vascular permeability.

Histamine is stored in mast cells, basophils and possibly in other cells. It has been shown to be released in vitro from human lung and is thought to cause increased vascular permeability and bronchoconstriction. Experiments with chemical histamine releasers in normal people show that endogenous histamine causes erythema, angioneurotic edema, a reduction in blood pressure, and a feeling of retrosternal oppression. In this experimental situation, pretreatment with antihistamine prevented the symptoms.

SRS-A is elaborated in large amounts when human lung tissue, obtained from patients with extrinsic asthma, is exposed in vitro to a specific pollen antigen. SRS-A also profoundly constricts the isolated human bronchiole in the presence of specific pharmacologic antagonists of histamine and serotonin. Bradykinin is known to be a powerful vasodilator. It has not been isolated in human tissue, but has been found in rabbit anaphylaxis. Serotonin is not thought to play a part in human anaphylaxis.

On the basis of minimal experimental data in man, it is possible to speculate that the pattern of laryngeal edema is mediated by histamine, the intractable bronchospasm by SRS-A and primary vascular collapse by brandykinin.

The antibody in human anaphylaxis appears to be primarily IgE. It is possible that other immunoglobulins, such as some subclasses of IgG, may mediate human anaphylaxis in some cases. In serum sickness and insect allergy, IgG is present in the sera of patients. Its role in human anaphylaxis is not clear. A nonimmunologic mechanism may account for the clinical picture suggestive of anaphylaxis in certain cases of reactions to insects. Reactions after ingestion of aspirin, injection of contrast media, dextran and gamma globulin may not be mediated by specific antibodies against these agents.

Physiologic Changes

The hypotension seen in human anaphylaxis may result from one or a combination of physiologic changes. Release of chemical mediators increases vascular permeability. Cardiac dysfunction may occur as a primary event or secondary to anoxia. There may also be a reduction in effective plasma volume.

A metabolic and hemodynamic study of two patients in anaphylactic shock showed that a critical reduction in plasma volume was primarily responsible for shock.[8] Hemoconcentration, a decrease in cardiac output, a reduction in peripheral blood flow and an increase in arterial vasoconstriction were documented. In both cases, there was evidence of acute myocardial and hepatocellular injury. The hemodynamic and metabolic defects were effectively reversed by the administration of large volumes of fluid.

Pathologic Findings

The pathologic findings in animal studies reflect the variable clinical picture of anaphylaxis in different species, the variation in organs primarily involved and possible difference in antibodies and mediators. Complete clinical and autopsy study was reported by James and Austen in six cases of fatal anaphylaxis in man. Antigens were penicillin (three cases), guinea pig hemoglobin, bee venom and a ragweed extract. All had been given subcutaneously or intramuscularly. Death occurred from 16 to 120 minutes after antigen challenge. The predominant abnormalities in five patients were in the respiratory system. Four of them had obstructing edema of the upper respiratory tract and three also demonstrated gross acute pulmonary emphysema, presumably due to outflow obstruction in the lower respiratory tract. The sixth case differed from the rest in that chest pain and shock without obvious respiratory distress predominated clinically. The post mortem examination did not reveal the mechanism of death. Barnard has reviewed pathologic findings in 50 insect sting fatalities [2]; 35 patients showed angiodema of the upper respiratory tract.

Differential Diagnosis

The differential diagnosis of human anaphylaxis is ordinarily not difficult because of the rapid onset of symptoms after antigen exposure. However, when the patient comes to the emergency room in shock, anaphylaxis should be considered in the differential diagnosis. A history of recent insect sting, administration of a drug or ingestion of a food would suggest a systemic allergic reaction. Accompanying signs of skin manifestations, laryngeal edema or asthma would suggest anaphylaxis. Anaphylaxis should be considered in a child or a young adult presenting with sudden vascular collapse, whereas in an older patient other factors become relatively more important. It is obvious that immediate supportive therapy must be initiated in such a patient, but treatment will be more rational if the correct diagnosis is made.

TREATMENT

A systemic allergic reaction requires immediate treatment. Epinephrine is the most important single agent in the treatment of anaphylaxis. It is a pharmacologic antagonist of the action of chemical mediators on smooth muscle and other effector cells.

First, 0.3 to 0.5 ml. of 1:1,000 aqueous epinephrine is injected intramuscularly into the upper arm and the area massaged. If possible, a tourniquet is applied above the site of antigen injection (such as allergy injection, penicillin administration or insect sting in an extremity) and 0.3 ml. of 1:1,000 aqueous epinephrine is injected into the site of the previous antigen injection. The last two steps will result in a reduction in the systemic absorption of the antigen.

The three steps mentioned above are often sufficient to stop a systemic reaction in its early stages. The aqueous epinephrine can be repeated every 15 minutes as needed. The tourniquet should be removed when the reaction seems to be under control or temporarily every 10 to 15 minutes and then discontinued. After the initial steps have been taken, a careful and continuing clinical appraisal is made. The pulse, blood pressure and state of respiration are monitored. The development of hypotension, whether on a cardiac basis or due to peripheral collapse, is an ominous sign. The development of respiratory distress, due either to bronchospasm or laryngeal edema or both, must be looked for.

If the reaction is not reversed rapidly by epinephrine, the use of an antihistamine intravenously should be considered next. Diphenhydramine chloride (50 to 75 mg. for an adult) intravenously over a 3 minute period may help prevent development of laryngeal edema and block the systemic effects of histamine released during anaphylaxis. For milder reactions, an oral antihistamine may be given as an adjunct. Epinephrine remains the drug of first choice, and the antihistamine should not be substituted for it.

If the reaction is accompanied by severe bronchospasm and shock is not present, intravenous aminophylline may be given to patients not responding to epinephrine; 250 to 500 mg. of aminophylline may be given slowly over a 10 minute period. Rapid infusion may cause severe hypotension.

If signs of upper airway obstruction develop (stridor, feeling of tightness in the throat), endotracheal intubation and/or tracheostomy may be essential, with oxygen administration. An adequate airway must be maintained while waiting for drugs to help.

Hypotension with signs of vasomotor collapse requires intravenous fluids with levarterenol bitartrate (Levophed) and metaraminol (Aramine). Measurements of the blood pressure and urinary output can be used as an index of response.

If there is no response to therapy, determination of the central venous pressure (CVP) becomes essential for further therapy. A low or normal initial CVP (0 to 12 cm. H_2O) suggests an ineffective plasma volume, and replacement of fluids may be lifesaving.[6] If the initial CVP is elevated (> 12 cm.), the primary cause of hypotension may well be due to myocardial insufficiency. Intravenous isoproterenol is the drug of choice in this situation. One milligram of isoproterenol is diluted in 500 ml. of 5 percent dextrose and infused at a rate of 1 to 2 μg. per minute.

TABLE 12-2
Treatment of Systemic Anaphylaxis

MANDATORY AND IMMEDIATE

1. Aqueous epinephrine, 1:1000, 0.3 to 0.5 ml. IM; may repeat in 15 minutes
2. Tourniquet above injection site
3. Local infiltration of aqueous epinephrine, 1:1000, 0.3 ml. at injection site of antigen

AFTER CLINICAL AND INDIVIDUAL APPRAISAL

1. Diphenhydramine, 50 mg., IV
2. Bronchospasm: aqueous epinephrine, aminophylline IV, intravenous fluids, corticosteroids
3. Hypotension: vasopressors, volume repletion, isoproterenol, corticosteroids
4. Laryngeal obstruction: tracheostomy and O_2
5. Cardiac arrest: cardiopulmonary resuscitation, $NaHCO_3$, further therapy dependent on ECG

Isoproterenol may induce cardiac arrhythmias and hypotension due to peripheral vasodilatation.

In case of cardiac arrest, cardiopulmonary resuscitation should be immediately undertaken. This would include external cardiac massage, assisted ventilation, use of sodium bicarbonate and further therapy depending on the electrocardiographic findings.

Corticosteroids may be useful agents for latter events in human anaphylaxis but do not help in the early stages because they take hours to take effect. Their mechanism of action is that of nonspecific anti-inflammatory agents. Because they may help, they should be given intravenously in severe reactions (e.g., hydrocortisone 100 mg. immediately or 300 mg. over 24 hours). They may help with asthma, laryngeal edema and hypotension. They may be especially worthwhile for the occasional prolonged reaction. Steroids should not be used first in treatment of human anaphylaxis, not because they are harmful but because they should not replace epinephrine as the drug of choice. Table 12-2 summarizes the treatment of anaphylaxis.

PREVENTION

Avoidance of Known Antigen

As in all treatment of allergic symptoms, avoidance of a known antigen is the single most useful prophylactic measure. Avoidance of a known food antigen is fairly easy. General measures can help avoid stinging insects. Avoidance of a drug antigen depends on a detailed history elicited from the patient by the physician.

History

Has the patient ever had the drug before? If so, has he experienced any allergic reaction to it? Here it is important to obtain a description of the reaction so as to ascertain whether it was an allergic manifestation or a side effect of the drug. Does the patient have a personal or family history of atopy? Severe anaphylactic drug reactions occur more frequently in atopic than in nonatopic patients.

When the history clearly suggests hypersensitivity, the agent or an antigenically related agent should not be used. In the rare situation where proper medical therapy demands use of a particular agent, "desensitization" may be attempted with great caution. This will be discussed later in this chapter.

Skin Testing

When the history of a previous allergic reaction is doubtful or if a substance is to be used which is known to be associated with anaphylaxis, particularly in an atopic patient, skin testing is useful only in limited instances. Skin testing must always be carried out with the customary precautions for all skin testing. Scratch tests should be done first, followed by intradermal tests, or, if initial intradermal tests are desirable the test antigen should be sufficiently diluted. Tests should begin with dilute solutions in either case. In addition, the physician should be ready to treat any systemic reaction.

Skin and conjunctival testing with heterologous serum has been done for a long time and may still be needed for therapy of snake bite, clostridial infections and use of antilymphocyte serum in organ transplantation. All patients, regardless of history, should be tested for cutaneous and conjunctival sensitivity prior to administration of serum. A scratch test should be performed first using the antitoxin or normal horse serum. If it is negative, testing may proceed with an intradermal test using 0.02 ml. of 1:100 dilution of the serum. If this is negative, 0.02 ml. of 1:10 dilution can then be used intradermally. When skin testing is questionable, conjunctival testing may be done using a 1:10 dilution. These dilutions may be used in the presence of a negative history. More dilute solutions should be used if the history is suspect for a previous reaction or if the patient shows atopic symptoms on exposure to horses. "Desensitization" may be necessary in the presence of a history of previous anaphylaxis.

Positive results of testing with penicilloyl-polylysine and the minor determinant mixture (MDM) of penicillin is predictive of an anaphylactic reaction. A negative test with the MDM generally predicts that anaphylaxis will not occur.[11] The proper antigens for penicillin are not yet commercially available, and there are problems involved in testing prior to penicillin injection. A patient who has a negative test for a particular drug may yet experience a reaction after administration of the drug. There is some danger of anaphylaxis after the skin test and even the scratch test.

Skin testing is also useful for protein antigens such as insulin and ACTH. Rarely, true allergic reactions occur after local anesthetic. A positive skin test is a helpful warning but it should be remembered that a negative reaction does not rule out the possibility of a systemic reaction.

Skin testing is not useful in determining sensitivity to most other drugs. Tests using iodinated contrast media are probably unreliable because many of these are histamine releasers. In addition, the reactions they produce may not be on an immunologic basis. Reactions after codeine and morphine may be the result of nonspecific histamine release. In vitro tests of drug allergy are not yet sufficiently clinically predictive to be generally useful.

General Rules to Lessen Incidence of Anaphylaxis

When a drug is to be administered, a definite medical indication should exist. If possible, the drug should be given orally instead of parenterally so as to decrease the likelihood of a severe reaction. A different drug should be substituted if a history of sensitivity exists.

After an injection of an allergy extract has been given in an extremity, the patient should be asked to wait in the physician's office for 15 to 20 minutes. Allergy injection therapy must be given in the presence of a physician, in case a systemic reaction develops. The patient must be made aware of the potential hazards of allergy injection treatment so that he will accept proper medical supervision in an intelligent manner.

Patients known to be sensitive to horse serum should maintain regular tetanus immunizations. Such a patient can now be given human tetanus antitoxin if necessary, thus avoiding the danger of horse serum. There are still clinical situations (snake bite for instance) where horse serum may be needed (see p. 328). Skin testing and "desensitization" are discussed elsewhere in this chapter.

The patient with systemic insect sting hypersensitivity can be immunized in the same way as the patient with hay fever or asthma. The current recommendation is that injection therapy be continued on a maintenance level for an indefinite period (see Chap. 11).

The patient's medical record should clearly show the presence of a history of anaphylaxis or other allergic reaction to an agent. The patient should carry on him at all times a statement to this effect, either on a necklace, bracelet or a card in his wallet.

"Desensitization"

"Desensitization" has been described with horse serum and penicillin.[13] Presumably it represents neutralization of antibodies without sufficient release of mediators to give a systemic reaction. This is accomplished by gradual increase in dosage of antigen.

"Desensitization" consists of scratch, then intradermal, then subcutaneous administration of gradually increasing doses of antigen every 15 to 20 minutes. The patient should have an intravenous infusion in place, with adrenalin, diphenhydramine chloride, vasopressors, steroids and oxygen available. Symptoms of a reaction should be treated, if mild, and the procedure continued very carefully. Disappearance of reaginic antibody against penicillin has been described with penicillin desensitization, together with disappearance of clinical sensitivity. However, a few months later, both clinical and skin test sensitivity had returned. It must be stressed that the clinical situation which demands this dangerous course of action is extremely rare and that the grave risks must be weighed against the potential benefits.

EMERGENCY DRUGS AVAILABLE TO THE PATIENT

The patient with a history of certain severe allergic reactions should have drugs needed to treat anaphylaxis available at all times. This should be done with insect sensitive patients and may be done in the rare cases where the antigen has not yet been identified.

The patient should have a tourniquet, an oral antihistamine such as diphenhydramine chloride and an injectable epinephrine. The availability of epinephrine in a prefilled syringe* makes this the drug of choice.

Emergency Materials Available to the Patient with a History of Anaphylaxis

1. Injectable epinephrine
   (as a substitute of second choice, epinephrine by inhalation)
2. Oral antihistamine
3. Tourniquet

As a substitute of second choice for the injectable epinephrine, epinephrine by inhalation may be provided. Recent work has shown less urinary excretion of inhaled epinephrine than of that administered parenterally.[9] It remains to be seen if this correlates with lower clinical effectiveness. For potential laryngeal edema, the local effect of the epinephrine spray may be useful. Isoproterenol given sublingually was used for many years, but the possible effect on blood pressure due to its peripheral action has raised some question concerning its use in cases in which hypotension might occur.

REFERENCES

1. Austen, K. F.: Systemic anaphylaxis in man. JAMA, *192*:108, 1965.
2. Barnard, J. H.: Allergic and pathologic findings in fifty insect-sting fatalities. J. Allerg., *40*:107, 1967.
3. Becker, E. L., and Austen, K. F.: Anaphylaxis. *In* Miescher, P. A.: Textbook of Immunopathology. vol. 1. New York, Grune and Stratton, 1968.
4. Booth, B. H., and Patterson, R.: Electrocardiographic changes during human anaphylaxis. JAMA, *211*:627, 1970.
5. Ellis, E. F., and Henney, C. S.: Adverse reactions following administration of human gamma globulin. J. Allerg., *43*:45, 1969.

* EPI-SIX, Center Laboratories.

6. Falleroni, A. E.: Treatment of allergic emergencies. Mod. Treat., 5:782, 1968.
7. Golbert, T. M., Patterson, R., and Pruzansky, J. J.: Systemic allergic reactions to ingested antigens. J. Allerg., 44:96, 1969.
8. Hanashiro, P. K., and Weil, M. H.: Anaphylactic shock in man. Arch. Intern. Med., 119:129, 1967.
9. Hoehne, J. H., Lockey, S. D., and Chosy, J. J.: Comparison of epinephrine excretion after aerosol and subcutaneous administration. J. Allerg., 46:336, 1970.
10. James, L. P., and Austen, K. F.: Fatal systemic anaphylaxis in man. New Eng. J. Med., 270:597, 1964.
11. Levine, B. B., Redmond, A. P., Voss, H. E., and Zolov, D. M.: Prediction of penicillin allergy by immunologic tests. Ann. N.Y. Acad. Sci., 145:298, 1967.
12. Patterson, R.: Allergic emergencies. JAMA, 172:303, 1960.
13. Reisman, R. E., Rose, N. R., Witebsky, E., and Arbesman, C. E.: Penicillin allergy and desensitization. J. Allerg., 33:178, 1962.
14. Richet, C.: Anaphylaxis. London, The University Press, Constable & Co., 1913.
15. Shehadi, W.: Clinical problems and toxicity of contrast agents. Amer. J. Roentgen., 97:762, 1966.
16. Van Arsdel, P. P.: The risk of penicillin reactions. Ann. Intern. Med., 69:1071, 1968.

13

Urticaria and Physical Allergy

Jordan N. Fink, M.D.

Although urticaria, or hives, and angio-edema may be fatal, they are usually self-limiting often occurring as a single episode and, thus, are not brought to a physician's attention. Acute urticaria may last up to 1 or 2 weeks. When the lesions persist for more than 3 weeks, the disorder is considered chronic. This type of urticaria may lead to morbidity and emotional distress, and patients with such recurrent episodes most often seek medical aid.

Urticarial lesions have been known since the time of Hippocrates. The term is thought to have been derived from the name of the common nettle plant *Urtica ureus,* which causes a rash when brushed. In Europe, urticaria and angio-edema are often called Quincke's edema, after the physician who described the disorder in 1882.

The incidence of urticaria in the general population is difficult to determine, but episodes have probably occurred at one time or another in up to 20 percent. Urticaria is more common in atopic individuals. Acute urticaria occurs frequently in young adults of either sex, while the chronic persistent form is more common in middle-aged women.

PATHOPHYSIOLOGY

The lesions of urticaria present as papular wheals surrounded by an erythematous base. Histologically there is dilatation of the superficial cutaneous blood vessels and lymphatics with edema and some eosinophilic infiltration of the surrounding area. Angio-edema may be associated with hives, but usually presents with more diffuse and deep seated swelling of the eyelids, lips, hands and feet and may involve the tongue, larynx, central nervous system, and gastrointestinal tract. The histologic appearance of angio-edema is similar to urticaria except that the deeper layers of the skin are involved; therefore, the edema tends to be more diffuse.

Certain evidence suggests that histamine released from mast cells and basophils plays the major role in the genesis of urticaria, although pharmacologic mediators such as the kinins may be important. Lesions of this type may be reproduced by the injection of histamine or histamine liberators such as morphine, codeine, meperidine and polymyxin B. Skin biopsies of urticarial lesions have demonstrated reduced amounts of histamine, as well as diminution in the number of basophils and tissue mast cells. Finally, hives often respond to moderate doses of antihistamines, suggesting a causal relationship of histamine to the lesions.

Although acute urticaria may be associated with the immunologic mechanism of the immediate type of hypersensitivity involving an IgE-antigen mediated reaction, the pathogenesis of chronic urticaria is often not clear and may be due to other immunologic or even nonimmunologic means. Therefore, it is important that in an investigation of the cause of a patient's urticaria or angio-edema, the physician must consider a variety of mechanisms which may result in the genesis of the lesions.

DIAGNOSIS

Urticaria can be diagnosed by the appearance of papular lesions surrounded by an erythematous flare, and fleeting in nature. They may be widespread or localized and tend to coalesce. Itching may be severe and is often associated with burning or tingling.

Angio-edema may occur alone or along with urticarial lesions. The swelling is nonpitting and may occur almost anywhere; most often it is found over the face. Pruritus is not as prominent as in urticaria, but burning or tingling of the skin is often present. Angio-edema may persist longer than urticaria, and when laryngeal involvement occurs, asphyxia and death may result.

Other conditions should be considered when entertaining the diagnosis of urticaria and angio-edema. *Urticaria pigmentosa,* found in systemic mastocytosis, consists of persistent tan pigmented macules and papules as well as transitory urticaria, which appears when the macules are stroked. The lesions are apparently due to histamine release from mast cells in the skin. *Erythema multiforme* may occur in a variety of underlying diseases and may resemble urticaria. Lesions seen in *serum sickness* may be identical to urticaria or angio-edema but are thought to be due to an IgG-antigen rather than an IgE-antigen mechanism. Angio-edema may be confused with any of the following: (1) the *superior vena cava syndrome,* due to mediastinal compression; (2) periorbital edema seen in *trichinosis;* (3) anasarca of *congestive heart failure* or *nephrotic syndrome;* or (4) the local lymphedema of *elephantiasis.*

Cholinergic urticaria is characterized by tiny blanched wheals surrounded by a narrow erythematous flare background. If the flares are confluent, the patient may appear to have a flush. The lesions occur after exposure to heat, or during emotional distress or exercise and are probably nonimmunologic in origin. It is thought that acetylcholine released from nerve endings results in the observed lesions. Often the particular type of hives may be reproduced in these patients by the intradermal injection of 1:5000 acetylcholine.

Dermographism, which is a wheal and flare reaction seen after stroking of the skin, develops in 5 to 20 percent of the population, depending on the degree of pressure applied in the stroke. It does not appear to be related to the atopic status of the patient but often accompanies chronic urticaria. The lesions usually occur under tight clothing, and scratching them increases their number.

ETIOLOGIC DIAGNOSIS AND TREATMENT

Successful therapy of urticaria is based on the demonstration and subsequent avoidance of the causative factor, if such a factor can be found. A systematic elimination and reintroduction of suspected antigens or events is necessary for establishment of the etiologic diagnosis and results in the most effective therapy. Once the offending agent has been eliminated, the urticaria will usually disappear within a few days. Lesions resulting from drug reactions such as penicillin, however, may persist much longer.

TABLE 13-1
Causes of Urticaria

	ACUTE (self-limiting)	CHRONIC (lasting over 3 weeks)
Drugs	+	+
Foods	+	+
Infection	+	+
Infestation	+	+
Inhalants	+	+
Insect bites	+	+
Connective tissue diseases	+	+
Neoplasia	−	+
Psychic factors	?	+
Light	+	+
Cold	+	+
Cholinergic	+	+

An etiologic diagnosis is made more often in acute urticaria, while the causative agent in chronic urticaria is usually not uncovered. This difficulty should not deter the physician from undertaking a thorough search for the cause of chronic urticaria. The annoyance of the recurring lesions and the risks of emotional distress and chronicity of illness certainly justify a thorough evaluation.

The offending agent must be uncovered in order to treat the patient by avoidance. This may be accomplished by serially eliminating and reintroducing suspected agents into the patient's environment. The causative agent may thus be uncovered when relief is induced by its elimination and urticaria returns by its addition. Therefore, the diagnosis and treatment of these lesions are interconnected and will be discussed together.

Drug Induced Urticaria

Drugs are the most common causes of allergic reactions resulting in urticaria and must be considered in every case of urticaria or angioedema. *Any* drug may cause a reaction, and, in order to discover what drugs a patient is taking, a careful and exacting history is required. Patients may take drugs by ingestion, inhalation, injection, rectal or vaginal insertion, or topical administration. Patients often misinterpret the examiners meaning of "drugs" and do not consider vitamins, laxatives, aspirin, birth control pills, and other proprietaries as drugs. These medications, therefore, are often overlooked in the history unless specific questions are asked. Because of difficulties in eliciting a history of drug use, thorough and specific questions must be asked, often requiring additional but necessary interviews. Persistence in questioning patients with urticaria is usually the most rewarding single diagnostic aid.

The temporal relationship of the onset of the lesions to the drug administration must be considered. Most drug induced urticaria occurs within minutes to a few hours or days after administration. In serum sickness, however, 10 to 14 days often elapse between the use of the drug and the onset of urticaria. Although a history of previous exposure to a drug is desirable for establishment of the diagnosis, many patients do not recall such exposure, and they do not know when the "sensitizing" dose of drug was given.

In diagnosis and therapy of suspected drug induced urticaria, the initial step is to stop the use of all drug or drug like preparations. If the urticaria disappears, a presumptive diagnosis of urticaria due to drugs can be made. In order to determine which drug is the offending one, the medications are reintroduced, one at a time, at intervals of

TABLE 13-2
Management of Urticaria and Angio-edema

I. DIAGNOSIS (AND POSSIBLE THERAPY) OF ETIOLOGY BY THOROUGH HISTORY AND ENVIRONMENTAL MANIPULATION

A. *Drugs*
1. Elimination
2. Skin tests (little value)

B. *Foods*
1. Elimination diet with stepwise introduction
2. Skin tests (questionable value)
3. Diet diary

C. *Infection or infestation*
1. Search for focus
2. Removal of focus
3. Empiric course of therapy

D. *Inhalant sensitivity or insect bites*
1. Skin tests
2. Hyposensitization

E. *Connective tissue disorders or neoplasia*
1. Search for disorder
2. Appropriate therapy

F. *Psychic factors*
1. Psychic evaluation
2. Control of psychic factors

G. *Physical factors*
1. Cautious testing with suspected agent
2. Elimination of contact

H. *Hereditary factors*
1. Possible familial history
2. Assay for abnormalities in serum components

II. SYMPTOMATIC THERAPY (SINGLE OR COMBINATIONS OF DRUGS)

A. Epinephrine
B. Ephedrine
C. Antihistamines
D. Hydroxyzine
E. Tranquilizers
F. Cyproheptadine
G. Corticosteroids

1 to 3 days. The return of urticaria after administration of a drug implicates that medication. This means of diagnosis, however, may entail some risk, since cessation of a drug followed by a period of no administration might result in an explosive reaction, possibly with laryngeal edema, when the drug is reintroduced. Therefore, it would be important to reduce the dose of the suspected drug to at least one half the previous dose when testing the patient. If urticaria is relieved when the drug is withdrawn and reappears when it is reintroduced, the diagnosis is confirmed, and continued avoidance of the drug is necessary.

Skin testing to drug allergy is useful only if the allergen is penicillin or some high molecular weight drug such as insulin or ACTH. In these cases, one may produce an immediate wheal and flare skin reaction, but the skin reactivity is confirmatory only in the presence of a significant history.

Food Induced Urticaria

Urticaria due to foods may be the result of hypersensitivity, or may follow the ingestion of a food such as strawberries, which acts as a histamine liberator. Reactions can occur within minutes after ingestion of the food, as is often the case with sensitivity to nuts or shellfish. In these cases, the offending foods are usually avoided by the patient, as he learns by experience that they result in urticaria.

In many cases, urticaria due to food sensitivity occurs some hours after ingestion of the offending food, or intermittent urticaria may occur depending on the quantity or number of allergenic foods ingested. Urticaria is likely to occur even if slightly allergenic foods are ingested on several successive days. Although any food may cause the acute explosive type of urticaria, the most common precipitating foods are nuts, berries, fish and shellfish. Cereals, milk, eggs, potatoes, beef, pork, legumes (such as peas and beans) and oranges usually cause reactions which begin some hours after ingestion.

The diagnosis and subsequent therapy of food induced urticaria usually depends on a thorough history. Sometimes the patient discovers the offending food and consciously eliminates it from his diet. In the case of multiple food sensitivities or in chronic hives, the history may be of lesser value, and other diagnostic measures may be needed.

Elimination Diets as Diagnostic Aids. The most widely used diagnostic measure for the evaluation of food induced urticaria is the elimination diet. During the dietary manipulations, symptomatic therapy should not be used, since such drugs may themselves account for improvement. In addition, during the use of diets only one change is made at a time in order to pinpoint the offending food.

One of the common elimination diets used is the rice and lamb diet (see p. 362). It consists basically of foods which are the least frequent causes of allergic reactions. Because such diets are nutritionally inadequate they should be used for no more than 10 to 14 days. It is also important that the patient eat no other foods and take no medications, such as vitamins, laxatives, etc. If no improvement occurs at the end of this period, the therapy may be abandoned or modified. If the urticaria disappears, new foods are added to the diet and the patient is observed for recurrence of urticaria. The eliminated foods are added one at a time, preferably at breakfast. Large amounts are given several times during the day before any particular food is ruled out as a possible cause of urticaria. If excluded, it is allowed to remain in the diet. The offending food usually produces urticaria within 24 hours of ingestion, and new foods may be added to the diet every second or third day.

If the addition of a food results in urticaria, no new foods are begun and the food most recently added is eliminated from the diet. The lesions should then disappear and return when the food is again ingested. That food is then avoided and the rest of the foods are systematically returned to the patient's diet. If there is no recurrence of urticaria, the food proven as the etiologic agent is no longer ingested by the patient. It is also important to remember that sensitivity to more than one food is common and therefore diagnostic diets must be used carefully.

In some patients with food induced urticaria, the sensitivity disappears after months of avoidance; careful reintroduction of the food into the diet, with observation of the patient, can then be tried. If the patient can tolerate the food, it can remain in his diet; if urticaria returns, the tested food is avoided for several months before reintroduction is again attempted.

Skin Tests. On occasion skin tests may be useful in the diagnosis of a specific food sensitivity, but prolonged elimination diets should not be undertaken on the basis of skin reactions alone. Wheal and flare reactions to specific foods may be of value in determining which foods may be added or eliminated from diet therapy. The *only* definite proof of a food as a cause of urticaria is not a positive skin reaction, but the disappearance and return of hives as suspected food is eliminated and returned to the patient's diet.

Food Diary. Sometimes a food diary may be of use in the evaluation of possible food sensitivity as a cause of urticaria. Using this method, the patient keeps an accurate written record of all substances eaten and indicates when his urticaria occurs. It may then be possible for the physician to correlate the onset of urticaria with the prior ingestion of one or more foods. Subsequent manipulation of the diet, with elimination and reintroduction of the suspected food, may make the diagnosis and lead to adequate therapy.

Infection and Infestation as Causes of Urticaria

Hives may accompany acute pyogenic infections, such as streptococcal infections in children. The role of chronic infection, especially infection in closed spaces such as the gallbladder, as a cause of urticaria is controversial. Although a search for a hidden focus of infection is often not rewarding, an occasional patient will respond to a short course of a broad spectrum antibiotic.

Urticaria may also accompany parasitic infestations such as pinworms, ascariasis, schistosomiasis, and echinococcosis, and may be associated with systemic absorption of antigen from parasitic focus. Appropriate diagnosis and therapy with the proper antiparasitic agent should result in a cure.

Inhalant-Sensitivity Urticaria

Hives or angio-edema rarely accompany seasonal rhinitis or asthma. They are more often associated with the inhalation of animal danders, flour, dispersed fish proteins, or cosmetics. The appropriate therapy would be hyposensitization with the common inhalant antigens and avoidance of the suspected allergens where practical.

Urticaria from Bites and Stings

Localized, or general hives, or angio-edema may be the result of reactions from certain stinging insects, especially of the Hymenoptera species. Appropriate therapy will depend on the degree and severity of the reaction. Hyposensitization with specific insect antigens is important to prevent more serious subsequent reactions.

Connective Tissue Diseases and Neoplasms as Causes of Urticaria

Urticaria may be associated with connective tissue disorders such as systemic lupus erythematosus or polyarteritis nodosa, or with neoplasms undergoing central necrosis. Treatment of the urticaria includes symptomatic therapy as well as specific therapy of the underlying disease.

Psychic Factors in Urticaria

Chronic urticaria, like most other chronic illnesses, can be aggravated by emotional stress. When uncovered, psychic disturbances should receive appropriate therapy. There is no evidence, however, that such factors alone cause urticaria. Therefore, the physician should not abandon a search for an etiologic agent when psychic disorders appear in the patient.

Hereditary Angioneurotic Edema

This form of angio-edema was first described by Osler in 1888 as a genetic disease transmitted in a mendelian dominant fashion but with irregular penetrance. Since then, over 500 patients in more than 60 families have been proven to have this disorder. Although the incidence of this disease may not be high, it must be considered in the differential diagnosis of angio-edema.

Hereditary angio-edema is characterized by recurrent episodes of circumscribed angio-edema of the skin or respiratory or gastrointestinal tracts, beginning in childhood and often precipitated by trauma. The lesions begin acutely and are usually quite transient, although areas of edema may persist for several days. Urticaria does not usually accompany the edema. Edema of the gastrointestinal tract may be associated with nausea, vomiting and severe abdominal pain, sometimes requiring surgical intervention. The most dangerous event occurring during an attack, however, is acute laryngeal edema. Almost 20 percent of patients with hereditary angio-edema have died in their third decade because of asphyxia due to laryngeal edema.

Recent histopathologic and ultrastructural studies of tissues from patients with the disorder have demonstrated several characteristic features. Skin changes during attacks consisted of capillary and venous dilatation with subcutaneous edema. In the upper respiratory tract, laryngeal, as well as labial, lingual and uvulal edema, were consistently detected. Examination of the gastrointestinal tract demonstrated edema of the lamina propria, submucosa and serosa. There was a paucity of inflammatory cells in these areas, in contrast to the prominent eosinophilic infiltration detected in tissues involved in acute allergic reactions. These findings suggest that nonimmunologic mechanisms are important in the genesis of this type of angio-edema.

Over the past few years, investigations by several groups have indicated that most individuals with hereditary angio-edema lack an alpha-2-globulin in their serum. This protein inhibits the action of C1 esterase, a component of the complement system, on its substrate C4 and C2. In addition, it may also inhibit the action of one of the vasoactive polypeptides, plasma kallikrein, on vessel walls. The presence of uninhibited C1 esterase presumably results in the release of a kininlike peptide which causes the vascular changes and the resulting angio-edema. The actual events which precipitate an episode of angio-edema, however, are not yet clear.

The diagnosis of hereditary angio-edema may be suspected when there is a history of recurrent attacks of angio-edema, usually without urticaria, in the patient as well as in his family. It may be confirmed by demonstrating the abnormality in serum proteins. The disorder should also be considered in children with early onset angio-edema, even in the absence of a family history, as well as in individuals with unexplained recurrent episodes of laryngeal edema.

The serum protein deficiency may be demonstrated by gel diffusion techniques using antiserum specific for C1 esterase inhibitor, by failure of the patient's serum to inhibit the esterolytic activity of C1 esterase, or by the failure of the patient's serum to inhibit immune hemolysis of red cells coated with C1. In addition, patients with this disorder have low serum levels of C2, especially during an acute attack. While most patients with hereditary angio-edema lack the C1 esterase inhibitor, certain families with this disorder have recently been described in whom the inhibitor is present in normal amounts but does not function.

Therapy of patients with hereditary angio-edema should be directed against the acute attack, especially when laryngeal edema occurs. Early hospitalization is important, and the attacks often subside within 3 to 4 days. Epinephrine, antihistamines, or steroids, although they are of limited effect, should be administered along with positive pressure breathing. When there is respiratory obstruction, tracheostomy may be necessary.

Prevention of the attacks is difficult. A number of drugs such as testosterone and epsilon-amino-caproic acid have been tried with limited success. Perhaps the use of fresh plasma or the administration of purified C1 esterase inhibitor, when made available, may be of value.

Urticaria Due to Light

Wheal and flare reactions due to exposure to light are not common but they must be considered in the differential diagnosis of urticaria. Although the ingestion of such drugs as phenothiazine or dimethylchlortetracycline prior to light exposure may also result in skin lesions, the mechanism of induction is more likely on a toxic rather than on a sensitivity basis. In these cases, it is usually not difficult to determine the etiology from careful history; avoidance therapy is then instituted.

Patients with true light induced urticaria may develop local or systemic manifestations including anaphylactic shock. Light with wavelengths between 2850 and 3200 angstroms is the most common sensitizer of these patients, but a smaller number of individuals may be sensitive to light with wavelengths between 4000 and 5000 angstroms. It may be necessary to expose patients to selected wavelengths in order to determine the type of sensitivity. Fluorescent lights may be used as the source of light, and special filters which allow passage of narrow spectra of

wavelengths can be interposed between the light and the skin.*
Small areas of the body can be exposed for varying times and at varying
light wavelengths and can then be observed for urticaria.

Therapy of this disorder is based on avoiding of exposure by wearing
protective garments. Light screening preparations are available for
topical administration. Compounds containing benzoic acid derivatives
will protect against light in the 2500 to 3200 angstrom range, and preparations containing titanium dioxide or benzophenone derivatives protect above 3200 angstroms.

Cold Urticaria

This form of urticaria is most often seen in healthy adults. The lesions
resemble urticaria or angio-edema and may be generalized or local.
They often occur after the part exposed to cold is rewarmed and may be
associated with systemic symptoms of headache, nausea, vomiting, tachycardia and syncope. Laryngeal edema may occur when very cold food
is eaten, and generalized edema may follow immersion in cold water.

The etiology of cold urticaria is usually not detected, but the lesions
have also been associated with underlying diseases such as cryoglobuli-
nemia, cryofibrinogenemia, or paroxysmal hemoglobinemia of the
Donath-Landsteiner type. In addition, this type of urticaria may be seen
in patients with Raynaud's phenomenon or multiple myeloma. In about
50 percent of the cases of the idiopathic form of cold urticaria, a serum
factor resembling IgE has been found. This suggests that mechanisms
similar to the more common inhalant hypersensitivity may play a
role in the pathogenesis of some forms of cold urticaria.

Cold urticaria may be difficult to control, but antihistamines may be
of some benefit. Successful desensitization by immersion of the affected
part in water, with gradually decreasing temperatures, for increasing
lengths of time has been reported. Some investigators have also reported
that relief may follow a course of injections of increasing amounts of
histamine; the rationale for this therapy, however, is unclear. In addition, protection of the exposed part or avoidance of exposure to cold
may afford relief, as will treatment of an underlying disease. Usually,
however, the sensitivity to cold gradually disappears and the patient is
relieved of symptoms.

DRUG THERAPY OF URTICARIA

As in other allergic disorders, the most important feature of therapy is
the elimination of the causative agent from the patient's external or internal environment. Since this is not always possible, drugs may be

* Such filters are made by Owens-Corning.

needed to control the urticaria. Drug therapy is most commonly
needed in cases of chronic urticaria, since the acute form of urticaria is
usually self-limited.

Antihistamines

These drugs antagonize the effects of histamine on smooth muscle
and blood vessels by competitive inhibition. They are thus quite useful in
urticaria therapy regardless of its etiology but the degree of symptomatic
relief they offer varies among patients. Primary among known side
effects is drowsiness. It may be necessary to try several different drugs
on a patient to determine which drug or combination is most effective
while producing no significant side effects.

As there are over 150 short- and long-acting forms of antihistamine
compounds available, the physician must use his judgment, experience
and often trial and error in choosing the proper drug. Compounds of
this class most useful in the control of urticaria include diphenhydramine (Benadryl), tripelennamine (Pyribenzamine), and chlorpheniramine (Chlor-Trimeton). Hydroxyzine (Atarax or Vistaril), used both as
a mild tranquilizer and an antihistamine, has become quite useful in
the therapy of chronic urticaria. This drug may often suppress the
pruritus, as well as the lesions, when other measures fail. It is of particular value in acute or chronic urticaria of undetermined cause. The drug
may be given in doses up to 400 mg. per day with little or no side
effects, except mild drowsiness. If this therapy is successful, the dose
should be reduced until the minimum effective dose is determined;
this could be as little as 10 mg. 2 to 3 times per week. If this drug is
not effective at the maximum dose, other compounds may be added
to the regimen of therapy.

Sympathomimetics

Epinephrine is extremely effective in controlling acute urticaria and
angio-edema except for the hereditary type. It is available in aqueous
solutions, suspended in oil, or in sodium thioglycolate (Sus-Phrine).
These latter forms prolong the absorption of the drug and thus prolong
its action. The disadvantage of these drug preparations is that they
must be injected and, therefore, are not useful for long term therapy.

Ephedrine may often control the lesions of urticaria and can be quite
effective when used in combination with the antihistamines or hydroxyzine. Small doses of barbiturates or larger doses of antihistamines may
be needed to suppress the sympathomimetic side effects of this drug.

Other Useful Drugs

Cyproheptadine (Periactin) may be effective in some cases of urticaria. It has as its major action an antiserotonin effect; however, the

role of serotonin in the genesis of hives has not been proven. This drug may be effective alone or may be used in combination with one or more of the above drugs.

Phenobarbital is one of the numerous sedatives or tranquilizers which may be of benefit when emotional factors seem to play a role in the genesis of the lesions.

Rarely, parasympatholytic drugs, such as belladonna, may have some benefit in controlling urticaria.

Finally, it must be emphasized that corticosteroids should be avoided for long term use because of their side effects and because the lesions usually can be controlled with other drugs or environmental manipulations. The corticosteroids, however, may be useful in controlling on a long-term basis urticaria which is a manifestation of serum sickness or other acute drug eruptions.

BIBLIOGRAPHY

1. Alexander, H. L.: Reactions with Drug Therapy. Philadelphia, W. B. Saunders, 1955.
2. Beall, G. N.: Urticaria. A review of laboratory and clinical observations. Medicine, 43:131, 1964.
3. Chester, A., Liebowitz, H., and Markow, M.: Causes of chronic urticaria including infection. New York J. Med., 59:1786, 1959.
4. Cohen, S. G., and Criep, L. H.: Urticaria and angio-edema in association with amebiasis. American Practitioner and Digestive Treatment, 1:246, 1950.
5. Eisenberg, B. C.: Management of chronic urticaria. JAMA, 169:14, 1959.
6. Epstein, S.: Urticarial hypersensitivity to light. American Practitioner and Digestive Treatment, 7:1326, 1956.
7. Feinberg, A. R., Pruzansky, J. J., Feinberg, S. M., and Fisherman, E. W.: Hydroxyzine (Atarax) in chronic urticaria and in allergic manifestations. J. Allerg., 29:358, 1958.
8. Graham, D. T., and Wolf, S.: Pathogenesis of urticaria. Experimental study of life situations, emotions and cutaneous vascular reactions. JAMA, 143:1396, 1950.
9. Horton, B. T., Brown, G. E., and Roth, G. M.: Hypersensitiveness to cold. JAMA, 107:1263, 1936.
10. Hansen, D. D., Arbesman, C. E., Ho, K, and Wicher, K.: Cold urticaria. Amer. J. Med., 49:23, 1970.
11. Johnson, T. J., and Cazort, A. G.: Dermographia—clinical observations. JAMA, 169:23, 1959.
12. Sheffer, A. L., Craig, J. M., Willms-Kretschmer, K., Austen, K. F., and Rosen, F. S.: Histopathologic and ultrastructural observation on tissues from patients with hereditary angioneurotic edema. J. Allerg., 47: 292, 1971.

13. Lauderman, N. S.: Hereditary angioneurotic edema: I. Case reports and review of the literature. J. Allerg., *33*:313, 1962.
14. Lewis, T.: The Blood Vessels of the Human Skin and Their Responses. London, Shaw and Sons, 1927.
15. Morgan, J. K.: Observations on cholinergic urticaria. J. Invest. Derm., *21*:173, 1953.
16. Sheldon, J. M., Lovell, R. B., and Mathews, K. P.: A Manual of Clinical Allergy. ed. 2. Philadelphia, W. B. Saunders, 1967.
17. Steinhardt, M. J.: Urticaria and angioedema. Statistical survey of five hundred cases. Ann. Allerg., *12*:659, 1954.
18. Winklemann, R. K.: Chronic urticaria. Proc. Staff Meet. Mayo Clin., *32*:329, 1957.

14

Food Allergy and Immunologic Diseases of the Gastrointestinal Tract

Thomas M. Golbert, M.D.

Food allergy is often erroneously diagnosed or inappropriately excluded from consideration because definitive evidence for many observations is difficult to obtain. Allergic etiologies have been suggested for certain diseases of undetermined pathogenesis. The first portion of this chapter will review the extraenteric and enteric manifestations of reaginic food allergy. Methods of diagnosis will be discussed. The second portion will review non-reaginic gastrointestinal disorders for which immunologic mechanisms have been postulated to participate in the pathogenesis.

FOOD ALLERGY

Food allergy is uncommon. Its incidence among children is estimated at 0.3 percent.[9] The incidence decreases with advancing age.[12] Food allergy causes a variety of cutaneous, gastrointestinal, and, rarely, respiratory manifestations.[13] The most common, urticaria and angioedema, occur immediately. Abdominal cramps, nausea, emesis, and diarrhea occur less frequently and are also immediate.

Certain characteristic relationships of food allergy can be described. These include consistent association of symptoms with specific foods and abrupt onset of reactions within 2 hours after ingestion. Onset of symptoms later than 48 hours after ingestion,[15] occult food allergy—(particularly in adults),[19] and respiratory disease caused by food allergy[46] are rare. Remission of symptoms follows abstinence from the causative allergen. The association of symptoms during exposure and remission during abstinence from a substance does not definitively establish an allergic pathogenesis because this association may be coincidental. Consistent association during several repetitions will establish a definite diagnosis of cause but not necessarily of an allergic mechanism.

Diagnosis of food allergy is frequently difficult. A detailed history is the

355

most important and productive single procedure. Diet diaries and elimination diets are helpful adjuncts. These procedures do not differentiate food allergy from nonimmunologic intolerance. Positive cutaneous tests neither establish nor confirm a definitive diagnosis of food allergy. Negative cutaneous tests in certain conditions do not conclusively exclude a diagnosis of food allergy. No laboratory or in vitro findings are, in themselves, diagnostic of gastrointestinal or food allergy.

Avoidance of the offending food is the only specific and practical treatment. Malnutrition resulting from dietary management is unjustifiable. Substitute foods and supplements of vitamins and minerals may be used when necessary. Food allergy often has spontaneous remission. Therefore, important foods should be cautiously reevaluated every 3 to 6 months.

Immunologic Considerations

The clinical manifestations of food allergy usually result from Type I (anaphylactic, reagin-dependent) hypersensitivity [12, 14] (See Chap. 1). This immunologic pathogenesis is considered to be identical to that of atopic diseases caused by other antigens. Reaginic antibody mediates the immediate wheal and erythema reaction and usually is of immunoglobulin class IgE.[25] In some patients antibodies from other immunoglobulin classes may also possess reaginic activity.[36] The immunochemical characteristics and immunologic mechanisms of immediate type allergy are discussed in detail in Chapter 2.

Reaginic antibody against food antigens can be detected by direct cutaneous wheal and erythema reactions and by passive transfer to the skin of subhuman primate [14] and human recipients.[14, 35] Passive transfer tests to human recipients are rarely, if ever, indicated for clinical purposes because of the risk of transferring infectious diseases such as viral hepatitis. Peripheral leukocytes from patients having anaphylactic sensitivity to foods may release measurable quantities of histamine when incubated in vitro with specific antigen.[14] This technique is useful only for experimental investigation because the diagnosis of clinical food allergy cannot be reliably made or excluded by histamine release. Diagnostic tests are discussed in detail in Chapter 3.

By use of the ammonium sulfate coprecipitation (Farr) technique, antibodies against beef serum albumin have been demonstrated to occur more frequently among allergic persons than among nonallergic persons. Postive cutaneous tests did not correlate with the presence or absence of this antibody.[1] Precipitating,[21, 33, 36] hemagglutinating,[33] and complement-fixing [30] antibodies against food proteins have been demonstrated in serum, and precipitating antibodies against food proteins have been demonstrated in feces.[21, 27, 28] The pathogenetic significance of these antibodies is unknown. These techniques do not measure reaginic antibodies and have no diagnostic value in food allergy at present.[16, 19, 26] Serum antibodies of immunoglobulin classes IgG and IgA and gastrointestinal antibodies of immunoglobulin classes IgA, IgM, and IgD have been demonstrated against bovine serum albumin in normal subjects and in patients with nonallergic disease.[28] Coproantibodies against milk proteins have been demonstrated in breast fed healthy infants and in infants having diarrhea not associated with allergic disease.[8]

Demonstration of antibodies against food proteins does not definitively establish or confirm a pathogenesis of food allergy. Antibodies against foods occur in normal subjects.[16] Antibodies can initiate the pathogenesis of diseases (see Chap. 1) by a reaginic mechanism,[25, 32] by tissue injury resulting from precipitating antibody-antigen complexes with participation of complement, and by complement mediated reactions.[7] More than one type of hypersensitivity mechanism may be operative in any clinical allergic state, including food allergy. At present, only the reaginic mechanism has conclusively been demonstrated in food allergy. Antibodies against foods or tissue can arise secondary to tissue injury from nonimmunologic causes. Theoretically, these antibodies might perpetuate tissue injury, might have no pathogenetic function, or might provide a protective mechanism. Absorption of antigenically active food protein occurs in certain diarrheal diseases [20] and in normal subjects.[30, 35] Antibodies may have a protective function in rapidly eliminating these proteins from the circulation.[16] Antibodies in gastrointestinal secretions might retard absorption of intact food proteins from the gut.[16]

Extraenteric Manifestations

Urticaria and angioedema are the most common extraenteric manifestations of food allergy.[19] Eczema is occasionally caused by food allergy, but no cause can be identified in most cases.[40] Asthma, rhinitis,[46] and anaphylaxis [14] are rare manifestations.

A syndrome of recurrent diarrhea and emesis, iron deficiency anemia, failure to thrive, and chronic pulmonary disease (often with infiltrates and atelectasis) has been described. Cutaneous tests and tests for precipitating antibodies are positive to milk.[22] Remission follows removal of milk from the diet. This syndrome occurs in infants and is rare. The signficance of the precipitating antibodies is unclear. Arthus-type hypersensitivity has not been demonstrated, and reaginic antibodies alone are not ordinarily associated with infiltrative disease.

Some cases of dermatitis herpetiformis have apparently benefited from treatment with a gluten free diet.[31] The significance of this observation relative to possible immunologic mechanisms is undetermined. Improvement was limited to cutaneous lesions and histological examination of small bowel. Malabsorption did not change, and improvement in skin lesions did not correlate with mucosal disease.

Some cot deaths in infancy have been attributed to anaphylaxis from milk allergy.[29] Most result from unknown causes and appear nonimmunologic. A single etiology will probably not account for all, or even most, of these deaths.

Food allergy has been reported as a cause of other syndromes. These include enuresis,[43] Henoch-Schönlein purpura,[48] migraine,[19] Meniere's disease,[6] idiopathic cyclic edema,[44] geographic tongue, and infantile cortical hyperostosis.[26] Various nonspecific manifestations include irritability, headache, malaise, fatigue, and mental and emotional symptoms. The evidence for associating these entities with food allergy is testimonial, and any true etiologic relationship is doubtful.

Foods occasionally cause respiratory allergic disease as inhalant antigens. "Baker's asthma" results from occupational exposure to flour. Wheat flour is most commonly the allergen but sensitization to rye or corn flour may also occur. Sensitization to soybean, green coffee, castor bean, cottonseed, [10] and potato also occurs from occupational inhalation. Ingestion of the cooked food does not produce symptoms in these patients. There is uncertainty whether chlorogenic acid or protein constituents are the significant antigens in green coffee and castor bean.[16]

The diagnostic approach to urticaria and angioedema must include causes other than food allergy. These are drug allergy, biologic medications containing heterologous protein; infection; parasitic infestation; emotional stress; certain collagen diseases; internal malignancies; direct cutaneous inoculation with antigen such as animal danders; physical or cholinergic factors such as heat, cold, light, or pressure; and, rarely, endocrine factors such as menopause, menstruation, and hypothyroidism. Hereditary angioedema must not be mistaken for an other type of angioedema because early tracheostomy is the only definitive treatment for the potentially lethal laryngeal edema which occurs in hereditary angioedema.[37] Hereditary angioedema is identified by the family history and by deficiency of C′ 1-esterase inhibitor.[37]

Asthma and rhinitis of allergic origin must be distinguished from nonallergic causes. Inhalant antigens are far more frequently the cause of allergic respiratory diseases than are foods. Inhalant factors must be controlled before and during evaluation of possible food allergy. Evaluation of food allergy requires observable changes in signs and symptoms when causative foods are eliminated or ingested. Persistence of symptoms resulting from uncontrolled infectious and inhalant factors may obscure variations caused by dietary manipulation.[16]

Anaphylaxis. Systemic reactions are immediate, explosive, potentially fatal manifestations of food allergy. Various combinations of urticaria, angioedema, dyspnea, cyanosis, chest pain, hypotension or shock, and abdominal distress including pain, nausea, emesis, or diarrhea develop shortly after ingestion and sometimes during ingestion of the causative agent. Nasal and conjunctival symptoms may be present. Cutaneous manifestations are almost invariably present.[14] Electrocardiographic changes may occur. These include sinus tachycardia, ST-T changes, atrial fibrillation,[14] T wave depression, T wave inversion, ST elevation, ST depression, and nodal rhythm.[2]

A reaginic mechanism is demonstrable. Direct cutaneous tests are positive. Passive transfer reactions with human or monkey recipients can be used experimentally. Peripheral leukocytes release histamine in vitro during incubation with the causative antigen. However, these immunologic techniques neither establish nor confirm a definitive diagnosis of food allergy.[14]

Diagnosis. The methods of establishing a diagnosis of food allergy are a comprehensive dietary history, elimination diets, diet diary, and cutaneous testing.

History. A careful history is the most important initial procedure in the diagnosis of food allergy. It should include foods ingested frequently, those avoided and reasons for avoidance, and foods which the patient suspects. Recurrent symptoms following repeated ingestion of a specific food are sometimes apparent. This history is most frequently obtained when explosive symptoms occur immediately after ingestion, particularly when the causative food is ingested only occasionally. Patients who recognize this relationship often do not consult a physician; they simply avoid the causative food.

A clear association of symptoms with the offending food may not be obtainable or immediately apparent. Highly antigenic and frequently ingested foods are most likely to cause allergic disease. Foods ingested daily are sometimes erroneously disregarded as causative agents or considered coincidental to symptoms.[12]

Several factors often make a diagnosis of food allergy difficult. Sometimes the onset of symptoms is delayed. Occasionally, symptoms may occur intermittently even though the food is ingested daily. The causative agent may be a contaminant, or the mechanism of symptoms might not be immunologic or even organic.[12] All of these factors can obscure the history and result in an incorrect omission of causative foods from consideration or an incorrect diagnosis of food allergy.

Symptoms usually occur immediately after ingestion and may be caused by antigenically unaltered protein.[35] These cases are associated with demonstrable cutaneous reactivity. Proteoses in various stages of digestion may also be absorbed from the gastrointestinal tract and are antigenic.[30, 41] Symptoms caused by partially digested food may occur hours after ingestion, depending upon the time required for absorption. The onset of symptoms rarely occurs more than 48 hours after ingestion,[15] but the causative food may become obscured by foods ingested during the interim.

The regularity with which symptoms occur depends upon: (1) the degree of the patient's sensitivity to the specific food, (2) additive effects of exposure to other antigens, and (3) the physical state of the proteins. Generally patients have symptoms every time the offending food is ingested. Patients who are only moderately sensitive might not have symptoms unless large quantities of the food are ingested. Ingestion of multiple foods to which the patient is moderately sensitive might cause symptoms. This relationship might be unrecognized if each food alone in usual quantity is tolerated. Some food processing methods denature protein, and foods so processed may cause symptoms intermittently in susceptible individuals. Cases are documented in which symptoms were produced by the raw or partially cooked food, but the same food, completely cooked, was well tolerated.[9, 12, 14] Other methods of processing foods which alter allergenicity include spray drying of cereals and dehydration of bananas.[12]

Contamination of foods by drugs and dyes may complicate the history. Milk from treated cattle has been contaminated with bacitracin, penicillin, and the tetracyclines.[12] Dyes approved by the Food and Drug Administration have caused asthma.[4]

Nonimmunologic intolerance to foods can mimic allergic disease. Contamination by bacteria or bacterial toxins is one example. Certain kinds of mushrooms, shellfish, and poisonous fish contain toxins which cause gastrointestinal and systemic illness. Prunes, onions, and soybeans are among foods which causes gastrointestinal symptoms by irritation or by pharmacologic activity. Various enzyme deficiency diseases may simulate allergic disorders; examples include favism, galactosemia, and the hemolytic anemia due to glucose-6-phosphate dehydrogenase deficiency.[12] Enzyme deficiencies may cause intolerance to lactose and other dissaccharides.[45] These diseases, like allergic diseases, are controlled by abstinence.

Nonorganic causes of intolerance to foods include food faddism, psychoneuroses, and functional gastrointestinal reactions. These entities must not be misdiagnosed as food allergy. This error causes many patients to resist the correct diagnosis and appropriate therapy.

Diet Diary. In cases with occasional symptoms the history can be augmented or clarified by a diet diary. All foods, beverages, and drugs taken within 48 hours before each recurrence are recorded in chronological order. Consistent appearance of the same antigen or related

Diet Diary

NAME —————————————————— NO. ——— RETURN DATE ————

Write down each day everything you eat or drink—at meals or between meals, including all medicines.

Bring these pages back to the Nutritionist on your next visit.

Day	*Day*
BREAKFAST	
BETWEEN MEAL	
NOON	
BETWEEN MEAL	
EVENING MEAL	
BED TIME	

antigens with exacerbations suggests a causal relationship. Unfortunately, this relationship is often absent or not apparent. The diet diary can also be used as a guide for cutaneous testing. Only foods which are temporally related to symptoms should be tested.

Elimination Diets. Elimination diets are useful for patients having symptoms daily or nearly every day. Diet No. 1 is usually used initially. It consists of lamb, rice, pineapple, and other foods ingested with relative infrequency. Substitutions may be made to include foods a particular patient eats frequently. Diet No. 2 is less restrictive and may be suitable for some patients who are unable or unwilling to observe Diet No. 1. Total elimination diets are *rarely* necessary, but synthetic milks are available for this purpose. These are amino acids from enzymatic digestion of

Allergy Diet No. 1

All fruits and vegetables, except lettuce, must be cooked.

FOODS AND BEVERAGES ALLOWED:

Lamb	Pineapple	Spinach	Any vegetable oil, such as
	Apricot	Celery	olive oil, Crisco, or Spry,
Poi	Cherries	Sweet Potatoes	EXCEPT oleomargarine *
	Blueberry		
Rice		Salt	
Rice cereals	Lettuce	Sugar, cane or beet	
Rice wafers	Artichokes	Synthetic vanilla extract	
	Beets	Tapioca	
Water			

AVOID:

Milk	
Tea	Chewing gum
Coffee	All medications except those prescribed by the doctor
Cola	All foods not listed under FOODS AND BEVERAGES ALLOWED
Soft drinks	

INSTRUCTIONS: *(Result)*

STAY ON BASIC DIET FOR _____ DAYS.

THEN, ON _____, ADD _____, ALONE, FIRST THING IN A.M., _____

NEXT, ON _____, ADD _____, ALONE, FIRST THING IN A.M., _____

NEXT, ON _____, ADD _____, " " " " " _____

NEXT, ON _____, ADD _____, " " " " " _____

NEXT, ON _____, ADD _____, " " " " " _____

NEXT, ON _____, ADD _____, " " " " " _____

NEXT, ON _____, ADD _____, " " " " " _____

NEXT, ON _____, ADD _____, " " " " " _____

KEEP A DIET DIARY AS INSTRUCTED

* Kosher pareve oleomargines and Mazola Margarine contain no milk.

Allergy Diet No. 2
(Cereal, Milk, Egg-Free Diet) *

Modified from Rowe's Cereal Free 1-2-3 Diet

All fruits and vegetables, except lettuce, must be cooked.

FOODS AND BEVERAGES ALLOWED:

Lamb
Chicken, Turkey
Beef, all beef wieners
Ham (boiled), bacon

Lettuce
Artichokes
Beets
Spinach
Celery
Carrots
Soy beans
Soy milk
Soy bean sprouts

Arrowroot
Potatoes, potato chips
Rice
Yams or sweet potatoes
Tapioca †

Lentils
Navy beans
Kidney beans
Asparagus

Water
Gingerale
White Soda
Poi

Olive oil
White vinegar
Vanilla extract

Any vegetable shortening or oleo-margine which contains *no milk solids* ‡

Salt
Cane or beet sugar
Maple syrup or maple flavored cane syrup

Pineapple
Apricot
Cherry
Blueberry
Plum
Prune
} and their juices

AVOID:

Tea
Coffee
Cola
Soft drinks

Chewing gum
All medications except those prescribed by the doctor

All foods not listed under FOODS AND BEVERAGES ALLOWED

INSTRUCTIONS: *(Result)*

STAY ON BASIC DIET FOR _____ DAYS.

THEN, ON _____, ADD _____, ALONE, FIRST THING IN A.M., _____

NEXT, ON _____, ADD _____, ALONE, FIRST THING IN A.M., _____

NEXT, ON _____, ADD _____,   "   "   "   "   "   _____

NEXT, ON _____, ADD _____,   "   "   "   "   "   _____

NEXT, ON _____, ADD _____,   "   "   "   "   "   _____

NEXT, ON _____, ADD _____,   "   "   "   "   "   _____

NEXT, ON _____, ADD _____,   "   "   "   "   "   _____

NEXT, ON _____, ADD _____,   "   "   "   "   "   _____

KEEP A DIET DIARY AS INSTRUCTED

* Modified from Rowe's Cereal-Free 1-2-3 Diet.
† Minute Tapioca may contain citric acid. Use whole or Pearl tapioca.
‡ Kosher pareve oleomargarines, Mazola Margarine, Crisco and Spry contain no milk.

casein [9] and include Nutramigen,* Amigen,† and Stuart Amino Acids.‡ None contains intact protein.

Nutramigen is the most adequate nutritionally. It provides 30 calories per fluid ounce and contains sucrose, arrowroot starch, corn oil, vitamins, and minerals. Infants take 1 measure of powder in 2 ounces of water. Adults take 8 ounces of powder in 1 quart of water. Five percent Amigen and 5 percent dextrose may be used in doses of 250 ml. 4 to 6 times daily. Stuart Amino Acids (3 tablespoonfuls or less dissolved in hot or cold liquid) are taken 6 times daily. Ginger ale, white soda, or sugar can improve the palatability of these preparations.

Certain foods, notably milk, egg, and wheat, might be difficult to avoid because of widespread use.§ Recipes which utilize milk substitutes and exclude wheat and eggs can be found in dietetic and standard cookbooks. These books also furnish necessary special instructions for preparation. Flours without wheat make satisfactory biscuits, muffins, and cookies but not bread. Kosher cookbooks provide recipes without milk products. Kosher pareve oleomargarines contain no milk.

The Allergy Diets 1 and 2 should be used for 7 to 10 days. (The author prefers not to exceed 7 days.) Synthetic milk diets should not exceed 3 to 7 days. If marked improvement does not occur, food allergy is unlikely, and a general diet may be reinstituted. Rarely, this may be followed by abrupt increase in symptoms; foods ingested during the preceding 48 hours may be eliminated for another 7 days. Foods returned to the diet earlier than 48 hours before the exacerbation need not be avoided. A diet diary is useful in this situation.

If improvement occurs during the elimination diet, individual foods may be introduced at two day intervals. Preferably, each new food is ingested alone in large quantity at breakfast the first day. At the next five meals it may be combined with any foods already in the diet. If exacerbation occurs, the last food returned to the diet is eliminated, and no new food is introduced until remission is established. Persistence of symptoms for 7 days suggests that the exacerbation was coincidental. Some authors suggest three or more separate exacerbations before eliminating an important food for a prolonged period.[15]

Extreme caution with direct, experienced medical supervision is mandatory during introduction of foods if a potential systemic reaction is suspected. In evaluating anaphylaxis, a presumptive diagnosis should

---

* Trademark of Mead Johnson Laboratories.
† Trademark of Baxter Laboratories.
‡ Trademark of The Stuart Company.
§ Names of grocers who sell dietetic foods are obtainable from several sources: Chicago Dietetic Supply House, Inc., 1750 West Van Buren Street, Chicago, Illinois 60612; National Dietary Foods Association, Cincinnati, Ohio 45224; and Ralston Purina Company, Checkerboard Square, St. Louis, Missouri.

be accepted. This can be based on historical certainty of ingestion or on parenteral administration of other temporally related antigens without adverse effect. If more than one important food has not been ingested since the reaction, cutaneous tests will provide additional information. These can be executed far more safely than ingestion, and the causative food will almost invariably produce a positive reaction.[14]

Improvement during an elimination diet does not definitively establish food intolerance. Other treatment is often initiated simultaneously with the diet. Many diseases, such as eczema, have spontaneous remissions and exacerbations. Improvement can be due to the diet, to the other measures, to both, or to neither.

Cutaneous Tests. Positive cutaneous tests neither establish nor confirm a definitive diagnosis of clinically significant food allergy; they merely demonstrate presence of reaginic antibody. Negative cutaneous tests do not necessarily exclude a diagnosis of food allergy. The reliability of cutaneous tests is influenced by the age of the patient, the food in question, and the allergic manifestations. The correlation between positive reactions and clinical sensitivity is generally greatest in young children and diminishes with advancing age. Foods giving the most reliable correlation include fish, shellfish, peanuts, nuts, and, to a lesser degree, eggs.[11] Cutaneous tests are usually positive with reactions occurring immediately, but they may be negative with reactions of delayed onset.

Selected cutaneous testing is sometimes valuable despite the problems of interpretation. Positive skin tests may provide evidence of atopy. When the history suggests possible food allergy but is unclear for specific foods, positive reactions may provide a guide for trial elimination diets. Patients must never be advised to eliminate foods indefinitely on the sole basis of positive skin tests.[14, 19, 30] Absence of cutaneous reactivity suggests that the suspected food may be ingested without significant risk of a systemic reaction.[14]

Testing is performed by the puncture or scratch technique on the forearm or back. Use of the forearm permits application of a tourniquet proximal to the test sites if a systemic reaction occurs. This precaution is mandatory when investigating anaphylaxis of undetermined cause. *The evaluation of any patient with a history of anaphylaxis following ingestion of a food must be performed with extreme caution by a physician experienced in this field.* When the etiology is obvious by history, skin testing for the obvious cause should be avoided. The intradermal technique should be used only for antigens which produced negative puncture tests. Many allergists do not employ intradermal tests for foods because of the risk of systemic reactions and the frequency of false positive reactions.[11]

Commercially prepared food extracts are used most commonly for skin testing. Raw foods and extracts freshly prepared from raw foods or frozen fruit juice may provide more reliable results [11] but must be used cautiously; skin tests with these have caused systemic reactions.[12] Certain substances are particularly dangerous and should not be used intradermally. These are walnut, pecan, cabbage, broccoli, mustard, onion, asparagus, cauliflower, coconut, glue, ginger, flaxseed, castor seed, cottonseed, chlorogenic acid, buckwheat, whitefish, smelt, salmon, perch, lobster, shrimp, clam, and oyster.

Other Tests. Other tests have been advocated for diagnosis of food allergy. These include the leukocytotoxic test, the basophil degranulation test, the leukopenic index, acceleration of pulse rate after ingestion, and the intracutaneous provocative food test with the so-called provoking dose and neutralizing dose. These methods have no proven value.[3, 5, 12, 19, 26]

Treatment of Extraenteric Manifestations. *Specific Treatment* Avoidance is the only specific treatment of food allergy.[13, 16] Most unessential foods are easily avoided, but some may be inadvertently ingested in concealed form. Nuts, for example, are often incorporated into cookies, cake, and candies. More importantly, eggs, milk, and wheat are contained in many prepared foods. Patients must examine the ingredients of commercially prepared food combinations. This precaution does not always obviate the possibility of inadvertent ingestion. For example, the term "flour" may include various combinations of wheat, rye, barley, oat, corn, and cottonseed. Immunologic cross-reactivity among biologically related foods may also cause recurrent inadvertent ingestion.

Biologically related foods contain antigens which may not be cross-reactive. While the casein fractions of goat's milk and cow's milk are immunologically similar or identical, the lactalbumin fractions of the two are relatively species-specific. Goat's milk is sometimes a suitable substitute for patients who are sensitive only to the lactalbumin fractions of cow's milk.[23] This observation is of limited usefulness because the lactalbumin fractions of cow's milk are also heat labile.[9] Patients who tolerate goat's milk may also tolerate cooked cow's milk.

Special processing of foods sometimes permits use of the food by denaturing the antigen. In addition to the lactalbumin fractions, the bovine serum albumin and gamma globulin in milk are heat labile. The β-lactoglobulin is incompletely denatured by boiling, and α-casein is heat stable.[16] Cooking and other methods of processing foods, including dehydration and spray drying, do not reliably achieve avoidance of the allergen. Reactions may occur if the food is incompletely cooked or if all of the allergen present is not otherwise denatured. If one or more of the allergens are stable under the conditions of processing, symptoms may follow ingestion of the food.

With the possible exception of "baker's asthma," hyposensitization—orally, sublingually, or parenterally—has not proven useful and is not indicated.[9, 12, 16, 19]

The complications of dietary avoidance may include stunting of growth, impairment of musculature, and vitamin deficiency disorders. These consequences of prolonged nutriment deprivation are preventable.[12] An erroneous diagnosis of food allergy can also cause psychological dependence on an unsound diet.

Prevention of malnutrition is not difficult in adults. Multiple food allergies in one patient are common but include relatively few foods. They rarely, if ever, preclude a balanced diet. Even the most restrictive elimination diets should not cause nutriment deficiency because 7 to 10 days' trial is adequate. If systematic return of foods is undertaken, resumption of a balanced diet can be completed within 2 to 3 weeks.

Compared to adults, children and infants have few staple foods and a relatively large number of food allergies. Nevertheless, malnutrition resulting from dietary management of food allergy is unjustifiable.[26] Numerous multivitamin and mineral supplements are available. Rotating diets may be beneficial for patients with mild sensitivities to numerous foods. These diets should be used cautiously and are rarely necessary. Food sensitivities are often lost spontaneously, with or without abstinence. This may result from maturation of the digestive system or by the immune system's preventing absorption of undigested antigens.[16] Nutritionally important foods may be cautiously re-evaluated at three- to six-month intervals.[19] However, with reactions of immediate onset, particularly with respiratory or hypotensive manifestations, permanent avoidance is recommended. These reactions are unusual. Sensitivity to nuts or fish is rarely lost.[12]

Specially processed milks or milk substitutes may be used for the infant with milk allergy. In order of increasing price, these include dried milk, boiled milk, evaporated milk, modified milks, soybean milks, meat milks, and synthetic milks. In general, the less expensive preparations should be tried first. With immediate systemic reactions, all milk preparations should be avoided. Poi [16] is also a suitable milk substitute.

Modified milk preparations containing vitamin and mineral supplements include: hypoallergenic whole milk powder, SMA,* Enfamil,† Similac,‡ and Baker's §. Side effects of these preparations include diarrhea, irritation of the buttocks, and, rarely, constipation. These symptoms are usually mild and require no specific treatment.[9]

* Trademark of Wyeth Laboratories.
† Trademark of Mead Johnson and Company.
‡ Trademark of Ross Laboratories.
§ Trademark of Baker's Milk.

Symptomatic Treatment. Symptomatic treatment for complications resulting from inadevertent ingestion is identical to treatment for the specific complication resulting from any other cause. The potentially fatal immediate systemic reaction with respiratory, hypotensive, and cutaneous manifestations, although rare, is the most serious complication; treatment of anaphylaxis is discussed in Chapter 12.

Gastrointestinal Allergy

Definition. Gastrointestinal symptoms frequently accompany systemic allergic reactions or may occur as the only clinical manifestation of allergy to ingested antigens. This type of reaction, termed gastrointestinal allergy, is analogous to the respiratory symptoms associated with inhalant allergy.[12] Gastrointestinal manifestations have been attributed to direct exposure of intestinal surface to antigen.[19] Plasma cells producing IgE immunoglobulins have been demonstrated in the mucosa and regional lymph nodes of the gastrointestinal tract as well as in those of the respiratory tract.[42] Reaginic antibody is demonstrable by cutaneous testing and passive transfer reactions.[12] Unlike inhalant allergy, gastrointestinal allergy is rare.[24]

Manifestations. The most common manifestations of gastrointestinal allergy are abdominal pain, nausea, emesis, and diarrhea.[19] Pruritus and edema of the lips and buccal mucosa occur.[12] Rare or unusual manifestations include pruritus ani,[12] hematochezia, occult fecal blood loss,[9, 15, 21] nonspecific colitis,[21] mucous colitis,[12] and protein losing enteropathy.[18] Nonallergic diseases must be considered before attributing these symptoms to gastrointestinal allergy.

Experimental Observations. Gastroscopic examinations of patients with food allergy have been performed after ingestion of offending antigens.[34] Hyperemia, nodularity, edema and thickening of the rugal folds, diminished peristalsis, excessive production of mucus, and rarely, submucosal hemorrhage were observed. Exposed, passively sensitized human ileum and colon [17] and rhesus monkey stomach, ileum, and colon [47] were examined after challenge with specific antigen. Edema, hyperemia, hypersecretion of mucus, increased peristalsis, and, sometimes, spasm and prolonged contractions occurred. Infiltration of eosinophils in the mucosa of small intestine has been demonstrated by biopsy during acute symptoms of gastrointestinal allergy associated with protein losing enteropathy.[18] Roentgenologic examinations have demonstrated delayed emptying and hypotonicity of the stomach and hypertonicity of the small intestine.[12]

Diagnosis. A diagnosis of gastrointestinal allergy must satisfy the following criteria: (1) symptoms caused by specific substances which are innocuous to normal persons, (2) evidence for an immunologic mechanism in the pathogenesis of symptoms, (3) demonstration of lesions or functional changes in the gut, and (4) exclusion of emotional and mechanical factors. Reproducible manifestations should consistently occur at a nearly constant interval, ordinarily within 2 hours after administration of the disguised food. Other foods given to the patient in the same manner should not produce adverse effects.[24]

History is the primary method of diagnosis. Recurrent gastrointestinal symptoms following ingestion of specific foods are characteristic of an allergic pathogenesis. Consistent remissions following withdrawal of certain foods and exacerbations of chronic symptoms following ingestion are suggestive of allergy. Neither observation is diagnostic. Nonimmunologic mechanisms must be excluded. These include toxic, pharamacologic, and irritative properties of the food and chemical and microbiological contaminants. Metabolic and structural disease can also cause an identical history. Collateral respiratory and cutaneous allergy in the personal and family histories may further suggest an allergic etiology but may be coincidental.

Occasionally, association of recurrent symptoms with repetitive ingestion of specific foods may not be apparent from the history, or a suggestive relationship may be incorrect. A diet diary or an elimination diet often clarifies these impressions. They are useful methods of augmenting the history.

Positive cutaneous tests provide evidence for a reaginic mechanism. Negative cutaneous tests suggest either a nonreaginic intolerance or coincidental association of foods with symptoms.

Treatment. The only specific treatment of gastrointestinal allergy is avoidance of the causative foods. Symptoms following inadvertent ingestion can be controlled by antihistaminic, sympathomimetic, or anticholinergic drugs. Which of these drug groups, alone or in combination, will be most beneficial for a specific patient cannot be predicted before treatment.

Antihistamines. Chlorpheniramine maleate is usually used in doses of 4 mg. 3 or 4 times daily for adults, 2 mg. 4 times daily for children under age 12 years, and 1 mg. 4 times daily for infants. Diphenhydramine HC1 may produce better therapeutic results than chlorpheniramine, but its sedative effects may be less well tolerated. Ordinary doses are 50 mg. 3 or 4 times daily for adults, 25 mg. 3 or 4 times daily for children under age 12 years, and 5 mg. to 10 mg. 3 or 4 times daily for children over 1 year of age. If necessary, dosage may be tripled for chlorpheniramine and doubled for diphenhydramine if the patient tolerates it. Other antihistamines may be equally or more useful in certain patients.

Sympathomimetics. Ephedrine sulfate (25 mg. 3 or 4 times daily) is sometimes administered to adults. Fifty milligram doses of ephedrine or 0.3 ml. of 1:1000 epinephrine may be used but are rarely necessary. Phenylpropanolamine may also be used. The dose for children is half the adult dose. Side effects include central nervous system excitation, tremulousness, tachycardia, palpitations, and gastrointestinal disturbances. These drugs must be used cautiously in the presence of cardiovascular disease, severe hypertension, hyperthyroidism, glaucoma, or prostatic hypertrophy. Addition of a sedative, such as phenobarbital or hydroxyzine HCl, can minimize many of the side effects. Patients should be instructed not to drive or operate other machinery while taking sedatives or antihistamines.

Anticholinergics. Propantheline bromide (15 mg. to 30 mg. 4 times daily) may be used for adults. Other parasympatholytic drugs, such as belladonna derivatives, may be used as well. Glaucoma and severe cardiac disease are contraindications for use of anticholinergic drugs. Usual precautions should be employed in patients having bladder outlet obstruction, such as prostatic hypertrophy. Side effects include mydriasis, dryness of the mouth, gastric fullness, and urinary hesitancy.

Adrenocorticosteroids. Prednisone has been used successfully in treating acute protein losing enteropathy accompanying food allergy.[18] The initial dose is 30 mg. daily. Other steroid preparations could be used in equivalent doses. These drugs are gradually withdrawn after elimination of the offending food and cessation of symptoms. Adrenocorticotropic hormone (ACTH) has no place in therapy of allergic disorders.

NONREAGINIC GASTROINTESTINAL DISORDERS

Nontropical Sprue

Synonyms for nontropical sprue are celiac disease, celiac sprue, idiopathic sprue, idiopathic steatorrhea, primary malabsorption, and gluten enteropathy. The disease is characterized by diarrhea, bulky malodorous stools, steatorrhea (fecal fat excretion exceeding 6 gm. in 24 hours), and weight loss with malabsorption of proteins, carbohydrates, vitamins, minerals, electrolytes, and water.[58] The pathology is characterized by villous atrophy, increase in depth of the intestinal glands, chronic inflammatory cell infiltration in the lamina propria, and degenerative changes in the surface epithelial cells. These cells become cuboidal or flattened instead of columnar. Electron microscopy demonstrates short, sparse, and distorted microvilli. The epithelial basement membrane is often disrupted, and inflammatory cells extend between the epithelial surfaces. Abnormalities of subcellular organelles have been described.[64] Exacerbations follow ingestion of gluten, and remissions are induced by abstinence from gluten.[58]

Relationship of Gliadin to Pathogenesis. Gluten is a mixture of proteins found in wheat, oats, rye, and barley. The 70 percent alcohol-soluble fraction, termed gliadin, contains the injurious factors. The crude fibers (carbohydrate, ash, fat fractions from wheat, and the alcohol insoluble fraction), termed glutenin, are innocuous in celiac patients. Local exacerbation of disease with typical histologic changes has been induced by instilling gliadin into a normal area of ileum in a celiac patient.[52]

Gliadin has been separated by electrophoresis and column chromatography into fractions of similar molecular weight and amino acid composition. These are termed α1-2, β1-4, and γ. Alpha gliadin has a molecular weight of 50,000 and contains the major concentration of antigen activity with precipitating antibodies in celiac sera. More than 50 percent of the peptide bound amino acids of gliadin are proline and glutamic acid. The disulfide bonds are largely intramolecular. Gliadin does not precipitate with antibodies in celiac sera after alkylation and reduction of these bonds.[52]

Theories of Pathogenesis. Two theories of the etiology of nontropical sprue have been proposed. One is an enzyme deficiency; the other, an immunologic mechanism. Neither is entirely satisfactory in view of present knowledge.

One hypothesis considers the primary defect to be a congenital or hereditary deficiency in the enzymatic processes of digestion. Absorption of gluten or gliadin peptides through the intestinal mucosa is impaired, and the accumulated indigestible peptides are toxic.[58] Exacerbation can be induced in celiac patients by pepsin, trypsin,[52] crude pancreatic enzyme,[58] and peptic-tryptic (fraction III) digests of gluten. The fraction III digest retains toxicity after being autoclaved. Digests prepared by papain,[52] hog intestinal peptidases, total acid hydrolysis, and deamidation with 1N HCl for 45 minutes,[58] inactivate gluten and its enzymatically derived peptides.

The ultrafiltrate of a peptic, tryptic, crude pancreatic enzyme digest of gliadin, eluted with water from a cation exchange resin yields two groups of polypeptides. Both are toxic to celiac patients but not to control subjects. One group contains 22 acidic polypeptides. Each polypeptide is rich in glutamic acid or glutamine, or both. The other contains 17 polypeptides, glutamic acid or glutamine, or both, and proline.[58] Another peptide containing six to seven amino acids, mainly glutamine and proline, has been postulated to be the celiac activating fragment.[52] Glutamine was proposed as the toxic component of gliadin, and elevated serum glutamine levels after ingestion of gluten or gliadin were demonstrated in celiac patients. This response was not consistent and was not demonstrable in all laboratories.[52] The jejunal mucosa of celiac patients has been demonstrated not to liberate proline from a peptic-tryptic digest of gliadin.[52] This apparent enzyme defect occurs in other disorders and reverts to normal, as do other jejunal enzyme activities, in celiac patients following remission associated with abstinence from gluten.[61, 63] These observations suggest that the enzymatic deficiencies are secondary to the disease. This situation may be analogous to the occurrence of lactase deficiency associated with intolerance of milk protein. These patients tolerate lactose during abstinence from milk protein.[52]

Other observations have suggested a possible immunologic mechanism. These are: (1) favorable response to adrenocroticosteroid therapy, (2) infiltration of the lamina propria with increased numbers of lymphocytes, plasma cells, eosinophils, and macrophages, (3) presence of humoral auto-antibodies to small intestinal epithelium in untreated celiac patients,[58] (4) occurrence of "acute gliadin shock" in a few celiac patients following ingestion of small quantities of gluten (this resembles anaphylactic reactions with forceful emesis, diarrhea, pallor, tachycardia, and shock, and manifestations are not alleviated by adrenocorticosteroids), (5) a higher incidence of precipitating and hemagglutinating[52] antibodies in sera from patients with nontropical sprue than in controls, (6) demonstration of precipitins to the peptic-tryptic digest of gluten in intestinal secretions of patients with celiac disease,[57] and (7) immunologic anomalies associated with steatorrhea responsive to a gluten free diet.[52]

The immunologic data do not establish the pathogenesis of nontropical sprue. The response to steroids and the histologic characteristics are not specific for immunologic disorders. Additional studies of the auto-antibodies in sera of celiac patients have not demonstrated reactivity against epithelial cell cytoplasm.[58] "Acute gliadin shock" is unusual, and celiac patients may require large quantities of wheat to produce acute symptoms.[52] Humoral antibodies in celiac patients are not limited to gluten; antibodies against other foods, such as milk proteins[54, 58] and eggwhite[58] also occur. These antibodies may be a result of increased permeability to food proteins by diseased intestine.

The relationship of precipitating antigluten antibodies in gastrointestinal secretions to the pathogenesis of nontropical sprue is unclear. These antibodies were postulated to be produced by the gut and were presumed to be IgA immunoglobulins.[57] Nontropical sprue has been reported in a patient with no IgA in the serum or duodenal secretions, and immunofluorescent staining of the small bowel biopsy specimen revealed absence of plasma cells containing IgA from the lamina propria.[59] The case suggests that intestinal antigluten IgA antibodies are unnecessary for development of nontropical sprue. Plasma cells containing IgG and IgM were present in the biopsy specimen, but antigluten antibodies were not sought. Jejunal biopsies have demonstrated more IgG- and IGM-containing plasma cells in the lamina propria from treated and untreated patients with nontropical sprue than from controls. Plasma cells containing IgA were present in similar numbers among all groups.[62] The antigluten antibodies in intestinal secretions remain to be classified, and a causal relationship has not been demonstrated.

Sera from celiac patients often contain elevated concentrations of IgA,[52] and many have isolated deficiency of IgM. These abnormalities disappear during abstinence from gluten. Steatorrhea and villous atrophy, often responsive to gluten free diet, occur in patients with absent or markedly decreased serum IgA,[52] in patients with depressed IgA and IgG levels,[55] and in patients with acquired and congenital hypoimmunoglobulinemia.[52] Patients with nontropical sprue have been described with atrophic lymphoid tissue, small fibrotic spleens, impaired antibody response to typhoid-paratyphoid vaccine, and Howell-Jolly bodies in circulating erythrocytes.[52] Steatorrhea is common in lymphopenic hypoimmunoglobulinemia.[51] Many diverse defects in the humoral immune system are associated with celiac syndromes, but none appears consistently. No specific humoral immune abnormality seems necessary for the pathogenesis of all cases of nontropical sprue. Antigen binding activity of intestinal lymphoid cells of patients with celiac disease has been studied by immunofluorescent techniques.[52] No binding of gliadin by inflammatory cells or by immunoglobulins within cells of the lamina propria was demonstrated. Lymphoma of the small intestine appears to be a complication of nontropical sprue.[53]

The possibility of a delayed hypersensitivity mechanism has been evaluated. Cutaneous tests with gluten are negative.[56] Lymphocytes from patients with nontropical sprue often have a subnormal blastogenic response when cultured in the presence of phytohemagglutinin. One study suggested that the defect was a serum factor, not an abnormality in the lymphocytes.[65] Another demonstrated increased blastogenic transformation in the presence of gluten fraction III.[66] This evidence for delayed hypersensitivity was considered a consequence of a primary mucosal lesion allowing abnormal access of antigenic gluten fragments to immunologically competent cells in the gut wall. This could also explain the production of antibodies. A chronic delayed hypersensitivity reaction, even though secondary, could possibly aggravate the primary mucosal lesion.

Some evidence suggests that nontropical sprue may be inherited through a dominant gene of incomplete penetrance.[60] Female monozygotic twins who are discordant for the disease have been reported.[58] This suggests that nongenetic factors are important.

Ulcerative Colitis

Ulcerative colitis is characterized by mucosal ulcerations in the colon and rectum with abdominal cramps, diarrhea, and hematochezia. Spread is in continuity. Crypt abscesses occur in any stage of the disease. Pseudopolyposis, shortening due to thickening of the colonic muscles and toxic megacolon occur in severe cases. Carcinomatous degeneration, benign strictures, and spontaneous free perforation are complications, and partial villous atrophy in small intestinal biopsies has been reported. Extracolonic manifestations include arthritis, uveitis, and involvement of the skin, liver, and biliary tract. Cutaneous lesions include erythema nodosum, pyoderma gangrenosum, papulonecrosis, and erythematous plaques on the shins. Liver and biliary tract diseases include fatty degeneration, hepatitis, cholangitis, and pericholangitis. Involvement of the entire portal triad and the hepatic parenchymal cells may simulate chronic active hepatitis. Bridging portal hepatofibrosis is apparently the most common form of cirrhosis, but postnecrotic cirrhosis has also been observed.[66]

Theories of Pathogenesis. Attempts to explain the etiology of ulcerative colitis include infection, mucolytic enzymes, allergy, autoimmunity, psychological factors, ischemia,[50, 66] and genetic predisposition.[49] The evidence supporting these hypotheses is inconclusive. Only the immunologic aspects will be discussed here.

The identification of allergy as the etiology of ulcerative colitis is based on the following observations. (1) Patients with ulcerative colitis may have a higher incidence of asthma, urticaria, and allergic rhinitis than members of the general population. (2) Eosinophilia is regularly observed in the colonic and rectal mucosa and in the inflammatory exudate. (3) The histamine content of the rectal mucosa has been increased in some patients. (4) Circulating antibodies against milk have been demonstrated in some patients. (5) Remissions and exacerbations in some patients seem associated, with removal and introduction, respectively, of dietary milk. (6) More patients receiving a milk free diet allegedly remained in remission than patients receiving a dummy diet during one year observation. (7) Titers of circulating antibodies against milk were reported higher among individuals who were weaned early and patients with ulcerative colitis than among individuals who were breast-fed.[50]

This evidence relating ulcerative colitis to allergy is circumstantial and inconclusive. Lactase deficiency is associated with milk intolerance and commonly occurs in ulcerative colitis. Other studies were unable to confirm the apparent benefit of dietary manipulation. The implication of early weaning in patients with ulcerative colitis has not been confirmed. Comparisons of dietary habits of ethnic groups with disparate incidences of ulcerative colitis demonstrated no correlation with consumption of milk.[50] Antibody titers do not correlate with activity of the disease. Antibodies against foods are of doubtful significance.[50, 66]

Autoimmunity is a controversial consideration in the etiology of ulcerative colitis. Antibodies reacting with colonic antigens have been demonstrated. *Escherichia coli* 014 and extracts of colon mucosa contain cross-reactive antigens. These observations suggest that lesions in colon mucosa might possibly result from antibodies against certain bacteria. However, antibodies reacting with colon antigen are sometimes indistinguishable from those reacting with group A substance. Anticolonic antibodies also occur in normal sera. The antibodies persist after colectomy and have no correlation with the clinical features of the disease. Sera containing anticolon antibodies are not cytotoxic for colon cells in vitro. A direct pathogenetic effect of these antibodies appears unlikely.[66] Other studies have suggested that a cytoxic factor in serum migrates in the alpha-2-globulin fraction by electrophoresis.[1] This factor would not be an immunoglobulin, and there seems to be another mechanism operative.

Rectal tissues of patients with ulcerative colitis commonly contain IgA in extracellular interstitial sites, and plasma cells containing IgA are fewer than in normal rectal tissues. The biologic significance of IgA in intestinal disease is undetermined. There is no evidence that immunologic reactions associated with IgE or IgA contribute to the pathogenesis of ulcerative colitis.[66]

Lymphocytes from some patients with ulcerative colitis have a cytotoxic effect upon fetal colon epithelial cells in tissue culture. This effect is rapidly lost after colectomy, suggesting against a delayed hypersensitivity response. This reaction may be a consequence of absorption of bacterial or colon antigen from a diseased intestine. Cytotoxicity for allogenic colon epithelial cells can be induced in lymphocytes from normal individuals by preliminary incubation of the lymphocytes with a lipopolysaccharide extract of *E. coli* 0 119:B 14. Evidence for a possible specific delayed hypersensitivity response to bacterial antigen has also been equivocal.[66]

Delayed hypersensitivity to dinitrochlorobenzene has been induced in the colons of guinea pigs and miniature swine. These lesions have some resemblance to ulcerative colitis. The possible relationship of these observations to the etiology of human ulcerative colitis is unknown.[66]

Although nontropical sprue and ulcerative colitis have features suggesting immunologic pathogeneses, the present evidence is inconclusive. The etiologies of these diseases remain undetermined.

REFERENCES

Food Allergy

1. Barrick, R. H., and Farr, R. S.: The increased incidence of circulating anti-beef albumin in the sera of allergic persons and some comments regarding the possible significance of this occurrence. J. Allerg., 36: 374, 1965.
2. Booth, B. H., and Patterson, R.: Electrocardiographic changes during human anaphylaxis. JAMA, 211:627, 1970.
3. Bronsky, E. A., Burkley, D. P., and Ellis, E. F.: Evaluation of the provocative food test technique. J. Allerg., [abstr.], 47:104, 1971.
4. Chafee, F. H., and Settipane, G. A.: Asthma caused by F. D. C. approved dyes. J. Allerg., 40:65, 1967.
5. Chambers, V. V., Hudson, B. H., and Glaser, J.: A study of the reactions of human polymorphonuclear leukocytes to various allergens. J. Allerg., 29:93, 1958.
6. Clemis, J. D.: Medical management of Meniere's disease. Arch. Otolaryng., 89:116, 1969.
7. Cochrane, C. G.: The role of immune complexes and complement in tissue injury. J. Allerg., 42:113, 1968.
8. Davis, S. D., Bierman, C. W., Pierson, W. E., Maas, C. W., and Iannetta, A.: Clinical nonspecificity of milk coproantibodies in diarrheal stools. New Eng. J. Med., 282:612, 1970.
9. Dees, S. C.: Allergy to cow's milk. Pediat. Clin. N. Amer., 6:881, 1959.
10. Freedman, S. O.: Allergic and toxic mechanisms in occupational lung diseases. Mod. Treatm., 3:838, 1966.
11. Freedman, S. S.: Skin testing for food sensitivity: Its clinical significance. Pediat. Clin. N. Amer., 6:853, 1959.
12. Fries, J. H.: Factors influencing clinical evaluation of food allergy. Pediat. Clin. N. Amer., 6:867, 1959.
13. Golbert, T. M.: Treatment of gastrointestinal and food allergy. Mod. Treatm., 5:852, 1968.
14. Golbert, T. M., Patterson, R., and Pruzansky, J. J.: Systemic allergic reactions to ingested antigens. J. Allerg., 44:96, 1969.
15. Goldman, A. S., et al.: Milk allergy. I. Oral challenge with milk and isolated milk proteins in allergic children. Pediatrics, 32:425, 1963.
16. Goldstein, G. B., and Heiner, D. C.: Clinical and immunological perspectives in food sensitivity. J. Allerg., 46:270, 1970.
17. Gray, I., Harten, M., and Walzer, M.: Studies in mucous membrane hypersensitiveness. IV. The allergic reactions in the passively sensitized

mucous membranes of the ileum and colon in humans. Ann. Intern. Med., *13*:2050, 1940.

18. Greenberger, N. J., Tennenbaum, J. I., and Ruppert, R. D.: Protein-losing enteropathy associated with gastrointestinal allergy. Amer. J. Med., *43*:777, 1967.
19. Grogan, F. T.: Food allergy in children after infancy. Pediat. Clin. N. Amer., *16*:217, 1969.
20. Gruskay, F. L., and Cooke, R. E.: The gastrointestinal absorption of unaltered protein in normal infants and in infants recovering from diarrhea. Pediatrics, *16*:763, 1955.
21. Gryboski, J. D.: Gastrointestinal milk allergy in infants. Pediatrics, *40*: 354, 1967.
22. Heiner, D. C., Wilson, J. F., and Lahey, M. E.: Sensitivity to cow's milk. JAMA, *189*:563, 1964.
23. Hill, L. W.: Immunologic relationships between cow's milk and goat's milk. J. Pediat., *15*:157, 1939.
24. Ingelfinger, F. J., Lowell, F. C., and Franklin, W.: Gastrointestinal allergy. New Eng. J. Med., *241*:303, 337, 1949.
25. Ishizaka, K., and Ishizaka, T.: Human reaginic antibodies and immunoglobulin E. J. Allerg., *42*:330, 1968.
26. Johnstone, D. E.: Food allergy in children under two years of age. Pediat. Clin. N. Amer., *16*:211, 1969.
27. Katz, J., Spiro, H. M., and Herskovic, T.: Milk-precipitating substance in the stool in gastrointestinal milk sensitivity. New Eng. J. Med., *278*:1191, 1968.
28. Kriebel, G. W., Kraft, S. C., and Rothberg, R. M.: Locally produced antibodies in human gastrointestinal secretions. J. Immunol., *103*:1268, 1969.
29. Lietze, A.: Laboratory research in food allergy. I. Food allergens. J. Asthma Res., *7*:25, 1969.
30. Lippard, V. W., Schloss, O. M., and Johnson, P. A.: Immune reactions induced in infants by intestinal absorption of incompletely digested cow's milk protein. Amer. J. Dis. Child., *51*:562, 1936.
31. Marks, R., and Whittle, M. W.: Results of treatment of dermatitis herpetiformis with a gluten-free diet after one year. Brit. Med. J., *4*:772, 1969.
32. Patterson, R.: Skin-sensitizing antibodies. Adv. Intern. Med., *16*:351, 1970.
33. Peterson, R. D. A., and Good, R. A.: Antibodies to cow's milk proteins— their presence and significance. Pediatrics, *31*:209, 1963.
34. Pollard, H. M., and Stuart, G. J.: Experimental reproduction of gastric allergy in human beings with controlled observations on the mucosa. J. Allerg., *13*:467, 1942.
35. Ratner, B., and Gruehl, H. L.: Passage of native proteins through the normal gastro-intestinal wall. J. Clin. Invest., *13*:517, 1934.

36. Reid, R. T., Minden, P., and Farr, R. S.: Biological and chemical differences among proteins having reaginic activity. J. Allerg., *41*:326, 1968.
37. Ruddy, S., Gigli, I., Sheffer, A. L., and Austen, K. F.: The laboratory diagnosis of hereditary angioedema. *In* Rose, B., *et al.*: Allergology. pp. 351-359. Amsterdam, Excerpta Medica Foundation, 1968.
38. Self, T. W., *et al.*: Gastrointestinal protein allergy. Immunologic considerations. JAMA, *207*:2393, 1969.
39. Sheldon, J. M., Lovell, R. G., and Mathews, K. P.: A Manual of Clinical Allergy. ed. 2. pp. 196-225. Philadelphia, W. B. Saunders, 1967.
40. Smith, R. E.: Treatment of atopic dermatitis. Mod. Treatm., *5*:866, 1968.
41. Stull, A., and Hampton, S. F.: A study of the antigenicity of proteoses. J. Immunol., *41*:143, 1941.
42. Tada, T., and Ishizaka, K.: Distribution of γ E-forming cells in lymphoid tissues of the human and monkey. J. Immunol., *104*:377, 1970.
43. Taub, S. J.: Enuresis is allergic in origin in many instances. Eye Ear Nose Throat Monthly, *48*:82, 1969.
44. Thorn, G. W.: Approach to the patient with "idiopathic edema" or "periodic swelling". JAMA, *206*:333, 1968.
45. Townley, R. R. W.: Disaccharidase deficiency in infancy and childhood. Pediatrics, *38*:127, 1966.
46. Van Metre, T. E., *et al.*: A controlled study of the effects on manifestations of chronic asthma of a rigid elimination diet based on Rowe's cereal-free diet 1, 2, 3. J. Allerg., *41*:195, 1968.
47. Walzer, M., Gray, I., Strauss, H. W., and Livingston, S.: Studies in experimental hypersensitiveness in the rhesus monkey. J. Immunol., *34*: 91, 1938.
48. Wintrobe, M. M.: Clinical Hematology. ed. 6. pp. 886-934. Philadelphia, Lea and Febiger, 1967.

Nonreaginic Gastrointestinal Disorders

49. Burch, P. R. J., de Dombal, F. T., and Watkinson, G.: Aetiology of ulcerative colitis. II. A new hypothesis. Gut, *10*:277, 1969.
50. de Dombal, F. T., Burch, P. R. J., and Watkinson, G.: Aetiology of ulcerative colitis. I. A review of past and present hypotheses. Gut, *10*:270, 1969.
51. Gitlin, D. and Craig, J. M.: The thymus and other lymphoid tissues in congenital agammaglobulinemia. I. Thymic alymphoplasia and lymphocytic hypoplasia and their relation to infection. Pediatrics, *32*:517, 1963.
52. Goldstein, G. B., and Heiner, D. C.: Clinical and immunological perspectives in food sensitivity. J. Allergy, *46*:270, 1970.
53. Harris, O. D., Cooke, W. T., Thompson, H., and Waterhouse, J. A. H.: Malignancy in adult coeliac disease and idiopathic steatorrhoea. Gut, *7*:710, 1966.
54. Heiner, D. C., and Rose, B.: A study of antibody responses by radioimmunodiffusion with demonstration of γ D antigen-binding activity in four sera. J. Immunol., *104*:691, 1970.

55. Hermans, P. E., Huizenga, K. A., Hoffman, H. N. II, Brown, A. L., and Markowitz, H.: Dysgammaglobulinemia associated with lymphoid hyperplasia of the small intestine. Amer. J. Med., *40:*78, 1966.
56. Housley, J., Asquith, P., and Cook, W. T.: Immune response to gluten in adult coeliac disease. Brit. Med. J., *2:*159, 1969.
57. Katz, J., Kantor, F. S., and Herskovic, T.: Intestinal antibodies to wheat fractions in celiac disease. Ann. Intern. Med., *69:*1149, 1968.
58. Kowlessar, O. D., and Phillips, L. D.: Celiac disease. Med. Clin. N. Amer., *54:*647, 1970.
59. Mann, J. G., Brown, W. R., and Kern, F. J.: The subtle and variable clinical expressions of gluten-induced enteropathy (adult celiac disease, non-tropical sprue). An analysis of twenty-one consecutive cases. Amer. J. Med., *48:*357, 1970.
60. MacDonald, W. C., Dobbins, W. O., and Rubin, C. E.: Studies on the familial nature of celiac sprue using biopsy of the small intestine. New Eng. J. Med., *272:*448, 1965.
61. Plotkin, G. R., and Isselbacher, K. J.: Secondary disaccharidase deficiency in adult celiac disease and other malabsorption states. New Eng. J. Med., *271:*1033, 1964.
62. Søltoft, J.: Immunoglobulin-containing cells in non-tropical sprue. Clin. Exp. Immunol., *6:*413, 1970.
63. Welsh, J. D., Zschiesche, O. M., Anderson, J., and Walker, A.: Intestinal disaccharidase activity in celiac sprue (gluten-sensitive enteropathy). Arch. Intern. Med., *123:*33, 1969.
64. Weser, E., and Sleisenger, M. H.: Pathophysiology of sprue syndromes. Adv. Intern. Med., *15:*253, 1969.
65. Winter, G. C. B., McCarthy, C. F., Read, A. E., and Yaffey, J. M.: Development of macrophages in phytohemagglutinin cultures of blood from patients with idiopathic steatorrhea and with cirrhosis. Brit. J. Exp. Path., *48:*66, 1967.
66. Wright, R.: Ulcerative colitis. Gastroenterology, *58:*875, 1970.

15

Atopic Dermatitis

Dale B. Sparks, M.D.

Atopic dermatitis is one of the most commonly diagnosed dermatoses presenting itself to family physicians, dermatologists and allergists. Its importance is emphasized by its severity and, at times, its long-term morbidity. Atopic eczema was first described by Besnier and Brocq in 1885 and became known in Europe as prurigo Besnier and is still described in European medical literature under this eponym. In 1934, Coca first used the name atopic dermatitis because of the observation that flexoral eczema, dermatitis, allergic rhinitis and bronchial asthma were frequently associated in a single patient. In Europe, the most frequently used name for the disease remains prurigo Besnier. It is also called flexoral eczema, infantile eczema, neurodermatitis, eczema pruriginosum allergicum, diathetic eczema and several other names. In the United States, the disease is most commonly called atopic dermatitis or neurodermatitis.

The derivation of the term neurodermatitis is interesting in that Brocq changed Besnier's first name for the disease of pruritus with lichenification to neurodermatitis, meaning by this that cutaneous receptors for itching sensation were particularly susceptible. It was not meant to imply that the disease was due to an emotional disturbance but rather to a difference in nerve end organ response in the skin.

The affected child frequently develops other atopic diseases in later years, and there is often a strong history of atopic disease in the family. Hellerstrom and Lidman [8] stated that 86 percent of the cases they studied occurred during the first five years of life, 60 percent of cases in the first year of life. The disease, rarely, if ever, starts before 1 month of age.

The actual incidence of atopic dermatitis in the general population is unknown because many cases are so mild that they never come to medical attention. It has been estimated that 1 to 3 percent of children in the first two years of life are affected by some degree of infantile eczema. Walker and Warin [12] estimated that 3.1 percent of children in Bristol, England, had eczema.

The incidence of atopic dermatitis in adults is also unknown but is certainly much less than that stated for infants and children. Hill [7] has stated that the incidence of atopic dermatitis may be decreasing. Hospital admissions to the Boston Children's Hospital for atopic eczema decreased from an average of 435 children in the period from 1930 to 1935, to 42 cases in 1959. This may not represent an actual decrease in incidence but rather may reflect the fact that more effective outpatient treatment was available in 1959 than in the 1930 to 1935 period. There may be a slight predominance of the number of males over females in the infantile group with reversal of the ratio in the older group and among adults.

Atopic eczema usually starts as an erythematous, dry eruption on the face that becomes pruritic. The patches of desquamation may spread into the scalp, forehead and neck, making the differential diagnosis of seborrheic dermatitis difficult, if not impossible in infancy. Some authors make no effort to separate the two diseases in infants and believe that they may be the same disease. Ultimate distinction between seborrheic dermatitis and infantile eczema depends on the subsequent course and clinical progress of the disease process. Characteristically, the patches of desquamation gradually turn from their early erythematous appearance to a brownish color, and with the passage of time, the skin becomes thickened, xerotic and lichenified. The disease may fluctuate in severity, clearing almost completely at times only to recur either spontaneously or subsequent to some local or systemic insult to the patient.

In a number of cases, the disease spontaneously improves about age three and becomes quiescent until age ten to twelve when in the prepubertal stage the disease again becomes active. At this time, the disease assumes the characteristics of adult atopic eczema characteristically located on the flexoral surfaces of the antecubital and popliteal spaces. It is, however, generally not limited to these areas and usually spreads to the nape of the neck, face, scalp, backs of the hands and chest. The abdomen is usually less severely involved. The skin of the palms and soles is generally spared from the disease. As the dermatitis becomes chronic, the skin is less apt to clear completely; once it has become lichenified and pigmented, it rarely clears completely.

ETIOLOGY

The etiology of atopic dermatitis is unknown. In the early 1930's it was generally recognized that there was a strong association between atopic dermatitis, allergic rhinitis and bronchial asthma. At that time, the atopic hypothesis of Feinberg was formulated as follows: "From previous contact with a specific allergen such as food, a specific reagin develops which attaches itself to tissue cells. Re-introduction of the specific antigen into the body causes an antigen-antibody reaction. When this reaction takes place in the cells of the capillary loop of the corium, subsequent inflammatory and exudative changes result in the entity recognized as atopic dermatitis. Wheal formation takes place beneath the epidermis with resulting irritation and thickening." [4]

The atopic hypothesis of the etiology of atopic eczema is not accepted currently because some 20 percent of the patients with atopic eczema do not have demonstrable reagin. The second major reason for rejection of the atopic hypothesis is that in a large majority of patients, the offending agent or agents cannot be identified and removed from the environment with clearing of symptoms. There is, however, general agreement that about 75 percent of patients with atopic eczema have a strong family history of other atopic diseases or themselves have or develop asthma or hay fever. Immunologically, the patients have reaginic antibody against a variety of antigens. Many authors over the years have denied any causal relationship between the presence of reagin and disease process. It is, however, striking that the patient may occasionally clear completely when he is removed from his usual environment. Engman, Weiss, and Engman [3] studied a child with atopic dermatitis who developed a severe exacerbation everytime he ate wheat. This was confirmed on several repeat observations. Subsequently, one side of the body was wrapped in an occlusive dressing so that the child could not scratch that half of the body. The lesions of atopic dermatitis did not develop on the half of the body under the occlusive dressing. That scratching is highly important in the development of atopic dermatitis is well established. Areas of the body inaccessible to scratching do not develop lichenification and are usually spared from the changes of atopic dermatitis.

Wheat, milk and eggs are usually cited as the most common foods producing exacerbations of atopic dermatitis. None of the foods, however, can be consistently incriminated as a causative agent. In the very young infant, cow's milk is frequently thought to be a causal agent and a change to soybean based food may yield great improvement. The presence of antibodies to cow's milk in infants is not closely associated with the development of atopic dermatitis. Infantile eczema is, however, reported in infants that have been fed mother's breast milk, supporting the view that sensitinogens other than food allergens are significant in the development of atopic eczema.

It has been suggested that sensitivity to human dander can precipitate atopic dermatitis. There is an increased incidence of positive skin test reactions to extracts of human dander in these patients. There is no definitive evidence that either autogenous or exogenous human dander is a true causative factor. The possibility of an auto-immune reaction to dermal cells has also been suggested but remains unproven.

DIAGNOSIS AND DIFFERENTIAL DIAGNOSIS

The diagnosis of atopic eczema in the severe case is usually obvious. The disease manifests itself by marked itching of the flexoral surfaces of the antecubital fossae and popliteal spaces. These areas rapidly become lichenified, and this is followed by pigmentation.

Characteristically, atopic eczema does not develop until after the first month of life, although the casual history obtained in the older child is one of "eczema all of my life."

Atopic eczema should be differentiated from other skin diseases of infancy and childhood. Diaper rash can be distinguished because of the obvious difference in location. Differentiation from seborrheic dermatitis and "cradle cap" is probably impossible during infancy, but the diagnosis usually becomes obvious with the passage of time.

There are other dermatoses of infancy and childhood that should be differentiated from infantile eczema because of the great difference in prognosis. Histiocystosis X (Letterer-Siwe syndrome) usually begins between 9 months and 1 year of age and presents as a diffuse eczema with petechiae, hepatosplenomegaly, lymph node enlargement and bone destruction. Biopsy of skin shows reticulum cells with large nuclei and eosinophilic cytoplasm. The course of histiocytosis X is progressive, nearly always leading to a fatal termination within months or years. The Aldrich syndrome consists of eczema, thrombocytopenia and recurrent infections. It is also characterized by petechial hemorrhages, diffuse eczema, and it usually appears before the first year of life. The disease progresses to death within the first five years of life; the cause of death is usually an infection such as pneumonia or otitis media.

The differentiation of atopic dermatitis from chronic dermatitis venenata is usually made on the basis of the distribution of the eruption. Dermatitis venenata most characteristically involves the hands and forearms while sparing the antecubital and popliteal spaces. Contact dermatitis from nickel or cadmium usually presents no serious problem in differential diagnosis because of the location of the dermatitis in an area of contact with metal. Shoe dye dermatitis should be considered when the areas involved are on the feet and lower legs, but, again, the characteristic locations of atopic dermatitis are spared. Fixed drug eruptions, such as those caused by phenobarbital and bromides, may create a problem in differential diagnosis in the adult. An adequate history of drug ingestion should alert the examiner to this possibility.

The chronicity of atopic eczema in the adult is helpful in the differential diagnosis. Symptoms generally are seasonally variable with a flare during the winter months and improvement during the summer. This is quite variable in individual patients, and when a definite season of exacerbation of symptoms can be identified, it may sometimes suggest a precipitating factor such as a pollen or contactant.

PATHOLOGY

The skin changes observed microscopically in atopic eczema depend solely on the acute or chronic state of the disease. They are not pathognomonic for the disease. The pathologist cannot differentiate chronic dermatoses such as contact dermatitis from atopic eczema. In acute atopic eczema there is exudation into the intracellular spaces of the stratum corneum with the formation of intra-epidermal vesicles leading to spongiosis. In addition, there is edema in the intracellular and intercellular spaces with dilated blood vessels. Multilocular vesicles separated by thin septa consisting of resistant walls of epidermal cells may be formed. The edema and vesicle formation is the cause of exudation onto the skin. As the disease becomes chronic, there is proliferation of the epidermal cells, leading to acanthosis, imperfect keratinization and hyperkeratosis with areas of parakeratosis with retention of nuclei in the cells of the horny layer. During the late stage, there is no vesicle formation and pigmentation occurs. During the chronic phase, the inflammatory cellular response usually consists of lymphocytes with occasional mast cells and eosinophils. Fibroblasts also occur in the late stages of the disease.

The gross pathological changes are those of papular or papulovesicular lesions measuring 1 to 2 millimeters without evidence of petechial hemorrhages. As the disease progresses, there is coalescence of lesions into plaques followed by lichenification and pigmentation.

IMMUNOLOGIC AND PHYSICAL MANIFESTATIONS

Patients with atopic eczema have serum levels of immunoglobulin E (IgE) significantly greater than the levels found in normal subjects or in patients with allergic rhinitis or bronchial asthma. Juhlin [9] has shown that patients with atopic eczema have serum concentrations which average 2,733 ng./ml. compared to the normal values of 248 ng./ml. IgE. The lowest values he reported were 240 ng./ml. and 460 ng./ml.

in two patients with negative intradermal skin tests. The highest level found was 31,750 ng./ml. There appeared to be no correlation between the level of IgE elevation and the severity of the disease. There was also no correlation between degree of lgE elevation and the presence of bronchial asthma or hay fever. Eighty-two percent of the patients with atopic dermatitis had levels of more than 1,000 ng./ml. of IgE and 93 percent of the patients with atopic dermatitis had levels in excess of 550 ng./ml. Gunnar and Juhlin [6] have shown that the IgE level is restored to normal when the patients have been free of eczema for 2 years. This is true even if eczema of the hand or nummular eczema persists. They have also shown that the treatment of atopic dermatitis with prednisone or azathioprine produces no significant change in the level of IgE. Screening tests of other common dermatoses, such as allergic contact dermatitis, nummular eczema, stasis dermatitis and non-specific chronic dermatitis, showed no significant elevation of IgE.

Fontana [5] has shown that the complement titers in children with atopic eczema are normal. He has also shown that gamma globulin levels are usually normal, except when superimposed infection is present.

Significant increases in catecholamine content of the skin have been noted in atopic dermatitis. The importance of this remains unknown. Blanchard [1] has shown that the level of catechol-o-methyl transferase is elevated in affected areas of skin and normal in unaffected areas of skin both in patients with atopic dermatitis and those with nonspecific dermatitis. Attempts to control symptoms with anti-catecholamine agents, however, have been unsuccessful.

Vascular changes, white dermagraphism and delayed blanching of skin have all been noted in atopic dermatitis. A decrease in skin temperature of the fingers with decreased blood flow in the fingers but normal blood flow elsewhere has been observed. Bystran [2] has shown that skin blood flow varied according to the presence and acuteness of skin lesions. When no skin lesions were present, the skin flow was low, but with the development of acute inflammatory lesions the skin blood flow increased to six times the normal value. Atopic individuals with chronic dermatitis had skin blood flow which was not significantly different from that of normal persons.

White dermographism and delayed blanching had long been clinically observed in atopic dermatitis. Normal skin reacts to rubbing by erythema which gradually pales and fades away. In atopic dermatitis, rubbing the skin produces immediate redness that is replaced in 15 to 30 seconds by pallor persisting for 1 to 3 minutes. Abnormal responses to intradermal acetylcholine or methacholine have been described and reproduced in patients with atopic dermatitis. In such patients, a flare develops around the injection site as in normal skin but is slowly replaced by pallor that persists for 15 to 30 minutes. In the past the cause of this pallor has been attributed to vasoconstriction, whereas in the normal individual, the erythema has been attributed to vasodilation. Ramsay [10] has demonstrated that the vasodilation response occurs in both normal and atopic eczematous skin as demonstrated with a photo-electric pulse meter. He and others have postulated that the white dermographism, then, is due to edema rather than the previously suggested vasoconstriction. Approximately 70 percent of patients with atopic dermatitis will show the delayed blanch to acetylocholine and related drugs. The delayed blanch, however, may not be present in unaffected "normal skin" of atopic individuals.

COMPLICATIONS

The most common complication of atopic eczema is bacterial infection of the skin in areas where it has been opened to the environment by persistent scratching. The infection is usually staphylococcal or streptococcal with the occasional formation of an erysipelas-type of fulminant lesion. Otitis externa is particularly common with exudation of dermal cells into the external canal leading to occlusion. Otitis media is also a common complication because of contiguous infection and occlusion of the external auditory canal. The development of respiratory infections with pneumonia is more common in this group of patients than in the general population and may lead to sudden death within days after the development of a febrile illness in children with atopic eczema. This complication as well as those of staphylococcal and streptococcal infections of the skin have become less of a clinical problem with the development of antibiotics.

The development of viral infections of the skin such as eczema vaccinatum or eczema herpeticum is a catastrophic event when it occurs. These lesions cannot be differentiated clinically but can be differentiated immunologically by acute and convalescent serological studies on serum. Vaccination of patients with atopic eczema for smallpox is extremely hazardous and is contraindicated. In instances of exposure to smallpox or for patients living in an endemic area of smallpox, the use of a special attenuated smallpox vaccine with the concomitant use of hyperimmune gamma globulin may be indicated. Vaccination of other members of the family also may be hazardous as the patient with atopic eczema, living in the same environment, may develop excema vaccinatum with systemic involvement from contact with the recently vaccinated person.

Cataract formation during the third decade of life is markedly more frequent in patients with atopic eczema than in the general population. The typical cataract is a dense, subcapsular plaque with radiating fibers in the anterior or posterior cortex, first occurring centrally in the pupil, then spreading through the periphery of the lens until it becomes opaque. A second type of cataract which occurs less frequently starts subcapsularly at the posterior pole and sends out striae which also involve the anterior cortex. These cataracts occur, characteristically, much earlier in life than do the usual cataracts. Their removal is accompanied by a much higher incidence of complications than the usual cataract surgery. Other eye complications consist of atopic keratoconjunctivitis, uveitis and conical cornea with cataract. Retinal detachment also occurs more commonly in the population of patients with atopic dermatitis.

TREATMENT

The principles of treatment of atopic dermatitis evolve into specific measures designed to elucidate and eliminate any precipitating factors involved in exacerbations of the disease and in the nonspecific local and systemic treatment of the dermatitis.

The physician primarily interested in allergy may well approach this type of patient with a careful allergy history to evaluate the importance of foods, animal danders, possible contactants, detergents and soaps in the environment. In addition, he should employ skin testing to detect the atopic state and to search for clues to any possible offending agent. This approach has been discarded by many dermatologists who feel that results are as good using nonspecific systemic and local therapy without an effort to demonstrate etiological agents.

The use of skin tests to evaluate the patient with atopic eczema may be helpful in establishing the diagnosis. They may suggest approaches which could help control the eczema by eliminating an offending antigen. Skin tests against some antigens will be positive in approximately 80 percent of the cases of atopic eczema, and these must be interpreted with caution. Carefully controlled elimination diets, however, for a period of 2 weeks appear to be appropriate to see if improvement can be obtained. In this disease, which has a high morbidity rate and chronicity spreading over many years and even a lifetime, efforts to find an etiological agents should be undertaken even though such efforts are often unsuccessful. To deny the patient such attempts because an etiological agent cannot be identified in all cases does not appear to be warranted.

The basic principle of specific treatment would be to avoid those antigens which may potentiate atopic eczema, such as wheat, milk, eggs, seafoods, as well as house dust and mold spores. Any effort at control of the environment to alleviate symptoms of atopic eczema should be continued for a period of at least 2 weeks and probably 1 month. Caution should be taken not to place a child or an adult on a deficient diet for long periods of time when no specific results are obtained from initial elimination of a food. It has been noted that contact with wool is often quite irritating to the patient with atopic dermatitis, however, usually no specific reaginic activity against wool can be demonstrated. While no evidence of wool as an antigen has been obtained, the physical irritation of skin in patients with atopic dermatitis by wool suggests that direct contact with skin is best avoided. If woolen sweaters are worn, a cotton shirt or blouse should be next to the skin. Silk has also been incriminated as a possible etiological agent in some cases, however, this too appears to be uncertain. Clinical findings show it to be very irritating to the typical patient with atopic dermatitis; it produces itching, perhaps by inducing perspiration. The fabric best tolerated is cotton, and it should be used next to the skin and for bedding.

The benefit of desensitization injections in atopic eczema remains unproven.

A hot, humid climate that promotes sweating aggravates the itching and the atopic dermatitis. Likewise a cold, dry climate that produces dryness and painful fissuring of skin similarly exacerbates the condition. The ideal climate for the patient with atopic eczema is a temperate, dry climate. This may not be feasible for socioeconomic reasons. Recommending a climate change is rarely indicated.

Soaps and detergents may be particularly irritating and the avoidance of all soap is essential in the acute and subacute phases. Infrequent bathing is generally recommended by most physicians. Baths should be tepid and of short duration. The use of special fatty soaps may be indicated for use with the limited bathing.

Topical treatment of atopic eczema consists of the application of adrenal cortical steroid creams, coal tar derivatives or both. The most spectacular advance in recent years in the management of atopic eczema has been the use of steroid creams and ointments. The application of steroid cream to large portions of the body may be associated with systemic absorption and subsequent adrenal suppression. This is particularly true where the skin is denuded which increases systemic absorption. The use of occlusive dressings (like Saran film) over an area of lichenified skin may be particularly helpful in clearing an area such as the antecubital space or popliteal fossa. The use of coal tar derivatives (such as 5 percent liquor carbonis detergens or 1 percent crude coal tar) may be used. These are less effective than the steroid creams but can be used with fewer complications. They are particularly useful in mild cases requiring therapy over many years.

The topical therapy of secondary infection can be accomplished with bacitracin or neomycin ointment. These can also be effectively combined with steroid cream. However, it is important to remember that these antibiotics may superimpose contact dermatitis. The use of topical penicillin or antihistamines should be avoided because of the frequent occurrence of contact dermatitis from these medications.

Systemic therapy of atopic dermatitis is directed at relief of the constitutional symptoms, extreme nervousness and tension, that accompany persistent itching. This can be accomplished most simply with an inexpensive sedative (phenobarbital) or with a mild tranquilizer (chlordiazepoxide hydrochloride, Diazepam).

Systemic steroid therapy may be necessary at times because of the severity of the dermatitis. Courses of systemic steroids should be of short duration and should be used only to control severe manifestations. Atopic eczema responds rapidly to systemic steroid therapy. The course of this disease is usually prolonged; and steroid therapy should not be used on a permanent basis because of the complications of long term steroid therapy. Psychotherapy and psychological counseling may, at times, be somewhat helpful in controlling anxiety and the hostility of the patient by allowing him to ventilate his emotions. In general, formal psychotherapy has not been particularly successful in controlling atopic eczema.

Radiation therapy and ultraviolet light have both been used in the past, and although superficial x-ray therapy does give some relief of the itching, its use is not recommended.

PROGNOSIS

The prognosis in atopic eczema is uncertain in any individual case. In general, symptoms tend to appear after the first month of life and to improve spontaneously by the second to fifth year of life. Many patients may later develop allergic rhinitis and bronchial asthma. The atopic eczema may return in adulthood. If the atopic eczema does reappear in adult life, the longer it persists, the more likely it is to develop into a chronic lifelong problem. Areas of severe lichenification and deep pigmentation rarely, if ever, return completely to normal. In the sixth and seventh decades. the disease usually becomes quiescent, leaving only the pigmented areas. Death from atopic eczema is rare except for the complications of eczema vaccinatum.

REFERENCES

1. Blanchard, J.: Catechol-o-methyl transference in skin patients with atopic dermatitis. J. Invest. Derm., 52:100-102, 1969.
2. Bystryn, J. S., *et al.*: Skin blood flow in atopic dermatitis. J. Invest. Derm., 52:189, 1968.

3. Engman, F. F., Weiss, R. S., and Engman, M. F. L.: Eczema and environment. Med. Clin. N. Amer., *20:*651, 1936.

4. Feinberg, S. M.: Seasonal atopic dermatitis: the role of inhalant atopens. Arch. Derm. Syph., *40:*200, 1939.

5. Fontana, V. J.: Complement titer C reactive protein and electrophoretic serum protein patterns in eczematous children. New York J. Med., *62:*2801, 1962.

6. Gunnar, S., Johansson, O., and Juhlin, L.: Immunoglobulin E in "healed" atopic dermatitis and after treatment with corticosteroids and azathioprine. Derm. *82:*10-3, Jan., 1970.

7. Hill, L. W.: Certain aspects of allergy in children. New Eng. J. Med., *265:*1298, 1961.

8. Hellerstrom, S., and Lidman, H.: Studies of Besnier's prurigo. Acta Dermatovener, *36:*11, 1956.

9. Juhlin, L., *et al.:* Immunoglobulin E in dermatoses. Levels in atopic dermatitis and urticaria. Arch. Derm., *100:*12, 1969.

10. Ramsay, C.: Vascular changes accompanying white dermographism and delayed blanch in atopic dermatitis. Brit. J. Derm., *81:*37, 1969.

11. Singh, G., *et al.:* Atopic erythroderma with bilateral cataract, unilateral keratoconus and iridocyclitis, and undescended testes. Brit. J. Opthal., *52:*61, 1968.

12. Walker, R. B., and Warin, R. P.: The incidence of eczema in early childhood. Brit. J. Derm., *68:*686, 1956.

16

Drug Allergy

Richard D. DeSwarte, M.D.

THE COMPLEXITY OF THE PROBLEM

A consequence of the rapid development of new drugs to diagnose and treat human illnesses has been the increased incidence of adverse reactions to these agents which may produce additional morbidity and, on occasion, mortality. Their occurrence violates a basic principle of medical practice, *primum non nocere* (above all do no harm). It is a sobering fact that adverse drug reactions are responsible for the majority of iatrogenic illnesses. Fortunately, most reactions are not severe, but the predictability of seriousness is usually not possible in the individual case or with the individual drug.

Prior to the introduction of the sulfonamides to medicine in the late 1930's, adverse drug reactions were estimated to occur in 0.5 to 1.5 percent of patients. The thalidomide catastrophe of 1961 focused increasing attention by physicians, the pharmaceutical industry, the public and government regarding the relative safety of those drugs in current use and other drugs which were planned for introduction into clinical practice. The magnitude and seriousness of the current problems are suggested by results of intensive hospital monitoring.[74, 33, 28] Up to five percent of all patients admitted to hospitals were suffering from drug reactions, and 30 percent of these patients develop a second reaction while hospitalized. Fifteen to 30 percent of all hospitalized patients develop drug reactions, doubling their hospital stay in many cases.

The frequency of drug reactions increases with the number of drugs given. The average hospitalized patient receives six to ten drugs simultaneously. Occasional patients receive more than 20 drugs simultaneously; here there is a 40 percent chance of developing adverse reactions to one or more drugs. Unfortunately, only a small proportion of adverse drug reactions occurring in outpatients are voluntarily reported to national registries by physicians and dentists. This is further complicated by the fact that it is often difficult to implicate with certainty a particular drug with observed symptoms. As drugs may be responsible for a wide variety of clinical manifestations, it is sometimes difficult to separate the drug reaction from the disease being treated. The simultaneous administration of multiple therapeutic agents further confuses the establishment of cause and effect. Despite these limitations, epidemiologic data have proved informative; an example of which was the discovery of an excess number of asthmatic deaths in the period 1961-1967, attributed by some to the injudicious use of pressurized bronchodilator aerosols.[81]

It is unlikely that the possibility of adverse reactions to a new drug can be eliminated prior to general clinical use. Preliminary animal testing is often carried out in inbred rodents where the response is often uniform for that strain of rats because of genetic homogeneity. Man, by contrast, is outbred. The metabolism and ultimate handling of drugs by man is influenced by a variety of individual differences. Some of these are genetically controlled, such as physiologic and immunologic differences. Others are not genetically controlled. Environmental factors and certain diseases being treated are examples. For the determination of the incidence and severity of reactions to a drug in man, the most definitive results are obtained from studies of man. Even here, the incidence of adverse reactions to a drug cannot be predicted on the basis of the usual types of clinical trial. A series of 200 patients treated without a reaction does not exclude the statistical possibility that one may occur in 1 out of 38 patients treated with that drug. Even a "safe" drug may bring ill effects to someone if it is used widely enough.

Although much attention has been given to adverse drug reactions as a medical problem, the economic consequences have been overlooked. Approximately one seventh of hospital days are devoted to the treatment of drug reactions, at an estimated cost of 3 billion dollars annually.[89] The direct costs of treating drug reactions, while at times formidable, are only a part of the picture.[91] Considerable expense is involved in efforts to detect and prevent such reactions. Detection costs are those involved in finding early evidence of a drug-induced problem; for example, monitoring blood counts of patients receiving cytotoxic drugs. Prevention costs are expenses incurred to reduce the possible occurrence of an adverse reaction; for example, the use of antacids by patients receiving corticosteroids or the administration of uricosuric agents and potassium supplements to patients on thiazide diuretics.

Although the intent of this chapter is to discuss *allergic* drug reactions, which probably account for only 25 percent of adverse drug reactions, preventative measures outlined later are applicable to all drug reactions, regardless of mechanism.

CLASSIFICATION OF DRUG REACTIONS

A *drug* may be defined as any substance used in diagnosis, treatment or prevention of disease. An *adverse drug reaction* may be considered as any unintended or undesired consequence of drug therapy. Although it may be difficult to classify a particular drug reaction, a useful classification, based on that of Brown,[11] is the following:

Classification of Adverse Drug Reactions

Adverse Reactions Occurring in Normal Patients
    Overdosage
    Side effects
    Secondary or indirect effects
    Drug interactions

Adverse Reactions Occurring in Susceptible Patients
    Intolerance
    Idiosyncrasy (Pharmacogenetics)
    Allergy or Hypersensitivity

Overdosage

The toxic effects of a drug are directly related to the systemic or local concentration of the drug in the body. Such effects are usually predictable on the basis of animal experimentation and may be expected in any patient provided a threshold level has been exceeded. Each drug tends to have its own characteristic toxic effect(s). Overdosage may result from an excess dose taken accidentally or deliberately. It may be due to accumulation as a result of some abnormality in the patient which interferes with normal metabolism or excretion of the drug. The toxicity of morphine is enhanced in the presence of liver disease (inability to detoxify the drug) or myxedema (depression of the metabolic rate). The toxicity of chloramphenicol in infants is due to immaturity of the glucuronide conjugating system allowing a toxic concentration to accumulate. In the presence of renal failure, drugs such as streptomycin, kanamycin, digitalis and potassium, normally excreted by this route, may accumulate and produce toxic reactions.

Side effects

A side effect can best be defined as a therapeutically undesirable, but often unavoidable pharmacologic action of a drug. These constitute the most frequent adverse drug reactions and often occur following normal drug doses. A drug frequently has several pharmacologic actions, and only one of these may be the desired effect. The others must be considered side effects. The dose of the drug can often be adjusted to produce the maximum desired pharmacological action with a minimum of undesired effects. Pertinent examples in the diagnosis and treatment of allergic disorders include the drowsiness associated with antihistamine therapy and the central nervous system and cardiac stimulation after sympathomimetics.

The development of minor side effects may be useful in adjusting the dose of a drug, since benign side effects may warn the physician about potentially more serious toxicity. The development of gastrointestinal symptoms after digitalis administration allows dosage manipulation to avoid serious cardiac arrythmias. Side effects may be alleviated by combining medications, such as the common practice of including barbiturates or tranquilizers with ephedrine (e.g., Tedral *, Marax †) to reduce central nervous system stimulation. However, one must be aware of the potential role of the additive in also producing side effects. Barbiturates rather than ephedrine may actually be responsible for stimulation in some patients, particularly the very young and older individuals.

An interesting and unusual side effect, which might even warrant separate classification, is the *nonimmunologic release of histamine* following administration of certain drugs such as morphine, codeine, Demerol,‡ strychnine, stilbamidine, polymyxin B, thiamine and d-tubocurarine. § It is possible that immediate reactions resulting from iodinated radiographic contrast media, aspirin and dextrans may be on this basis. This group of reactions are particularly confusing as they resemble established immunologic allergic reactions in which histamine is released as a result of an antigen-antibody interaction with consequent development of flushing, pruritis, urticaria, angioedema, bronchospasm and, occasionally, hypotension. A differential point is that these reactions often occur in nonatopic patients without prior exposure to these substances.

Secondary or Indirect Effects

These are indirect effects of a drug which are unrelated to its primary pharmacological action and which may not occur in all patients. Of concern is the fact that some of these secondary effects may be interpreted as the appearance of another naturally occuring disease, rather

* Trademark, Warner Chilcott.
† Trademark, Roerig.
‡ Trademark, Breon.
§ Trademark, Upjohn.

than being associated with administration of a drug. There are a variety of examples of this. The ecologic disturbance of the normal interrelationships among gastrointestinal microorganisms by the administration of broad spectrum antibiotics may result in overgrowth of drug resistant staphylococci and the development of psuedomembranous enterocolitis. The same mechanism may permit the overgrowth of monilia and destruction of intestinal bacteria responsible for vitamin B synthesis, thus producing moniliasis and vitamin B deficiency. Gout may develop as a consequence of treatment of myeloproliferative disorders with antimetabolites. The Herxheimer reaction is attributed to flooding of the body with large quantities of dead organisms and their products as a result of antimicrobial therapy, producing clinical manifestations. Drug addiction may be an indirect consequence of narcotic therapy.

Drug Interactions

Multiple drug therapy is therapeutically beneficial in the treatment of certain disorders such as tuberculosis, hypertension and neoplastic diseases, especially acute leukemia. However, the response to multiple drug therapy is not necessarily equal to the sum of the known responses to the separate administration of each drug. As a consequence of combined therapy, dramatic manifestations such as hemorrhage, severe hypoglycemia and hypertensive crises have occurred. These perplexing responses to multiple drug therapy have become known as "drug interactions," which are defined as the action of an administered drug upon the effectiveness or toxicity of another drug administered earlier, simultaneously or later. Hospitalized patients receive an average of ten drugs, whereas outpatients receive only six. As the number of drugs taken concurrently increases, the chance of an important drug interaction follows a curve of geometric progression. The danger of a drug interaction is greatest when several physicians are treating a patient, each for a separate condition. It is the responsibility of a physician to determine what other medications his patient is taking. An increasing number of recent publications have dealt with this problem.[80, 8, 55] Some of the more important mechanisms whereby drugs can influence the action of others will be explained briefly with representative examples.

Drug Interactions in Vitro. Interactions of drugs mixed in bottles for intravenous infusion are well known. Kanamycin and methicillin inactivate each other. Levarterenol should be given in solutions containing dextrose to prevent oxidation. Tetracyclines are photo-oxidized by the riboflavin in vitamin B complex and rendered inactive.

Interference with Drug Absorption. Many drugs interact in the gastrointestinal tract before absorption. Antacids will lower the rate of absorp-

tion of acidic drugs, such as aspirin, phenylbutazone (Butazolidin *),
nitrofurantoin (Furadantin †), nalidixic acid (NegGram ‡), some sulfonamides, oral anticoagulants, penicillin G and barbiturates. The antacids
enhance the absorption of basic drugs such as alkaloids and amphetamines. Drugs may be complexed in the gut lumen to retard their absorption. For example, aluminum and calcium salts in antacids bind
with tetracyclines, kaolin preparations bind lincomycin, and cholestyramine reduces the amount of thyroxine absorbed.

Diphenylhydantoin (Dilantin §) administration may produce a folate-
deficient megaloblastic anemia in susceptible individuals. This results
from inhibition of intestinal wall conjugase enzymes required to convert
poorly absorbed polyglutamate to the more readily absorbed monogluta-
mate form. Other drugs which may produce a similar effect include
nitrofurantoins, oral contraceptives and triamterene (Dyrenium ||).

Drugs with anticholinergic properties, such as the tricyclic antidepressants and many other tranquilizers, may retard absorption of drugs by
decreasing intestinal motility. Cathartics may have the same effect by
speeding the passage of drugs through the gastrointestinal tract.

Protein Binding. Following absorption, most drugs are bound to tissue
and plasma proteins (particularly serum albumin) and, in this form,
are pharmacologically inert. Only the free form can exert a pharmacologic action. For this reason, any second drug with a higher affinity for
the mutual binding site may displace another drug, thus resulting in more
unbound drug which may then exert its pharmacologic action and
produce untoward effects.

The most important interactions of this type involve the displacement
of anticoagulants with resultant hemorrhagic complications. Warfarin anticoagulants may be displaced by phenylbutazone (Butazolidin **), oxy-
phenbutazone (Tandearil **), indomethacin (Indocin ††) and clofibrate
(Atromid-S ‡‡). Salicylates can displace protein-bound penicillin analogs,
long-acting sulfonamides and chlorpropamide (Diabinese §§); the latter
resulting in hypoglycemia. Methotrexate can be displaced by salicylates
and sulfonamides, thereby resulting in pancytopenia.

Interference with Metabolism. Drugs may interact through interference

---

* Trademark, Geigy.
† Trademark, Eaton.
‡ Trademark, Winthrop.
§ Trademark, Parke, Davis.
|| Trademark, Smith Kline & French.
** Trademarks, Geigy.
†† Trademark, Merck Sharp & Dohme.
‡‡ Trademark, Ayerst.
§§ Trademark, Pfizer.

with metabolism, thus enhancing or inhibiting each others' breakdown. Most drugs are metabolized by enzymes located in the hepatic endoplasmic reticulum. Certain drugs, notably phenobarbital, stimulate the increased production of these hepatic microsomal enzymes, a process referred to as enzyme induction, resulting in more rapid metabolism of the drug itself or of other drugs administered simultaneously. The most familiar example of this interaction is between phenobarbital and the warfarin anticoagulants, frequently given simultaneously after myocardial infarction. Due to phenobarbital's effect on the liver microsomal enzymes, much larger doses of anticoagulant are required to maintain therapeutic efficacy. Sudden withdrawal of the sedative may then result in increased anticoagulant activity and hemorrhage. In addition to barbiturates, the metabolism of warfarin anticoagulants is accelerated by glutethimide (Doriden *), chloral hydrate, meprobamate, ethchlorvynol (Placidyl †), griseofulvin and diphenylhydantoin (Dilantin ‡).

Enzyme induction by drugs may be useful, as phenobarbital also stimulates the production of another hepatic enzyme, bilirubin glucuronyl transferase, which converts bilirubin to a more rapidly excreted form. Infants with kernicterus are given phenobarbital to hasten elimination of bilirubin.

Some drugs may impede the metabolism of others, resulting in increased activity of the latter. Dicumarol interferes with the metabolism of Dilantin and Orinase §, resulting in toxicity of the latter. Severe bone marrow depression has resulted from simultaneous administration of allopurinol to patients receiving azathioprine or 6-mercaptopurine to control hyperuricemia. Allopurinol inhibits the enzyme, xanthine oxidase, which is required for metabolism of these antimetabolites.

Enzyme systems other than those in the hepatic endoplasmic reticulum are affected by drugs. The most dramatic example concerns monoamine oxidase (MAO). This enzyme is inhibited by antidepressants such as isocarboxazid (Marplan ||), nialamide (Niamid #), phenelzine (Nardil **) and tranylcypromine (Parnate ††), and by the antihypertensive agent, pargyline (Eutonyl †). Such inhibition results in a build-up of various biogenic amines within the adrenergic neuron. Subsequent administration of drugs that release norepinephrine from the adrenergic

* Trademark, Ciba.
† Trademark, Abbott.
‡ Trademark, Parke, Davis.
§ Trademark, Upjohn.
|| Trademark, Roche.
Trademark, Pfizer.
** Trademark, Warner Chilcott.
†† Trademark, Smith Kline & French.

neuron may produce a hypertensive crisis. Such drugs as ephedrine, amphetamine, phenylephrine, phenylpropanolamine, guanethedine, reserpine and alpha methyldopa should not be given to patients receiving MAO inhibitors. Even naturally occurring amines, such as tyramine, found in aged cheese, wines, canned figs, chicken livers and pickled herring, may release norepinephrine and should be avoided by such patients.

Interference with Drug Excretion. As many drugs are weak acids, they compete for renal weak-acid-secreting sites. Thiazide diuretics compete for uric acid-secreting sites and result in elevation of the plasma uric acid level. Other drugs with a similar capacity include low doses of salicylates, penicillin and acetylated sulfonamides. Low dose salicylates in particular are apt to increase the concentration of other simultaneously administered acidic drugs.

A drug may modify the excretion of another by altering the urine pH. Acidic drugs, for example salicylates, phenylbutazone and phenobarbital, are excreted more rapidly in an alkaline urine; basic drugs, for example, amphetamines and chloroquine, are more promptly excreted at an acid pH. Acetazolamide (Diamox *) alkalinizes the urine and enhances excretion of acidic drugs.

The activity of a drug may be enhanced by blocking tubular secretion of that substance by another drug. Probenecid, by retarding the tubular secretion of penicillin, may be useful in raising the serum concentration of the antibiotic. Phenylbutazone interferes with the renal clearance of hydroxyhexamide, a metabolite of acetohexamide (Dymelor †), often resulting in hypoglycemia.

Finally, electrolyte disturbances produced by one drug may affect the toxicity of another. Diuretic therapy, resulting in potassium loss, may make the patient more susceptible to digitalis intoxication and may increase the effect of curariform drugs.

Interference at the Adrenergic Neuron. Following an appropriate stimulus, norepinephrine is released from postganglionic adrenergic neurons to exert an effect on alpha or beta receptors. However, most is taken up again by the nerve terminal, and its activity terminates. This uptake mechanism is shared by other amines such as ephedrine, amphetamines and guanethedine, and is blocked by the tricyclic antidepressants, such as imipramine (Tofranil ‡) and amitriptyline (Elavil §). Guanethidine (Ismelin ||) must be taken up by the nerve terminal to exert its anti-

* Trademark, Lederle.
† Trademark, Lilly.
‡ Trademark, Geigy.
§ Trademark, Merck Sharp & Dohme.
|| Trademark, Ciba.

hypertensive effect. This effect may then be negated by the tricyclic antidepressants.

Interactions at the Receptor Site. To be effective, a drug must bind to a receptor site in sufficient quantity to exert its activity. D-Thyroxine increases the affinity between warfarin and its receptor site in the liver, thereby enhancing the anticoagulant effect.

Drugs are used excessively often without adequate indications. It is expected that there will be increasing problems with drug reactions, due to both the increased number of drugs available and the problem of drug interactions. The physician will have great difficulty keeping up, but he must do so, and he must be aware of all agents prescribed for his patients. The trend should be toward more cautious use of polypharmacy and limitation of the number of agents prescribed to those that are truly indicated.

Intolerance

A characteristic pharmacologic effect of the drug is produced by an unusually small dose. Most patients develop tinnitus on large doses of salicylates or quinine, but a few experience this after a single dose of average or smaller amounts than usual. It is likely that this does not represent a qualitative difference in the susceptible individual but merely one extreme of normal biologic variation.

Idiosyncrasy

This term is used to describe a qualitatively abnormal response to a drug, differing from its pharmacological effects and thus resembling allergy or hypersensitivity (See below). However, the reaction does not involve an immunologic mechanism. Susceptible patients often possess an inherited enzyme abnormality, not expressed under normal conditions, but aggravated by the administration of certain drugs. The study of these problems has been termed "pharmacogenetics." [20]

The most familiar example of this is the hemolytic anemia occurring in about 13 percent of Negro American males (sex-linked dominant) receiving oxidant drugs. The erythrocytes of such individuals lack glucose-6-phosphate dehydrogenase (G-6-P-D), an enzyme necessary for aerobic metabolism of glucose and, consequently, cellular integrity. Enzyme deficient cells cannot protect themselves against oxidant drugs and are hemolyzed. Although the original observations of this phenomenon were among susceptible individuals receiving primaquine, a large number of oxidant drugs can produce hemolysis and include other antimalarials, sulfonamides, sulfones, nitrofurans, acetanilid, aminopyrine, antipyrine, phenacetin, aminosalicylic acid, probenecid, phenylhydrazine, methylene blue and vitamin K. Contact with naphthalene and fava beans has produced a similar reaction. This problem is of particular concern as many of the "over the counter" cold remedies, antipyretics and analgesics contain some of these substances. Fortunately, susceptible individuals can be identified by finding increased amounts of reduced glutathione in their red cells after incubation with acetylphenylhydrazine.

Other examples would include the prolonged apnea after administration of suxamethonium compounds among certain patients with an inherited abnormality of the enzyme psuedocholinesterase; the development of peripheral neuritis after isoniazid among patients lacking acetyl transferase, an enzyme that normally inactivates the drug; the development of hemolysis and severe methemoglobinemia among patients with a rare hemoglobin type—hemoglobin Zurich—following administration of sulfonamides.

It is reasonable to expect that many drug reactions, classified or unclassified, may eventually be proven to have a genetic basis.

Allergy or Hypersensitivity

Like idiosyncratic reactions, allergic drug reactions occur in only some patients, are qualitatively abnormal and are unrelated to the pharmacologic action of the drug. Unlike idiosyncrasy, they are the result of an immune response to a drug following prior exposure to the same drug or to a chemically related substance leading to production of specific antibodies or sensitized cells, or both. Ideally, the term should be reserved for those reactions known or presumed to be the result of an immunologic mechanism.

Drug allergy requires separate consideration from allergic reactions in general. Although drugs may produce the spectrum of the common allergic manifestations discussed elsewhere in this book, many manifestations of drug allergy—drug fever, a variety of skin rashes, hepatic and hematologic reactions and collagen disorders—are rarely, if ever, produced by naturally encountered allergens, such as pollens. It is not possible to demonstrate an immunologic mechanism in most allergic drug reactions, and very frequently the diagnosis is inferred on clinical grounds using some of the following criteria:

1. The observed manifestations do not resemble the known pharmacological actions of the drug.

2. The presence of a latent period during which the drug has been taken with no ill effects. This latent period may vary from a few days to many years, but is commonly 7 to 10 days after initiation of drug administration. Once allergic sensitization has occurred, the reaction upon reexposure to the drug may be immediate and explosive.

3. Once a reaction has occurred, it generally recurs upon readministra-

tion of the same, or a closely related, drug often in minute doses and even after long intervals.

4. Such reactions may occur only in a minority of persons receiving the drug.

5. At times, the reaction is characteristic of other classical allergic reactions—anaphylaxis, serum sickness, urticaria and angioedema, asthma and contact dermatitis; but often, as noted above, it is not.

6. Because pathologic changes are rarely characteristic, these, eosinophilia, and the response to antiallergic measures may be helpful but generally do not give a specific diagnosis of a reaction from a particular drug.

This classification of adverse drug reactions must be considered tentative. At times, it is difficult to place a drug reaction under one of these headings. The common practice of labeling any drug reaction as "allergic" should be discouraged. With the development of better diagnostic techniques, more accurate classification seems likely. However, the rapid introduction of new synthetic drugs provides an ever-changing picture.

FACTORS INFLUENCING THE DEVELOPMENT OF DRUG ALLERGY

Although the exact reasons why a patient develops hypersensitivity to a drug often remain unknown, certain factors do seem to influence the likelihood of sensitization.

Factors Influencing the Development of Drug Allergy

Drug Factors
Nature of the drug
Route of administration
Degree of exposure

Patient Factors
Age and sex
Presence of atopy
Prior drug reactions
Underlying diseases

Drug Factors

Nature of the Drug. Some drugs, such as milk of magnesia, rarely produce reactions; whereas others, such as Nirvanol *, do so in the majority of those exposed. It is difficult to predict the sensitizing capacity of a drug prior to widespread clinical use on the basis of its chemical

---

* 5-Ethyl-5-phenylhydantoin

structure. The capacity to sensitize depends on the ability of the drug itself or one or more of its reactive metabolites to bind firmly with circulating and tissue proteins and function as haptens. Once sensitization to a drug has occurred, the possibility of reactivity to related drugs is present because of antigenic similarity. Much information on cross-sensitization has come from studies on allergic contact dermatitis (Type IV reaction) in animals and is probably not as generally applicable to allergic drug reactions in man mediated by other immunologic mechanisms.[19]

The range of cross-sensitization varies so greatly between individuals that it is often difficult to predict. However, certain commonly used drugs have similar chemical structures, and it is safest to substitute drugs of an entirely different chemical composition once a suspected hypersensitivity reaction has occurred. Familiar examples include chemical similarity between procaine, aminosalicylic acid, sulfanilamide and sulfadiazine; between sulfonamides and related compounds such as sulfonylurea hypoglycemic agents, thiazide diuretics and carbonic anhydrase inhibitors; and among the phenothiazine derivatives such as chlorpromazine, promazine, trifluoperazine and thioridazine.

Although numerous drugs have been implicated in the production of allergic reactions, particularly common drug allergens are listed below, and some will receive special attention at the end of this chapter. Penicillins, aspirin and sulfonamides account for 80 to 90 percent of allergic drug reactions.

Common Drug Allergens

Aspirin	Barbiturates	Organ extracts (ACTH, insulin)
Penicillins	Anticonvulsants	Heavy metals
Sulfonamides * †	Local anesthetics	Sera and vaccines
Antituberculous drugs	Phenolphthalein	Tranquilizers
Nitrofurans	Quinine and quinidine	Antithyroid drugs
	Iodides and bromides	Aminopyrine

* Includes antibacterials, diuretics and oral hypoglycemics.

† The term sulfonamides will include the antibacterials, the oral hypoglycemic agents tolbutamide, (Orinase °), chlorpropamide (Diabenese), etc., the thiazide diuretics chlorothiazide (Diuril), chlorthalidone (Hygroton) etc., and the carbonic anhydrase inhibitors acetazolamide (Diamox).

° Trademark, Upjohn; Pfizer; Merck Sharp & Dohme; Geigy; Lederle, respectively.

Route of Administration. Topical application of a drug is associated with a high sensitization risk and should be avoided with certain agents, especially on inflamed skin. Certain drugs, such as penicillin and sulfonamides are no longer used topically because of this risk. Oral administration of a drug is generally safer than any type of parenteral administration; however, severe reactions have followed this mode of administration.

Degree of Exposure. There is some evidence to suggest that sensitization is more likely with higher drug doses and prolonged administration, but clinically this does not appear to be important. Of greater importance are intermittent courses of therapy which clearly predispose to sensitization. The incidence of penicillin reactions among patients receiving long term prophylaxis is extremely low.

Patient Factors

Age and Sex. The incidence of drug allergy in children is considerably less than in adults; a circumstance which has never been satisfactorily explained. One possibility is that children have not had the repeated exposure to drugs necessary to result in sensitization. There is some evidence suggesting that older adult patients are not as readily sensitized. Sex does not appear to be an important factor.

Presence of Atopy. It has been suggested that allergic reactions to drugs occur more frequently in atopic persons. It appears that this is true of penicillin but is less convincing for other drugs.[51] If indeed this were true for all drugs, it might simply reflect an increased exposure to medications by atopic individuals. The atopic state does not predispose to development of contact sensitivity to topically applied medications.

Prior Drug Reactions. There is some evidence that patients who have demonstrated drug hypersensitivity in the past may have an increased tendency to develop sensitivity to new drugs, and one should be more cautious in medicating such patients.

Underlying Diseases. Patients with systemic lupus erythematosus are reported to have a higher incidence of allergic drug reactions than other chronically ill patients requiring similar medications, but this has never been well substantiated. It has been suggested that such is possible because of increased immunologic responsiveness of such patients. On the other hand, patients with some immunologic impairment, such as hypogammaglobulinemia, sarcoidosis and Hodgkin's disease would be expected to be less prone to allergic reactions.

IMMUNOCHEMICAL BASIS OF DRUG ALLERGY

Only a few drugs in current usage, such as foreign antisera, papain, insulin and other organ extracts, are complete antigens in the usual sense and are capable of inducing sensitization. All of these are high molecular weight proteins of animal or plant sources. The vast majority of drugs implicated in allergic reactions are simple chemicals with a relatively low molecular weight, usually less than 1000. Landsteiner first showed that low molecular weight compounds become antigenic only after forming firm (covalent) bonds with circulating or tissue proteins, thus forming a hapten-protein conjugate. The resultant conjugate then induces antibody formation, cellular sensitization, or both. The simple chemical, nonantigenic by itself, now directs the specificity of sensitization as a chemical-protein conjugate. The immunologic response is primarily directed against the simple chemical group which serves as the antigenic determinant, although some reactivity may be elicited against the protein carrier. The reason for the need of a carrier protein is not known, but a minimal molecular size may be required for appropriate antigen processing.

The understanding of the immunochemistry and reactivity of simple chemical-protein conjugates derived from this experimental work has been applied to human allergic drug reactions. This application remains theoretical in most human allergic drug reactions because neither the actual drug-protein conjugates nor the antibodies or sensitized cells have been isolated. The use of this concept in considering certain drug allergic reactions is useful and logical.

To further complicate the picture, most drugs do not appear capable of binding irreversibly with protein to form the necessary conjugate to produce sensitization. Here, it appears that a degradation product or metabolite of the drug may be more reactive and capable of firm binding with tissue and serum proteins to form the complete antigen. Such chemical derivatives formed by the metabolism of penicillin have been demonstrated by Parker [51] and Levine [42] and will be discussed later under the section dealing with this drug. The use of the unaltered drug for testing to detect sensitivity would not be expected to detect immunologic responses resulting from a drug metabolite. Such haptenic determinants for drugs other than penicillin have not been identified, but it appears likely that allergic reactions to many of these drugs are also produced by metabolites. Even if the appropriate haptens were known, they must be combined to a suitable macromolecule for testing. The information gleaned from the penicillin work is a good foundation for expanded investigation, but it also emphasizes the complexity of the problem.

In summary, several steps are presumed to be required in the induction and elicitation of an allergic response to a simple chemical drug:

1. The chemical reaction of the drug, or more likely a degradation product or metabolite of the drug, to form covalent bonds with tissue or serum proteins resulting in a hapten-protein conjugate.

2. The induction of antibodies, sensitized lymphocytes, or both, by the hapten-protein conjugate acting as a complete immunogen or antigen.

3. Upon readministration of the drug and reformation of the conjugate, an allergic reaction may occur.

Gell and Coombs have proposed a useful classification of immunopathologic mechanisms by which cellular or tissue injury may occur after contact with an antigen, once the sensitized state has developed.[24] This was discussed in Chapter 1 and may be applied to allergic drug reactions. Although this cannot be done with certainty, it may aid in selecting tests that would be helpful in diagnosis and also the most appropriate therapy. Types I and IV reactions may be detected by a skin test, providing the appropriate haptenic determinant is available, while Types II and III may be detected by the classic serologic methods of antibody detection. Regarding treatment, Type I reactions would be expected to respond to antihistamines and sympathomimetics, while the other types may require corticosteroids.

The immunologic response to a given antigen may be quite diverse, and drugs are no exception. Penicillin serves to illustrate this point. Anaphylactic or urticarial reactions due to penicillin are an example of Type I reactions; the hemolytic anemia due to penicillin is Type II; the serum sickness-like reaction, now most commonly due to penicillin, is Type III; while the contact dermatitis from topically applied penicillin is an example of a Type IV reaction.

CLINICAL PATTERNS OF DRUG ALLERGY

The clinical manifestations of drug allergic reactions are protean and not specific or unique for drug hypersensitivity. Similar clinical patterns may be produced by other allergens or on a nonimmunological basis. It is likely that many such reactions are not recognized and are attributed to the illness for which the drug(s) were prescribed, and vice versa. As syphilis was once considered the great imitator, drug allergy has now become the great mimic of disease. A minor drug reaction may progress, if unrecognized, to a more severe, even fatal, reaction. As was pointed out for penicillin, some drugs may produce a wide spectrum of clinical manifestations, further complicating the situation. On occasion, certain types of reactions are more apt to be related to certain drugs, for example, the fixed drug eruption due to phenolphthalein.

A discussion of the more common manifestations generally thought to be allergic in nature is presented here. For most of these reactions, definite immunological proof of an allergic mechanism is lacking. A brief description of these manifestations follows with a listing of the more familiar drugs known to be associated with them. For more detailed information, the monographs by Alexander and Martin [46a] and periodic literature reviews by Meyler [50] are available.

Clinical Manifestations of Drug Allergy

CUTANEOUS
Contact dermatitis
    Allergic eczematous contact dermatitis
    Systemic eczematous "contact-type" dermatitis
Dermatitis medicamentosa
    Pruritis
    Urticaria and angioedema
    Exanthematic eruptions
    Exfoliative dermatitis
    Erythema-multiforme-like eruptions
        Stevens-Johnson syndrome
    Erythema-nodosum-like eruptions
    Fixed drug eruptions
    Purpuric eruptions
        Henoch-Schönlein (Anaphylactoid) purpura
    Photosensitivity
Other drug-induced dermatoses (possibly allergic)
    Eczematous eruptions
    Vesiculobullous eruptions
    Toxic epidermal necrolysis
    Lichen-planus-like eruptions
    Vasculitis
Other drug-induced dermatoses (not allergic)
    Acneiform eruptions
    Tumors
    Pigmentary changes
    Alopecia

SYSTEMIC
Anaphylaxis
Serum sickness syndrome
Pulmonary manifestations
    Bronchial asthma
    Hypersensitivity lung disease
    Loeffler's-type syndrome
    Interstitial fibrosis
    Vasculitis
Drug fever
Hematological manifestations
    Eosinophilia

Thrombocytopenia
Hemolytic anemia
Agranulocytosis
Hepatic manifestations
Cholestasis
Hepatocellular damage
Collagen-vascular manifestations
Vasculitis
Polyarteritis
Reactions simulating systemic lupus erythematosus
Lymphadenopathy
Nephropathy
Neurologic reactions

CUTANEOUS MANIFESTATIONS

The most frequent manifestations of drug allergy are dermatalogical. Drugs may produce almost any kind of skin eruption, although contact dermatitis, urticaria and exanthematous eruptions are the most common. The majority of drug eruptions are of mild or moderate severity and pose no threat to life or subsequent health. On occasion, they may be severe and even life-threatening such as exfoliative dermatitis, toxic epidermal necrolysis and Stevens-Johnson syndrome. Further, an innocent-looking eruption may progress to a more disturbing one if the cause is not recognized and the drug continued. Unfortunately, the appearance of the eruption is usually not characteristic enough to implicate a drug as the most likely etiology. However, some eruptions are characteristic enough to suggest drug etiology, for example, the fixed drug eruption due to phenolphthalein. Some more typical features of drug eruptions include an acute onset usually within 1 to 2 weeks after drug exposure, symmetric distribution, predominant trunk involvement, brilliant coloration and pruritus. Systemic features, such as fever, may also be present.

As a maxim, any eruption appearing in a patient receiving drugs should be scrutinized for a possible association. However, one should be cautious in automatically labeling any eruption as drug-induced, as it may be due to the disease itself. A good example is the exanthem due to a viral illness, arising during penicillin or antibiotic therapy which frequently results in incorrectly branding that particular patient as "allergic" to the drug.

Contact Dermatitis

Allergic Eczematous Contact Dermatitis is produced by medications applied topically to the skin and mucous membranes sensitized by the same or a chemically similar drug previously applied to it. The clinical picture resembles contact dermatitis from other causes discussed in Chapter 17. This diagnosis should be suspected when the condition for which the topical preparation is being applied fails to respond or becomes worse. Some individuals develop contact sensitivity merely by handling materials in their occupation. Nurses are prone to develop such reactions on the hands by handling penicillin and streptomycin, while dentists may develop a similar problem from local anesthetics. Commonly incriminated topical medicaments include: local anesthetics, antihistamines, mercurials, penicillin, parabens, sulfonamides, streptomycin, neomycin, and Furacin.*

Topical penicillin and sulfonamides are so highly sensitizing that this route of administration has been largely abandoned. A problem of increasing magnitude relates to contact dermatitis to the paraben esters (methyl- ethyl-, propyl- and butyl parahydroxybenzoate) used as preservatives in most dermatologic and cosmetic creams and lotions. Patients with chronic dermatitis may develop paraben sensitivity due to repeated applications of various topicals, particularly corticosteroid creams. Females may become sensitized through use of cosmetics containing these substances. Paraben allergy should be suspected in any patient with intractable dermatitis not responding to, or even worsening on, local therapy. The diagnosis may be established by patch testing using 5 percent paraben esters in petrolatum. Once the diagnosis has been established, there are several choices of treatment. If the dermatitis will tolerate a greasy preparation, corticosteroid ointments, may be used, as they do not contain preservatives. If more acute, corticosteroid creams or lotions may be necessary and selection of one utilizing other preservatives is indicated. Such preparations include Hytone,† Valisone,‡ and Synalar-E §. It is possible to develop contact sensitivity to preservatives in these preparations, but there is no cross-reactivity with the paraben esters. When these alternatives are substituted, the dermatitis generally subsides promptly.

Systemic Eczematous "Contact-Type" Dermatitis describes the eruption developing in some patients by the systemic administration of a drug to which the patient has been previously sensitized by topical application of that drug or an antigenically related substance. A partial list of commonly used topical sensitizers with immunochemically similar drugs that may produce such an eruption upon systemic administration would include:

* Trademark, Eaton.
† Trademark, Hytone.
‡ Trademark, Schering.
§ Trademark, Syntex.

Topical	Systemic
Neomycin	Kanamycin, streptomycin
Para-amino compounds (e.g., local anesthetics)	PAS, sulfonamides
Mercurials (e.g., ammoniated mercury and merthiolate)	Mercurial diuretics
Hydroxyquinolines (e.g., Vioform)	Diodoquin, Vioform

A more detailed review of this problem is available in the excellent monograph by Fisher.[22] The diagnosis of drug-induced contact dermatitis by patch testing is identical to other forms of contact dermatitis described in Chapter 17.

Dermatitis Medicamentosa

Pruritus is often a conspicuous feature of many drug eruptions; in fact, its absence raises doubt that drug allergy is causative in a case of dermatitis. On occasion, it may be the only manifestation or it may precede other cutaneous or systemic manifestations. The earliest indication of gold toxicity may be transient pruritus and should be considered in any patient receiving gold therapy. As many rheumatologists now consider this preparation second to salicylates in treatment of rheumatoid arthritis, the incidence of this problem may increase. Sulfonamides may also produce pruritus as an isolated symptom.

Urticaria and Angioedema frequently occur alone, but are also common features of the serum sickness-like reaction discussed later under systemic manifestations (Fig. 16-1). The eruption does not significantly differ from urticarias of diverse etiologies discussed in Chapter 13. However, wide distribution of giant urticaria should raise the suspicion of a drug etiology. A drug etiology must be considered in the evaluation of any patient with chronic urticaria. Although a long list of drugs have been incriminated, particularly common drug allergens include: penicillin, salicylates, organ extracts, foreign antisera, sulfonamides, and allergy extracts. Histamine release by a nonimmunologic mechanism resulting in urticaria and angioedema was discussed earlier under the section dealing with side effects.

Exanthematous Eruptions are often difficult to distinguish from the common viral exanthems (Fig. 16-2). This is confusing because some of the common offending drugs may have been used to treat these viral diseases. The appearance of the drug-induced rash may be erythematous, macular, papular, morbilliform or scarlatiniform and is usually acute in onset and widespread, particularly involving the trunk. Although pruritus is a conspicuous feature of eczematous allergic dermatitis discussed earlier, it is more variable in this group. On occasion, the lesions may have a cyanotic tint, a feature suggesting drug etiology. If they are not recognized as such and the drug is continued, exfoliative dermatitis may ensue (see below). Virtually any drug may produce an eruption of this type, but particularly common offenders include: barbiturates, sulfonamides, penicillin (especially ampicillin), streptomycin, pyrazolones (aminopyrine, etc.), anticonvulsants, antituberculous drugs (especially PAS), and novobiocin.

Exfoliative Dermatitis is characterized by extensive erythema and scaling in which, as the name implies, the superficial skin is shed (Fig. 16-3). Often the hair and nails are similarly shed. Fever, chills, malaise are often prominent, and secondary infection frequently develops. On occasion, glomerulitis has developed. Death is frequent, particularly among debilitated or elderly patients. This lesion may follow a number of dermatoses including psoriasis, seborrheic dermatitis and lymphomatous skin involvement. It may appear abruptly in patients receiving certain drugs; frequently it follows a drug-induced exanthematous eruption. The process may continue for weeks or months after withdrawal of the offending drug. Commonly involved drugs are: heavy metals, barbiturates, sulfonamides, quinacrine, phenothiazines, phenylbutazone, hydantoins, and penicillin.

Erythema Multiforme-like Eruptions are often due to drug allergy (Fig. 16-4). The eruption is often considered a more severe variant of the basic underlying process resulting in urticaria. It has been observed in cases of serum sickness and allergic purpura. The lesions are often variable in size, configuration and appearance; hence the term erythema multiforme. The typical eruption is acute, polymorphous, dull red, often sharply circumscribed, at times with central clearing to produce an annular or iris lesion. The distribution is usually symmetrical on the dorsal surfaces of distal extremities. The lesions may become vesiculobullous—erythema multiforme bullosum. Constitutional symptoms of fever, malaise, gastrointestinal upset and arthralgias occur frequently, particularly in the bullous variant. The lesions heal completely, unless complicated by secondary infection. Laboratory studies may indicate leukocytosis; eosinophilia is unusual. Commonly implicated drugs include: sulfonamides, penicillin, barbiturates, salicylates, anticonvulsants, phenothiazines, phenylbutazone, and pyrazolones (antipyrine, etc.).

Stevens-Johnson Syndrome (erythema multiforme exudativum) is a fulminant, primarily bullous variant of erythema multiforme with ocular, oral and genital mucous membrane involvement, often occurring in children. The disease may last 4 to 6 weeks and, before the availability of steroids, the fatality rate was in excess of 30 percent. In addition to the skin and mucous membrane involvement, fever and sepsis are present and lesions of the respiratory tract may result in bronchitis and pneumonia, sometimes with pleural effusion; renal damage may be severe; ocular damage may cause blindness. Long-acting sulfonamides, particularly sulfadimethoxine (Madribon *) and sulfamethoxypyridazine (Kynex ,† Midicel ‡), and barbiturates have been implicated most often where drug etiology was suspected, but often it is difficult to assess the role of drugs.[12] As the short-acting sulfonamides are as useful, they should be given precedence over the long-acting preparations. Other drugs occasionally implicated include penicillin, quinine, antipyrine, hydantoins, phenylbutazone, heavy metals, amithiazone, chlorpromazine and possibly others. In many instances, no causal agent is discovered or even suspected.

Erythema Nodosum-like Lesions may be classified as a deeper variant of erythema multiforme (Fig. 16-5). The lesions are usually bilateral, symmetrical, ill-defined, nodular, warm and tender, involving the anterior aspects of the legs. The lesions are red or, at times, resemble a bruise and persist for a few days to several weeks. They do not ulcerate or suppurate and usually resemble contusions as they involute. Mild constitutional symptoms of low fever, malaise, myalgia and arthralgia may appear. Iodides and bromides are most often implicated, but occasionally sulfonamides, penicillin, antipyrine and salicylates have been suspected. Sulfones used to treat leprosy have produced an increased incidence of erythema nodosum in this condition. The author has observed numerous asthmatics receiving iodides and has seen this complication on only one occasion.

Fixed Drug Eruptions in contrast to most other drug-induced dermatoses, are virtually pathognomonic of drug hypersensitivity (Fig. 16-6). These lesions recur in the same site(s) each time the specific drug is given. On occasion, the dermatitis may flare with antigenically related and even unrelated substances. The characteristic lesion is well delineated, round or oval, varying in size from a few millimeters to 25 to 30 centimeters. Edema appears first, followed by erythema which then darkens to a deeply colored, reddish-purple, dense, raised lesion. On occasion, the lesions may be eczematous, urticarial, vesiculobullous, hemorrhagic or nodular. Mucous membrane involvement, particularly of the mouth and penis, has been occasionally observed. The lesions are occasionally mildly pruritic or may produce a burning sensation. Usually only one or two lesions are present, but they may be more

* Trademark, Roche.
† Trademark, Lederle.
‡ Trademark, Parke, Davis.

numerous. Additional lesions may develop with subsequent administration of the drug. Constitutional signs are rarely present. The lesions usually subside within 2 to 3 weeks after drug withdrawal, leaving transient desquamation and residual hyperpigmentation.

Patch testing at the site with the drug may occasionally be positive. Skin graft exchanges with normals does not transfer this susceptibility, suggesting the "shock organ site" is in deeper structures, possibly the vasculature. Common causative drugs include: phenolphthalein, barbiturates, sulfonamides, tetracyclines, analgesics-antipyretics, phenylbutazone, heavy metals, and quinine.

Purpuric Eruptions may occur as the sole expression of drug allergy, but are often seen in association with other severe eruptions, notably erythema multiforme (Fig. 16-7). Purpura associated with drugs typically is symmetric, at times pruritic, and other lesions may be present which are often maculopapular, eczematous, urticarial or vesicular. Purpuric lesions do not blanch on pressure or become brownish in color as they resolve. Purpura due to drug hypersensitivity may be due to thrombocytopenia. This will be discussed under hematologic systemic reactions; immunological mechanisms appear to be important. Nonthrombocytopenic or simple purpura due to drugs has been reported, but no immunological mechanism has been demonstrated. Some reported offending drugs include sulfonamides, barbiturates, gold salts, carbromal, iodides, antihistamines and meprobamate. A few drugs may produce both simple and thrombocytopenic purpura; phenylbutazone is an example. A very severe purpuric eruption, often associated with large sloughs, has been associated with the coumarin anticoagulants. The histologic appearance resembles an Arthus (Type III) reaction, and some have considered this to be the pathogenesis.[52]

When articular and gastrointestinal involvement occur with non-thrombocytopenic purpura, the condition is referred to as Henoch-Schönlein (anaphylactoid) purpura. Although occurring most often in children, its presence in an adult should alert one to the possibility of a drug etiology. Initially, the skin lesions are often pruritic, maculopapular or urticarial. Within a day, the lesions become dusky, red macules of variable size that do not blanch on pressure and are more prominent on the buttocks and lower extremities. Gastrointestinal symptoms include abdominal pain, emesis and bleeding which may be slight or severe, producing melena and hematemesis. Intussusception may occur. Articular symptoms are usually pain and periarticular swelling and often involve many joints. Fever and leukocytosis are common. Glomerulonephritis, resembling lupus erythematosus, occurs in 30 to 50 percent of cases and may be a fatal complication. Serum complement is usually normal. The etiology often remains unknown, but antecedent

Cutaneous Drug Reactions

Photographs courtesy of Rudolf L. Baer, M.D., Department of Dermatology, New York University School of Medicine. From Baer, Rudolf and Harris, Harriet: Types of cutaneous reactions to drugs. JAMA, *202*:710, 1967.

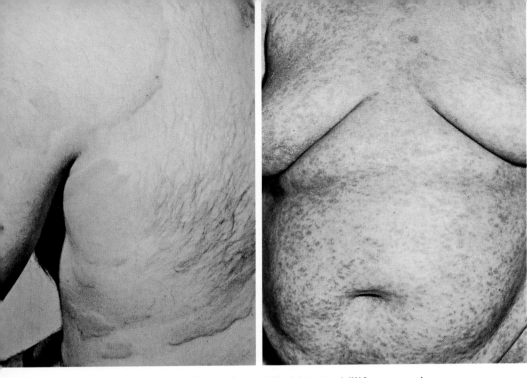

Fig. 16-1. Urticarial eruption.   Fig. 16-2. Morbilliform eruption.

Fig. 16-3. Exfoliative dermatitis.   Fig. 16-4. Erythema multiforme-like eruption.

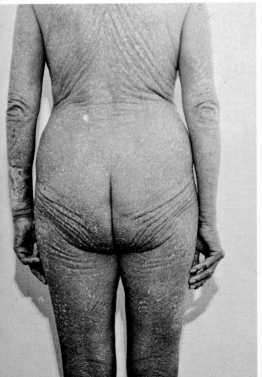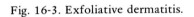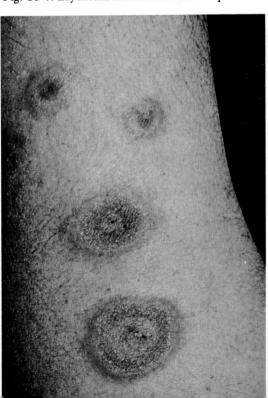

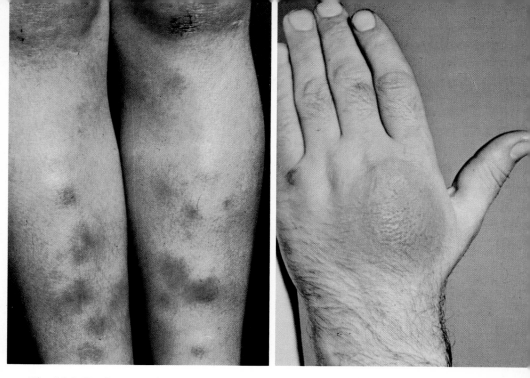

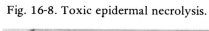

Fig. 16-5. Erythema nodosum-like eruption. Fig. 16-6. Fixed eruption.

Fig. 16-7. Purpuric eruption. Fig. 16-8. Toxic epidermal necrolysis.

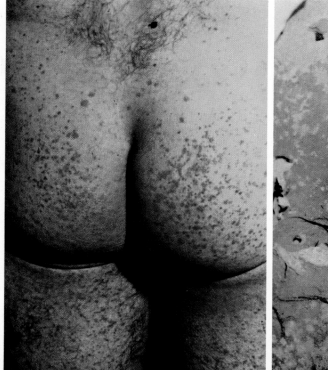

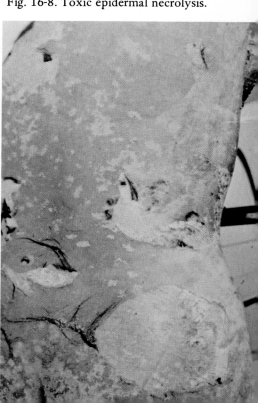

respiratory infections, foods and drugs, notably salicylates, have been incriminated. Despite occasional drug suspects, the proof of a definite relationship is usually inadequate. Of interest is the fact that corticosteroids may modify the arthritic symptoms and the gastrointestinal bleeding, but have little effect on the renal lesion. Despite uncertainties regarding drug etiology, all drugs should be discontinued, if possible.

Photosensitivity Reactions are produced by the interaction of a drug and light energy (Fig. 16-8). The drug may be administered topically, orally or parenterally. Although direct sunlight (ultraviolet spectrum 2800-4300Å) is usually required, filtered or artifical light may produce such reactions. The eruption is limited to light-exposed areas, such as the face, neck, V-area, arms, backs of hands and anterior aspects of women's legs. Often, a triangular area on the neck is spared due to shielding by the mandible, as well as infranasal areas and the groove of the chin. Unilateral distribution may result from activities such as driving a car.

Drugs increase the sensitivity of the skin by two mechanisms: phototoxic and photoallergic. *Phototoxic reactions* are nonimmunologic, occurring in a significant number of persons upon first exposure when adequate light and drug concentration are present. The drug absorbs light and this oxidative energy is transferred to tissues, resulting in damage. The light absorption spectrum is specific for each drug. Clinically, the reaction resembles an exaggerated sunburn developing within a few hours after exposure; on occasion, some vesiculation occurs. Hyperpigmentation remains in the area. Topically applied coal tar derivatives may result in this type of reaction. Approximately 40 percent of patients receiving demethylchlortetracycline (Declomycin *) will develop this reaction if conditions are appropriate. Other tetracyclines do not produce this reaction. Most phototoxic reactions are prevented if the light is filtered through ordinary window glass.

Photoallergic reactions, in contrast, generally go through an eczematous phase and more closely resemble allergic contact dermatitis. Here, the radiant energy presumably alters the drug to form a hapten which combines with cutaneous proteins to form a complete antigen, to which an immunological response is directed. Features differentiating photoallergic eruptions from phototoxic reactions are as follows: (1) They occur in only a small fraction of patients exposed to the drug and light. (2) The incubation period is days or months. (3) The concentration of drug needed to elicit the reaction is often much lower. (4) There is cross-reactivity to immunochemically related allergens. (5) The lesion often resembles allergic contact dermatitis. (6) Flareups

* Trademark, Lederle.

may occur at lightly covered, unexposed and at distant, previously exposed sites. (7) The reaction may recur over a period of days or months after each exposure to light, even without further drug administration. (8) The sensitivity may be detected by a positive photo-patch test. Photo-patch testing involves application of the suspected drug as an ordinary patch test for 24 hours, followed by exposure to a light source.

Drugs most commonly implicated are the phenothiazines, particularly chlorpromazine (Thorazine *), and promethazine (Phenergan †), the sulfonamides (antibacterial, hypoglycemics, diuretics) and griseofulvin. Bithional and halogenated salicylamides, bacteriostatic agents used in many topical preparations such as soaps, antiseptics and acne medications, are responsible for contact photoallergic reactions. Some drugs, notably chlorpromazine and sulfanilamide, have been reported to produce both phototoxic and photoallergic reactions. The agents responsible for photosensitivity reactions are summarized in Table 16-1. Although treatment of drug allergic reactions is considered elsewhere, it is to be noted that some patients with photosensitivity reactions must avoid sun exposure or use a sun-screen, such as Pre-Sun lotion, during the spring and summer long after the drug has been discontinued.

* Trademark, Smith Kline & French.
† Trademark, Wyeth.

TABLE 16-1
Photosensitivity Due to Drugs

	PHOTOTOXIC	PHOTOALLERGIC
Topical	Coal tar derivatives (Anthracene, phenanthrene)	Bithional
	Furocoumarins (in perfumes and lime juice)	Halogenated salicylamides
Systemic	Demethylchlortetracycline (Declomycin)	Phenothiazines
	Chlorpromazine (Thorazine) (occasionally)	Chlorpromazine (Thorazine) Promethazine (Phenergan)
	Sulfanilamide (occasionally)	Sulfonamides
		Antibacterials
		Hypoglycemics Tolbutamide (Orinase) Chlorpropamide (Diabinese)
		Diuretics Thiazides
		Griseofulvin

Other less frequent drug-induced dermatoses, possibly allergic, are considered here, but the eruptions presented thus far are the more common ones suspected to have an immunologic basis. *Eczematous eruptions* are characteristically the result of topically applied medicaments described earlier. On occasion, it has developed as the sole manifestation following oral or parenteral administration of penicillin, streptomycin, sulfonamides, heavy metals, phenothiazines, antihistamines, local anesthetics and quinine. *Vesiculobullous eruptions* are generally considered a variant of erythema multiforme. There are occasional patients who develop bullous lesions on a nonerythematous base and are free of constitutional symptoms. The drugs producing this are quite different from those commonly associated with erythema multiforme and include the halogens, especially bromides and iodides, heavy metals, barbiturates and occasionally phenothiazines, sulfonamides and hydantoins.

Toxic epidermal necrolysis (Lyell's syndrome, Fig. 16-8) is often considered as another severe, at times fatal, variant of erythema multiforme. This syndrome is characterized by the rapid development of generalized erythema followed by extensive desquamation, resembling scalding of the skin. Generally, healing occurs in about 2 weeks and results in no scarring. However, the mortality rate approximates 25 percent, usually as a result of sepsis or electrolyte imbalance. Infection with phage group 2 staphylococcus has been associated with this syndrome in infants and young children, while drug reactions have been suspected in older children and adults. Implicated drugs include hydantoins, phenylbutazone, barbiturates, isoniazid, phenolphthalein, penicillin, sulfonamides, sulfones, antipyrine and aminopyrine.

Lichen planus-like eruptions were first observed during World War II in association with quinacrine administration. The lesions are pruritic, violaceous, flat-topped papules distributed primarily over the ankles and wrists. Mucous membrane lesions may also occur. In addition to antimalarials, other drugs have been incriminated and include thiazides, gold salts, arsenicals, quinidine, PAS and thiouracils.

Drug-induced allergic vasculitis often results in multisystem involvement, cutaneous involvement being frequent. The condition is characterized by a variety of cutaneous manifestations including purpura, papules, vesicles, urticaria, nodules and ulcerations. The lesions occur principally on the lower extremities and are usually symmetric and bilateral. Commonly implicated drugs include penicillin, sulfonamides, thiouracils, phenylbutazone, busulfan, iproniazid and iodides.

Additional drug-induced eruptions, nonallergic in mechanism, are mentioned briefly for completeness. *Acneiform eruptions* induced by drugs superficially resemble acne vulgaris; however, there are some differences: No age is exempt; eruption is not limited to sebaceous

areas; no comedones are present; onset of the eruption is generally
abrupt; additional side effects due to the drugs being administered
may be present. Commonly involved drugs include the halogens, notably
iodides and bromides, and the steroid hormones. On occasion, *granulomatous skin involvement* and *benign tuberous lesions* have developed following the use of halogens.

Skin tumors have resulted from the prolonged administration of arsenic found in Fowler's and Gay's solutions. Keratoses develop on the
palms and soles and later become squamous cell carcinoma, while basal
cell epitheliomas may develop on the trunk. *Acanthosis nigricans,*
usually associated with internal malignancies, has resulted from large
doses of nicotinic acid. *Pigmentary changes* have been associated with a
variety of drugs, including heavy metals (particularly silver and lead),
high doses of chlorpromazine, alkylating agents (particularly busulfan)
and antimalarials. Tetracyclines administered to a pregnant woman or
to children under age 7 or 8 may stain permanent teeth. *Alopecia* has
been associated with the administration of antineoplastic agents, tri-
paranol (MER 29), and rarely heparin.

SYSTEMIC MANIFESTATIONS

Certain drug-induced systemic reactions, such as anaphylaxis, a serum
sickness-like illness, and bronchial asthma, have features similar to reactions known to be the result of classical protein allergy. It is reasonable
to accept such reactions as allergic in nature even though, for reasons
to be cited later, it is often impossible to demonstrate an immunological
mechanism, such as positive wheal and flare skin test reaction to the
suspected drug. In contrast, there are other systemic manifestations of
drug allergy, such as drug fever, and hematologic and hepatic reactions, which have no counterpart in classical protein allergy and, in
many instances, are considered allergic strictly on clinical features suggesting hypersensitivity outlined previously.

Anaphylaxis

Anaphylaxis is the most acute, potentially fatal reaction and, hence,
the most important allergic drug reaction which is a constant hazard
to the practicing physician. The term is used to describe an immediate
systemic allergic reaction (Gell and Coombs' Type I reaction) occurring
within seconds or minutes after exposure to an agent to which the patient is specifically sensitive, which characteristically involves in varying
degrees four major organ systems: the skin, respiratory system, gastrointestinal tract and cardiovascular system. Although most anaphylactic reactions do not terminate fatally, the potential for such an outcome

must be borne in mind and the attending physician must respond almost reflexly with appropriate therapy.

Although anaphylaxis is not limited to atopic individuals, there is a distinct impression that such reactions, particularly to penicillin, are increased in this group. Although anaphylaxis is discussed fully in Chapter 12, some features bear repetition.

Within seconds or minutes following drug administration (usually parenteral), syncope, collapse and hypotension may occur. Such rapid reactions are more apt to terminate fatally without the development of other manifestations. More slowly evolving reactions are usually not immediately life-threatening. They often result in cutaneous manifestations such as pruritus (most pronounced over face, upper chest, palms, axillae and groin), erythema, urticaria and angioedema; respiratory distress (hoarseness, stridor, tightness in chest and wheezing) due to angioedema of the hypopharynx or larynx and bronchospasm; and gastrointestinal symptoms of nausea, vomiting, abdominal pain and diarrhea. Uterine cramping may occur with vaginal spotting. Cardiac manifestations such as arrythmias and ischemic ECG changes may develop. The point to be made is that the reaction may initially appear minor, such as the development of slight pruritus, a "strange" feeling, dizziness, slight hoarseness or a "lump in the throat" or substernal tightness; if ignored, more severe or less reversible manifestations may ensue. As the outcome is uncertain, it is best to treat with expectancy, rather than simply let the mild symptoms subside. Death from anaphylaxis is due to airway obstruction, especially of the upper airway, or shock or a combination of these factors.

Anaphylaxis must be differentiated from other common causes of syncope or collapse. Many patients experience vasovagal syncopal reactions following an injection or any traumatic procedure. Helpful differential points that indicate the reaction is vasovagal include rapid recovery in the recumbent position, normal blood pressure and pulse (even bradycardia) and lack of other signs of anaphylaxis. When there is doubt, it is safer to assume the reaction is anaphylaxis and treat accordingly. For patients prone to such vasovagal reactions, it is advisable to administer injections to them while they are seated or recumbent.

Penicillin is the most common cause of anaphylaxis, possibly owing in part to its widespread use. Less frequent causes of anaphylaxis include foreign antisera and allergy extracts. Reactions to allergy extracts are not a major problem, because of cautious administration. Occasional reactions have been reported to a wide variety of agents—streptomycin, demethylchlortetracycline, hormones, enzymes, vaccines, local anesthetics, salicylates and diagnostic agents such as Bromsulpha-lein,* Decholin † and iodinated radiographic material.

As approximately 10 percent of anaphylactic reactions are fatal, it is this type of reaction that one would like to be able to predict in advance. The problems arising in this regard are discussed under the sections dealing with allergic emergencies and penicillin allergy.

Serum Sickness Syndrome

Serum sickness-like reactions, virtually indistinguishable from true serum sickness [92] resulting from the administration of heterologous (usually equine) serum, are produced by a number of nonprotein drugs. Serum sickness was quite common in prechemotherapy days when large amounts of foreign sera were used to treat infectious diseases —for example, pneumococcal antisera to treat pneumococcal pneumonia. The quantity of foreign sera used was important in the incidence of this reaction. Ninety percent of patients developed serum disease when given 100 ml. or more sera, while only 10 percent had difficulties when given 10 ml. With adequate immunization procedures, effective antimicrobial therapy and the use of human gamma-globulin preparations—for example, human tetanus antitoxin—serum disease has declined. Currently, penicillin is most frequently responsible for production of a clinical entity identical to that produced by foreign antisera. However, equine antitoxins are still necessary to treat rabies, venomous snake and black widow spider bites, gas gangrene, botulism and diphtheria. Fifteen percent of patients receiving rabies antitoxin develop serum sickness. Antihuman lymphocyte antisera, usually of equine origin, has played an increasing role in the prevention of organ graft rejection.

Primary serum sickness occurs 6 to 21 days, typically 7 to 12 days, after administration of the causative agent, the initial dose serving both to sensitize and to elicit symptoms. The cardinal manifestations include skin eruptions, fever, joint symptoms and lymphadenopathy. The onset of symptoms may be heralded by the development of pruritus, erythema and swelling at the injection site; a point of diagnostic value. Skin eruptions occur in 90 percent of patients and often are the earliest manifestations. Although variable, urticaria and angioedema are commonest, on occasion, they may be morbilliform, scarlatiniform, erythema multiforme or purpuric. The skin eruptions are usually pruritic. A diagnosis of this syndrome without a skin eruption must be questioned. Fever is usually slight to moderate, but may be considerable in more severe cases; here, headache and malaise may be present.

Joint symptoms develop in about 50 percent of patients. Arthralgia is

---

* Trademark, Hynson, Westcott and Dunning.
† Trademark, Dome.

usual, although an inflammatory joint effusion may occur. Multiple joints are usually involved, particularly the larger joints such as the knees, ankles, wrists and rarely the small joints of the hands and feet. Occasional involvement of the temporomandibular joint may provide confusion with clinical tetanus. Tender lymphadenopathy usually affects regional lymph nodes draining the injection site; on occasion, generalized lymphadenopathy and even splenomegaly may be present. Less frequently observed symptoms include generalized edema, weight gain, abdominal pain, nausea, vomiting and diarrhea. All the cited manifestations may be present, or only one or two. The symptoms may be very mild, lasting a few days, or quite severe, persisting for several weeks or longer. The average duration is approximately 1 week. The protracted urticaria following penicillin is not well understood.

More serious manifestations are fortunately infrequent and usually develop with or after the development of more typical symptoms cited above. Peripheral neuropathy, especially effecting the brachial plexus (fifth and sixth cervical nerves), is commonest, resulting in a scapulo-humeral paralysis. Although involvement is primarily motor, sensory changes resulting in pain and hyperesthesias in the nerve distribution may be present shortly before the onset of paralysis. Cranial nerves have been rarely involved. The most severe neurological involvement is the Guillain-Barré syndrome.[7] Recovery from neurologic involvement, although slow, is usually complete within 6 months. Although glomerulonephritis is a prominent feature of experimental serum sickness,[88] clinically evident renal involvement in man is unusual. However, actual glomerulonephritis accounted for three deaths following administration of horse antihuman-cancer serum.[16] Vasculitis has been described in the myocardium, kidneys, liver, pancreas, adrenals, muscles and skin. Indeed, any vascular bed may be involved.

Accelerated serum sickness develops within a few days (usually 2 to 4) after administration of the agent, indicating prior sensitization of the host. The clinical manifestations, although similar to primary serum disease, are often more severe. Anaphylaxis, described earlier, may develop particularly among patients atopically sensitive to horse dander and among some patients sensitized by prior exposure to horse serum products.

Laboratory signs during acute serum sickness include a normal or slightly elevated sedimentation rate and slight leukocytosis; during recovery, slight eosinophila may be present but is not an invariable feature of the disease. Atypical lymphocytosis and plasmacytosis may be present. Serum sickness is one of the few illnesses where plasmacytosis may occasionally be seen. Occasionally albuminuria and a few casts may be present, but nitrogen retention is rare. Serum complement may be reduced. An electrocardiogram may be compatible with myocardial infarction or ischemia.

The immunopathology of experimental serum sickness is well understood and there is little reason to doubt the similarity of drug-induced serum sickness-like reactions in man. Skin sensitizing antibodies (IgE), circulating antigen-antibody complexes, or both are probably responsible for the cutaneous manifestations; while the other manifestations result from a vasculitis produced by toxic antigen-antibody complexes (Gell and Coombs' Type III Reaction). The lymphadenopathy probably reflects increased antibody production. The IgG antibodies against heterologous serum proteins may be shown by the hemagglutination (HA) test. This sensitive test uses red blood cells coated with serum protein as the test material. Patients may have low titers of HA antibodies against horse serum even prior to injection of foreign serum, and a pretreatment elevated titer indicates greater likelihood of development of serum disease.[68] Following the onset of symptoms, HA titers may rise to 10,000 or higher and often persist for long periods after other antibodies have disappeared. Such high titers may help differentiate whether the clinical reaction was due to serum or penicillin, where both agents have been simultaneously administered. The presence of precipitating IgG antibodies is less constant and may appear after the onset of symptoms. Forssman antibodies may appear after large amounts of horse serum and are distinguished from the heterophil antibody observed in infectious mononucleosis by differential absorption studies with guinea pig tissues.

The prognosis for complete recovery is excellent. As this reaction usually follows the initial administration of an agent, it cannot be predicted in advance by any prior skin or laboratory testing. However, in view of its usual benign course, the concern here is less than for anaphylactic reactions. Management will be discussed later, using this syndrome as a model for symptomatic treatment of allergic drug reactions. In addition to penicillin, other nonprotein drugs occasionally implicated include the sulfonamides, streptomycin, thiouracils, hydantoins and, rarely, others.

Pulmonary Manifestations

The lung is infrequently the primary organ involved in suspected allergic drug reactions. *Bronchial asthma* is the most common pulmonary manifestation of a drug reaction. It may occur as a pulmonary manifestation of anaphylaxis. It may also occur as a result of inhalation of a drug used for therapy or accidentally. Patients treated with aerosolized antibiotics, especially penicillin, have developed asthma. Occupational exposure of nurses and pharmacists to penicillin by inhalation has also caused asthma. Bronchial asthma and rhinitis have followed the inhalation of pituitary snuff for treatment of diabetes insipidus.

The most common drug resulting in severe paroxysms of asthma is acetylsalicylic acid (aspirin). Most patients so affected have chronic intractable asthma and, commonly, nasal polyps that had been present for many years prior to the precipitation of asthma by aspirin. Hence there is some merit to warning such patients about the potential of this drug reaction or even recommending that aspirin be avoided. Usually, there is no allergic explanation for the asthma or nasal problem. Similarly, there is no satisfactory explanation for the aspirin-induced asthmatic episodes, but immunologic or allergic mechanisms do not appear to be involved. Skin testing with aspirin gives negative results and involves a great risk of inducing severe asthma. The diagnosis is based on clinical history. A suspect patient should never be given even a small dose of aspirin, as it may result in a violent, even fatal, attack of asthma. Asthma induced by aspirin may also be precipitated by indomethacin (Indocin *) and tartrazine (FD&C yellow No. 5), a commonly used dye in foodstuffs and some drugs. Further discussion of aspirin-induced asthma is in the chapter on asthma.

A form of *hypersensitivity lung disease* (discussed in detail in Chap. 18) has been produced by the inhalation of powdered extracts of bovine or porcine pituitary glands for treatment of diabetes insipidus. After sensitization, symptoms develop within 4 to 6 hours of exposure and include fever, chills, headache, malaise, and a nonproductive cough, and disappear, usually without bronchospasm. The dyspnea is often out of proportion to physical findings, which may include basilar crepitant rales and, on occasion, wheezes. The chest x-ray may be normal or show diffuse nodulation. Pulmonary function studies reveal a restrictive defect. Leukocytosis and minimal eosinophilia are often present. A high titer of precipitating IgG antibodies against the offending antigens, in this case, bovine and porcine serum proteins and pituitary antigens, can be demonstrated. The atopic individual may also develop reagins or skin sensitizing antibodies (IgE) to these antigens and, upon exposure, promptly develop asthma (Type I reaction), followed in 4 to 6 hours by the later response described above. Current evidence suggests that this delayed reaction, mediated by precipitating antibodies, belongs to Gell and Coombs' Type III category.[61] In chronic forms of this drug-induced illness, the symptoms are more persistent and less reversible, ultimately resulting in chronic pulmonary interstitial fibrosis. Recently, synthetic lysine vasopressin has become available and pituitary snuff is no longer required.

* Trademark, Merck Sharp & Dohme.

An unusual pulmonary reaction produced by the administration of nitrofurantoin (Furadantin°) [29] has some features of hypersensitivity pneumonitis. Initial symptoms develop 3 to 4 days after the drug is started and consist of fever, chills, cough and dyspnea. Occasionally cyanosis and pleuritic chest pain are present. Physical findings often consist of widespread crepitant rales of the type usually attributed to pulmonary edema. The chest x-rays may be normal or indicate interstitial changes more characteristic of pulmonary edema. A pleural effusion may be present. The symptoms and physical signs often exceed the radiographic findings. Eosinophilia, when present, is usually modest. Pulmonary function studies are compatible with a restrictive defect. Subsequent readministration of the drug following recovery (not recommended) results in recurrence of the clinical picture, often more severe, within hours or within the same day. Prompt cessation of the clinical manifestations often within a day, occurs upon withdrawal of the drug, although chronic interstitial fibrosis has developed in a small percentage of cases.

The precise genesis of this pulmonary lesion is not understood. Careful studies have concluded that it is not of cardiac origin. It also differs from the Loeffler's syndrome evoked by certain drugs described below. Although there are some features suggesting hypersensitivity lung disease, no immunological mechanism has been demonstrated. As patients treated with nitrofurantoins are often elderly and more likely to have heart disease, it is important to recognize this syndrome to avoid unnecessary, long term treatment for cardiac failure. Inferior vena caval ligation has been carried out on the theory that those drug-induced episodes were the result of septic pulmonary emboli.[56]

A *Loeffler's-type syndrome* (pulmonary infiltrates with eosinophilia) has been reported following the administration of para-aminosalicylic acid, penicillin, sulfonamides and mephenesin. The onset is usually abrupt; the infiltrates are flocculent, nodular and often migratory; significant eosinophilia is present; and these findings may persist for weeks after withdrawal of the offending drug. *Chronic pulmonary interstitial fibrosis* occurs in a small percentage of patients receiving busulfan and several antihypertensive preparations (hexamethonium, mecamylamine), and may develop as a complication of hypersensitivity lung disease induced by drugs as described above. The lung may also be involved in *allergic vasculitis,* to be discussed later under systemic manifestations of drug allergy.

Drug Fever

Fever is a well-known accompaniment of drug hypersensitivity reactions, but is rarely seen in allergic reactions to naturally encountered

° Trademark, Eaton.

allergens. Fever may occur alone as the sole manifestation of drug hypersensitivity and is particularly perplexing in a clinical situation where a patient is being treated for an infection. Drugs given regularly and in fairly high doses are more often incriminated. The patient developing drug fever when treated for the first time has gradually increasing fever beginning on the seventh to tenth day of treatment. The fever has a sustained or remittent course, often as high as 104° to 105,° and usually persists as long as the drug is continued. Leukocytosis, often 20,000 to 30,000, mostly polymorphonuclear leukocytes rather than eosinophils, may add further to confusion regarding the differential diagnosis between infection and drug fever. Prompt defervescence, usually within 2 to 3 days, occurs following withdrawal of the offending drug. Subsequent administration of the same drug produces fever, occasionally chills, in a matter of hours.

A distinguishing feature of drug fever is often the disparity between the degree of the recorded febrile response and the relative well-being of the patient. On occasion, a mild maculopapular or urticarial eruption may be present to provide a clue, but often there are no additional indications of drug allergy. As drug fever commonly precedes development of more serious manifestations—for example, hematologic reactions, vasculitis, hepatic reactions, exfoliative dermatitis and anaphylaxis—its recognition is imperative. Tissues of patients dying during drug fever show arteritis and focal necrosis in many organs, such as the myocardium, liver, lung and spleen, attesting to the systemic nature of the reaction. The mechanism of fever is probably the result of release of endogenous pyrogens from granulocytes by the hypersensitivity reaction. A detailed analysis of the problem is provided by Cluff.[14]

Sulfathiazole and sulfadiazine were the most notorious causes, but their use has been largely abandoned. Drugs more commonly implicated now include: para-aminosalicylic acid, sulfonamides, iodides, thiouracils, quinidine, procaine amide, mercurial diuretics, streptomycin, isoniazid, anticonvulsants, barbiturates, salicylates, and other antibiotics (except tetracyclines and chloramphenicol).

Hematological Manifestations

Eosinophilia may be present as the sole manifestation of drug hypersensitivity, but is more often associated with other cutaneous and systemic manifestations of drug allergy. Its presence should alert one to consider this possibility. The function of eosinophils is not definitely established, but they appear to be attracted to sites of antigen-antibody interactions. Contrary to expectation, eosinophilia is found infrequently in serum sickness-like reactions. *Leukocytosis* is present less frequently and produces confusion, particularly in the differential diagnosis of drug fever described above.

Drug-induced blood dyscrasias are basically of three types:

1. Direct toxicity upon the bone marrow due to cytotoxicity, for example benzol, or by blocking metabolic pathways essential to cell replication, for example antimetabolites.

2. Related to an inborn metabolic defect, the most common being a glucose-6-phosphate dehydrogenase deficiency described earlier under idiosyncratic or pharmacogenetic reactions. Patients with the unusual hemoglobin Zurich have red cells that are more vulnerable to certain drugs. Phenothiazine-induced agranulocytosis may fall into this category.

3. Related to proven or, at least, suspected immunological mechanisms, notably Gell and Coombs' Type II reactions.

This discussion deals with drug-induced hematopoietic manifestations where immunological mechanisms are considered operative. Many instances of drug-induced thrombocytopenia and fewer cases of drug-induced hemolytic anemia have been unequivocally shown by methods in vitro to be mediated by antigen-antibody interactions. There is less certainty regarding drug-induced agranulocytosis and evidence for such a mechanism in aplastic anemia is largely circumstantial. Characteristics of drug-induced blood dyscrasias include an abrupt onset with rapid recovery upon withdrawal of the offending drug.

Several immunological mechanisms are proposed, and one alone or, possibly, all may be responsible, depending upon the drug involved.

1. Hapten Type. In this type, the drug reacts with a carrier protein on the cell surface to form a complete antigen capable of initiating antibody production (IgG). The resultant antigen-antibody reaction on the cell surface causes agglutination or, in the presence of serum complement, cell lysis. Usually the cell destruction is mild, mostly extravascular due to phagocytosis. Sedormid * thrombocytopenic purpura is an example. On occasion, the drug hapten may bind firmly to the cell surface, but the antibodies are directed primarily against the hapten alone and not against any carrier protein on the cell surface. Penicillin immunohemolytic anemia is an example of this, resulting in a mild reaction that usually disappears in a few days or a week or so after discontinuance of the drug.

2. Innocent-Bystander Type. The interaction of the drug and its specific antibody occurs in the fluid phase, resulting in activation of serum complement, components of which are adsorbed to the cell membrane producing damage. The term innocent arises from the fact that the cells are passively involved and do not take part in binding the antigen or the antibody. In many cases, the type of antibody involved (IgG, IgM) is not known. The reaction is usually abrupt and often severe. It is likely that many drug-induced blood dyscrasias are of this

* No longer available in the United States.

type. Quinidine or quinine-induced thrombocytopenic and chlorpropamide-induced hemolysis are familiar examples. Why certain cells are selected for injury with certain drugs is unknown.

3. Autoimmune Type. Although the incidence of hemolytic anemia among patients receiving alpha-methyldopa (Aldomet *) is quite low (less than 1 percent), up to 20 percent receiving the drug for 3 months or more have a positive Coombs' test. The IgG antibody is directed against normal red cell membrane constituents, probably the Rh locus.[45] Hemolysis is usually not acute but may persist for weeks or months after withdrawal of treatment, in contrast to other drug-induced hematologic reactions where recovery is more rapid.

Exactly how this drug induces autosensitization remains speculative, but the long latency period is compatible with the hypothesis that the drug may act upon formation of the red blood cell membrane at a point during the maturation process, thus rendering it auto-antigenic. Recently, a similar phenomenon has been reported with the use of mefenamic acid (Ponstel †).[73] In the hapten and innocent-bystander types, the involved cells must be incubated with the drug and the patient's serum to induce the reaction. In the Aldomet or autoimmune type, the patient's serum will react with normal erythrocytes, even in the absence of the drug. Most of these hematologic reactions involve increased phagocytosis of cells, rather than lysis.

Thrombocytopenia is a well-known complication of drug therapy. The usual clinical manifestations are those of petechiae and, rarely, hemorrhage. On occasion, there may be associated fever, chills and arthralgia. Prompt recovery is expected upon withdrawal of the drug. Readministration of the drug, even in small amounts, usually produces prompt recrudescence of thrombocytopenia, often within a few hours. Much work has been carried out on the immunological mechanism of drug-induced thrombocytopenia.[2] The plasma or serum of the patient contains an antibody which causes agglutination or, in the presence of complement, lysis of platelets in the presence of the drug. Most forms of drug-induced thrombocytopenia are of the "innocent bystander" type.

Drugs producing thrombocytopenia are generally not the same as those resulting in simple purpura (nonthrombocytopenic) described under cutaneous manifestations. Quinidine and its isomer quinine are most commonly implicated. Sedormid (allyl-isopropyl-acetylcarbamide), upon which much of the original investigative work was carried out, is no longer available. Other common offenders include sulfonamides, sulfonamide derivatives (diuretics, hypoglycemic agents), chlorampheni-

* Trademark, Merck Sharp & Dohme.
† Trademark, Parke, Davis.

col, meprobamate and phenylbutazone. Less frequently involved drugs are digitoxin, thiouracils, procainamide, penicillin and cephalothin.

Hemolytic anemia due to drugs on an immunologic basis must be differentiated from drug-induced hemolytic reactions on a genetic basis, for example a glucose-6-phosphate dehydrogenase deficiency. Drug-induced immunohemolytic anemias (hapten type, "innocent bystander" type, Aldomet type) all have a positive Coombs' test, reacting with nonspecific Coombs' antiglobulin antiserum. Drugs commonly implicated include stibophen (Fuadin *), penicillin, para-aminosalicylic acid, phenacetin, quinidine and quinine, mephenytoin and alpha-methyldopa. A positive direct Coombs' test has been detected in 65 percent of patients receiving cephalothin sodium and cephaloridine, but to date only two cases of hemolysis have been reported.[26] A recent case report implicated methysergide in production of a hemolytic anemia.[79]

Agranulocytosis, as an expression of drug hypersensitivity, became familiar when aminopyrine was widely used. The sera of affected individuals contained an antibody which agglutinated or lysed leukocytes in the presence of aminopyrine. Readministration of minute amounts of the offending drug would result in a precipitous fall in the leukocyte levels, often within hours. For most other implicated drugs, the immune mechanisms are less clear. As a rule, this complication does not develop until the patient has been receiving the drug for 2 to 8 weeks. Its presence is often heralded by severe pharyngitis. Recovery usually occurs within several weeks after withdrawal of the drug, providing the patient does not succumb to an intercurrent infection. The reported mortality rates vary from 20 to 50 percent. Treatment is usually directed at the complicating infection. Of drugs commonly used today phenothiazines, phenylbutazone, chloramphenicol, thiouracils, sulfonamides and anticonvulsants are among the more frequent offenders. Again, an "innocent bystander" type of immunological mechanism is suspected.

Aplastic anemia induced by a drug is usually insidious in onset and early symptoms reflect the combined effects of a decrease in all three cellular elements. As a rule, the implicated drug has been administered over a long period of time. Unlike other hematologic reactions due to drugs, many cases continue for many weeks or months after withdrawal of the offending agent. It is unlikely that immunological mechanisms are responsible. However, there are reports of individuals who, after having tolerated a course of drug therapy, promptly developed this complication after only a small dose upon subsequent retreatment. Chloramphenicol is most frequently implicated, but other drugs have also been associated with this complication and include phenylbutazone, sulfonamides and sulfonamide derivatives, anticonvulsants, thiouracils and

---

* Trademark, Winthrop.

heavy metals, particularly gold salts. Treatment is that of the complications, for example, transfusions and antibiotics, to prevent death while recovery of the cellular elements takes place.

Hepatic Manifestations

Jaundice and other signs of hepatitis may result from a variety of drugs and are less frequent manifestations of drug hypersensitivity. Direct chemical injury to liver cells results from hepatotoxins, notably carbon tetrachloride, chlorinated hydrocarbons such as chloroform and tetrachloroethylene, and occasionally gold salts and 6-mercaptopurine. Following administration of drugs parenterally, hepatitis may be transmitted by the syringe. Some drugs, such as the C 17- alkyl substituted testosterones (methyl testosterone, methandrostenolone (Dianabol *), norethisterone and norethynodrel) induce simple cholestatic jaundice in all patients providing they receive the drug for a long interval, usually several months. A similar response has been observed in a few patients receiving sulfadiazine and methimazole.

There are a number of drugs which produce hepatic reactions in only a small percentage of patients receiving them. There is often no constant relationship between the dose and severity of the reaction and the latent period is highly variable. The occasional presence of fever, skin rash, arthralgia, lymphadenopathy and eosinophilia suggests a hypersensitivity mechanism, but none has been demonstrated. Further, prompt exacerbation of symptoms has followed readministration of the drug.

The hepatic involvement is bacically of two types; intrahepatic cholestasis and hepatocellular injury and necrosis. Recovery is expected unless irreversible cell damage has developed. *Intrahepatic* cholestasis is primarily associated with phenothiazines, but has occasionally developed with chlorpropamide (Diabinese †), erythromycin estolate (Ilosone ‡), triacetyloleandomycin (TAO §), nitrofurantoins and thiouracils. The clinical picture resembles biliary obstruction and the prognosis is excellent. Occasionally, the jaundice is more prolonged and may resemble biliary cirrhosis. Treatment is nonspecific and corticosteroids are of no value. *Hepatocellular reactions* resemble viral hepatitis and are most often due to monoamine oxidase inhibitors, such as iproniazid (Marsilid) and phenylzine (Nardil ||). Other less frequently implicated drugs include para-aminosalicylic acid, sulfonamides, hydantoins, isonia-

---

* Trademark, Ciba.
† Trademark, Pfizer.
‡ Trademark, Lilly.
§ Trademark, Roerig.
|| Trademark, Warner-Chilcott.

zid, and alpha-methyldopa. This reaction is more serious, with a less favorable prognosis, and must be treated as acute viral hepatitis.

Collagen–Vascular Manifestations

Vasculitis has been demonstrated in patients with serum sickness and drug fever. Drugs have also been implicated in more severe forms of acute vasculitis with widespread organ involvement. The lesions occur in small vessels—arterioles, venules, capillaries and small arteries. Commonly involved are the skin, musculoskeletal system, kidneys, lungs and peripheral nerves. The gastrointestinal system and heart are less commonly involved. Fever is usually present. Cutaneous manifestations are usually purpuric, but may be erythematous, nodular or urticarial, and tend to involve the lower legs and feet. Arthralgia is quite frequent. Less common manifestations include pneumonitis, asthma, myositis, coronary arteritis, gastrointestinal bleeding and peripheral neuropathy. Laboratory studies often demonstrate an elevated sedimentation rate, eosinophilia, microscopic hematuria and proteinuria. Renal failure is the usual cause of death. The outcome of drug-induced vasculitis is usually favorable, but prolonged treatment with corticosteroids may be necessary. Drugs most frequently implicated in severe vasculitis include penicillin, sulfonamides, thiouracils, hydantoins, phenylbutazone, iodides and allopurinol.

Polyarteritis nodosa primarily involves medium sized arteries, for example, large muscular arterioles near bifurcations or at hilar regions of viscera. The pulmonary circulation and spleen are usually spared. Necrotizing and aneurysmal arterial changes result in cerebral, coronary, mesenteric, renal and other vascular infarctions. The prognosis is ominous. Initially, sulfonamides no longer in use were incriminated in this type of reaction. However, the incidence of polyarteritis has not appreciably lessened with the declining use of these sulfonamides. Although one should consider the possibility of a drug etiology in polyarteritis, drugs appear to be more commonly implicated in acute or subacute vasculitis described above.

The best evidence implicating drug hypersensitivity in vasculitis or, rarely, in polyarteritis is the similarity of lesions to those of serum sickness and a history of drug ingestion or, rarely, exacerbation of the process upon readministration of the drug in question. It should be noted that the suspected drug may have been given to the patient to treat early symptoms of vasculitis, for example fever, and therefore one may assume guilt by association. On occasion, the implicated drug has been administered later without adverse effect.

Other vascular involvement such as Wegener's granulomatosis, allergic granulomatosis and temporal arteritis rarely are associated with drug administration. In general, granulomatous changes are less suspect in drug allergy than angiitic changes, especially allergic vasculitis described earlier.

Drug-induced lupus erythematosus syndrome has been described following prolonged treatment with the hydrazides hydralazine (Apresoline *), isonicotinic acid hydrazide (isoniazid) and procainamide (Pronestyl †). From 8 to 13 percent of hypertensives receiving Apresoline in moderate to large doses for several months develop clinical, serological and pathological features indistinguishable from systemic lupus erythematosus—fever, skin rash, arthritis, hepatomegaly, splenomegaly, lymphadenopathy and, in the more severe cases, the lupus cell phenomenon in the blood. During antituberculous isoniazid therapy, up to 20 percent of patients develop antinuclear antibodies, but only a few actually develop clinical manifestations. Currently, procainamide appears to be the most frequent drug inducing lupus erythematosus symptoms. Serological abnormalities develop in a high percentage of individuals taking this drug even without associated symptoms. Although anticonvulsants occasionally are related to this syndrome, it should be recalled that convulsions may be an early symptom of lupus and antedate other manifestations by many years. Other drugs sporadically implicated include sulfonamides, thiouracils, penicillin, oral contraceptives and alpha-methyldopa (Aldomet).

There are some differences between the spontaneously occurring disease and that which is induced by drugs. Generally, affected individuals are older in the drug-related syndrome and significant renal involvement is less common. Fever and rash are less common in drug-induced forms, and the degree of anemia and leukopenia is less. More pleural involvement has been described in the procainamide-induced cases. The symptoms usually subside upon withdrawal of the drug, but a surprising number of patients have had manifestations persisting for years following withdrawal of the suspected drug.[32] After recovery, there are occasional reports of exacerbation after small doses of the drug.

Whether the drug-induced syndrome merely "unmasks" a latent immunologic disease or represents an allergic drug reaction is unknown. Early manifestations of lupus may have been present in many patients prior to their receiving hydralazine.[4] The use of the implicated drugs may then merely exacerbate the condition, much as sunlight often does. On the other hand, these drugs may alter nucleoprotein to render it autoantigenic, giving rise to antinuclear antibodies.

The other connective tissue diseases have not been regularly associated with drug allergy and the immunological relationship here is even more tenuous. An acute rheumatoid state has been described with

* Trademark, Ciba.
† Trademark, Squibb.

thiouracil derivatives. Symmers suggested a causal relationship between polymyositis and penicillin therapy on two occasions and further
questioned whether thrombotic thrombocytopenic purpura may be produced by drug allergy.[84] Again, one must recall that some implicated drugs may have been given for early symptoms of the particular
connective tissue disease.

Recently an association has been noted between methysergide
(Sansert *) therapy and fibrosclerotic disorders, particularly retroperitoneal fibrosis.[79] This develops in only a small percentage of patients
receiving the drug and is usually reversible upon withdrawal of the
agent, thus raising the possibility of hypersensitivity. On the other hand,
it may simply unmask a collagen-like disease as suggested for drug-
induced lupus syndromes.

Lymphadenopathy

Lymphadenopathy is a common feature of the serum sickness syndrome and may be present in drug-induced lupus erythematosus.

Lymphadenopathy associated with prolonged treatment with anticonvulsants (hydantoins—Dilantin †, Mesantoin ‡, occasionally the
oxazolidines—Tridione §, Paradine ‖), is a rare, but well established
disorder that may mimic clinically and pathologically a malignant
lymphoma.[34] Cervical lymphadenopathy is most frequent, but it may
be generalized; hepatomegaly and splenomegaly are uncommon. Fever,
an erythematous skin eruption and eosinophilia are frequently present.
The reaction subsides within 2 to 3 weeks after discontinuation of
therapy and reappears upon readministration of the drug.

Pathologically, lymph node architecture is often partially obliterated
by a polymorphic cellular infiltrate composed of reticulum cells and
lymphocytes. The differentiation of anticonvulsant lymphadenopathy
from malignant lymphomas of the reticulum cells or poorly differentiated
lymphocytic types is not difficult, as the infiltrate in the latter is mono-
morphic. Greater difficulty arises in differentiation from Hodgkin's
disease; less atypicality of the reticulum cell, lack of Reed-Sternberg
cells, less fibrosis and matting of lymph nodes are points against this
diagnosis.

The pathogenesis of anticonvulsant lymphadenopathy is unknown.
The presence of rash, eosinophilia and "blast" transformation of the
patient's lymphocytes in the presence of the drug suggests a hypersensitivity reaction.[98] It may be that anticonvulsants stimulate the

* Trademark, Sandoz.
† Trademark, Parke, Davis.
‡ Trademark, Sandoz.
§ Trademark, Abbott.
‖ Trademark, Abbott.

lymphoreticular system, unmasking lymphomas. Regardless of patho-genetic mechanisms, the knowledge of the association between this therapy and atypical lymphoid hyperplasia is necessary to avoid an erroneous diagnosis of lymphoma with its therapeutic and prognostic implications. However, it should be noted that not all patients experi-ence a regression after drug withdrawal, with some progressing to a fatal outcome indistinguishable from malignant lymphoma.[23]

Nephropathy

Glomerulonephritis is a prominent feature of experimental serum sickness, but is infrequently described in man. In all probability it is a transient, completely reversible phenomenon in man. A similar renal lesion occurs in drug-induced vasculitis. Tubular necrosis may follow anaphylactic shock or drug-induced immunohemolysis. A relatively small percentage of patients have developed chronic interstitial nephritis after prolonged use of analgesics, notably phenacetin; proof of an immunologic mechanism is lacking. Similarly, a few patients receiving the oxazolidine anticonvulsants (Tridione, Paradione) for prolonged periods develop a nephrotic syndrome indistinguishable clinically and pathologically from the idiopathic type.[31] Although discontinuation of the drugs generally results in complete recovery, this is not always the case. Readministration of these drugs after recovery has resulted in prompt recurrence.

Interstitial nephritis and tubular damage leading to renal failure have developed following treatment with high doses of the penicillins, particularly methicillin.[9] Fever, rash and eosinophilia are frequently present and suggest a hypersensitivity reaction. Although the drug hapten and gamma-globulin were detected in the glomerulus, no com-plement was noted, and glomerular damage was absent, indicating that this is not an immune complex (Gell and Coombs' Type III) disease. The damage may be due to delayed hypersensitivity.

Neurologic Reactions

Drug-induced anaphylactic shock may be accompanied by convulsions and encephalopathy. Postvaccinal encelphalomyelitis resembles experi-mental allergic encephalomyelitis produced in animals. A peripheral neuritis has been described in patients receiving gold salts, colchicine, nitrofurantoins and sulfonamides, but such reactions have not been an-alyzed sufficiently to strongly suggest a hypersensitivity mechanism. The neurologic features occasionally seen in serum sickness were de-scribed in that section.

SUMMARY

This list of manifestations attributed to, or at least suspected of being, allergic drug reactions must be considered tentative. With the proliferation of new drugs and more information forthcoming regarding mechanisms, it is reasonable to assume that there will be additions to and deletions from the current compilation. Levine has suggested another classification based upon the time of onset of symptoms.[41] Immediate allergic reactions occur within 30 minutes after drug administration and include manifestations of anaphylaxis. Accelerated reactions occur up to 3 days after the start of drug therapy and include urticaria and angioedema. Late reactions begin after 3 days and include most skin eruptions, serum sickness and drug fever. Unusual reactions, occurring late, include the hematologic reactions, hepatic reactions and nephropathy. It is likely, if these are all immunologic reactions, that the mechanism may vary and include the spectrum of known hypersensitivity mechanisms and possibly additional mechanisms not yet described.

DIAGNOSIS OF DRUG ALLERGY

The investigation and identification of a drug responsible for a suspected hypersensitivity reaction still depends largely upon circumstantial evidence. Proof that a drug is the actual offender is usually lacking since, with few exceptions, conventional methods used to diagnose allergic disorders are not useful in determining a drug etiology. A knowledge of the varied manifestations ascribed to drug allergy and syndromes commonly associated with certain drugs is of great value in evaluating these situations. On a practical level, the physician would like to ascertain with reasonable certainty that a particular reaction appearing during therapy is due to the drug, whether he must discontinue its administration and whether he can administer it again safely in the future. There is an urgent need for reliable and safe methods for detecting susceptible patients before drug administration. The list below summarizes what is currently known about this problem.

Evaluation of Patients with Suspected Drug Allergy

I. HISTORY—basis of diagnosing most allergic drug reactions.

II. SKIN TESTS—limited value in most cases
   A. Immediate (wheal and flare) prick or intradermal tests
      Reliable for high molecular weight compounds (complete antigens)
      Unreliable for low molecular weight compounds (haptens); partial exception: penicillin skin testing.
      False positive reactions:
         Nonspecific irritation, e.g. too concentrated
         Histamine liberators, nonimmunologic

B. Delayed (tuberculinlike) tests
Little correlation with clinical picture;
possible exception: procaine

C. Patch or photopatch tests
Useful for diagnosis of allergic contact dematitis

D. Skin window
Investigational

III. *TESTS IN VITRO*—limited value

A. Serologic tests for specific antibodies
1. Passive hemagglutination
Little correlation with clinical state.
2. Hematologic reactions—generally useful.
a. Thrombocytopenic purpura
* Agglutination and lysis (in presence of complement) of platelets by drug-patient's serum mixture.
* Inhibition of clot retraction of patient's blood by suspected drug—good screening test.
* Complement—fixation reaction of platelets, drug and patient's serum—most sensitive test.
Liberation of platelet factor 3 by drug-patient's serum mixture—promising new test.
Precipitate formation in drug-serum mixture ⎫
Antihuman globulin consumption test ⎬ rarely observed
b. Hemolytic anemia
* Coomb's antihuman globulin test—agglutination or lysis of erythrocytes in presence of drug, patient's serum and antihuman globulin.
* Aldomet reaction—agglutination or lysis of erythocytes in presence of patients serum without the drug.
Agglutination and lysis (in presence of complement) of erythrocytes by drug patients serum mixture—rarely observed.
c. Agranulocytosis
* Agglutination of leukocytes in presence of patient's serum, even in absence of the drug.
3. Radioallergosorbent test (RAST)—a promising in vitro method to detect reaginic (IgE) antibodies.

B. Biologic tests—investigational
1. Reactions involving histamine release
a. Basophil degranulation test.
b. Leukocyte histamine release.
2. Lymphocyte transformation

IV. PROVOCATIVE TEST DOSING—controversial

---

* Tests of greatest demonstrated value.

History

The clinical history is the most important aid in evaluation. When patients present with suspected drug-induced manifestations, it is essential to identify all drugs the patient is currently taking or recently has received. The physician must suspect all drugs including apparently innocent medications which the patient has taken for some time without difficulty. The patient may not admit to taking certain drugs unless specifically questioned about them. This usually is not intentional withholding of information, as many patients do not consider frequently used nonprescription items as drugs. Further, many patients have not been appraised of medications that they have had in the past and many have simply forgotten about the treatment. Table 16-4 provides a list of commonly encountered drug allergens. In addition, it is often helpful to routinely review with the patient the medications listed below, as these substances are often ignored by the patient. At times, relatives may be questioned about drugs used by the patient and asked to inspect the contents of the medicine cabinet at home. It cannot be overstressed that *all* medications used by the patient must be identified.

Medications Often Implicated in Drug Reactions

Aspirin	Sulfa	Ointments
Nose drops	Penicillin	Contraceptives
Cold tablets	Other antibiotics	Douches
Headache remedies	Tonics	Suppositories
Sedatives	Vitamins	Lozenges
"Pain relievers"	Hormones	Dysmenorrhea tablets
Cathartics	Biologicals	

Recognition of drug allergy may be relatively easy when: 1. the manifestations are sufficiently distinctive to arouse a suspicion of drug allergy, for example urticaria or a fixed drug eruption; 2. the temporal relationships between administration of the drug and onset of symptoms is appropriate 3. the presenting complaints are known to occur as features of a reaction to the drug being taken 4. the patient has previously received the drug in question with impunity (sensitizing exposure) 5. the patient has had an allergic reaction to a drug in the past and now has similar manifestations. When some or all of these features are present, it is likely that the patient is experiencing drug hypersensitivity.

The clinical evaluation is often complicated by the fact that many patients believe they have had a hypersensitivity reaction to a drug to which, in fact, they are not allergic. A thorough analysis of the circumstances described above and other tests, if available, may help to clarify this situation. On occasion, the manifestations strongly suggest hypersensitivity in a patient receiving several drugs and the real offender cannot be identified for certain. At times, certain manifestations produced by allergic drug reactions resemble symptoms of the disease and vice versa, making evaluation even more complex. *As a general rule, it is helpful to consider that a drug may be responsible for any clinical finding the cause of which is not immediately apparent or differs from the usual course of the illness being treated.*

The further clinical evaluation of the role of a drug in causation of an illness depends upon its prompt subsidence, usually a few days or weeks after therapy has been discontinued. This is presumptive evidence of drug allergy and suffices for most clinical purposes. Occasionally the reaction may persist for long periods, weeks or months, in cases in which elimination of the drug is slow, for example depot preparations, or where less reversible tissue damage has occurred. Also, continued exposure may result from occult sources, for example, penicillin in dairy products, or from cross-reactions with chemically related substances that are not drugs. When several drugs are involved, it is generally impossible to determine which one was the offender.

Direct challenge of the patient with a test dose of the drug (provocative test dosing) remains as the only absolute method to establish an etiological relationship between most suspected drugs and the clinical manifestations produced. In certain cases it is essential to determine whether a patient is reactive to a drug. This is because of the necessity of that drug as a therapeutic agent and the lack of an acceptable non-cross-reacting substitute. Such provocative testing for academic interest alone is not justified. This procedure is potentially dangerous and not advisable without appropriate consultation and considerable experience in management of hypersensitivity phenomena. This subject will be discussed in more detail later on.

It is apparent that additional safe and reliable methods are urgently needed to confirm or predict drug allergy, particularly for high risk patients and where the drug is of major importance to the patient. The next sections on skin tests and methods to detect drug allergy in vitro emphasize that conventional methods used to diagnose other allergic illness are generally unsatisfactory.

Skin Tests

Scratch (prick) and intracutaneous immediate-type skin tests are widely used to detect reaginic (IgE) hypersensitivity to inhalants and foods (see Chap. 3). In general, this technique to detect reagin-mediated drug hypersensitivity has limited value. As suggested earlier, for most drugs it is a metabolic or degradation product which combines with tissue proteins to form the immunogenic hapten-protein conjugate. The drug alone would not be expected to elicit a wheal and flare skin test reaction. Unfortunately, very little information is available about the metabolism and degradation of most drugs and suitable skin testing materials are not available. Further, prick testing would not be useful for detecting allergic drug reactions of immunologic mechanisms other than the reagin-mediated type.

In contrast, persons experiencing immediate type allergic reactions to *high molecular weight compounds* frequently have positive wheal and flare skin test reactions that correlate with the clinical picture. Such testing is useful in evaluating suspected allergy to such agents as equine and bovine antisera, ACTH, insulin, liver extract and vaccines containing egg. Suggestions for testing with these materials are often included in package inserts and will be discussed later.

Most drugs in current use are low molecular weight compounds and, for reasons cited earlier, would not be expected to elicit immediate skin test reactions. There are occasional exceptions in some patients to such simple chemicals as quinine, sulfonamides, tannic acid, chlorogenic acid, halazone and chloramine T. However, correlation of such testing with clinical hypersensitivity to these agents is usually uncertain. Penicillin is a partial exception to the general statement regarding the ineffectiveness of skin testing with simple chemical drugs and is discussed more fully later in this chapter.

False-Positive Skin Tests. Skin tests to drugs may be positive in the absence of hypersensitivity if the drug solution is too concentrated, if the drug is a histamine releaser, or if the solution in which the drug is dissolved is unphysiologic. When recommended concentrations of a drug for skin testing are unavailable, normal controls must be tested to rule out irritant responses.

Delayed (tuberculin-like) skin test reactions have been observed infrequently in drug allergy. There is evidence that occasional delayed clinical reactions (swelling) to procaine are associated with a positive delayed skin test response and this form of hypersensitivity has been transferred by leukocytes.[48] Delayed skin test reactions to the Merthiolate preservative in allergen testing and treatment solutions have been described.[66] Observations of such skin test reactions to penicillin and a few other drugs have not correlated with clinical hypersensitivity.

Patch tests commonly are of value in cases of contact hypersensitivity to topically applied medicaments, even if the eruption was provoked by systemic administration of the drug. In photosensitivity reactions, the patch test may become positive only after subsequent exposure to an erythemic dose of ultraviolet light (photopatch testing).

In some patients who have recovered from purpura due to drugs such as quinidine and quinine, patch testing with these substances may result in the appearance of purpura in the area of skin exposed to the drug. If the patch test is negative, a Rumpel-Leeds test should be applied to detect increased capillary fragility in the skin area exposed to the drug compared to a control site. Before such testing, the platelet count should be normal and checked at intervals while the patch is on as percutaneous absorption of the drug is possible.

The skin window technique, used initally to study inflammatory exudates induced by injury to the skin, has been applied to the investigation of drug allergy. Although there are reports of a correlation between a suspicion of drug hypersensitivity and a positive skin window response,[75] this technique has not received widespread application and remains investigational.

With exceptions already noted, skin testing for detection of drug allergy is unreliable. Negative skin test reactions do not exclude hypersensitivity. As this approach represents a modified form of direct challenge with the drug, it could produce a severe reaction. Aspirin-sensitive asthmatics invariably have negative skin tests to aspirin, yet the procedure may precipitate severe asthma. A fatality has followed intradermal skin testing with penicillin. If such testing is contemplated, prick or scratch tests must precede intracutaneous testing. Passive transfer (Prausnitz-Küstner) testing would avoid risks to the patient, but the procedure carries the threat of hepatitis to the recipient and no more positive results are obtained than in direct testing for the same reasons. The development of penicillin skin test reagents, discussed later, does represent an important potential advance in the diagnosis of drug allergy and may serve as a model for development of similar conjugates for many other drugs.

Tests in Vitro

Testing in vitro to detect drug hypersensitivity would avoid the inherent dangers in challenging patients with the drug. Although some of the tests currently available may be helpful, many are technically difficult to perform and may not correlate with the clinical state.

Serologic testing for specific antibodies to drugs is generally not available or helpful. To determine hemagglutinating antibody (HA) titers, sera of individuals with suspected drug allergy are reacted with red cells previously incubated with the drug so that it is attached by covalent bonds to the red cell membrane. Unfortunately, most drugs do not bind to erythrocytes. Under appropriate conditions, HA antibodies (IgG, IgM) can be detected in virtually all individuals who have received penicillin and many who receive cephalothin, regardless of the clinical state of the patient. These antibodies may be involved in the rare hematologic reactions due to penicillin and cephalothin. More important is the fact that the presence of HA antibodies is of no aid in the diagnosis of IgE-mediated drug reactions, for example immediate or accelerated reactions to penicillin. However, it has been suggested that IgG antibodies may be protective, serving as "blocking antibodies" competing for antigen with reaginic (IgE) antibodies among some patients with immediate penicillin hypersensitivity.[21]

Hematologic reactions afford an opportunity to test affected tissues in vitro. The summary on page 435 provides a list of diagnostic tests for drug-induced immune cytopenias; exact details are provided in Ackroyd.[1]

Drug-induced immune thrombocytopenic purpura has received most attention. Only one or two of the suggested tests may be positive in a particular case, but all should be performed, if available. Although antibodies may persist for months, these tests should be performed as early as possible in case the antibodies disappear rapidly after the drug is discontinued. For this reason, a negative group of tests may not always mean that an immune reaction has not occurred. If limited to a choice of one test, the complement fixation test is the most sensitive. For *drug-induced immunohemolytic anemias,* a positive Coombs' test is a most useful screening procedure, but should be followed by tests for specific antibodies (hemagglutinating) to suspected drugs, if available. In the Aldomet reaction, the drug is not necessary to produce the reaction, as the antibody appears to be directed against a locus on normal red cell membranes. This problem must be differentiated from hemolytic anemias occurring on a genetic basis, for example the glucose-6-phosphate dehydrogenase deficiency. Tests in vitro have been less successful in the detection of *drug-induced immune agranulocytosis.* The antibodies in the patient's serum may cause leukocyte agglutination even in the absence of the drug and disappear rapidly as the patient recovers. As leukoagglutinins are occasionally found in cases of agranulocytosis where no drug is involved, this test is of less value in establishing an etiologic diagnosis. On occasion, the leukoagglutinin activity may be increased by adding the suspected drug to the leukocyte-patient's serum mixture.

The radioallergosorbent test (RAST) is a method to detect reaginic antibodies to allergens in vitro.[94] Reaginic antibodies (IgE) in serum are reacted with an allergen that has been chemically coupled to an insoluble matrix. The allergen-bound reagins are then detected by their ability to bind radioactively labeled antibodies directed against IgE. This method has been applied to the detection of reagins to the penicilloyl determinant, and the results correlate favorably with those of skin and provocative testing in the investigation of penicillin hypersensitivity of the immediate type.[95] With further experience, this technique may provide a valuable alternative to skin testing for detection of drug allergy of the immediate type, probably mediated by IgE antibodies.

A number of *biologic tests* have recently been proposed for the diagnosis of drug allergy and must be considered investigational. One group of tests is based on the release of histamine from granules in circulating basophils as a result of the interaction between antibody and the suspected drug.

The basophil degranulation test involves mixing the patient's serum with a fresh preparation of human (direct test) or rabbit (indirect test) basophils which are stained supravitally. A solution of the drug is then added and the test considered positive if over 30 percent of the basophils become degranulated. Shelley recommends this procedure to detect immediate hypersensitivity states to penicillin and other drugs.[77] The interpretation depends largely upon the personal judgment of the technician. Varying results have been obtained in different laboratories, and the technique is not in common use. To reduce the subjective interpretive element, histamine release from rabbit platelets in the presence of the drug and patients serum has been fluorometrically assayed.[78] This procedure requires considerable experience to obtain consistent results and awaits further confirmation. Recently, rat peritoneal mast cells have been incubated with the patient's serum followed by the suspected drug.[61] The migration of granules to the cell periphery or occasional degranulation is considered significant. The value of this test for drug studies awaits confirmation.

Direct histamine release from leukocytes of human peripheral blood is a correlate in vitro of immediate (Type I) hypersensitivity. It is less sensitive for detection of IgE-mediated reactions than skin testing. Although it has shown significant changes in certain reactions, such as the rare case of hypersensitivity to tetanus toxoid, it has not been used successfully in other drug reactions.

The lymphocyte transformation test has received considerable attention for its possible application to the diagnosis of drug allergy. The initial observation that phytohemagglutinin could induce blast cell formation in tissue-cultured small lymphocytes was followed shortly by finding that a similar phenomenon could be induced by antigens including various drugs. Halpern [30] regularly found good correlation between a significant number of small lymphocytes into blast cells when lymphocytes from sensitized individuals are cultured in the presence

of the suspected drug; others are more cautious in their interpretation.[72]
As in the basophil degranulation test, much depends on subjective interpretation of the cellular response. The application of radiometric methods using measurement of the uptake of a DNA precursor, tritiated
thymidine, by the transformed lymphocytes has overcome this objection.
Other criticisms include the complexity of the procedure, delay in obtaining results and the fact that lymphocyte transformation does not
necessarily indicate a deleterious immunologic response. Further, the
test appears to be a better correlate in vitro of delayed type (Type IV)
reactions and may not correlate with circulating antibodies. These objec-
tions would militate against its widespread use in the investigation of
drug hypersensitivity. It has been suggested that the virtue of this
procedure and the skin window previously described is that they may
simulate more closely conditions in vivo by permitting development of
degradation products or metabolites of the drug which appear to be
more important in hypersensitivity reactions. However, most drugs are
metabolized by the liver, and the likelihood of peripheral degradation
seems remote.

SUMMARY

It is apparent that no test has been uniformly successful in the investigation of drug hypersensitivity. Table 16-2 is an attempt to correlate the reaction with the classification of hypersensitivity, the tests
expected to be positive, and the current state of such testing. Further,
the timing of these tests may have much to do with the results. The
time elapsed since the allergic reaction is important. Tests may be negative immediately after a severe reaction, suggesting that available antibody may have been utilized by the antigen-antibody reaction. Later,
the tests may become positive once again. As might be expected, without exposure to the drug, either directly or through occult sources, the
tests may again become negative.

Most testing procedures have limits of sensitivity and very small
amounts of antibody may remain undetectable; however, readministration of the drug may result in a significant reaction despite negative tests.
In spite of this, gradually a group of tests are being developed which
may eventually provide much needed answers. Considering the complexity of antigens, the variety of allergic responses (Types I to IV) and
other variables, it is not surprising that a single test may not be adequate
for diagnosis. Hopefully, a battery of tests in vitro may become routine
in the evaluation of a case of suspected drug hypersensitivity, thus
sparing the patient the discomfort and occasional danger of skin tests
and possibly provocative test dosing. Until then, one must rely almost

Table 16-2
Summary of Tests In Vivo and In Vitro for Drug Hypersensitivity

Type of Clinical Manifestation	Proposed Immunologic Mechanism	Test System In Vivo or In Vitro	Correlation with Clinical State
Immediate Reactions	*Type I (Anaphylactic)*	Cutaneous testing	Useful for high molecular weight substances; not for most drugs, penicillin being a partial exception (See text)
	Antibody: Reagin (Probably IgE)		
	Antigen: (A) Protein (B) Hapten-protein		
	Cell: Mast cell and basophils	Basophil degranulation	Difficult to reproduce with drugs
	Mediators: Histamine, SRS-A, Kinins	Leukocyte histamine release	Few correlations with drugs
Examples: Anaphylaxis Urticaria Asthma		Radioallergosorbent test (RAST)	Correlation with immediate-type penicillin hypersensitivity
Drugs: * (A) Horse serum * (B) Penicillin			
Late Reactions	*Type II (Cytotoxic) Hapten Type* (A and B)		
Examples: Hematologic reactions (A) Hemolytic anemia (B) Thrombocytopenia * (C) Agranulocytosis	*Antibody:* IgG *Antigen:* Hapten-protein *Cells:* Erythrocytes (Penicillin) Platelets (Sedormid)		
Drugs:	"Innocent bystander"		

* A, B, and C correlate the type of reaction, drugs involved and proposed mechanism.

TABLE 16-2 (*Continued*)

Summary of Tests In Vivo and In Vitro for Drug Hypersensitivity

[444]

TYPE OF CLINICAL MANIFESTATION	PROPOSED IMMUNOLOGIC MECHANISM	TEST SYSTEM IN VIVO OR IN VITRO	CORRELATION WITH CLINICAL STATE
Late Reactions (*cont.*)			
Penicillin (A) Stibophen (A) (B) PAS (A)	*type (A, B, C)* Antibody: IgG, IgM Antigen: Hapten-protein Cells: Erythrocytes (Stibophen)	Available tests listed on p. 435. Details in Akroyd [1]	Generally good correlation with clinical state provided testing is carried out soon after the reaction. May need to carry out multiple tests, if available.
Sulfonamides (A, B, C) Quinidine (A, B, C) Hydantoins (A, C) Alpha methyldopa (A)	Platelets (quinidine) Leukocytes (aminopyrine) *"Autoimmune Aldomet" type (A)* Antibody: IgG		
Sedormid (B)	Antigen: Altered red cell membrane, Rh locus Cell: Erythrocyte (Aldomet)		
Aminopyrine (B, C)			
Phenylbutazone (C)			
Example:	*Type III (Toxic antigen antibody complexes)* Antibody: IgG	A. Passive hemagglutination to detect IgG antibodies to horse serum	Practical diagnosis is by history and physical examination. Little clinical application for current testing in vitro.
Serum sickness-like	Antigen: (A) Protein		

TABLE 16-2 (*Continued*)

Summary of Tests In Vivo and In Vitro for Drug Hypersensitivity

TYPE OF CLINICAL MANIFESTATION	PROPOSED IMMUNOLOGIC MECHANISM	TEST SYSTEM IN VIVO OR IN VITRO	CORRELATION WITH CLINICAL STATE
Drugs: (A) Horse serum (B) Penicillin	*Cell:* PMN's (B) Hapten-protein *Mediator:* Serum complement	B. For penicillin, none	
Example: Contact Dermatitis	Type IV (*Delayed reactions*) *Antibody:* none		
Drugs: Nonprotein drugs, eg. local anesthetics	*Antigen:* Hapten-protein *Cell:* Lymphocyte *Mediators:* MIF, cytotoxic factor, chemotactic factors	Patch and photopatch testing	Good correlation with clinical state
Other late reactions Many skin eruptions (morbilliform, etc.)	*Toxic antigen-antibody complexes* (Type III)	None	None
Drug fever Hepatic reactions	*Delayed hypersensitivity* (Type IV)	Intradermal (tuberculin-like) testing	Rarely successful
Pseudolymphoma Vasculitis Other	Both Other	Lymphocyte transformation	Reactivity reported. Clinical correlation and predictability uncertain at this time.

entirely on careful history taking and experience in evaluating patients with suspected drug allergy.

Provocative Test Dosing

When a patient presents with a history compatible with drug allergy and cutaneous tests and tests in vitro are negative or, more likely, unavailable, readministration of the drug when the patient is asymptomatic is the only way to establish allergy or tolerance. Among patients who are highly sensitized and who may have had a life-threatening reaction, for example anaphylaxis or a hematologic reaction, this procedure may be dangerous and should be considered only when there are no acceptable, immunochemically unrelated substances available for treatment and when the probable benefit of the drug clearly outweighs the risk. The principle is to give sufficiently small doses initially and increase the dosage by safe increments until a therapeutic dose is achieved. Before proceeding, informed consent must be obtained from the patient or the patient's family; this information should be recorded in the medical record. It is advisable to point out the risks of giving as well as withholding the drug. Hospitalization and appropriate specialty consultation to underscore the need for proceeding in this manner are desirable. Emergency equipment should be immediately available.

What follows is an approach used by various competent and experienced specialists familiar with the risks and management of allergic reactions. It has been used primarily in situations where the manifestations were often dermatologic, for example morbilliform, erythematous or urticarial; where the patient or his physician were convinced that "allergy" to a drug was present regardless of the clinical manifestations; and where the symptoms may have been on a nonimmunologic basis, for example a vasovagal reaction following an injection. It is likely that most of these patients could have tolerated the drug in question at full dose without significant risk. However, for safety and medicolegal reasons, it is prudent to approach this problem cautiously.

If the drug is to be given parenterally, skin testing with the drug in question is the initial procedure. Details for the cautious administration of penicillin are outlined later. For other drugs, such as local anesthetics, the initial dilution used is 1:10,000 of the full strength material. If the drug reaction of suspected allergic origin was unusually severe, a 1:100,000 or a millionfold dilution would be more appropriate; if the reaction was dubious, a 1:1,000 dilution is reasonable. For some injectables, an irritant reaction may develop and it may be advisable to test several normals to provide controls.

Prick or scratch tests (see Chap. 3) are used for the initial dilutions to detect the potentially anaphylactic reactor. If negative, further skin tests are intradermal using 0.02 ml. of the material. Appropriate controls using the diluent are required with initial prick and intradermal skin tests. Providing no local or systemic reactions develop, skin testing is continued at 15-minute intervals, using more concentrated materials at tenfold increases in strength as suggested in Table 16-3. A positive skin test or development of symptoms is strong presumptive evidence that the patient is allergic to the drug and further testing should be abandoned. A negative skin test does not mean the patient is not allergic to the drug, but does suggest that he can tolerate that dose of material without an immediate type reaction, and should a reaction develop with the next higher dose, it is apt to be mild. Following a negative response to full strength material, the drug is then given by

TABLE 16-3

METHOD	DILUTION	RESULT	CONTROL RESULT
Prick test	1:10,000	Negative	Negative
Prick test	1:1000	Negative	—
Intradermal test	1:10,000	Negative	Negative
Intradermal test	1:1000	Negative	—
Intradermal test	1:100	Negative	—
Intradermal test	1:10	Negative	—
Intradermal test	Full strength	Negative	—

whatever route is necessary for therapeutic administration. Using local anesthetics as an example, one then may give 0.10 ml. full strength material subcutaneously and repeat this at 15- to 30-minute intervals using tenfold increments until therapeutic doses are achieved. Such an approach may not be applicable to iodinated contrast media, which will be discussed later. During parenteral challenge, it is desirable to have an intravenous infusion established and the patient's vital signs monitored carefully. Using this approach with the necessary precautions, it has been gratifying to evaluate dental patients who have been subjected to the risks of general anesthesia or allowed to suffer because they are presumably allergic to all local anesthetics, only to find after provacative test dosing that they are able to tolerate one of these preparations.

For oral preparations, such as isoniazid, an example of a schedule for administering the drug is as follows. The initial oral dose is 0.1 mg. Subsequent doses are increased by 5 to 10 times and given at 12- to 24-hour intervals until one reaches 50 mg., after which 50 mg. is added to each successive dose until the daily therapeutic level is attained.

Using this approach it has been possible to administer isoniazid, Dilantin, erythromycin and tetracycline safely to patients with questionable hypersensitivity to these substances. Where a hematologic reaction has occurred, Ackroyd [1] recommends starting with an oral dose of 1 μg. and increasing the dose on successive days to 10 μg., 0.1 mg., 1.0 mg., 10 mg., 50 mg. and finally 100 mg., providing appropriate laboratory tests are acceptable before the next dose is given.

This approach is an attempt to determine practically and safely whether a patient presumed allergic to a drug may now receive that material where it is essential and there are no acceptable substitutes. The decision to initiate such an approach depends on the training and experience of the physician. Although the above does provide certain guidelines, the initial dose and rapidity of increases in dose depends on the drug in question, the nature of the previous reaction and the urgency for readministration. It cannot be overstressed that caution must be exercised in the implementation of such a procedure and informed consent must be obtained from the patient.

It has been suggested that such an approach, and others like it, represent desensitization to the drug. There is controversy as to whether such is actually possible, and more will be said about this in sections dealing with penicillin and foreign antisera. It is likely that this procedure only demonstrates that the patient is no longer, or perhaps never was, allergic to the drug. One should not ignore the possibility that the patient may become sensitized during test dosing; hence, caution must be exercised in future use of the drug. Reisman [67] reported successful "desensitization" to penicillin in a subject allergic to the drug. Subsequently, repeat administration of penicillin produced a reaction.

PREVENTION OF DRUG REACTIONS

Although treatment of drug allergy is generally satisfactory, prevention is more desirable. The physician would be advised to consider carefully the points outlined here:

Prevention of Allergic Drug Reactions

Before administration of the drug
1. Evaluate the need for drug therapy.
2. Determine whether there is a previous history of drug allergy.
3. Consider whether the patient has an increased risk of drug allergy.
4. Consider the availability of diagnostic tests to detect or predict reactions.

During administration of the drug

    5. Methods of drug administration
        a. Route of administration—oral preferred.
        b. Administer allergy suppressants simultaneously.
        c. Avoid intermittent treatment courses.
        d. Keep patient for observation after an injection.
        e. Label all prescriptions.
        f. Inform patients and/or relatives about potential reactions.
    6. Have emergency treatment equipment available.
    7. Provocative test dosing or "densensitization."

Following administration of the drug

    8. Detect early evidence of an allergic reaction.
    9. Encourage active immunization procedures.
   10. Patient and physician education after an allergic drug reaction. Instruct patient in avoidance after an allergic reaction.

Considerations of Drug Use

The simplest way to reduce or prevent allergic drug reactions is to prescribe medication only when clearly indicated. Medications, especially antibiotics, are often used inappropriately, too frequently and over a prolonged period of time. Self-discipline is necessary to refuse patients' demands for "a penicillin shot" to treat the common cold. Of a group of 30 penicillin anaphylactic deaths, only 12 subjects had a clear indication for penicillin therapy.[70]

The number of drugs prescribed should be limited because adverse drug reactions increase when more drugs are administered. Should a reaction develop, there may be uncertainty as to which drug was the cause. It is a common practice for patients to receive a penicillin injection, presumably to achieve more rapid blood therapeutic levels, followed by continued therapy with an oral broad spectrum antibiotic. In addition to the undesirability of such practice, the agent responsible for a subsequent drug reaction may be difficult to determine.

The physician must be well informed regarding adverse reactions to drugs commonly used and be particularly cautious with newly introduced drugs to be sure of known drug reactions and be prepared for reactions which may not have been reported. Penicillin was initially thought to be of very low risk and only with time and a certain degree of misuse did reactions begin to appear. Lastly, drugs with a reputation for producing allergic reactions should be avoided if possible.

The Drug History

The patient must be questioned carefully about prior administration of the drug and whether there was any adverse reaction. This information should be obtained about other drugs as well as the drug about to be given. It is often helpful to suggest common allergic manifestations that may result from that drug to aid the patient's memory. In a report of fatal anaphylaxis after parenteral penicillin, about one third of patients or their relatives could have provided information about a prior allergic reaction to penicillin had this information been solicited.[70]

The responsibility for evaluating drug safety is that of the physician prescribing the drug. Overdiagnosis may be a problem; however, *when a patient believes he is allergic to a drug or was so advised, it is advisable to accept this information and select a drug of different immunochemical composition if possible.* When one member of a class of closely related substances has produced an allergic reaction, other members are likely to produce a similar reaction. A patient allergic to penicillin may react to semisynthetic analogues and even cephalothin. In most situations, the large number of available drugs allows the physician to prescribe a suitable alternative. Examples of suitable substitutes include acetaminophen (Tylenol,* Nebs †) for aspirin-sensitive patients and lidocaine (Xylocaine ‡) for procaine (Novocain §)-sensitive patients. Human tetanus antitoxin should be used preferentially in place of equine antitoxin. Norman [53] has provided a frequently updated list of commonly used drugs, common reactions attributable to them and suggested therapeutic alternatives.

High Risk Patients

Certain patients appear more prone to allergic drug reactions. Patients with a personal history of atopic disease (eczema, allergic rhinitis and bronchial asthma), if not more prone to such reactions, appear to experience more serious allergic reactions, especially to penicillin. Anaphylactic reactions occur 3 to 10 times more frequently in atopic individuals. The risk of allergic reactions appears greater among patients with chronic illnesses, in part owing to the increased frequency and number of drugs administered, which heightens the risk of eventual sensitization. Patients who have experienced drug hypersensitivity in the past may be more prone to developing sensitivity to newly administered drugs.

In these particular groups of patients the suggestions made thus far are even more pertinent. In treating infectious episodes among asthmatics in the Northwestern University Allergy Clinic, penicillin is rarely given, in part due to increased concern over the development of serious hypersensitivity.

* Trademark, McNeil.
† Trademark, Norwich.
‡ Trademark, Astra.
§ Trademark, Winthrop.

Availability of Predictive Tests

As emphasized in the section dealing with diagnosis, there are no reliable predictive tests except for skin tests with protein antigens. These can be used under special circumstances to be described later. Penicillin skin testing is a partial exception to the general statement that such testing is of no value for simple chemical drugs and will be discussed later.

Methods of Drug Administration

At the time of drug administration, certain precautions may lessen the likelihood of a significant allergic reaction: 1. *Route of administration.* When there is a choice, the oral route is preferable, as it is least apt to sensitize the patient and allergic reactions are less frequent and generally less severe. However, it is not safe to use a drug orally to which the patient is known or suspected to be hypersensitive. If the medication is given intramuscularly, use an extremity for the initial dose rather than the buttocks to allow placement of a tourniquet should a reaction occur. Topical application of certain drugs (e.g., penicillin, antihistamines) carries such a high risk of sensitization that they should never be administered in this way.

2. *Simultaneous administration of several antiallergic agents.* The efficacy of antihistamine, sympathomimetic, and corticosteroid prophylaxis in drug allergy is controversial.[47, 48, 69] These preparations may confer some degree of protection against certain disagreeable, nonfatal reactions or even modify to some extent more serious reactions (e.g., anaphylaxis); but they cannot be relied upon to prevent fatal reactions. Further, as milder reactions may be followed by more serious reactions in subsequent administration, the routine attempt to modify them is probably inadvisable.

3. *Unduly prolonged or intermittent exposure* to a drug should be avoided whenever possible, as this increases the likelihood of sensitization.

4. *Patients should remain under observation* a minimum of 15 to 20 minutes after an injection of a drug, as most serious allergic reactions develop within this period. If the patient has a history of vasovagal snycopal reactions following injections, the material can be administered while he is in the recumbent position.

5. The safety of drug treatment could be increased if all physicians would insist that pharmacists *label all drug containers* and inform patients about their medications. Where there are medical reasons not to do so, a relative or another responsible person should have this information. Should the patient report to another physician with early

symptoms that might represent drug allergy, there will be little difficulty in obtaining a drug history.

6. Patients or responsible persons should be informed about potential
reactions so that they may be alerted to, and can report, early symptoms.

Emergency Kit

A drug should never be administered parenterally unless appropriate
medication, equipment and trained medical personnel are immediately
available to treat anaphylaxis. As seconds may count, it is advisable
to have these materials gathered in an emergency kit, and personnel
should be instructed to react to this situation without confusion and
hesitation. Available medication and equipment ideally should include:

* 1. A tourniquet
* 2. Aqueous epinephrine 1:1000
* 3. Assorted syringes and needles
* 4. Injectable antihistamines, e.g., diphenhydramine (Benadryl †) or chlorpheniramine (Chlor-trimeton ‡)
* 5. Intravenous aminophylline
* 6. Water soluble corticosteroid, e.g., hydrocortisone succinate (Solu-
  Cortef §)
  7. Injectable vasopressor, e.g., metaraminol (Aramine ‖) or levarterenol
  bitartrate (Levophed #)
  8. Intravenous fluids, e.g., 5 percent dextrose in saline
  9. I-V infusion set
* 10. Sphygmomanometer
* 11. Stethoscope
  12. Lifesaving tube or oropharyngeal airway
  13. Surgical equipment for tracheostomy or venesection
  14. Source of oxygen
  15. Equipment for suctioning and resuscitation

* Those items marked with an asterisk are the basic minimum necessary to suc-
cessfully treat most severe reactions.
† Trademark, Parke, Davis.
‡ Trademark, Schering.
§ Trademark, Upjohn.
‖ Trademark, Merck Sharp & Dohme.
Trademark, Winthrop.

The details of treatment are outlined in Chapter 12.

Provocative Test Dosing

Provocative test dosing has been discussed as an approach to the administration of a drug to a patient presumed sensitive to that preparation. Desensitization is described later under discussions of penicillin,
hormones and foreign antisera. *These procedures are dangerous and*

should only be considered where the clinical need for the drug is appropriate and no adequate substitutes are available; where appropriate consultation, if available, has been obtained; where medicolegal protection has been obtained; and preferably where advice may be obtained from physicians experienced in handling hypersensitivity. Although these approaches may avoid anaphylaxis and other immediate allergic reactions, they are no protection from later reactions such as many drug eruptions, fever, serum sickness-like reactions and hematologic reactions. They do not insure against anaphylactic reactions on subsequent administration after an interruption in therapy.

Early Diagnosis

Following administration of a drug, the physician should advise patients to report promptly any minor symptoms such as slight fever, skin eruption, pruritus or any manifestation not previously present. After an injection, the patient experiencing early symptoms of anaphylaxis may simply "feel strange." Obviously, the sooner drug allergy is suspected and appropriate management begun, the more likely is a favorable outcome. Where indicated, laboratory studies must be monitored to detect early evidence of drug hypersensitivity, for example in hematologic reactions.

Prophylactic Immunization

Encouraging active immunization with tetanus toxoid will reduce the need for passive immunization with equine antisera. Allergic reactions to tetanus toxoid are fortunately rare and will be discussed later. Further, hyperimmune human tetanus antitoxin (Hyper-Tet °) is now available and is the treatment of choice when passive immunization is required. This material is more effective and no preliminary skin testing is necessary, although allergic reactions have occasionally developed, probably as a result of aggregated gamma globulin.

Patient and Physician Education

The responsibility to a patient who has sustained a drug reaction does not end with discontinuation of the preparation and treatment of the reaction. The patient or responsible persons must be informed that a drug reaction has occurred and what agent is presumed responsible. The patient should be informed of suitable alternative drugs and advised regarding hidden sources of the preparation, for example the presence of acetylsalicylic acid in many cold and headache remedies. They should be instructed to read labels on proprietary drugs and be certain that other physicians are advised about a previous drug reaction

° Trademark, Cutter.

if they fail to inquire about this before prescribing medication. To afford additional protection, the patient should carry a card or wear a tag (Medic-Alert Emblems, Turlock, California 95380) designating the drugs to be avoided. All medical records and hospital charts must display the patient's drug sensitivities in a conspicuous location.

It should be the responsibility of physicians to promptly report adverse drug reactions to the respective manufacturer and other responsible agencies such as The Registry on Adverse Reactions, Council on Drugs, American Medical Association, 535 No. Dearborn Street, Chicago, Illinois, 60610 or to the Bureau of Medicine, Adverse Reactions Branch, Food and Drug Administration, Washington, D.C., 20202.

TREATMENT

The treatment of drug-induced allergic reactions is symptomatic. Obviously, the drug is discontinued except for very unusual circumstances. Frequently, no additional therapy is required, and the clinical manifestations often subside within a few days. Where several medications are involved, all should be discontinued. If such is impossible, the most likely offender(s) must be withdrawn; certainly those with a reputation for producing drug hypersensitivity, for example antimicrobials, aspirin, barbiturates and anticonvulsants. If treatment is still necessary for the primary illness, drugs of a different immunochemical structure must be substituted.[53]

A possible exception to this relates to infants and small children who develop nonurticarial eruptions (often morbilliform) during antibiotic therapy for a febrile illness. Commonly the rash is due to the viral illness and not the drug. Here, particularly where the child has not received the drug previously, it seems advisable to continue therapy for a few days and observe closely, rather than label the child as allergic to penicillin or another antibiotic. After a penicillin reaction, particularly if prolonged, the patient should be instructed to avoid dairy products as they may be contaminated with small amounts of penicillin.

Attempts to hasten elimination and degradation of the drug may be of value. Dimercaprol (BAL °) is of value in heavy metal reactions such as exfoliative dermatitis due to gold. BAL is given as a 10 percent solution intramuscularly. The dosage is 2.5 mg. per kilogram body weight given at 4-hour intervals for 2 successive days; then every 6 hours on day three; then once or twice daily for about 10 days, depending upon the severity of symptoms. Therapy must continue until the urinary secretion of the metal is negligible. BAL is a good antidote for gold, arsenic, mercury, nickel, and antimony but is less effective for silver and may be

° Trademark, Hynson, Westcott & Dunning.

contraindicated for lead. The material is toxic and may produce lacrimation, salivation, nausea, emesis, headache, myalgias and burning paresthesias about the face. Diphenhydramine (Benadryl), 25 to 50 mg. orally every 4 to 6 hours, may prevent or modify these side effects. An exacerbation of rheumatoid arthritis has followed the use of BAL, giving rise to the suggestion that corticosteroids be used to treat gold reactions, reserving BAL for unresponsive cases.[46] Attempted enzymatic degradation of the drug is exemplified by the use of penicillinase (Neutrapen *) in the treatment of penicillin reactions. Aside from its ineffectiveness, the material is costly, extremely painful to inject and, because it is a protein, has produced severe allergic reactions. Therefore, the use of this material is not recommended.

Managing the Symptoms

Symptomatic treatment of allergic drug reactions is aimed at alleviating the symptoms until they subside spontaneously. For mild reactions, therapy is usually unnecessary. Treatment of more severe reactions depends upon the nature of the skin eruption and the degree of systemic involvement, and is similar to therapy applied to these manifestations whatever the etiology. In the latter circumstance, hospitalization may be advisable for more careful observation. Treatment of anaphylaxis (Chap. 12), urticaria and angioedema (Chap. 13), eczema (Chap. 15) and contact dermatitis (Chap. 17) is considered in detail elsewhere.

For most cutaneous drug eruptions, topical therapy is unnecessary. In life-threatening eruptions, such as Stevens-Johnson syndrome, exfoliative dermatitis and toxic epidermal necrolysis, systemic treatment with corticosteroids is mandatory using an initial dose of at least 60 mg. prednisone or its equivalent daily. For most other drug-induced cutaneous eruptions, local therapy, if required at all, is designed to be soothing and provide symptomatic relief until the lesion heals. Recommendations for local therapy include the following:

1. For widespread eruptions, colloid baths may be cleansing, soothing, antipruritic, and decongestive. Tepid water (90° to 96° F) should be used. Common additives include:

a. Linit starch (pulverized cornstarch). Dissolve 1 cup in a saucepan and add to a half full tub of water.

b. Oatmeal. Cook two cups of oatmeal in one quart of water in a double boiler for 30 to 45 minutes. Allow to cool for 15 minutes and add one half cup of baking soda. Place the contents into a gauze bag and tie securely. Fill the tub one half to three fourths full with tepid water. Express the oatmeal mash through the gauze and apply it over the body. The mash is rinsed off thoroughly before leaving the tub.

* Trademark, Riker.

A shortcut to this is the use of commercially available colloidal oatmeal (Aveeno °). One cup is combined with 2 cups of cool water, and the mixture is poured into a tub half full of tepid water.

These oatmeal preparations are quite slippery and patients must be cautioned about this. If too drying, Oilated Aveeno may be used.

These soothing baths may be taken two to four times daily, with the patient soaking for 30 to 60 minutes each time. The patient should not remain in the bath long enough to allow the skin to become soggy or macerated. Upon leaving the tub, chilling should be avoided and the patient should dry himself by gently blotting the skin with a soft towel to allow some of the solution to dry on his skin.

2. Between cutaneous hydrotherapy and at bedtime, a bland "shake" lotion may be applied to provide a protective, drying and cooling effect. Calamine lotion, U.S.P., may be used or another inexpensive basic shake lotion. A cooling or antipruritic effect may be obtained by adding 0.25 percent menthol to the shake lotions. These lotions may be applied liberally to large areas with fingers, hands or even a soft paint brush. Shake lotions should not be used in hairy areas and frequently are not well tolerated in the anogenital region; here one may use a mixture of equal parts of olive oil and aqua calcis (lime water) or calamine liniment U.S.P.

3. As the skin becomes drier or in situations where the dermatitis is primarily a dry one, for example morbilliform eruptions, liquid emulsions or liniments may be used if necessary. Calamine liniment with 0.25 percent menthol, Keri Lotion, † and Lubriderm ‡ lotion are useful. These may be applied liberally as needed to control symptoms. For more sensitive areas, corticosteroid creams may be thinly applied four or five times daily until the dermatitis subsides. The more expensive corticosteroid creams (Cordran, § Kenalog, ‖ Synalar # Valisone °°) may be diluted with 1 to 3 parts of hydrophilic ointment U.S.P., Neobase ‡‡ or Acid Mantle §§ without impairing efficacy. *If the areas requiring topical steriods are widespread, systemic corticosteroids are advisable.* For very dry, scaly eruptions, more lubricating creams and ointments are preferable.

4. For localized lesions, wet dressings may be advisable in the more

---

° Trademark, Cooper.
† Trademark, Westwood.
‡ Trademark, Texas Pharmeceutical.
§ Trademark, Lilly.
‖ Trademark, Squibb.
Trademark, Syntex.
°° Trademark, Schering.
‡‡ Trademark, Burroughs Wellcome.
§§ Trademark, Dome.

acute weeping phase. In addition to cleansing the area, this affords temporary relief of pruritus and reduction of inflammation. The technique of applying wet dressings is of greater import than medicaments added to water. Two or three layers of gauze, Kerlix, or soft linen are moistened, loosely wrung out and applied to the area. The dressing should be removed and remoistened every 5 minutes to prevent drying and sticking to the lesion. The total treatment is carried out for 20-30 minutes four times daily if necessary. Commonly used solutions include:

Burow's solution (aluminum acetate)—one Domeboro * tablet or packet in one quart of cool water makes a 1:40 solution.

Saline—one teaspoonful of salt to one pint of cool water produces an isotonic solution.

$KMnO_4$ (potassium permanganate)—add 0.3 g. to 1½ quarts water to make a 1:4000 solution. It is excellent if infection is present, but it stains.

Milk—is an excellent, frequently overlooked preparation, but is not as drying as others.

Between applications of wet dressings, shake lotions may be applied. As the lesions become drier, one progresses to liniments, creams, and ointments as previously described. As the areas are limited in size, topical corticosteroids are very effective. To enhance penetration of the fluorinated corticosteroid creams and ointments, the treated area may be covered by a thin plastic film occlusive dressing, for example Saran Wrap, held in place by tape for up to 12 hours.

5. For mucous membrane lesions, especially those in the mouth, Xylocaine Viscous † helps to reduce the pain when used before eating. A soft or liquid diet is desirable.

6. For secondary infections, appropriate systemic antibiotics are of greater value than those applied topically. Prophylactic antibiotic usage is not indicated.

7. While the skin lesion heals, bathing frequently should be decreased and mild soaps (Basis, Oilatum) and lubricating oils (Lubriderm, Alpha-Keri) used. Cetaphil ‡ lotion may be used as a nonlipid cleansing agent. Harsh clothing, for example woolens and starched linens, are irritating and should not be worn. High environmental temperatures and excess humidity may also aggravate the condition. Local skin care must be continued for several weeks after healing to avoid aggravation of the eruption long after the offending drug has been eliminated.

8. Often, long after a photosensitivity reaction, the patient must continue to avoid sunlight as much as possible and use topical sunscreens

---

* Trademark, Dome.
† Trademark, Astra.
‡ Trademark, Texas Pharm.

(Pre-Sun, * Uval, † Solbar, ‡ Pabafilm §). At times, an oral antimalarial such as chloroquine phosphate (Aralen ||), 250 mg. twice a day, may be beneficial. When treatment with this preparation is prolonged, the eyes must be examined every few months for the development of retinopathy.

Systemic Therapy

Systemic therapy may not be necessary in mild reactions. If indicated, the type depends upon the clinical manifestations. Commonly used medications include antihistamines, sympathomimetics, salicylates and corticosteroids. Serum sickness will be discussed in detail, as this reaction is the result of a definite immunologic mechanism, and therapeutic principles may be applied to many aspects of other drug hypersensitivity reactions. For children, age and size must be considered for the doses prescribed, as those suggested here are for treatment of adults. Examples of selected agents such as antihistamines are given. Other similar agents may be equally effective.

Antihistamines are especially useful in treatment of urticarial dermatoses and angioedema and moderately effective for pruritus associated with other drug-induced allergic dermatoses. Initially, large doses may be required. Diphenhydramine (Benadryl), 50 to 100 mg. every 4 to 6 hours, is desirable if sedation is not a serious objection. The associated sedation may be an asset during the more acute pruritic stage of the illness. For ambulatory patients where sedation is undesirable, chlorpheniramine (Chlor-trimeton) and brompheniramine (Dimetane #) may be used. Initially, the short acting antihistamines are advisable as they allow greater dosage flexibility, for example 4 to 8 mg. 3 to 4 times daily. The longer-acting antihistamines, for example Chlor-trimeton Repetabs, Teldrin Spansules, Dimetane Extentabs, 8 to 12 mg. may be used every 8 to 12 hours. Promethazine hydrochloride (Phenergan), 12.5 to 25 mg., may be substituted at night as it has a soporific effect and more prolonged duration of action.

If pruritus persists despite the above measures, cyproheptadine hydrochloride (Periactin **), 4 mg. every 4 to 6 hours or trimeprazine (Temaril ††), 2.5 to 5.0 mg. every 4 hours may be substituted. For the anxious

* Trademark, Westwood Pharmaceuticals.
† Trademark, Dome.
‡ Trademark, Person & Covey.
§ Trademark, Owen.
|| Trademark, Winthrop.
Trademark, Robins.
** Trademark, Merck Sharp & Dohme.
†† Trademark, Smith Kline & French.

patient, hydroxyzine hydrochloride (Atarax °), 10 to 50 mg. 3 to 4 times daily is often useful.

If one antihistamine is ineffective, substitution of an antihistamine with a differing chemical structure may be tried. It is likely that the change in antihistamine may not prove beneficial, but it allows the physician an out while the reaction spontaneously subsides or becomes severe enough to warrant the use of corticosteroids. An excellent review of antihistamines has been provided by Wilhelm.[96]

Sympathomimetic amines are drugs of choice in the treatment of anaphylaxis and drug-induced asthma. In serum sickness-like reactions epinephrine has limited usefulness because of its brief duration of action; however, it may provide immediate relief of rapidly developing, uncomfortable urticaria and angioedema. Subcutaneous injections of 0.3 ml. 1:1000 aqueous epinephrine, repeated, if necessary, after 5 minutes, can be given on such occasions. A more prolonged effect results with Sus-Phrine † (a long-acting 1:200 suspension of epinephrine tannate in glycerine and distilled water), 0.20 ml. subcutaneously every 8 hours. Oral ephedrine, 25 mg. every 4 to 6 hours, may sustain the effect, but is usually not required. Combination therapy utilizing an antihistamine and sympathomimetic amine, for example Actifed, ‡ Co-Pyronil, § or Pyribenzamine || with ephedrine, may be of value.

Salicylates are used to control fever, tender lymphadenophathy and joint discomfort.

Corticosteroids will completely or partially suppress the clinical manifestations of most allergic drug reactions when given in full therapeutic dosage. Such therapy is justified because of the severity and duration of symptoms and the failure of other medications to control them. In addition to severe serum sickness reactions, corticosteroids are often required in treatment of other drug hypersensitivity such as severe hematologic reactions, vasculitis, and severe cutaneous reactions, such as Stevens-Johnson syndrome, exfoliative dermatitis, and toxic epidermal necrolysis.

Prednisone (or its equivalent), 40 to 80 mg. daily, is administered orally in divided doses until the manifestations are suppressed. The prednisone should be tapered as rapidly as possible consistent with control of the reaction. A suggested tapering schedule is a dosage reduction of 10 mg. daily or every other day until reaching a daily dose of

° Trademark, Roerig.
† Trademark, Cooper.
‡ Trademark, Burroughs Wellcome.
§ Trademark, Lilly.
|| Trademark, Ciba.

20 mg., after which the dose is reduced by 5 mg. increments daily or every other day until discontinuance. If symptoms recur, the dose may be temporarily increased and then reduced more slowly. Frequently, concomitant antihistamine administration will obviate the need to prolong steroid therapy. Parenteral administration of steroids does not produce a significantly more rapid response, and depot steroid preparations provide less predictable dosage control. ACTH is not recommended.

The duration of treatment of serum sickness and most other allergic drug reactions with corticosteroids is usually brief (1 to 2 weeks). Because of their usual self-limited nature, the risk of using these agents is minimal. Occasionally, more prolonged use may be necessary. Then, all the usual precautions of steroid therapy must be considered.

Other therapy may be necessary, especially for drug-induced hematologic reactions. Transfusions are occasionally required in severe hemolytic anemia and frequently in aplastic anemia. The hemoglobin levels should not be brought to normal but only to a level (8 to 10 g. hemoglobin) at which symptoms are relieved, in order to preserve the natural stimulus to blood formation. Prophylactic antibiotic therapy is not recommended; but when infections do occur, they must be vigorously treated with appropriate chemotherapy.

SPECIAL CONSIDERATION OF ALLERGIC DRUG PROBLEMS

THE PENICILLINS

Incidence

Penicillin and its homologues are the most frequent causes of anaphylaxis in man. The reported incidence of penicillin allergy ranges from 1 to 10 percent. The incidence of anaphylactic reactions ranges between 10 and 40 per 100,000 injections. The risk of fatal anaphylaxis is approximately 2 in 100,000.[35] The lower reported incidence probably applies to an ambulatory population, while the higher figure reflects reactions occuring among hospitalized patients. The latter include chronically ill patients receiving multiple courses of penicillin therapy. As is generally true of drug allergy, penicillin reactions appear less frequently among children. Some reactions attributed to penicillin in children are misdiagnosed. They may be the result of the disease for which penicillin was given. An example would be morbilliform, nonurticarial viral exanthems. Using currently available tests in vivo and in vitro, Bierman and Van Arsdel found that many hospitalized children with a previous diagnosis of penicillin allergy were able to tolerate penicillin.[10] Among atopic subjects, there appears to be an increased risk, especially for the development of anaphylactic reactions.

The widespread, often indiscriminate use of penicillin, especially administered by injection, is an important problem in creating penicillin allergy. Almost everyone has had exposure to penicillin even without receiving the drug therapeutically. There are reported allergic reactions to penicillin among patients who deny previous exposure to it. Potential sources of contact include food products and milk from animals treated with penicillin. Many of these sources have been controlled by reduction of penicillin in milk, use of other antimicrobial agents in vaccines, the decreased use of glass reusable syringes, and better controls in the pharmaceutical industry. Medical personnel may become sensitized by topical contact or inhalation of the drug during preparation and administration. Small amounts of penicillin may be synthesized from the ubiquitous parent Penicillium molds in the environment; however, atopic patients with Penicillium hypersensitivity generally can tolerate penicillin.

Clinical Manifestations

Allergic reactions to penicillin may be diverse and may be classified according to the time of onset.[92] Immediate reactions occur within an hour after penicillin administration. The most serious is anaphylaxis. Pruritus, urticaria and angioedema may constitute the entire reaction. However, hypotension and death may occur without other symptoms. Less commonly rhinitis, asthma and laryngeal edema develop. Accelerated reactions begin 1 to 72 hours after penicillin therapy as urticaria and angioedema. Occasionally laryngeal edema is present, but hypotension and death are unusual. Late reactions appear more than 3 days after penicillin administration and usually appear as a variety of benign skin eruptions, such as exanthems involving the trunk and proximal extremities. Other erythematous rashes may appear and rarely the Stevens-Johnson syndrome may develop. Penicillin and its homologues are the most common causes of serum sickness-like reactions. Another late reaction begins 3 to 21 days after penicillin is discontinued and results in a syndrome of recurrent urticaria and arthralgia that may persist for up to 4 months. In contrast to serum sickness-like reactions, there is no fever, lymphadenopathy or splenomegaly. Renal and cardiac abnormalities are not present. Relatively unusual late reactions include drug fever, hemolytic anemia, thrombocytopenia and renal failure.[67] Vasculitis has been described, but the causal relationship to penicillin is less clear.[63]

Antigenic Determinants

Penicillin is a low molecular weight substance (molecular weight of 300) and does not bind firmly enough with tissue or serum proteins to form an antigenic complex. Benzylpenicillin is degraded mostly into benzylpenicillenic acid, a chemically reactive metabolite which combines with proteins to form benzylpenicilloyl (BPO) haptenic groups. Approximately 95 percent of penicillin in vitro is handled in this way; hence, the benzylpenicilloyl (BPO) group is referred to as the "major" antigenic determinant. To a much lesser degree, benzylpenicillin may react directly with proteins to form this haptenic group. BPO conjugates for skin testing may be prepared by reacting benzylpenicillin with proteins, such as human serum albumin, or with synthetic polypeptides such as polylysine. As the former may induce penicillin hypersensitivity in man, the latter is used as it lacks immunogenicity, particularly the poly-D-lysine.

Several other antigenic determinants are formed in relatively small amounts and are designated as "minor" antigenic determinants. Their chemical nature and mechanism of formation are not as well defined as for the BPO determinant. However, they are of considerable importance clinically as they are frequently responsible for severe, immediate reactions. Levine has used a combination of benzylpenicillin, benzylpenicilloate, benzylpenilloate and a-benzylpenicilloyl-amine as a "minor" determinant mixture (MDM) for skin testing.

Penicillin, although refined for clinical use, may contain traces of impurities. These include protein or polypeptide complexes remaining from molds used in the manufacturing process or developing from penicillin in solution as a result of polymerization. It has been suggested that these contaminants may sensitize patients and result in allergic reactions,[82] but their significance in penicillin allergy has not been established.

Immunologic Response

Penicillin elicits formation of antibodies in several of the immunoglobulin classes. Most individuals studied, even those with no prior history of penicillin treatment, have low titers of IgM antibodies to penicillin, possibly due to exposure to sources described earlier. Following administration of penicillin, there is a rise in antibody titer, particularly in IgG and IgE (reaginic) antibodies. Atopic patients appear more likely to form reaginic antibodies. The mere presence of anti-penicillin antibodies does not denote clinical sensitivity.

Reaginic antibody, presumptively IgE like most other reaginic antibody, mediates immediate and accelerated allergic reactions to penicillin. The antibodies are usually directed against "minor" determinants in the case of anaphylaxis, while the "major" determinant is usually involved in the accelerated urticarial reactions. A retrospective study indicated reagins to "minor" determinants in the syndrome of recurrent urticaria and arthralgia.[92]

IgG and IgM antibodies with BPO specificity may be detected by the hemagglutination technique in virtually all patients treated with penicillin. High titers of IgG antibodies are associated with the Coombs'-positive immunohemolytic anemia which occasionally develops in a few patients receiving high doses of penicillin. BPO-specific IgG antibodies may also serve as "blocking" antibodies competing with BPO-specific reaginic antibodies. If BPO-specific blocking antibody titers are low, a severe, immediate penicillin reaction to BPO-specific reagins may occur.[45] Conversely, some patients developing accelerated urticarial reactions on intravenous penicillin therapy had these manifestations subside as the BPO-specific IgG titer rose with continued therapy. Prior knowledge of this titer may be useful in assessing a patient's risk regarding development of immediate or accelerated reactions mediated by BPO-specific reagins. To date, blocking (IgG) antibodies have not been detected to minor determinants which are more frequently associated with anaphylaxis.

BPO-specific IgM antibodies in high titer have been associated with late maculopapular and diffuse erythematous eruptions developing during penicillin therapy and fading with some scaling 3 to 21 days after the drug has been discontinued. This is particularly common with ampicillin therapy. The mechanism of this reaction and prognosis for future reactions is unknown. When an infectious exanthem is in the differential diagnosis, the finding of BPO-specific IgM antibodies in high titer (over 1:1000) is presumptive evidence that penicillin is the culprit.

Skin Testing

As anaphylactic and accelerated penicillin reactions are mediated by skin sensitizing or reaginic antibodies, skin testing to detect a wheal and flare reaction is logical. Penicilloyl-polylysine (PPL), a conjugate of benzylpencilloyl moieties attached to a polylysine chain, and a minor determinant mixture (MDM) of benzylpenicillin, benzylpenicilloate, benzylpenilloate and a-benzylpenicilloyl amine have been studied extensively as skin test reagents. A negative skin test reaction to both reagents significantly reduces the likelihood of an immediate (anaphylactic) reaction to penicillin. The likelihood of accelerated urticarial reactions is reduced.[43] The rare false negative reactions are probably due to antigenic determinants not present in either reagent. A positive skin test to only PPL is associated with a decreased likelihood of anaphylaxis, but such patients do have an increased risk of accelerated urticarial reactions. A positive skin test with the MDM is predictive of anaphylactic sensitivity. Skin testing with these agents is not predictive of late reactions such as various rashes, hemolytic anemia or serum sickness. As the initial administration of penicillin serves to sensitize and elicit symptoms in primary serum sickness-like disease, the skin tests would be of no value. In one prospective study, routine skin testing with these penicillin reagents significantly reduced serious penicillin reactions and allowed safe administration of penicillin to many patients with histories of penicillin allergy who otherwise would have been denied the use of the drug.[3] The PPL and MDM skin test reagents are not available except for experimental study, and clinicians are forced to use benzylpenicillin G for scratch (prick) and intradermal skin testing.

When penicillin administration is being considered in spite of a questionable history of penicillin allergy, a skin test should be done first, using freshly prepared dilutions of the drug. It has been recommended that older solutions of benzylpenicillin be used for testing because they may contain benzylpenicilloate and would be more apt to identify "minor" determinant sensitivity, but this has not been uniformly accepted. Prick tests on a distal extremity using aqueous benzylpenicillin G in increasing concentrations of 10, 100, 1,000, and 10,000 units per milliliter are performed. If severe penicillin allergy is suspected, the initial prick test should be done with even more dilute solutions, for example 1 unit or less per milliliter. If prick tests are negative, intradermal skin tests, using 0.02 ml. of solutions containing 100, 1,000, and 10,000 units per milliliter are performed. The tests are done at 15 to 30 minute intervals using an initial saline control. A positive immediate skin test must be considered sufficient warning that anaphylaxis is likely if the drug is given. In effect, this graded skin test system is simultaneously administering doses of penicillin, for example 200 units will have been given with the intradermal skin test of 0.02 ml. of the solution containing 10,000 units per ml. Discussion of further cautious administration of penicillin follows later.

Table 16-4 is an attempt to depict the role of skin testing in the prevention of penicillin anaphylaxis. In general, the usefulness of skin testing with penicilloyl-polylysine, penicillin itself and "minor" determinants may be summarized as follows: [58] (1) Among patients with a positive history, there is an increased incidence of positive skin test reactions; (2) in patients with a negative history, a positive skin test indicates an increased risk of a subsequent allergic reaction; (3) among patients with a history of penicillin allergy, negative skin tests minimize, but do not completely exclude, the risk of a serious reaction upon subsequent penicillin administration; (4) the incidence of immediate or accelerated penicillin reactions decreases if patients with positive skin

TABLE 16-4
Prevention of Penicillin Anaphylaxis

HISTORY OF PENICILLIN ALLERGY		IDEAL	ACTUAL
No	*Best:*	Skin test with PPL and MDM prior to penicillin administration	Reagents not available
	Second best:	Skin test with penicillin G Prick test 500,000 u/ml. Intracutaneous 10,000 u/ml.	Not standard practice
Yes	*Best:*	Substitute other antibiotics	Often appropriate
	Second best:	Skin test with PPL and MDM	Reagents not available
	Next best:	Graded skin test — test dose system	Clinically useful

tests are not treated with the drug. One must remember that skin tests may induce penicillin sensitivity and testing has produced serious reactions.[43]

Management of Patients with Histories of Penicillin Allergy

Current practice is variable in managing a patient with a history compatible with penicillin allergy and an illness for which penicillin is the usual drug of choice. Therapeutic alternatives include the use of semisynthetic penicillins, cephalosporin C derivatives or some other antibiotic.

Multiple semisynthetic penicillins have been produced by modification of the side chain (R) attached to the 6-aminopenicillanic (6-APA) nucleus (Fig. 16-9). The 6-aminopenicillanic acid nucleus is responsible for most of the antigenic activity of the penicillins by reacting with host proteins to form hapten-protein conjugates. Therefore, a variation in the side chain (R) would not have a marked effect in decreasing cross allergenicity between penicillin and other homologues containing the 6-APA nucleus. The oral penicillins, oxacillins, nafcillin, ampicillin and carbenicillin produce the same types of allergic reactions as penicillin G, although the incidence of immediate or accelerated reactions appears to be lower.

Of special interest are the rare reactions associated with renal failure, particularly among patients receiving methicillin.[67] The clinical state

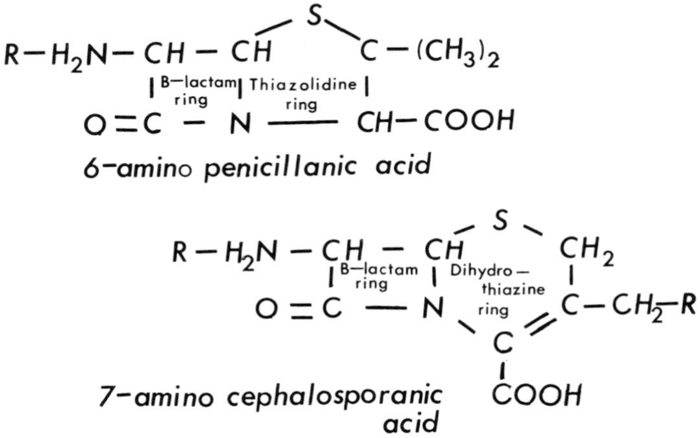

$$R-H_2N-CH-CH \overset{S}{\diagup}\diagdown C-(CH_3)_2$$

| B—lactam | Thiazolidine |
ring | ring

$$O=C - N \longrightarrow CH-COOH$$

6-amino penicillanic acid

$$R-H_2N-CH-CH \overset{S}{\diagup}\diagdown CH_2$$

| B—lactam | Dihydro—
ring | thiazine

$$O=C \longrightarrow N \underset{ring}{\diagdown}\diagup C-CH_2-R$$

C
|
COOH

7-amino cephalosporanic acid

Figure 16-9.

includes fever, skin eruptions, eosinophilia, proteinuria, hematuria and a variable degree of azotemia. Renal biopsy shows tubular damage and interstitial nephritis without glomerular abnormalities or arteritis. One patient studied was found to have gamma globulin and the hapten (BPO) in glomerular tissue, but no complement was detected and glomerular abnormalities were not evident, suggesting these antigen-antibody complexes were not tissue damaging. It is possible the lesion was due to delayed-type hypersensitivity, and the patient did exhibit delayed skin reactivity to methicillin. In these cases, the renal failure is usually reversible after stopping the drug.

Ampicillin is associated with a higher incidence (7.7 percent) of drug rash than are other penicillins (2.7 percent).[76] During the first week of therapy, the incidence of rash due to ampicillin is no more than that produced by other penicillins. Most of the excess rash with ampicillin occurs at least a week after institution of therapy and occasionally as late as the end of the third week, even after treatment has been discontinued. Also, many patients with infectious mononucleosis treated with ampicillin develop this drug eruption.

Drug eruptions due to ampicillin fall into two major categories: urticarial and erythematous. Urticaria represents true penicillin hypersensitivity and ampicillin is no more likely to produce this eruption than other penicillins. Erythematous reactions associated with ampicillin may not be associated with penicillin allergy as it is currently understood in terms of risk of progressive hypersensitivity and fatality. The eruption subsides after stopping the drug. It may even disappear with stopping

TABLE 16-5
Alternate Antimicrobials for Patients Allergic to Penicillin

INFECTION	ANTIBIOTICS
Pneumococcal pneumonia	Erythromycins or lincomycin
Streptococcal pharyngitis	
Minor staphylococcal infection (skin, soft tissue)	
Streptococcal prophylaxis	Erythromycins or sulfonamides
Severe staphylococcal infections (pneumonia, meningitis, osteomyelitis, septicemia)	Vancomycin
Purulent meningitis (*D. pneumoniae, N. meningitis, H. influenzae*)	Chloramphenicol
Diphtheria	Erythromycin
Gonorrhea	
Syphilis	Erythromycin or tetracyclines
Actinomycosis	
Clostridial infections	Tetracyclines
Listeriosis	
Bacterial endocarditis—	
S. *viridans*	Erythromycin plus streptomycin
Staphylococcal	Vancomycin
Enterococcal	Vancomycin, or penicillin "desensitization"

the drug. The nature of this erythematous eruption is not known and its relationship to penicillin allergy not definitely established. Patients developing this nonurticarial eruption with ampicillin probably should not be labeled penicillin sensitive.

Results of preliminary skin testing with major and minor determinant reagents prepared from the semisynthetic penicillins have shown marked variability in patterns of reactivity; a positive skin test to one penicillin drug is not necessarily associated with positive reactions to all penicillin drugs.[90] With additional experience, such testing may be helpful in selecting which penicillin a patient may safely receive. Until then, it is advisable to consider a history of penicillin allergy as a contraindication to the administration of semisynthetic penicillins. If, for reasons to be cited later, one must administer one of these agents, preliminary skin testing and cautious administration may be considered as outlined later.

Method for Cautious Administration of Increasing Doses of Penicillin °

A. Preparation of solutions, using aqueous crystalline penicillin G

Dilute 20,000,000-unit vial to 20 ml = 1,000,000 units/ml (solution 1).

Dilute 1 ml of solution 1 to 10 ml = 100,000 units/ml (solution 2).

Dilute 1 ml of solution 2 to 10 ml = 10,000 units/ml (solution 3).

Dilute 1 ml of solution 3 to 10 ml = 1,000 units/ml (solution 4).

Dilute 1 ml of solution 4 to 10 ml = 100 units/ml (solution 5).

B. Application

1. Administer scratch test (15 min) with 1 drop of solution 3 on forearm.

2. Administer intradermal test (15 min) with 0.02 ml of solution 5.

3. Proceed with penicillin administration as outlined in C. Record blood pressure, pulse, and respiration at frequent (5-min) intervals and have antianaphylactic equipment † always at hand.

4. Immediately begin continuous therapy with intravenous penicillin G.

C. Details of penicillin administration for Step B-3.

Penicillin Solution

Solution Number	Concentration	Injected Each 15 min	Injected Subcutaneously
	units/ml	ml	units
5	100	0.05	5
		0.1	10
		0.2	20
		0.4	40
		0.8	80
4	1,000	0.15	150
		0.3	300
		0.6	600
		1.0	1,000
3	10,000	0.2	2,000
		0.4	4,000
		0.8	8,000
2	100,000	0.15	15,000
		0.3	30,000
		0.6	60,000
		1.0	100,000
1	1,000,000	0.2	200,000
		0.4	400,000
		0.8	800,000

° From Green, G. R. *In* Stewart, G. T. and McGovern, J. P.: *Penicillin Allergy.* Courtesy of Charles C Thomas, Springfield, Ill., 1970.

† Syringes, hypodermic needles, alcohol, sponges, and drugs for injections: epinephrine (aqueous, 1:1,000) and ephedrine; intramuscular chlorpheniramine (Chlor-Trimeton; metaraminol or phenylephrine; levarterenol (Levophed); sodium bicarbonate; aminophylline; corticosteroids.

Equipment for intravenous infusion and tracheostomy, including tourniquet, venous cutdown equipment, and 5% glucose: sphygmomanometer and stethoscope; oxygen tank, with mask or intranasal tube, or bag and valve equipment; endotracheal tube.

Cephalosporins have a similar spectrum of antibacterial activity and do differ in structure from benzlpenicillin (Fig. 16-9). It initially appeared that they would be logical substitutes for penicillins, except in treatment of enterococcal endocarditis where cephalosporins are ineffective. However, both do contain a beta-lactam ring and may form antigenic determinants through beta-lactam carbon-protein conjugation. Consequently, patients with a history of penicillin allergy have four times as many allergic reactions to cephalothin therapy as those with no history of penicillin allergy; this figure approaches 50 percent among patients with a history of penicillin allergy and a positive penicilloyl-polylysine (PPL) skin test.[85] Although administration of cephalosporins may entail less risk in a patient with a history of penicillin allergy, it is advisable to consider such patients potentially allergic to cephalosporins and either select another alternative drug or, if the drug is absolutely necessary, carry out preliminary skin testing. Cephalothin for injection is prepared by adding 4 ml. sterile water to 1 gram, resulting in approximately 250 mg./ml. Several tenfold dilutions using saline as the diluent are prepared, resulting in solutions containing 25 mg./ml., 2.5 mg./ml. and 0.25 mg./ml. Prick tests are done using successive solutions containing 0.25 mg./ml 2.5 mg./ml. and 25 mg./ml.; if negative, intradermal tests follow using 2.5 and 25 mg./ml. successively. If these tests are negative, one may proceed with cautious administration of the drug by successive increases in dose as outlined later for cautious administration of penicillin.

In general, substitution of an equally effective antibiotic, non-cross-reactive with penicillin, is recommended for treatment of infections in patients allergic to penicillin.[97, 93] Generalizations can be made regarding what constitutes adequate substitution therapy, but it is imperative to secure precise antibiotic susceptibility data (Table 16-5).

Bacterial endocarditis deserves special mention in that the penicillins are superior to all other antimicrobials for penicillin sensitive organisms. Any alternative drug must be bactericidal at blood levels that can be easily maintained for prolonged periods. Bacteriostatic drugs, such as erythromycins and tetracyclines, should never be given alone. For endocarditis caused by sensitive viridans streptococci, combined treatment with erythromycin and streptomycin has been successful. Vancomycin is the drug of choice in treatment of staphylococcal endocarditis in patients allergic to penicillin. The treatment of endocarditis due to enterococci in patients allergic to penicillin is a more difficult problem. Cephalosporins are of no value therapeutically. Vancomycin is the recommended drug, but experience with it is limited and prolonged intravenous administration frequently results in thrombophlebitis. In this situation, cautious administration of penicillin as described (p. 468) may be advisable.

After considering alternatives to using penicillin, there may be occasions when penicillin is mandatory, for example, enterococcal endocarditis or other serious infections where there is failure of the patient to respond to the suggested antimicrobial alternatives. Here, the cautious administration of penicillin must be considered despite a history and skin tests indicating the likelihood of penicillin allergy. As discussed under provocative test dosing, medicolegal aspects must be considered. That the procedure may be fatal is attested to by a report of a case of laryngeal edema and death during penicillin desensitization.[27] No uniform procedure has been followed, but the basic principle is to start at a dose low enough not to produce a reaction and then increase the dose at short term intervals.

Simultaneous administration of antihistamines, sympathomimetics and corticosteroids has been advocated.[67, 47, 64] These drugs do not offer protection from anaphylaxis and may suppress milder allergic manifestations that could portend more serious consequences. In our opinion, it is best to withhold these agents during the period of increasing doses of penicillin until symptoms of a reaction occur. At that time, they are used depending upon the severity of the reaction. After reaching therapeutic levels of penicillin, they may be necessary to control mild or even more severe reactions.

Evaluation of the risk and methods of penicillin desensitization has been hampered by the small number of cases so treated and the unpredictability of the natural history of penicillin allergy. Patients with histories of penicillin allergy have received increasing doses of penicillin without any local or systemic reactions. It is likely that many of these patients never were penicillin-sensitive or that they had lost their sensitivity. Desensitization implies gradual neutralization of available antibodies by giving small, nonreacting doses, with a gradual increase until full dosage is reached. It is possible that patients with "minor" determinant skin reactivity or positive skin tests to penicillin G cannot be desensitized in the time necessary to control the clinical infectious emergency.

OTHER ANTIBACTERIAL AGENTS

The older sulfonamides were responsible for many drug-induced hypersensitivity reactions, notably drug fever, pruritus and rashes (particularly exanthematous) developing between the seventh and tenth day of treatment. The newer sulfonamides are less likely to produce allergic reactions. Among newer preparations, the long-acting types, for example sulfamethoxypyradizine (Kynex,* Midicel †) and sulfadimethoxine (Madribon ‡) have been more frequently associated with Stevens-Johnson syndrome especially in children.[13] As short-acting sulfonamides are as effective for similar conditions, their use should be considered before long-acting preparations are employed. Sulfonamides have been frequently implicated in precipitating hypersensitivity vasculitis.

Topical application of sulfonamides results in such a high incidence of contact sensitization that this route of administration has been largely abandoned, except in ophthalmic preparations. Further, topical sensitization may preclude future systemic administration.

The risk of cross-sensitization among sulfonamides and related com-

* Trademark, Lederle.
† Trademark, Parke, Davis.
‡ Trademark, Roche.

pounds (sulfonylurea oral hypoglycemic agents, thiazide diuretics and carbonic anhydrase inhibitors) varies greatly between individuals. However, whenever possible, it is advisable to select drugs of an entirely different chemical composition once a patient has suspected hypersensitivity to one of the sulfonamides or related compounds. Some patients allergic to sulfadiazine or sulfanilamide may react to other compounds containing the p-aminophenyl group, for example local anesthetics of the procaine type discussed later.

The aminoglycosides, streptomycin, kanamycin, neomycin, paramycin and gentamycin, have similar structures, pharmacology and toxicology. Allergic reactions to streptomycin occur following injection and after contact, the latter exposure produces an eczematous eruption, particularly among nurses and other persons handling the drug. Other allergic reactions include drug fever and other cutaneous eruptions, occasionally exfoliative dermatitis. Although rare, anaphylaxis has been reported.

The extensive use of neomycin in dermatological preparations has resulted in an increase in allergic contact dermatitis which may not be recognized, as the neomycin is often used in combination with topical corticosteroids. Among patients sensitized to neomycin, cross sensitization is frequently observed to kanamycin and gentamicin, but not to streptomycin, as determined by patch testing.

The clinically important macrolide antibiotics include erythromycins and oleandomycin. Allergic reactions to this group, especially erythromycin, are infrequent and consist mainly of benign skin eruptions. This group is considered to be the safest form of antimicrobial therapy for atopic patients. Erythromycin estolate (Ilosone *), unique among the salts of erythromycin, and triacetyloleandomycin (TAO †, Cyclamycin ‡) have resulted in cholestatic hepatitis in some patients after prolonged (two weeks or more) treatment. Fortunately, recovery is usually spontaneous upon withdrawal of the drug, but may be prolonged up to a month or longer.

Novobiocin produces a high incidence (7 to 20 percent) of adverse reactions, many of which are potentially serious. The most frequent suspected allergic reactions are skin eruptions, but drug fever, serum sickness-like reactions, hematologic reactions, Stevens-Johnson syndrome, allergic pneumonitis and myocarditis have been reported. As bacterial resistance develops rapidly, use of this drug probably should be abandoned.

Allergic reactions to the tetracyclines and lincomycins are uncommon, but drug fever, rash, urticaria and angioedema and a few deaths from anaphylaxis have been documented. Demethylchlortetracycline (De-

* Trademark, Lilly.
† Trademark, Roerig.
‡ Trademark, Wyeth.

clomycin *) has been more frequently implicated in the fairly common phototoxic reactions and the rare anaphylactic reactions.

Hypersensitivity reactions to the polymyxins, colistins, nalidixic acid and vancomycin are quite infrequent, with reports of drug fever and erythematous or urticarial skin eruptions. The infrequent pulmonary reaction to the nitrofurans was described earlier under systemic manifestations. Chloramphenicol has been most frequently implicated in the production of aplastic anemia, but the immunologic nature of this reaction is questionable.

A discussion of hypersensitivity reactions to antituberculous drugs is limited to isoniazid (INH), streptomycin (mentioned earlier) and aminosalicylic acid because of frequent usage and because reactions to the second line drugs are usually of the toxic, nonallergic type. Clinical manifestations of hypersensitivity usually appear within 3 to 7 weeks after initiation of therapy and most commonly include drug fever and rash. Any febrile episode occurring during this interval without obvious cause should be suspect as a hypersensitivity reaction to one or more of the drugs. Often fever may appear alone for a week or more before other manifestations develop. The rash is usually morbilliform, but may be urticarial, purpuric and rarely exfoliative. Less common manifestations include arthralgia, lymphadenopathy, hepatitis, myocarditis, leukopenia, eosinophilia and rarely a syndrome resembling systemic lupus erythematosus (especially with INH). Fatalities may occur when hepatitis is present. Hypersensitivity reactions may occur with any of these agents, but especially with the aminosalicylates. However, in a given situation, it may be difficult to determine which drug is the cause, or possibly all three may be responsible.

A common approach is to discontinue all drugs to avoid more serious difficulties such as hepatoxicity and exfoliative dermatitis. After the reaction has subsided, each drug is reintroduced in small doses (see provocative test dosing) to identify the responsible agent. Another drug may then be substituted for the causative agent. Ethambutol (Myambutol *) is a very satisfactory substitute for aminosalicylates and is gradually replacing them as a first line drug. Second line drugs available to replace isoniazid and streptomycin are less effective and more toxic, for example ethionamide for isoniazid and viomycin for streptomycin. Cycloserine frequently produces central nervous system toxicity, while pyrazinamide is responsible for hepatotoxicity.

Isoniazid remains the most effective and most economical antituberculous agent. When it appears to be responsible for a hypersensitivity reaction, an attempt to orally "desensitize" the patient is often considered (see provocative test dosing). An alternative to slow "desensi-

---

* Trademarks, Lederle.

tization" proposed by some is more rapid administration under cover of corticosteroids to allow one to reach therapeutic doses in 8 or 9 days and minimize the risk of developing drug resistance. Another suggested approach has been the simultaneous administration of corticosteroids, 40-60 mg. prednisone daily, while the drugs are continued and maintained at therapeutic levels.[86] This has resulted in prompt clearing of the hypersensitivity reaction and, with adequate chemotherapy, steroids do not appear to unfavorably affect the course of the tuberculosis. It should be noted that this latter suggestion has not been widely accepted.

ASPIRIN

More than 13 million pounds of aspirin are consumed by the American public annually, contributing to the fact that this agent ranks second or third to penicillin in producing allergic drug reactions. The most commonly reported allergic reaction to aspirin is urticaria and angioedema; the most serious reaction is bronchial asthma. Many of these patients have no other stigmata of an allergic diathesis. Although urticaria and asthma may be induced by aspirin in the same patient, more commonly this is not true, as patients with aspirin-induced asthma belong to a rather distinctive group.

The prevalence of aspirin intolerance among asthmatics is 2 to 4 percent. A composite type of the patient with aspirin disease is a middle-aged female with preexisting vasomotor rhinitis, nasal polyps (in over 50 percent), peripheral eosinophilia and intrinsic bronchial asthma.[25] The nasal symptoms usually appear during the second or third decade of life, often many years before asthma develops, although both may appear simultaneously. Nasal polyps occur in over 50 percent of cases and may require frequent polypectomies.

Usually asthma first appears in the fourth or fifth decade and sometimes follows a nasal polypectomy. The nasal and bronchial symptoms continue and, typically, the first aspirin-induced asthmatic episode may not occur until respiratory manifestations have been present for months or years, though rarely it may occur concomitant with or before respiratory symptoms. Typically, aspirin-induced asthmatic attacks begin within 20 to 30 minutes (up to 2 hours) after ingestion, are commonly severe and prolonged, and occasionally have a fatal outcome. Infrequently, syncope and severe cyanosis accompanies the aspirin-induced reactions.

Although certain clinical features of aspirin intolerance resemble other well-defined allergic reactions, convincing evidence for an immunologic mechanism in aspirin intolerance is lacking.[100] Skin tests with aspirin are negative and are contraindicated, as the absorption of small amounts from the skin test site may induce bronchospasm and hypotension. Tests in vitro, discussed previously, have been uniformly unrevealing. For this reason, nonimmunological mechanisms in susceptible individuals have been suggested, but these must be considered speculative. One theory suggests that aspirin stimulates altered kinin receptors in the lungs and capillaries, inducing symptoms similar to those produced by the kinins.[71] Other hypotheses include activation of complement by aspirin which releases anaphylatoxin which, in turn, releases histamine with resultant symptoms; patients may lack an inhibitor of an enzymatic reaction that allows release of an active mediator of bronchospasm.[100]

Patients with aspirin intolerance must permanently avoid acetylsalicylic acid and check for its presence in the commonly available over-the-counter cold, headache or analgesic remedies. As nasal polyps and asthma usually precede the initial aspirin-induced asthmatic episode, it seems advisable to caution such patients of this possibility and encourage them to avoid aspirin. Aspirin intolerant patients frequently do not tolerate indomethacin (Indocin), pyrazones (antipyrine and aminopyrine) and mefenamic acid (Ponstel). Approximately 25 percent also react to the coal tar dyes, particularly tartrazine (F.D.&C. yellow #5), used to color foods (Tang, yellow-colored candies, soft drinks, vegetables) and medications (Decadron, Deronil, Paracortil, Premarin and Povan tablets). The wide variation in molecular structure of these drugs which produce a similar reaction is further evidence against an immunologic mechanism. All these preparations have an analgesic property, and perhaps analgesic-induced asthma might be a more appropriate designation. Acetominophen (Tylenol, Nebs) and other salicylates provide suitable substitutes for aspirin in such patients.

LOCAL ANESTHETICS

Adverse reactions to local anesthetics fall into three main categories: toxic, vasovagal and allergic. Contrary to popular belief, true allergic reactions to local anesthetics are relatively infrequent. Toxic symptoms arise from overdosage due to rapid absorption of the drug or inadvertent intravascular injection and involve primarily the central nervous and cardiovascular systems. Initially, central nervous system stimulation produces talkativeness, slurred speech, euphoria, restlessness, dizziness, excitement, nausea, emesis, disorientation and convulsions followed by depression characterized by coma, respiratory and cardiac failure, and occasionally death. Shock results from myocardial depression and peripheral vasodilatation.

Systemic sympathomimetic symptoms such as anxiety, tremor, diaphoresis, tachycardia, hypertension may be due to epinephrine which is mixed with local anesthetics to reduce systemic toxicity by reducing systemic absorption by producing local vasconstriction. This differs from local anesthetic toxicity as convulsions do not occur and tachy-cardia rather than bradycardia is present.

Vasovagal reactions are the most common cause of snycope with dental anesthesia. Symptoms commonly include apprehension, hyper-ventilation, hysteria and syncope accompanied by bradycardia. This quickly responds to placing the patient in a recumbent position.

Among allergic reactions, contact dermatitis is most frequent particu-larly among dentists, nurses and physicians who handle these agents. Also these agents are frequently incorporated in ointments. Methyl-paraben and other parabens used as preservatives in local anesthetics may also be responsible for contact dermatitis. Patch testing will con-firm this form of delayed hypersensitivity. The delayed local swelling at the site of injection of a local anesthetic, usually due to trauma of the procedure, may occasionally be due to delayed hypersensitivity to the agent. Immediate-type hypersensitivity reactions resulting in urticaria, angioedema, bronchospasm and anaphylactic shock are extremely rare.

Local anesthetics may be divided into two groups based upon the presence of the *p*-aminophenyl group. Group I local anesthetics, often referred to as the procaine group, are para-aminobenzoic acid esters that frequently cross-react with each other. Group II includes mostly amides that may not be chemically related to each other and generally do not cross-react with each other and do not appear to cause reactions in persons sensitive to the procaine group. Although studies of cross-reactivity among local anesthetics are based on allergic contact sensitiza-tion, there appears to be some relevance to parenteral administration.

Antigenic Grouping of Local Anesthetics

GROUP I (contain p-aminophenyl group)	GROUP II (lack p-aminophenyl group)
Procaine (Novocain)	Xylocaine (Lidocaine)
Benzocaine	Carbocaine (Mepivacaine)
Pontocaine	Nupercaine
Tantocaine	Holocaine
Larocaine	Metycaine
Monocaine	Alypine
Butyn	Stovaine
Borocaine	Diothane
Butesin	Apothesine
° Procaine amide	Cocaine
	Intracaine

° Not used for local anesthesia, but should be avoided in procaine-sensitive patients.

When confronted with a patient suspected of being allergic to local anesthetics, the clinical details of the previous reaction are often unavailable, making evaluation on historical grounds difficult. Commonly, when any unusual response has occurred, patients are incorrectly labeled as "allergic" to all local anesthetics. If one has knowledge of the local anesthetic used, a representative from the other group may be considered. In practice, this usually involves substitution of xylocaine or carbocaine for procaine. Xylocaine has proven to be a very safe local anesthetic, as attested to by its increased use intravenously in treatment of cardiac arrhythmia without reported allergic reactions.

When hypersensitivity to all available local anesthetics is suspected, other courses of action may be considered. Antihistamines have local anesthetic properties and may be injected for minor procedures. General anesthesia may be required for major procedures. The use of skin tests to determine whether a patient will react adversely to a given local anesthetic agent has met with variable enthusiasm for the same reasons cited earlier regarding the use of such tests in the diagnosis of drug allergy. There are reports of success using intracutaneous tests to determine which drug may be tolerated, but more work needs to be done in skin testing with these agents.[5] The author has used the method of provocative test dosing described earlier to determine whether a local anesthetic may be tolerated, thus sparing the patient of less than optimal local anesthesia or the risk of a general anesthetic.

Iodides And Iodinated Contrast Media

Iodism is a common side effect of iodine administration and includes acneiform skin lesions, salivary gland enlargement and tenderness, conjunctivitis, swelling of the eyelids, coryzal symptoms, sore mouth and excessive salivation. There is no evidence of an immunological mechanism. On the other hand, hypersensitivity may be responsible for the infrequent development of drug fever, eosinophilia, urticaria and angioedema, exanthematic eruptions, bullous eruptions, exfoliative dermatitis, erythema nodosum, thrombocytopenic purpura, vasculitis and a serum sickness-like syndrome. Weber-Christian disease has also been reported, but a causal relationship is less certain.

Reactions to the iodinated contrast media deserve special consideration, particularly those administered intravascularly. The estimated incidence of such dye reactions is approximately 1 in 1,000, with one death resulting every 10,000 to 100,000 examinations, depending somewhat on the nature of the procedure, for example, the route of administration, speed of injection and state of hydration of the subject. There are fewer reactions following intra-arterial administration than to media given intravenously,[38] and if the material is given slowly. Generalized pruritus; urticaria; angioedema, especially of the face, pharynx and larynx; sneezing and rhinorrhea; asthma; and, rarely, shock and death developing rapidly during or after the injection of contract media suggest an allergic (Type I) reaction.

Features of reactions to the iodinated contrast media which are inconsistent with an allergic mechanism include the following: (1) adverse reactions often occur during the first exposure; (2) the incidence of reaction does not appear to increase among patients previously exposed to the dye; (3) following a reaction, some patients have tolerated subsequent administration of the same material; (4) there is conflicting evidence that such reactions are more common among patients with a history of allergy of some kind; (5) the agents used are not very reactive with proteins, a prerequisite to the formation of drug (hapten)-protein complexes; (6) attempts to demonstrate antibodies, with one exception,[39] have failed.

The precise mechanism of such reactions is unclear, but it has been suggested that these agents are capable of non-immunologic histamine release in susceptible individuals. Using dogs, one study found an elevation of plasma histamine in blood draining organs with high histamine content following injection of contrast media; particularly with methylglucamine media (76 percent Reno-M *), (52 percent Cholografin Meglumine †); less so with sodium contrast media (50 percent sodium Hypaque ‡).[40] Although this work suggests that direct histamine release is responsible for these contrast media reactions, other mechanisms cannot be ruled out.

At present, there is no satisfactory method to predict serious, at times fatal, reactions. A history of iodism is not a contraindication to the use of these media, although several instances of salivary gland enlargement have been reported following pyelography.[83] A history of allergy of some kind is also not a contraindication. Intradermal skin tests, ocular and oral tests have generally been discarded as misleading. The widely used intravenous "test" dose of 1 ml. is not without hazard because deaths have resulted from this precedure. Further, severe reactions have followed negative sensitivity tests while others have tolerated the procedure despite positive predictive tests. Routine premedication with antihistamines has been advocated.[62] The administration of 6 to 10 mg. of chlorpropamide intramuscularly 5 minutes before intravenous cholangiograms significantly reduced to one quarter the incidence of reactors to Cholografin. It appears that this procedure may reduce minor annoying reactions, but cannot be relied upon to avert major reactions

* Trademark, Squibb.
† Trademark, Squibb.
‡ Trademark, Winthrop.

and may provide a false sense of security. Slower infusion, if possible, of the contrast media and better hydration of patients appear to further reduce the likelihood of such reactions.

The approach to a patient with a compatible history of a prior reaction is difficult. If an allergic, Type I mechanism was clearly implicated, one would be hesitant to administer the dye regardless of the indication(s) for the procedure. With the knowledge that some patients will tolerate subsequent dye administration despite previous difficulties under certain conditions, specialists seeing patients who have had previous reactions to contrast media, and require repeat radiographic evaluation, have cautiously repeated the administration of the agent. At this time, the risk of such a procedure cannot be stated and such an approach must depend upon the necessity of the examination and the experience of the physician. Among patients who have had a reaction following intravenous urography, retrograde pyelography cannot be considered a safe alternative, as there is no assurance that the mucosal barrier effectively prevents systemic absorption.

It cannot be overemphasized that emergency equipment must always be at hand to promptly treat reactions during routine contrast media examinations.

Hormones

Immediate (Type I) allergic reactions, commonly urticaria and angioedema, have followed the administration of foreign protein hormones, notably ACTH and insulin, rarely of pituitrin, parathormone and thyrotrophic hormone. Anaphylaxis and occasional deaths have resulted. A case of anaphylaxis to parathormone has recently been described.[54] Although many of these reactions are probably due to the specific animal protein source or a contaminant introduced during the manufacturing process, it is likely some are directed to the hormone molecule itself. Skin tests, scratch (prick) and intradermal, are frequently helpful in detection of this hypersensitivity reaction.

Allergic reactions to adrenocorticotrophic hormone (ACTH) have frequently been reported since 1950, some of the most alarming episodes following intravenous administration. Patients allergic to ACTH from one source are likely to react similarly to ACTH derived from any source.[69] As ACTH appears to possess no advantages over available glucocorticoids and glucocorticoids rarely, if ever, result in allergic reactions, use of ACTH should be restricted to that of a diagnostic agent for adrenal disorders. However, there still is a clinical impression that ACTH may be more effective than glucocorticoids in certain conditions such as ulcerative colitis, multiple sclerosis and some cases of intractable asthma. Objective evidence of this is lacking. The effectiveness of intermittent ACTH administration to restore or maintain adrenal responsiveness during treatment with or withdrawal from corticosteroids has not been substantiated. Alternate day cortocosteroid therapy is a more logical approach. ACTH has the additional disadvantage of increasing the secretion of mineralocorticoids and analogues, possibly resulting in additional side effects.

Circulating antibodies (IgG, IgA, IgM) to insulin can be demonstrated, at least in low titer, in the serum of most diabetic patients within a few months after starting insulin treatment. These antibodies may bind insulin rendering it biologically inactive. Usually the insulin binding capacity of serum remains low, often less than 10 units per liter.[99] In some cases of insulin resistance (defined as an insulin requirement in excess of 200 units daily for at least several days in the absence of acute complication, e.g. acidosis, infection), the sera may bind from 50 to 1,000 times this amount of insulin and high titers of insulin binding antibodies are present. This phenomenon occurs more commonly in patients over age 40 and among those in whom insulin was discontinued and then reinstituted. Most patients experience insulin resistance for periods of less than 6 to 12 months. Insulin resistance and allergy may coexist. Resistance to other hormones, for example growth hormone, thyrotrophic hormone, parathormone, may have a similar immunologic basis. Treatment of immunologic insulin resistance most commonly involves the use of corticosteroids, for example at least 40 mgm prednisone daily. A dramatic decline in the insulin requirement may occur within the first few days, with a more gradual decline over the next few weeks. The dose of prednisone is gradually reduced, but many patients require 10 mg daily for at least one month, often as long as 6 to 12 months. After steroids are discontinued, the diabetes may be subsequently controlled with diet and oral hypoglycemic agents, presumably related to a change in the insulin binding activity of the serum.

Local and systemic immediate allergic reactions are occasionally seen in patients receiving insulin injections for the first time or upon reinstitution of therapy. IgE is believed to play a major role in insulin allergy.[59] The majority of reactions are of the mild local type characterized by redness, swelling and pruritus at the injection site developing within the first two weeks of treatment. The local response appears immediately after the injection, reaches a maximum in several hours, and subsides in 24 to 48 hours. These local responses generally disappear within 3 to 4 weeks despite continuing insulin treatment and generally do not require any therapy. If the reactions persist or are annoying, antihistamines may be helpful. If this fails and the reactions persist, one may boil the insulin, use recrystalized insulin or switch to pure porcine insulin which is less antigenic than beef insulin. (Pork insulin differs from human insulin by only one amino acid, while beef insulin differs by three.)

Systemic allergic reactions to insulin characterized by urticaria, angio-edema and manifestations consistent with anaphylaxis are uncommon. One may anticipate such a reaction in the face of gradually increasing local reactions. In most cases there has been an interruption in insulin therapy. The acute management of this reaction is discussed in the chapter dealing with anaphylaxis. Following a systemic reaction to insulin, control of diabetes with diet and oral hypoglycemic agents should be attempted. Even if successful, one must be cognizant of the fact that such patients may develop acute complications, for example, acidosis, infection, a need for surgery, where insulin may temporarily be required. Therefore, it is of some value to predetermine which insulin may be used with less risk. Skin testing with insulins of several species and types, for example recrystallized, boiled, etc., may provide a useful alternative. However, patients may react to all available insulins, thus suggesting that the reactivity is directed against the insulin molecule itself. The acid-alcohol extraction process used in preparing commercial and synthetic insulins probably accounts for its allergenic properties and explains why such patients would not react to their own endogenous insulin.[44]

Desensitization may be cautiously attempted in the patient with systemic insulin allergy, but only if such therapy is mandatory. In addition to precautions for treatment of anaphylaxis, one must be prepared to treat hypoglycemia, which may complicate the frequent doses of insulin required for desensitization. Where no emergency exists, slow desensitization over several days may be used. Following successful desensitization, it would seem reasonable to maintain that patient on such therapy even though it might be possible later to manage the diabetes on diet with or without oral hypoglycemics; thus obviating future repetition of the process.

The insulin least reactive by skin test titering, usually pure pork insulin, is used. The initial dose is based on intradermal skin testing, starting with a concentration one tenth as strong as the most dilute preparation giving a positive skin test. A representative schedule has been provided by Lieberman et al.[44] Rapid desensitization may be required if ketoacidosis is present. Corcoran suggests starting with 0.2 units of crystalline insulin subcutaneously (less if the patient is extremely sensitive by skin test) and doubling the dose every 15 to 30 minutes until a therapeutic dose is achieved.[15] Successful desensitization has been associated with a decline in skin reactivity suggesting gradual antibody neutralization.[44] Alternatively, there is reported a decline in skin reactivity with a rise of IgG antibody producing a "blocking" or protective effect.[17] Both mechanisms of decreased reactivity may occur in different patients or in the same patient and may also depend on the dosage and rapidity of desensitization.

Rhinitis and bronchial asthma due to inhalation of powdered extracts of porcine and bovine pituitary glands for treatment of diabetes insipidus has long been known, but the development of allergic alveolitis is a more recent observation, as discussed earlier, with systemic manifestations of drug hypersensitivity. Allergic reactions after administration of vaso-pressin are uncommon, but have included fever, urticaria, asthma and shock. Allergic reactors to thyroid hormone preparations, corticosteroids, estrogens and androgens are rare. Androgens have been implicated in producing jaundice, but hypersensitivity is unlikely. Aggravation of rhini-tis, asthma and eczema has followed the use of oral contraceptives, but the mechanism for this is unknown.

IMMUNIZATION MATERIALS

The two major allergic reactions that may follow an injection of *heterologous immune sera* are anaphylaxis and serum sickness. Current immunization procedures and the availability and greater efficacy of

Foreign Serum Hyposensitization *

1. Initial dose is determined by scratch and intradermal testing (dilutions are made with normal saline)
   a. Scratch test with 1:1000
   b. If the result is negative, perform an intradermal test with same dilution (1:1000)

NUMBER DOSE	AMOUNT OF SERUM IN ML.	DILUTION
1	0.1	1:1000
2	0.2	1:1000
3	0.4	1:1000
4	0.7	1:1000
5	0.1	1:100
6	0.2	1:100
7	0.4	1:100
8	0.7	1:100
9	0.1	1:10
10	0.2	1:10
11	0.4	1:10
12	0.7	1:10
13	0.1	Undiluted
14	0.2	Undiluted
15	0.4	Undiluted
16	0.7	Undiluted
17	1.0	Undiluted

* From Siegel in Gellis and Kagan: *Current Pediatric Therapy.* Philadelphia, W. B. Saunders, 1966.

c. If the result is positive, begin treatment with 1:1000 as initial concentration

d. If the result is still negative, perform intradermal test with 1:100 dilution. Unless a large reaction is observed, this concentration may be used for the first dose

2. Start an intravenous infusion with 100 mg. of cortisol succinate (Solu-Cortef) and 25 mg. of diphenhydramine (Benadryl) (or their equivalents) in 500 ml. of 5 per cent glucose and saline. One-tenth to 0.2 cc. of Sus-Phrine, a suspension of epinephrine in thioglycolate, glycerin and chlorbutanol, is administered subcutaneously.

3. The first dose of diluted serum is then injected subcutaneously at a site in an extremity where a tourniquet could be placed proximally if a reaction should occur. Subsequent injections are given every thirty minutes, approximately doubling the dose each time until the full dose is administered.

4. When a dose of 1 ml. of undiluted serum has been reached, additional injections are best administered intramuscularly, particularly when large doses of antitoxin are necessary as in the treatment of diphtheria. As with the subcutaneous route, the dose is doubled every thirty minutes until the desired amount of antiserum has been administered. Use of the intravenous route for administering serum is best avoided unless massive amounts of antiserum are required in critically ill patients. For this purpose the serum should be diluted one hundredfold in saline and given slowly.

human tetanus antitoxin have virtually eliminated the need for heterologous tetanus antitoxin. Equine antitoxins may still be required in the management of snakebites, black widow spider bite, botulism, gas-gangrene and rabies. Antilymphocyte antisera also appears to be useful in the prevention of graft rejection.

Prior to the administration of horse serum products, skin testing must be performed on a distal extremity. This is particularly important where the patient has received this material in the past or is atopically sensitive to horses. All patients should be tested regardless of history. A scratch or prick test using undiluted serum with a saline control is the initial test. A positive skin test indicates the likelihood of anaphylaxis upon subsequent administration. If the prick test is negative, proceed with an intradermal test using 0.02 ml. 1:100 dilution of the serum and a saline control. If the history suggests a prior reaction or the patient has atopic symptoms upon horse exposure, begin intradermal testing with a 1:1,000 dilution. A intradermal skin test with a 1:10 dilution follows when the previous tests are negative. If negative, this excludes horse serum sensitivity and the patient may be given the full dose of antiserum. It is to be remembered that this approach is to predict the anaphylactically sensitive patient and does not exclude the possibility of developing serum sickness for reasons cited earlier in the discussion of this systemic manifestation.

When the history and skin tests indicate a very real likelihood of horse serum allergy, it is desirable to use antisera from another species, for example bovine. However, patients must be similarly tested with the substitute materials. Where there is no alternative to equine antisera, desensitization may be attempted as outlined by Siegel (pp. 481-482) who warns that the procedure is extremely hazardous and should be carried out in a hospital. (See dose schedule p. 481). As suggested, this procedure is apt to be more difficult to accomplish and less likely to succeed in patients with a history of atopic sensitivity to horse dander. Because of extreme sensitivity, one may not be able to proceed as rapidly as suggested in the schedule. The possibility exists that the antitoxin may be removed at an accelerated rate without achieving satisfactory therapeutic levels.

Infrequent allergic reactions to *human immune globulin* have been reported. It seems likely that these reactions are the result of biologically active aggregated gamma globulin molecules which release histamine and other vasoactive mediators from tissue mast cells and circulating basophils.

Allergic reactions may follow the administration of *agents given for active immunization.* In addition to the immunizing agent, the vaccine may contain allergenic material in small amounts derived from the manufacturing process, for example egg protein and other media on which the viruses are grown, silk used in filters, penicillin and other preservatives such as phenol and mercurials. With improvements in preparation techniques and elimination of some of these substances, the incidence of hypersensitivity reactions has declined. The only routine prophylactic immunization contraindicated in allergic disease is smallpox vaccination in patients with atopic dermatitis or any other eczematous dermatitis. If absolutely necessary, such immunization may be carried out if the patient receives hyperimmune vaccinia gamma globulin simultaneously. Also, an attenuated smallpox vaccine has been used by Kempe with success. Patients may be vaccinated if they remain free of the dermatitis for several months. However, the risk of smallpox in the United States is so small that routine vaccination is no longer indicated in this country.

D.P.T. is occasionally responsible for mild allergic reactions, usually urticarial; rarely anaphylactic. Encephalopathic reactions have occurred in one out of one million immunizations and are attributed to pertussis. The mechanism of this reaction is unknown. As it occurs more commonly after age 6, pertussis is routinely excluded from the triple antigen after that age.

Tetanus toxoid deserves special mention. The effectiveness of this immunization procedure has led to the overzealous administration of additional booster doses without consideration of the prior immunization status of the patient.[18] Allergic reactions to tetanus toxoid were first reported in 1940 and were attributed to the Witte peptone in the culture broth. Subsequently, with improvement in preparation techniques, the incidence of allergic reactions became negligible. Although no statistics are available, there is a general consensus that allergic reactions to tetanus toxoid, some quite severe, are again increasing, particularly in older children and adults. Such reactions are generally associated with greatly elevated tetanus antitoxin titers, a condition associated with hyperimmunization. Excessive booster doses of tetanus toxoid not only enhance the antitoxin titer, but may lead to a qualitative change in the spectrum of antibodies produced, with an increased frequency of IgE type skin sensitizing antibodies, responsible for Type I reactions.[37] Reported reactions include urticaria and angioedema, exaggerated local reactions with fever and malaise persisting up to a week (resembles an Arthus, Type III reaction), and rarely peripheral neuropathy. Positive wheal and flare skin test reactions to tetanus toxoid are not uncommon in such patients.

To reduce the incidence of these reactions, routine practices such as automatic tetanus toxoid boosters for camp, etc., should be abandoned. Tetanus boosters may be spaced at least 10 years apart and emergency boosters need not be given oftener than once a year, possibly even further apart. Where doubt about the prior immunization status exists, it would be helpful to have an available method to determine the patient's tetanus antitoxin titer.

Where it is necessary to administer tetanus toxoid to an individual with a history of a previous reaction or a positive skin test, desensitization may be considered.[37] Tetanus toxoid is diluted 1:10, 1:100 and 1:1000. Successive test doses of 0.10 ml. of 1:1,000, 1:100 and 1:10 are given intradermally or subcutaneously, and the strongest dilution that fails to produce a reaction is used. Subsequently, injections are given once or twice a week increasing the dose by 0.05 to 0.10 ml. depending upon the extent and duration of the local reaction, until the limit of tolerance or 0.10 ml. undiluted toxoid is attained. This dose can then be repeated once a month until the patient is adequately immunized. Adequate immunization can be determined by sending serum to an appropriate state lab to assay the antitoxin titer to be certain it is in excess of 0.01 unit. A booster of the top tolerated dose is given in one year and then at five-year intervals.

Allergic reactions to *Salk poliomyelitis vaccine* may be due to the addition of small amounts of penicillin (1 to 20 units/ml.) and other antibiotics as preservatives; a fact which has prompted manufacturers to decrease the amount of penicillin or use another antibiotic in vaccines. The use of Sabin oral polio vaccine should eliminate this potential.

Influenza virus vaccines are derived from viruses grown in embryonated chicken eggs and may contain a small amount of egg protein. More highly purified vaccines recently have become available and contain much less egg protein. There will be available soon a vaccine prepared on chick embryo tissue cultures. As a rule, if the patient can eat eggs without developing allergic symptoms, the vaccine is not contraindicated, even in the presence of a positive skin test reaction for egg. In the latter circumstance, one might give a small test dose first. The same criteria would apply to the administration of vaccines for typhus, yellow fever, and Rocky Mountain spotted fever.

Some of the more recent viral vaccines, for example, rubeola, rubella and mumps, are prepared in cell cultures of various mammalian and avian sources, and their content of host tissue proteins are almost negligible. Measles (rubeola) vaccine, prepared in tissue cultures of chick embryo cells, was administered to 22 children highly allergic to egg without any subsequent allergic reaction.[36] For some of these vaccines, for example rubella, preparation is carried out on several different cell sources (duck embryo cells, canine renal cells, rabbit renal cells) allowing one a choice of vaccines if there is some concern. There are no reports of allergic reactions to any of these vaccines prepared on canine cells in patients sensitive to dog hair. Although it is suggested that patients sensitive to feathers not receive these egg-related vaccines, there is no evidence of cross reactivity causing allergic reactions to these vaccines. Local reactions have followed typhoid and cholera immunization, but have not been particularly troublesome. Urticarial reactions, often on the contralateral arm, have been a problem with plague vaccine.[65]

Approximately one in 2500 patients who receive *rabbit brain tissue type rabies vaccine* (Semple) develops encephalomyelitis. This represents an immunologic reaction to heterologous brain antigen, probably myelin, contained in the vaccine and is classified as a delayed, Type IV reaction. Duck embryo type rabies vaccine is preferable, although urticaria and serum sickness have been reported among patients receiving this material, many of whom also had received tetanus antitoxin, thus complicating the picture.

DRUG ALLERGY I.Q.

The following is a series of true or false statements that may be useful as a guide to understanding of drug allergy. It is not inclusive but is intended to emphasize certain concepts as a teaching aid.

1. Adverse reactions to drugs are responsible for the majority of iatrogenically induced illnesses.
2. Allergic drug reactions account for the majority of adverse drug reactions.
3. Drug allergy is usually suspected on clinical grounds as in vivo and in vitro tests are generally unavailable.

4. Penicillins, aspirin and sulfonamides (includes oral sulfonylureas, thiazides and carbonic anhydrase inhibitors) are the drugs most commonly implicated in allergic drug reactions.
5. Topical application of medicaments and intermittent exposure to a drug are associated with the highest sensitization risk.
6. The commonest allergic drug reactions are dermatologic in nature.
7. The outcome following anaphylaxis generally relates to the rapidity of onset of the reaction.
8. The diagnosis of a serum sickness-like reaction is easily established without a skin eruption.
9. Although glomerulonephritis is a prominent feature of experimental serum sickness, clinically evident renal disease in serum sickness in man is unusual.
10. Penicillins are now the commonest cause of serum sickness-type reactions.
11. There is no place for the use of equine or other foreign antisera in modern medicine.
12. Furadantin has been responsible for a suspected hypersensitivity pulmonary edema.
13. Drug fever is often associated with a marked disparity between the recorded febrile response and the relative well-being of the patient.
14. An immunological basis for drug-induced hematologic reactions is reasonably well defined for agranulocytosis and aplastic anemia, but speculative for thrombocytopenia and hemolytic anemia.
15. Hepatic drug reactions on a hypersensitivity basis may mimic biliary obstruction or viral hepatitis.
16. Drugs incriminated in collagen-vascular disorders (e.g., vasculitis) often assume guilt by association.
17. Drug-induced lupus erythematosus often differs from spontaneous appearing lupus by having less impressive renal involvement.
18. Dilantin-induced lymphadenopathy always regresses following discontinuation of the drug.
19. Most commonly used drugs bind firmly to tissue and circulating proteins; thus forming a necessary hapten-protein conjugate to induce sensitization.
20. Drugs are capable of producing the entire spectrum of immunologic reactions (Gell and Coomb's Types I to IV); in fact, a single drug may produce the entire spectrum of such reactions.
21. The clinical history provides the greatest help in the diagnosis of drug allergy.
22. For Type I allergic reactions (e.g., urticaria, anaphylaxis, etc.) skin testing with suspected drugs is as useful as in the diagnosis of pollen allergy.
23. Tests in vitro to diagnose most allergic drug reactions must be considered investigational at this time.
24. In the final analysis, readministration of the suspected drug, after the reaction has subsided, is the only way to be certain of a cause and effect relationship. This approach is generally not recommended.
25. Simultaneous administration of antihistamines, sympathomimetics and corticosteroids can be relied upon to protect the patient from serious immediate allergic drug reactions, e.g., anaphylaxis.

26. Safe, alternative antimicrobial therapy for penicillin sensitive patients would include:
    a. Semisynthetic penicillins
    b. Cephalosporins
    c. Other non-cross-reacting antibiotic based on microbial sensitivity studies.
27. Currently, the only illness for which penicillin is probably a *must* is sub-acute bacterial endocarditis due to streptococcus viridans.
28. Patients sensitive to antibacterial sulfonamides may be similarly allergic to the oral sulfonylureas, thiazide diuretics and carbonic anhydrase inhibitors.
29. Ampicillin is associated with a higher incidence of drug rash than other penicillins.
30. The macrolide antibiotics (erythromycins and oleandomycins) are among the safest to use from the standpoint of allergic reactions.
31. Patients with asthma aggravated by acetylsalicylic acid may have similar difficulties with Indocin,° aminopyrine, mefenamic acid (Ponstel †) and foods and drugs containing F.D. & C. #5 yellow dye (tartrazine).
32. Most adverse reactions to local anesthetics are allergic in nature.
33. Iodism is a contraindication to the use of iodinated contrast media.
34. Predictive tests—skin, conjunctival and an I.V test dose—are good ways to screen out the potential iodinated contrast dye reactor.
35. There is good clinical support for the continued use of ACTH in place of oral corticosteroids, despite occasional episodes of anaphylaxis with the former.
36. Pork insulin is less antigenic in man than beef insulin.
37. Most local reactions following insulin administration are predictive of future, more serious reactions and contraindicate the continued use of that insulin preparation.
38. Skin testing of patients who receive equine antitoxins will reduce the likelihood of serum sickness.
39. Tetanus toxoid allergic reactions appear to be increasing in number and severity.
40. Patients who tolerate egg ingestion can safely receive egg source vaccines, e.g., influenza, measles, etc.

ANSWERS AND PAGE REFERENCE

1. True	p. 393	15. True	p. 429	27. False	p. 469
2. False	p. 394	16. True	p. 430	28. True	p. 471
3. True	p. 402	17. True	p. 431	29. True	p. 466
4. True	p. 404	18. False	p. 433	30. True	p. 471
5. True	p. 404	19. False	p. 406	31. True	p. 474
6. True	p. 409	20. True	p. 407	32. False	p. 475
7. True	p. 419	21. True	p. 436	33. False	p. 478
8. False	p. 420	22. False	p. 437	34. False	p. 478
9. True	p. 421	23. True	p. 439	35. False	p. 479
10. True	p. 420	24. True	p. 446	36. True	p. 480
11. False	p. 420	25. False	p. 451	37. False	p. 480
12. True	p. 424	26. a. False	p. 467	38. False	p. 482
13. True	p. 425	b. False	p. 467	39. True	p. 484
14. False	p. 426	c. True	p. 467	40. True	p. 485

° Trademark, Merck Sharp & Dohme.
† Trademark, Parke, Davis.

REFERENCES

1. Ackroyd, J. F.: The diagnosis of disorders of the blood due to drug hypersensitivity caused by an immune mechanism. *In* Ackroyd, J. F. (ed): Immunological Methods. Philadelphia, F. A. Davis, 1964.
2. Ackroyd, J. F.: The immunological basis of purpura due to drug hypersensitivity. Proc. Roy. Soc. Med., 55:30, 1962.
3. Adkinson, N. F., Jr., Thompson, W. L., Maddrey, W. C., and Lichtenstein, L. M.: Routine use of penicillin skin testing on an impatient service. New Eng. J. Med., 285:22,2 1971.
4. Alarcon-Segovia, D., Waki, K. G., Worthington, J. W., and Ward, L. E.: Clinical and experimental studies on the hydralazine syndrome and its relationship to systemic lupus erythematosus. Medicine, 46:1, 1967.
5. Aldrete, J. A., and Johnson, D. A.: Evaluation of intracutaneous testing for investigation of allergy to local anesthetic agents. Anesth. and Analg., 49:173, 1970.
6. Alexander, H. L.: Reactions with Drug Therapy. Philadelphia, W. B. Saunders, 1955.
7. Arbesman, C. E., Hyman, I., Danzier, G., and Kantor, S. Z.: Immunologic studies of a Guillain-Barre syndrome following tetanus antitoxin. New York J. Med., 58:2647, 1958.
8. Azarnoff, D. L., and Hurwitz, A.: Drug reactions. Pharmacol. Physicians, 4:1-7, 1970.
9. Baldwin, D. S., Levine, B. B., McCluskey, R. T., and Gallo, C. R.: Renal failure and interstitial nephritis due to penicillin and methicillin. New Eng. J. Med., 279:1245, 1968.
10. Bierman, C. W., and Van Arsdel, P. P., Jr.: Penicillin allergy in children: the role of immunological tests in its diagnosis. J. Allerg., 43:267, 1969.
11. Brown, E. A.: Problems of drug allergy. JAMA, 157:814, 1955.
12. Bukantz, S. C.: The Stevens-Johnson Syndrome. *In* Disease-a-Month. Chicago, Year Book Medical Publishers, October, 1968.
13. Carroll, O. M., Bryan, P. A., and Robinson, R. J.: Stevens-Johnson syndrome associated with long-acting sulfonamides. JAMA, 195:691, 1966.
14. Cluff, L. E., and Johnson, J. E.: Drug fever. *In* Kallós, P., and Waksman, B. H.: Progress in Allergy. vol. 8, Basel, S. Karger, 1964.
15. Corcoran, A. C.: Note on rapid desensitization in a case of hypersensitiveness to insulin. Am. J. Med. Sci., 196:357, 1938.
16. DeLaPava, S., Nigogosyan, G., and Pickren, J. W.: Fatal glomerulonephritis after receiving horse anti-human-cancer serum. Arch. Intern. Med., 109:391, 1962.
17. Dolovich, J., Schmatz, J. D., Reisman, R. E., Yagi, Y., and Arbesman, C. E.: Insulin allergy and resistance. J. Allerg., 46:127, 1970.
18. Edsall, G., Elliott, M. W., Peebles, T. C., Levine, L., and Eldred, M. C.: Excessive use of tetanus toxoid boosters. JAMA, 202:111, 1967.
19. Eisen, H. N.: Hypersensitivity to simple chemicals. *In* Lawrence, H. S.: Cellular and Humoral Aspects of the Hypersensitive States. New York, Paul B. Hoeber, 1959.

20. Evans, D. A. P.: Pharmacogenetics. Am. J. Med., *34:*639, 1963.
21. Fellner, M. J., Redmond, A. P., Levine, B. B., and Baer, R. L.: Immediate penicillin reactions associated with penicilloyl-specific skin sensitizing antibodies and low titers of blocking (IgG) antibodies. J. Allerg., *39:*106, 1967.
22. Fisher, A. A.: Contact Dermatitis. Philadelphia, Lea and Febiger, 1967.
23. Gams, R. A., Neal, J. A., and Conrad, F. G.: Hydantoin-induced psuedopsuedolymphoma. Ann. Intern. Med., *69:*557, 1968.
24. Gell, P. G. H., and Coombs, R. R. A.: Classification of allergic reactions responsible for clinical hypersensitivity and disease. *In* Gell, P. G. H., and Coombs, R. R. A.: Clinical Aspects of Immunology. ed. 2, p. 575. Blackwell Scientific Publications, Oxford, London, and Edinburg, 1968.
25. Giraldo, B., Blumenthal, M. N., and Spink, W. W.: Aspirin intolerance and asthma. A clinical and immunological study. Ann. Intern. Med., *71:*479, 1969.
26. Gralnick, H. R., McGinniss, M., Elton, W., and McCurdy, P.: Hemolytic anemia associated with cephalothin. JAMA, *217:*1193, 1971.
27. Grieo, M. H., Dubin, M. R., Robinson, J. L., and Schwartz, M. J.: Penicillin hypersensitivity in patients with bacterial endocarditis. Ann. Intern. Med., *60:*204, 1964.
28. Haddinett, B. C., Gowdy, C. W., Coulter, W. K., and Parker, J. M.: Drug reactions and errors in administration on a medical ward. Canad. Med. Ass. J., *97:*1450-1457, 1967.
29. Hailey, F. J., Glascock, H. W., Jr. and Hewitt, W. F.: Pleuropneumonia reactions to nitrofurantoin. New Eng. J. Med., *281:*1087, 1969.
30. Halpern, B., Ky., N. T., and Amache, N.: Diagnosis of drug allergy in vitro with the lymphocyte transformation test. J. Allerg., *40:*168, 1967.
31. Heymann, W.: Nephrotic syndrome after use of trimethadione and paramethadione in petit mal. JAMA, *202:*893, 1967.
32. Hildreth, E. A., Biron, C. E., and McCreary, J. A.: Persistence of "hydralazine syndrome." A follow up study of 11 cases. JAMA, *173:*657, 1960.
33. Horwitz, N.: Admissions to hospital due to drugs. Brit. Med. J., *1:*539-540, 1969.
34. Hyman, G. A., and Sommers, S. C.: The development of Hodgkin's disease and lymphoma during anticonvulsant therapy. Blood, *28:*416, 1966.
35. Idsoe, O., Guthe, T., Wilcox, R. R., and De Weck, A. L.: Nature and extent of penicillin side-reactions, with particular reference to fatalities from anaphylactic shock. Bull. WHO, *38:*159, 1968.
36. Kamin, P. B., Fein, B. T., and Britton, H. A.: Use of live, attenuated measles virus vaccine in children allergic to egg protein. JAMA, *193:*1125, 1965.
37. Kuhns, W. J.: Relationship of immediate wheal reactions to the repeated administration of diphtheria and tetanus toxoids. J. Immun., *89:*652, 1962.
38. Lang, E. K.: Clinical evaluation of side-effects of radiopaque contrast

media administered via intravenous and intra-arterial routes in the same patient. A preliminary report. Radiology, 85:666, 1965.

39. Lasser, E. C.: Basic mechanisms of contrast media reactions. Theoretical and experimental considerations. Radiology, 91:63, 1968.

40. Lasser, E. C., Walters, A., Reuter, S. R., and Lang, J.: Histamine release by contrast media. Radiology, 100:683, 1971.

41. Levine, B. B.: Immunochemical mechanisms of drug allergy. *In* Miescher, P. A., and Muller-Eberhard, H. J.: Textbook of Immunopathology. vol. I. New York and London, Grune & Stratton, 1968.

42. Levine, B. B.: Immunologic mechanisms of penicillin allergy. A haptenic model system for the study of allergic diseases of man. New Eng. J. Med., 275:1115, 1966.

43. Levine, B. B., and Zolov, D. M.: Prediction of penicillin allergy by immunological tests. J. Allerg., 43:231, 1969.

44. Lieberman, P., Patterson, R., Metz, R., and Lucena, G.: Allergic reactions to insulin. JAMA, 215:1106, 1971.

45. LoBuglio, A. F., and Jandl, J. H.: The nature of the alpha-methyldopa red-cell antibody. New Eng. J. Med., 276:658, 1967.

46. Lockie, L. M., Norcross, B. M., and Riordan, D. J.: Gold in treatment of rheumatoid arthritis. JAMA, 167:1204, 1958.

46a. Martin, Eric: Hazards of Medication. Philadelphia, J. B. Lippincott, 1971.

47. Maslansky, L., and Sanger, M. D.: Method of decreasing penicillin sensitivity. Antibiot. Chemother., 2:385, 1952.

48. Mathews, K. P.: Drug Allergy. *In* Sheldon, J. M., *et al.:* A Manual of Clinical Allergy. ed. 2. Philadelphia, W. B. Saunders, 1967.

49. Mathews, K. P., Hemphil, F. M., Lovell, R. G., Forsythe, W. R., and Sheldon, J. M.: Controlled study on use of parenteral and oral antihistamines in preventing penicillin reactions. J. Allerg., 27:1, 1956.

50. Meyler, L., and Herxheimer, A.: Side Effects of Drugs. Amsterdam, Excerpta Medica Foundation, 1968. vol. VI and previous volumes.

51. Miller, F. F.: History of drug sensitivity in atopic persons. J. Allerg., 40:46, 1967.

52. Nabandian, R. M., Moder, I. J., Barrett, J. L., Pearce, J. F., and Rapp, E. C.: Petechiae, ecchymosis, and necrosis of skin induced by coumarin congeners. JAMA, 192:603, 1965.

53. Norman, P. S.: Adverse drug reactions and alternative drugs of choice. *In* Modell, W.: Drugs of Choice 1970-1971. St. Louis, C. V. Mosby, 1970.

54. O'Rourke, J. N., Booth, B. H. III, and Patterson, R.: Anaphylactic reaction to parathormone. Submitted for publication.

55. Palmer, R. F.: Drug interactions. Med. Clin. N. Am., 55:495, 1971.

56. Pankey, G. A.: Unusual antimicrobial toxic reactions. Med. Clin. N. Am., 51:925, 1967.

57. Parker, C. W.: Immediate skin reactions in penicillin hypersensitivity. *In* Stewart, G. T., and McGovern, J. P.: Penicillin Allerg. Springfield, Ill., Charles C Thomas, 1970.

58. Parker, C. W., Shapiro, J., Kern, M., and Eisen, H. N.: Hypersensitivity to penicillenic acid derivatives in human beings with penicillin allergy. J. Exp. Med., *115*:821, 1962.
59. Patterson, R., Lucena, G., Metz, R., and Roberts, M.: Reaginic antibody against insulin: demonstration of antigenic distinction between native and extracted insulin. J. Immun., *103*:1061, 1969.
60. Pepys, J., Jenkins, P. A., Lachmann, P. J., and Mahon, W. E.: An iatrogenic autoantibody: immunological response to pituitary snuff in patients with diabetes insipidus. Clin. Exp. Immun., *1*:377, 1966.
61. Perelmutter, L., and Khera, K.: A study on the detection of human reagins with rat peritoneal cells. Int. Arch. Allerg., *39*:27, 1970.
62. Peters, G. A., Hodgson, J. R., and Donovan, R. J.: "The effect of premedication with chlorpheniramine on reactions to methylglucamine iodipamide. J. Allerg., *38*:74, 1966.
63. Peters, G. A., Moskowitz, R. W., Prickman, L. E., and Conger, H. M.: Fatal necrotizing angiitis associated with hypersensitivity to penicillin O and iodides. J. Allerg., *31*:455, 1960.
64. Raper, A. J., and Kemp, V. E.: Use of steroids in penicillin-sensitive patients with bacterial endocarditis. A report of three cases and review of the literature. New Eng. J. Med., *273*:297, 1965.
65. Reisman, R. E.: Allergic reactions due to plague vaccine. J. Allerg., *46*:49, 1970.
66. Reisman, R. E.: Delayed hypersensitivity to Merthiolate preservative. J. Allerg., *43*:245, 1969.
67. Reisman, R. E., Rose, N. R,. Witebsky, E., and Arbesman, C. E.: Penicillin allergy and desensitization. J. Allerg., *33*:178, 1962.
68. Reisman, R. E., Rose, N. R., Witebsky, E., and Arbesman, C. E.: Serum sickness. II. Demonstration and characteristics of antibodies. J. Allerg., *32*:531, 1961.
69. Rosenblum, A. H., and Rosenblum, P.: Anaphylactic reactions to adrenocorticotropic hormone in children. J. Pediat., *64*:387, 1964.
70. Rosenthal, A.: Follow up study of fatal penicillin reactions. JAMA, *167*:1118, 1958.
71. Samter, M., and Beers, R. F., Jr.: Concerning the nature of intolerance to aspirin. J. Allerg., *40*:281, 1967.
72. Sarkary, I.: Clinical and laboratory aspects of drug allergy. Proc. Roy. Soc. Med., *61*:891, 1968.
73. Scott, G. L., Myles, A. B., and Bacon, P. A.: Autoimmune haemolytic anaemia and mefenamic acid therapy. Brit. Med. J., *3*:534, 1968.
74. Seidl, L. G., Thornton, C. F., Smith, J. W., and Cluff, L. E.: Studies on the epidemiology of adverse drug reactions. III. Reactions in patients on a general medical service. Bull. Hopkins Hosp., *119*:299-315, 1966.
75. Seinfeld, B. M., and McCombs, R. P.: Skin window: an aid in the diagnosis of drug allergy. J. Allerg., *38*:156, 1966.
76. Shapiro, S., Victor, S., Slone, D., Lewis, G. P., and Jick, H.: Drug rash with ampicillin and other penicillins. Lancet, *2*:969, 1969.

77. Shelley, W. B.: Indirect basophil degranulation test for allergy to penicillin and other drugs. JAMA, *184:*171, 1963.
78. Shelley, W. B., and Comaish, J. S.: New test for penicillin allergy: fluorometric assay of histamine release. JAMA, *192:*36, 1965.
79. Slugg, P. H., and Kunkel, R. S.: Complications of methylsergide therapy. JAMA, *213:*297-298, 1970.
80. Solomon, H. M.: Clinical disorders of drug interaction. Advances Intern. Med., *16:*285, 1970.
81. Speizer, F. E., Doll, R., Heaf, P., and Strang, L. B.: Investigation into use of drugs preceding death from asthma. Brit. Med. J., *1:*339, 1968.
82. Stewart, G. T.: Allergenic residues in penicillin. Lancet, *1:*1177, 1967.
83. Sussman, R., and Miller, J.: Iodide "mumps" after intravenous urography. New Eng. J. Med., *255:*433, 1956.
84. Symmers, W. St. C.: The occurrence of angiitis and of other generalized diseases of connective tissues as a consequence of the administration of drugs. Proc. Roy. Soc. Med., *55:*20. 1962.
85. Thoburn, R., Johnson, J. E., III, and Cluff, L. E.: Studies on the epidemiology of adverse drug reactions. IV. The relationship of cephalothin and penicillin allergy. JAMA, *198:*345, 1966.
86. Thompson, J. E.: The management of hypersensitivity reactions to antituberculous drugs. Med. J. Aust., *36:*1058, 1969.
87. Tuft, L.: Allergic reactions following immunization procedures. Arch. Environ. Health, *13:*91, 1966.
88. Unanue, E. R., and Dixon, F. J.: Experimental glomerulonephritis: immunological events and pathogenetic mechanisms. *In* Dixon, and Humphrey: Advances in Immunology. vol. 6, pp. 1-90. New York and London. Academic Press, 1967.
89. United States Department of Health, Education and Welfare, Task Force on Prescription Drugs: Final report. Washington, D.C. Government Printing Office, 1969.
90. Van Dellen, R. G., Walsh, W. E., Peters, G. A., and Gleich, G. J.: Differing patterns of wheal and flare skin reactivity in patients allergic to penicillins. J. Allerg., *47:*230, 1971.
91. Visconti, J. A., and Smith, M. C.: Economic consequences of adverse drug reactions. Hospitals, *43:*85, 1969.
92. vonPirquet, C. F., and Schick B.: Die Serum Krankheit. Leipzig, Weir, 1905. English trans. Serum Sickness. Baltimore, Williams and Wilkins, 1951.
93. Westenfelder, G. O., and Paterson, P. Y.: Life-threatening infection: Choice of alternate drugs when penicillin cannot be given. JAMA, *210:*845, 1969.
94. Wide, L., Bennich, H., and Johnasson, S. G.: Diagnosis of allergy by an in-vitro test for allergen antibodies. Lancet, *2:*1105, 1967.
95. Wide, L., and Juhlin, L.: Detection of penicillin allergy of the immediate-type by radioimmunoassay of reagins (IgE) to penicilloyl conjugates. Clin. Allerg., *1:*171, 1971.

96. Wilhelm, R. E.: The newer anti-allergic agents. Med. Clin. N. Am., *45:*887, 1961.
97. Winterbauer, R. H., Ronald, A. R., Belcher, D. W., and Truck, M.: Antimicrobial therapy in patients sensitive to penicillin. J. Chronic Dis., *20:*407, 1962.
98. Wood, T. A., and Frenkel, E. P.: The atypical lymphocyte. Am. J. Med., *42:*923, 1967.
99. Yalow, R. S., and Berson, S. A.: Immunologic aspects of insulin. Am. J. Med., *31:*882, 1961.
100. Yurchak, A. M., Wicher, K., and Arbesman, C. E.: Immunologic studies on aspirin. J. Allerg., *46:*245, 1970.

17

Allergic Contact Dermatitis

Raymond G. Slavin, M.D.

A skin condition commonly seen by all physicians is allergic contact dermatitis, or dermatitis venenata. With new chemical sensitizers being introduced into our environment constantly, we will undoubtedly be seeing more instances of this disease. To diagnose allergic contact dermatitis and especially to elicit the inciting cause, requires all of the patience, thoroughness and acumen of the physician. The introduction of corticosteroids into our therapeutic armamentarium has been a two-edged sword. Although these agents are almost uniformly successful in treating allergic contact dermatitis, they have perhaps dulled the interest and desire of the physician to take the necessary time to discover, through history, physical examination and diagnostic patch testing, the offending agent. In addition, fatalities and serious systemic complications of allergic contact dermatitis are rare, and this, too, may diminish the physician's interest.

To the patient with allergic contact dermatitis such disinterest is unjustified. He is frequently extremely uncomfortable and at times disabled. The chronicity may be quite depressing. Frequent hospitalization and inability to pursue employment or recreational activity are common. Few patients exist in medical practice more grateful than the patient with allergic contact dermatitis whose physician has found the inciting cause. In addition, the intellectual satisfaction for the physician who has tracked down the offending allergen in a difficult case is great indeed.

IMMUNOLOGIC BASIS

Allergic contact dermatitis seems indistinguishable in its immunologic mechanism from other classical forms of the delayed, or cellular, type of hypersensitivity. Most clinical allergic problems are related to diseases associated with the immediate type of hypersensitivity, dependent on humoral antibody (see Chap. 2). In contrast, delayed or cellular hypersensitivity is dependent on sensitized lymphocytes.

495

Sensitization

Contact sensitivity can be acquired or induced by topical application to the skin of chemically reactive substances. These substances may be organic or inorganic and are generally of low molecular weight. Examples are the catechol of poison ivy leaves and many synthetic chemicals found in industry and the home. The simple chemical is not the immunogenic agent. It is a hapten, and, as such, its ability to sensitize depends on forming a conjugate in vivo with a tissue protein. In the case of the commonly used skin sensitizer, dinitrochlorobenzene, the union of the chemical hapten and the tissue protein occurs in the malpighian layer of the epidermis, with the amino acid sites of lysine and cysteine being most reactive.[1] It has been suggested that skin lipids might exert an adjuvant effect comparable to the mycoside of *Mycobacterium tuberculosis.*

The specificity of the contact sensitivity response resembles that of delayed hypersensitivity (cellular) rather than immediate hypersensitivity (humoral). When a hapten-protein complex is used to induce an immune response, the circulating antibody produced is directed toward, or is specific for, the hapten. The delayed hypersensitivity specificity is usually directed toward the protein carrier as well. This "carrier specificity" is clearly evident in contact sensitivity.[8]

It has been suggested that the type of protein with which the hapten links will determine whether immediate or delayed sensitivity results. The union of the contact allergen with an insoluble fibrous protein, such as keratin collagen, will result in delayed hypersensitivity. Conjugation of the chemical with a serum protein, such as albumin, results in the immediate response with production of humoral antibodies.

Experiments on skin transplants between identical twins have demonstrated the importance of organ systems other than the skin in the induction of contact sensitivity.[9] An area of skin from a sensitized donor loses its sensitivity when transplanted to a nonsensitive host. On the other hand, nonsensitive skin transplanted to a sensitized host acquires contact sensitivity. The sensitivity develops as long as the regional lymph nodes and lymphatic pathways between the nodes and the cutaneous sites of allergen application remain intact. If the pathways are cut or the nodes removed within 48 hours after application of the allergen, sensitization will not occur.[7] The lymph nodes are necessary for the induction, but not for the maintenance, of sensitivity.

A final comparison of contact dermatitis to delayed hypersensitivity in terms of sensitization is seen in the response of anergic patients. Patients with lymphoma or sarcoidosis who have lost their delayed hypersensitivity response to tuberculin, for example, also show a diminution in their sensitization to simple chemical contact allergens. Sensitization in anergic patients may be the same as in normal subjects with a potent sensitizer such as poison ivy, but it is diminished in response to a less powerful sensitizer, such as dinitrochlorobenzene.[4]

Histopathology

The histologic picture in allergic contact dermatitis closely resembles the delayed tissue response. The dermis is invaded by mononuclear inflammatory cells, especially about blood vessels and sweat glands. The epidermis appears somewhat different, probably due to the method of allergen application. It is hyperplastic with mononuclear cell invasion. Frequently intraepidermal vesicles form which may coalesce to form large blisters. The vesicles are filled with serous fluid containing granulocytes and mononuclear cells.

Transfer

Successful transfer of immediate and delayed hypersensitivity can be accomplished, but by completely different modes. The immediate type response is readily transferred with serum, either locally to the skin, as in the Prausnitz-Küstner reaction, or systemically (see Chap. 2). The delayed type of hypersensitivity cannot be transferred with serum under ordinary circumstances but can only be transferred with sensitized lymphocytes. It has been further shown in man that a cell-free dialyzable fraction obtained from sensitized lymphocytes can transfer delayed hypersensitivity.[13] In this respect, allergic contact dermatitis again resembles delayed hypersensitivity. Successful transfer of contact sensitivity can be accomplished with viable lymphoid cells both in the experimental animal [12] and in man,[3] although not as easily as with tuberculin or other types of bacterial sensitivity. Peripheral blood lymphocytes, exudative cells from the vesicles of contact dermatitis, and cell-free blister fluid have all successfully transferred contact sensitivity in man.

Lymphocyte Response in Vitro

Lymphocytes in tissue culture will transform into blast cells in a nonspecific fashion in response to phytohemagglutinin and in a specific fashion in response to antigen stimulation. The antigen-induced lymphocyte transformation is strongly correlated with delayed hypersensitivity,[15] although not exclusively so. It has been shown [16] that lymphocytes of guinea pigs sensitive to dinitrofluorobenzene (DNFB) show significant uptake of tritiated thymidine, indicative of stimulation, in the presence of DNFB-skin protein conjugates.

In summary, allergic contact dermatitis does seem to be a cutaneous manifestation or analogue of delayed or cellular hypersensitivity. Sensitization, immunologic specificity, histopathology, passive transfer and cellular response in vitro are common to both allergic contact dermatitis and delayed hypersensitivity; these facts emphasize their close resemblance, if not complete identity.

CLINICAL FEATURES

History

Allergic contact dermatitis occurs most frequently in the middle-aged and elderly, although it may appear at any age. In contrast to the classical atopic diseases, contact dermatitis is as common in the population at large as in the atopic population, and a history of concomitant or family allergy is of no help. No familial tendency in man towards the development of allergic contact dermatitis has been demonstrated.

The interval between exposure to the responsible agent and the occurrence of clinical manifestations is usually 12 to 48 hours, although it may be as early as 4 hours and as late as 72 hours. The incubation or sensitization period between initial exposure and the development of skin sensitivity is at least five days and may take several years. One may see, both experimentally and clinically, a situation analogous to serum sickness. If sufficient allergen from the sensitizing exposure remains to react with the sensitized skin after the incubation period has elapsed, a spontaneous flareup may occur at the site of the sensitizing exposure. In addition, a previously involved site may flare up weeks to years later after exposure to the allergen or a closely related allergen at a distant site. Once the sensitivity is established, it generally persists for many years. There are, however, instances in which the sensitivity has been lost after several years.

The patient will usually note the development of erythema followed by papules and then vesicles. Pruritus follows the appearance of the dermatitis and is uniformly present in allergic contact dermatitis.

Physical Examination

The appearance of allergic contact dermatitis depends on the stage at which the patient presents. In the acute stage, erythema, papules, and vesicles predominate with edema and occasionally bullae. The boundaries of the dermatitis are generally sharply marginated. Edema may be profound in areas of loose tissue such as the eyelids and genitalia. Acute allergic contact dermatitis of the face may result in a marked degree of periorbital swelling that resembles angioedema (Fig. 17-1). The presence of the associated dermatitis should help the physician make the distinction easily.

In the subacute phase, vesicles are less pronounced; and crusting,

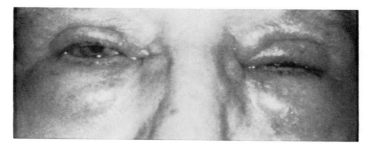

Fig. 17-1. Contact dermatitis of face and eyelids due to hair dye containing paraphenylene diamine. (Photo courtesy of Dr. Louis Keller.)

scaling and the beginning of lichenification may be present. In the chronic stage, few papulovesicular lesions are evident, and thickening, lichenification, and scaliness predominate.

The dermatitis is usually localized to the sites of the major exposure; however, lesions may be seen in areas that are not conspicuously exposed.

Differential Diagnosis

The skin conditions most frequently confused with allergic contact dermatitis are seborrheic dermatitis, atopic dermatitis, and primary irritant dermatitis.

In seborrheic dermatitis there is a general tendency to oiliness of the skin and a predilection of the lesions for the scalp and the nasal labial folds. Pruritus is not a prominent feature, and the lesions are irregular and covered with a greasy coating.

Atopic dermatitis (see Chap. 15) generally has its onset in infancy or early childhood. The skin is dry, and, while pruritus is a prominent feature, it appears before the lesions and not after as in the case of allergic contact dermatitis. The areas most frequently involved are the flexural surfaces. The margins of the dermatitis are indefinite, and the progression from erythema to papules to vesicles is not seen.

The dermatitis due to a primary irritant is one of a simple chemical or physical insult to the skin. An example of this is the familiar housewives' dermatitis of the hands due to household detergents. A prior sensitizing exposure to the primary irritant is not necessary, and the dermatitis develops in a large number of normal individuals. The dermatitis begins shortly after exposure to the irritant in contrast to the 12 to 48 hours after exposure to the allergen in allergic contact dermatitis. The eruption begins with mild dryness, redness and scaling. On continued exposure, fissuring, crusting and lichenification may result. Primary irritant dermatitis is usually confined to the hands and may be virtually indistinguishable in its physical appearance from allergic contact dermatitis.

It should be emphasized that skin conditions may coexist. It is not unusual to see allergic contact dermatitis due to topical ointments applied for the treatment of atopic dermatitis and other dermatoses.

IDENTIFYING THE OFFENDING AGENT

History and Physical Examination

Once the diagnosis of allergic contact dermatitis is made, vigorous efforts should be directed toward determining the cause. A careful, thorough history is absolutely mandatory. The period from exposure to clinical manifestations must be kept in mind and an exhaustive search made for exposure to any sensitizing allergen in the patient's occupational, home or recreational life. The location of the dermatitis most often relates closely to direct contact with a particular allergen. At times this is rather straightforward, such as dermatitis of the feet due to contact sensitivity to shoe materials or dermatitis from jewelry appearing on the wrist, the ear lobes or the neck. The relationship of the dermatitis to the direct contact allergen may not be as obvious at other times, and being able to associate certain areas of involvement with particular types of exposure is extremely helpful. Contact dermatitis of the face, for example, is often due to cosmetics directly applied to the area. One must, however, keep in mind other possibilities such as hair dye, shampoo and hair tonics. Contact dermatitis of the eyelids, while often due to eye shadow, mascara and eye liner, may also be caused by nail polish. Involvement of the thighs may be due to keys or coins in pants pockets. It is, therefore, vital that the physician familiarize himself with various patterns of distribution of contact dermatitis that may occur in association with particular allergens.

Frequently, the distribution of the skin lesions may suggest a number of possible sensitizing agents, and patch testing (to be described later) is of special value. Certain allergens may be airborne, and exposure may occur by this route. Dermatitis in farmers due to ragweed oil sensitivity is a common example. Smoke from burning the poison ivy plant may contain the oleoresin as particulate matter and thus expose the sensitive individual. Another route of acquiring poison ivy contact dermatitis without touching the plant is by indirect contact with clothing or animal fur containing the oleoresin.

Patch Testing

Principle. Patch testing is the diagnostic technique of applying a specific substance to the skin with the intention of producing a small area of allergic contact dermatitis. It can be thought of as reproducing the disease in miniature. The patch test is generally kept in place for 48 to 72 hours (although reactions may appear after 24 hours in markedly sensitive patients) and then observed for the gross appearance of a localized dermatitis which resembles the primary lesion. The same principles of proper interpretation of a positive patch test apply as in the case of the immediate wheal and erythema reaction (see Chap. 2). A positive patch test is not absolute proof that the test substance is the actual cause of presenting dermatitis. The positive patch test must always correlate with the patient's history and physical examination.

Testing with the Appropriate Substance. The patient is exposed to a myriad of chemical and plant substances in his everyday life, a great number of which have a potential of causing allergic contact dermatitis. Frequently, the history and physical examination may reveal the cause of the dermatitis, and the patch test serves only as corroborative evidence. On other occasions the history and location of the dermatitis will suggest a particular category of exposure, and then patch testing should be performed that will be appropriate to the particular category. This includes the patient's occupation, hobbies, household articles, clothing, cosmetics, plant exposure and topical medications. Several interviews and exhaustive questioning may be necessary before a clue to the particular exposure is revealed. In some instances there may be little or no suggestion of the offending agent; then, application of a standard group of substances known to be common causes of allergic contact dermatitis is indicated. Fisher's experience [5] is that the five most common causes of allergic contact dermatitis, in order of decreasing frequency, are Rhus (poison ivy, oak or sumac), paraphenylene diamine, nickel compounds, rubber compounds and the dichromates.

The following list includes the most common sensitizers and can be used as a survey or screening series:

1. Paraphenylene diamine (2% in petrolatum)
2. Turpentine (25% in olive oil)
3. Mercury bichloride (0.1% aqueous solution)
4. Pyrethrum powder (as is)
5. Nickel sulfate (5% aqueous solution)
6. Formalin (5% aqueous solution)
7. Lanolin (as is)
8. Potassium dichromate (0.5% aqueous)
9. Ethylamino benzoate (benzocaine-5% in petrolatum)
10. Copper sulfate (1% aqueous)
11. Procaine (1% aqueous)
12. Resorcin (5% aqueous)
13. Ammoniated mercury (10% in petrolatum)
14. Linseed oil (as is)
15. Methylparaben (5% in petrolatum)

16. Sodium hypochlorite (5% aqueous)
17. Carbowax 1500 (as is)
18. Potassium iodide (25% in petrolatum)
19. DDT (50% in olive oil)
20. Phenyl-beta-naphthylamine (1% in petrolatum)
21. Mercaptobenzothiazole (1% in petrolatum)
22. Ragweed oil (1:1000 in olive oil)
23. Poison ivy oil (1:5000 in acetone)
24. Eosin dye (powder)
25. Para-red (powder)

The physician should familiarize himself with the potent sensitizers and with the various modes of exposure. It is important to keep in mind the possibility of cross reactivity to other allergens because of chemical similarities. Sensitivity to paraphenylene diamine, for example, may also indicate sensitivity to para-amino-benzoic acid and other chemicals containing a benzene ring with an amino group in the "para" position.

CONTACTANT	EXPOSURE
Paraphenylene diamine	Hair dye, fur dye, black, blue and brown clothing
Pyrethrum	Insecticides
Mercury	Topical ointments, disinfectants, insecticides
Nickel	Coins, jewelry, buckles, clasps, door handles
Formalin	Cosmetics, insecticides, wearing apparel (drip-dry, wrinkle resistant, water repellant)
Potassium dichromate	Leather (chrome tanning), yellow paints
Copper	Coins, alloys, insecticides, fungicides
Resorcin	Hair tonics, tanning, cosmetics
Linseed oil	Furniture polishes, paints, varnishes
Sodium hypochlorite	Bleach, cleansing agents
Carbowax	Cosmetics
Potassium iodide	Photography (emulsions) table salt
Mercaptobenzothiazole	Rubber compounds (accelerator)
Phenyl-beta-naphthylamine	Rubber compounds (antioxidant)
Para-red dyes	Colored sections of newspapers and magazines

Above is a list of some of the most potent sensitizers and their most frequently presenting forms. It is by no means complete, and is not intended as a general survey. More detailed information on other sensitizers, environmental exposures, and preparation of testing material can be found in several standard texts.[18, 20, 6]

Techniques. Since contact dermatitis is a systemic sensitivity, it should be possible to use any area of the skin for patch testing. In rare instances of small, isolated areas of dermatitis, patch testing at a far distant sight may give negative results. Generally the back is used for patch testing. After washing with alcohol or acetone, the skin is allowed to dry. The test materials are applied in rows either directly to the skin and covered with a small gauze flat or placed on the gauze portion of a Band-aid. Inert materials should be moistened with a drop of saline. The gauze is held in place by adhesive tape. There may be indications for so-called open testing in which the test substance is not covered by gauze or tape. Plant oils generally adhere to the skin without tape. In order to determine whether a substance is a photosensitizer, open testing must be employed. Other substances may be primary irritants when occluded and should only be tested by the open method. These include hair tonics, perfumes, antiperspirants, shaving creams, toothpastes and strong medications, such as tincture of iodine and ammoniated mercury and salicylic acid combinations.

After 48 hours the patches are removed, and after a wait of 20 to 30 minutes to allow nonspecific mechanical irritation to subside, the reactions are read. Generally, the site of a positive patch test itches. As was stated earlier, the disease is reproduced in miniature and in a positive reaction, vesicles on an erythematous, edematous base are present (Fig. 17-2). A true allergic reaction persists for several days. Irritative skin reactions subside in a few hours; so, when there is doubt, the area should be examined the following day. Positive patch test reactions often show an increase in the next 24 hours. Therefore, all test sites should be routinely reexamined at 72 hours. The reading should be directed to the center of the patch, where the skin was not in contact with the tape. Arbitrary grading of patch test results is $+$ erythema; $++$ erythema and papules; $+++$ erythema, papules and vesicles; $++++$ erythema, papules, vesicles and severe edema.

Materials to be used in testing may be obtained from commercial allergy supply houses. It should, however, be remembered that the patient himself is an excellent source and that the materials he may bring from his home or place of work may be extremely valuable.

Precautions. Several precautions must be observed in patch testing. The application of the test material itself may sensitize the patient. Potent materials which may sensitize on the first application include poison ivy extract, picryl chloride, and methyl salicylate. In testing, one has to avoid provoking nonspecific inflammation. The testing material must be dilute enough to avoid a primary irritant effect. This is especially important when testing with a contactant not included in the standard patch test materials. In order to be significant, a substance must elicit a reaction at a concentration which will not cause reactivity in

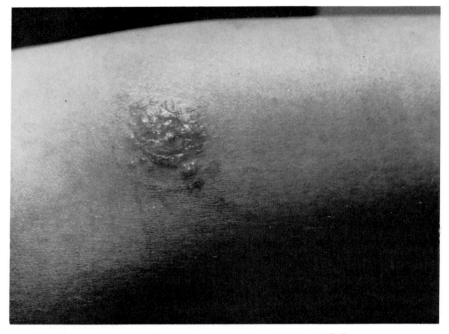

Fig. 17-2. Positive patch test reaction to nickel.

a suitable number of normal controls. Patch tests should never be performed in the presence of an acute or widespread contact dermatitis.
False positive reactions may be obtained because of increased reactivity of the skin. In addition, a positive patch test reaction with the
offending agent may cause a flareup of the dermatitis. The patient
should be carefully instructed at the time of patch test application to
remove any patch which is causing severe irritation. If left on for the full
48 hours, such an area may actually slough. Systemic corticosteroids or
ACTH will, in sufficient doses, decrease or ablate a delayed skin reaction. These substances should also mask or cause a decrease in the
patch test reaction. It is felt by some that the clinically significant reaction is not affected by small doses of corticosteroids and that only
the weak or borderline reaction is affected. Attempts should be made to
eliminate the use of corticosteroids or to decrease to the lowest possible
dose before patch testing is carried out. Antihistamines or sympathomimetic amines do not, of course, affect the delayed skin response
or the patch test reaction.

Intradermal Testing

Several investigators in recent years have emphasized the importance
of intradermal testing in allergic contact dermatitis.[2, 14] In some

instances, intradermal testing has been found to be positive in patients with a negative patch test. These cases are usually represented by papular dermatitis, and the abnormality is thought to be in the dermis. The chemicals that have been reported to result in such a reaction are nickel, neomycin and the dichromates. Proponents of the dermal delayed sensitivity theory believe that transepidermal absorption of the antigen sets up the allergic reaction in the corium. In these cases therefore, a negative patch test does not rule out the material as the offending agent, and the hypersensitivity can be demonstrated only by intradermal testing. Others have found that patch testing with higher concentrations will elicit a positive reaction in such cases. Further investigation on a larger scale is needed to determine the relative value of the intradermal test versus the patch test.

COMPLICATIONS

The most common complication of allergic contact dermatitis is secondary infection due to the intense pruritus and subsequent scratching. An interesting but poorly understood complication is the occasional occurrence of the nephrotic syndrome and glomerulonephritis in severe generalized contact dermatitis due to poison ivy or poison oak.[17]

SYMPTOMATIC TREATMENT

The inflammation and pruritus of allergic contact dermatitis necessitate symptomatic therapy. In the acute stage accompanied by weeping lesions, cold wet dressings are indicated. Burow's solution in a dilution of 1:20 saline, or cold tap water may be used. An alternative would be 6% white vinegar in water (2 oz. vinegar to 1 qt. water). In mild cases, systemic antihistamines may be helpful in relieving the pruritus. In the subacute and chronic stages, topical corticosteroids usually prove quite effective. It probably makes little difference as to the preparation used, since the response is generally excellent. When the dermatitis is particularly acute or widespread, systemic corticosteroids may have to be employed. In instances when further exposure can be avoided, such as poison ivy dermatitis, there should be no hesitation in administering systemic corticosteroids. This is a classic example of a self-limited disease which will respond to a five- to ten-day course of oral corticosteroid therapy. There seems to be no need for prolonged antihistamine therapy in such instances. The response to systemic corticosteroids is generally dramatic with improvement apparent in only a few hours. Three rules which might be applied to systemic corticosteroid therapy in acute contact dermatitis are: (1) use the least expensive preparation (prednisone), (2) use enough, (3) avoid prolonged administration.

For secondary infection resulting from scratching due to the pruritus of allergic contact dermatitis, antibiotics may be needed. Because of the risk involved in sensitization from topical antibiotics, the oral or injectable forms are preferred.

PROPHYLAXIS

The physician has a responsibility to his patients, not only to treat disease but also to prevent it. For that reason one should avoid topical application of medications which have a high index of sensitization. Included in this group are benzocaine, furacin, antihistamines, neomycin, penicillin, sulfonamides, and ammoniated mercury.

When the offending agent causing allergic contact dermatitis is discovered, careful instruction must be given to the patient so that he may avoid it in the future. The physician should discuss all of the possible sources of exposure. In the case of chemical sensitivity this list may be quite extensive. When dealing with a plant dermatitis, the patient should be instructed in the proper identification of the offending plant.

There may be instances in which exposure cannot be avoided either through occupation or the ubiquitous nature of the allergen. In such cases hyposensitization may be considered. While there is some laboratory and clinical evidence to suggest effectiveness, the actual benefit obtained from hyposensitization in allergic contact dermatitis is often difficult to evaluate and this type of treatment should be used only in exceptional circumstances.

There is experimental work which points to the possibility of desensitization in delayed hypersensitivity reactions. In the laboratory animal with delayed hypersensitivity to a particular allergen, several intradermal skin tests performed simultaneously elicit a less intense reaction than a single test. The same is seen with application of multiple contact skin tests. Desensitization to tuberculin can be accomplished in both the experimental animal and in man by repeated injections of gradually increasing doses of tuberculin. On a clinical basis, the American Indian has long chewed poison ivy leaves as a form of prophylaxis or treatment of poison ivy dermatitis. A spontaneous type of desensitization resulting from natural exposure may occur, termed the "hardening" process. This is especially common in industrial exposures to chemicals.

A large amount of experience in hyposensitization to contact allergens has been obtained with poison ivy, poison oak and poison sumac. However, the errors in evaluation of these hyposensitization procedures have led to great confusion. The criterion for success in most studies has been simply a decrease in the subsequent development of dermatitis. This does not take into account such variables as the degree of exposure to the offending allergen. There is a definite need for more controlled studies which will detect changes in sensitivity as measured by quantitative patch testing.

Attempts to hyposensitize to poison ivy have been reported using both parenteral injection and oral preparations. Kligman [11] found that repeated intramuscular injections of a specially prepared hapten, 3-n-pentadecyl catechol, over five to nine months was necessary to decrease skin reactivity. Oral administration of a commercially available oleoresin resulted in a decrease in skin reactivity in one half of the patients treated, but only after an average of 25 weeks of treatment. [10] This is a small series, and further studies are indicated. It would appear from the information available that an approximate total of 3000 mg. of the oleoresin should be given over a six month period to obtain maximum effect. The extracts should never be given to an individual with the active dermatitis because of the possibility of exacerbating the condition. Treatment must be repeated yearly and the patient should still be cautioned to avoid the plant. Side effects of the hyposensitization are numerous including fever, stomatitis, dermatitis, pruritus ani, urticaria and glomerulonephritis. [19] For these reasons, attempts at hyposensitization to poison ivy should be directed at only two groups. The first would be those in whom a change of occupation would be necessary for complete avoidance. The second group would be individuals who are exquisitely sensitive and for whom careful avoidance has simply not been enough.

The same precautions observed in hyposensitization to poison ivy, poison oak and poison sumac should also be applied to other plant dermatitides, such as ragweed contact dermatitis. The side effects are the same, and prolonged therapy with commercially available materials in excess of that recommended by the supplier may be necessary.

REFERENCES

1. Eisen, H. N., and Belman, S.: Studies of hypersensitivity to low molecular weight substances. II. Reactions of some allergenic substituted dinitrobenzenes with cysteine or cystine of skin proteins. J. Exp. Med., 98: 533, 1953.
2. Epstein, S.: Contact dermatitis due to nickel and chromate: observation on dermal delayed (tuberculin-type) sensitivity. Arch. Derm., 73:236, 1956.
3. Epstein, W. L., and Kligman, A. M.: Transfer of allergic contact-type delayed sensitivity in man. J. Invest. Derm., 28:291, 1957.
4. Epstein, W. L., and Mayock, R. I.: Induction of allergic contact dermatitis in patients with sarcoidosis. Proc. Soc. for Exp. Biol. Med., 96:786, 1957.

5. Fisher, A. A.: Contact Dermatitis. p. 10. Philadelphia, Lea and Febiger, 1967.
6. ———.: Contact Dermatitis. pp. 257-307. Philadelphia, Lea and Febiger, 1967.
7. Frey, J. R., and Wenk, P.: Experimental studies on pathogenesis of contact eczema in guinea pigs. Int. Arch. Allerg., *11*:81, 1957.
8. Gell, P. G. H., and Benacerraf, B.: Studies on hypersensitivity. IV. The relationship between contact and delayed sensitivity: a study on the specificity of cellular immune reactions. J. Exp. Med., *113*:571, 1961.
9. Haxthausen, H.: Allergic dermatitis: studies in identical twins. Acta Dermatovener., *23*:438, 1943.
10. Kanof, N. B., and Baer, R. L.: Attempts to hyposensitize with poison ivy extracts. Ann. Allerg., *22*:161, 1964.
11. Kligman, A. M.: Hyposensitization against Rhus dermatitis. Arch. Derm., *78*:47, 1958.
12. Landsteiner, K., and Chase, M. W.: Experiments on transfer of cutaneous sensitivity to simple compounds. Proc. Soc. Exp. Biol. Med., *49*:688, 1942.
13. Lawrence, H. S.: The transfer in humans of delayed skin sensitivity to streptococcal M substance to tuberculin with disrupted leukocytes. J. Clin. Invest., *34*:219, 1955.
14. Marcussen, P. V.: Comparison of intradermal test and patch test using nickel sulfate and formaldehyde. J. Invest. Derm., *40*:263, 1963.
15. Mills, J. A.: The immunologic significance of antigen-induced lymphocyte transformation in vitro. J. Immuno., *97*:239, 1966.
16. Milner, J. E.: In vitro lymphocyte responses in contact dermatitis. J. Invest. Derm., *55*:34, 1970.
17. Rytand, D. A.: Fatal anuria, the nephrotic syndrome and glomerular nephritis as sequels of the dermatitis of poison oak. Amer. J. Med., *5*:548, 1968.
18. Schwartz, L., Tullipan, L., and Peck, S. M.: Occupational Diseases of the Skin. ed. 3. Philadelphia, Lea and Febiger, 1957.
19. Shaffer, B., Burgoon, C. F., and Gosman, J. H.: Acute glomerulonepritis following administration of Rhus toxin. JAMA, *146*:1570, 1951.
20. Sheldon, J. M., Lovell, R. G., and Mathews, K. P.: A Manual of Clinical Allergy. ed. 2. pp. 268-295. Philadelphia, W. B. Saunders, 1967.

18

Miscellaneous Topics in Allergy

RELATION OF HEADACHES TO ALLERGY

John D. Holloman, M.D.

Headache is so common that few escape it in the course of their lives. Abdominal discomfort is probably the only rival of headache for numbers of people affected and frequency of occurrence. Fortunately, most head pain is of trivial importance and only a small percentage of these events are relayed to the physician's attention. The majority of headaches are of the *tension type,* rarely alleged to be of allergic origin. Most laymen are aware that headache, though usually insignificant, can be the harbinger of severe disorders and even disaster. The intent of this chapter is to clarify the relationship between allergy and headache seen commonly in clinical practice. Some headache mechanisms are still but partially understood and stubbornly defy medical treatment. The cyclic recurrence of headache has led researchers to postulate allergic mechanisms of both food and inhalant types. Such a connection has been most frequently associated with migraine and sinus headaches. The focus of this chapter will be on these two types of headaches.

MIGRAINE HEADACHE

Head pain was described in ancient medical writing. Aretaeus of Cappadocia,[10] in the first century A.D., described a severe, paroxysmal type of headache consistent with the diagnosis of migraine. Galen introduced the term hemicrania a half century later emphasizing the unilateral nature of this condition.

According to H. G. Wolff,[19] over the centuries the term evolved from hemigranea through emigranea, migranea, megrim, and now migraine. Migraine and its variants are a common disorder. The incidence may be as high as five percent of the general population in a two to one ratio of women to men. In contrast, one type of migraine variant called cluster headaches has a strong predilection for males.

Migraine is a problem of significance because of its frequent extreme severity and its occasional recurrence throughout an entire lifetime. Other types of headache may rival migraine in severity, but their course is of shorter duration. They are generally diagnosed by the nature of their underlying cause, for example, brain tumor or subarachnoid hemorrhage.

The most significant feature of migraine headaches is periodic recurrence especially unilateral, but often becoming generalized. The patient is always irritable, usually nauseated, and often has vomiting and photophobia. Many note a prodome of scotoma, paresthesia, or even hemianopia and speech defect. Commonly a family history of similar headaches exists. The pain can include both face and neck.

Several generalized dysfunctions frequently occurring with the headache include cold extremities, tremors, vertigo, pallor, abdominal distention, sweating and "chilly sensations." The sensation of tight rings on fingers and edematous appearance suggest an acute, but poorly understood disturbance of water metabolism. Patients with migraine headaches may appear markedly ill.

Such migraine attacks may last from several minutes to days, and on occasion may exceed one week. Great variation of intensity during an attack and from one episode to another may occur. The duration of attacks tends to be predictable in the individual patient as does site of onset. Migraine, like all vascular headaches, is characterized by depth, diffusion, aching, and rhythmic throbbing and pulsating. Sometimes the headache phase is preceded or followed by a sense of euphoria. If vomiting and dehydration occur during the headache, this euphoria is absent during the postheadache period. Anorexia always accompanies the headache phase.

At this point it is appropriate to consider what constitutes a classical migraine attack and to attempt to correlate the phases with the presumptive pathophysiology. The phases of a typical attack have been identified as three: preheadache, headache, and postheadache phenomena. All have been well described by Wolff.[19]

During the preheadache phase pain is not yet apparent, but several of its portents are. These may be scotomata, tinnitus, scintillations and other hallucinations of light, sound, and color. This period lasts from minutes to over an hour. Less commonly, hemianopia and paresthesias occur unilaterally. About one tenth of those afflicted with migraine headaches note this phase, and occasionally these symptoms are not followed by headache.

Evidence for vasoconstriction of the internal carotid system as the cause of the preheadache symptoms has been obtained from subjects given amyl nitrite or carbon dioxide-oxygen mixtures. These drugs promptly relieved preheadache symptoms. More recently, angiograms done during a preheadache episode clearly demonstrate marked constriction of the internal carotid branches. What mediator causes this constriction still provokes debate.

The above prodrome gives way to the painful headache phase. This is usually a deep aching, throbbing pain felt behind the eye on the affected side. This pain will then progress to involve the entire side and sometimes the entire head. Photophobia, tearing and blurred vision are frequent. Dilatation of conjunctival vessels is common. Edema of the lids and face is not unusual. The duration is from hours to days. Toward the end of the attack vomiting often occurs. If edema was present during the preheadache phase, diuresis begins during the headache with urine of low specific gravity.

In contrast to the constriction of the internal carotid system during the preheadache phase, the headache phase is associated with a marked dilatation of the external carotid systems sometimes observable on the patient's forehead. It is believed that local tissue factors, probably of humoral nature, cause and sustain this vasodilatation. Again, what these substances are remains controversial. Histamine has almost certainly been eliminated as a participant.

With the ultimate disappearance of the headache, the third, or postheadache phase occurs. This is much less dramatic than the other phases and might go unnoticed except for a few indicators which reveal that a return to normalcy has not yet occurred. There may be a subjective feeling of euphoria or total apathy. Dehydration is frequently apparent, and the normal physiologic reactivity of the cerebral arteries and their branches to vasoactive drugs like noradrenalin and histamine are usually reduced. This phase of the syndrome is thought to be a disorder of functions, not structures, and has no morbid anatomy.

Etiology

The preceding description of phases and the pathophysiology of blood vessels in the migraine syndrome is generally accepted. The ultimate biochemical causes inciting these events is a problem that generates much debate. Two biochemical substances may be significant in this disorder. They are serotonin and tyramine, both vasoactive agents. They may, in turn, interact with noradrenalin or one of the vasoactive kinins, but the system has yet to be elucidated.

Serotonin could be directly involved. Recent literature appears to have established an increased blood level of this substance during the preheadache or phase I part of the syndrome. An abrupt drop in blood level occurs with the onset of pain, phase II. Between attacks, blood levels remain within the normal range.[13] This sequence of events has gained further support from investigations showing that intravenous injection of reserpine promptly lowers blood serotonin levels and precipitates a typical migraine headache in migrainous subjects. Of further interest is the action of methysergide, the only effective drug for migraine prevention that is commercially available. It is a potent serotonin antagonist.

The possible role of tyramine in migraine headache has stirred recent interest. Attention was pointed to this vasoactive amine, which is derived from tyrosine, by the recent elucidation of the headache syndrome caused by monamine oxidase (MAO) inhibitors. These headaches closely resemble typical migraine attacks. It was originally noted that certain patients on MAO inhibitor drugs would undergo migraine-type headache attacks when eating certain foods high in tyramine. MAO inhibitors blocked the enzymatic deamination of tyramine to relatively inert p-hydroxyphenylacetic acid (HPAA) thus allowing elevation of the blood level of tyramine, a toxic vasoactive amine. Severe, transient hypertension was also a frequent concomitant. Both free and conjugated tyramine were found to be reduced in the urine of migraine subjects compared with controls when fed measured amounts of tyramine. Migraine attacks were regularly induced by such oral intake in these patients of known migraine predisposition.[12]

These data strongly suggest the possibility of an enzyme dysfunction or block particularly in the migraine syndrome associated with dietary factors. From the above data two possible types of genetic enzyme malfunction or mutation leading to headaches may be suggested: deamination and conjugation of tyramine. The pathway of tyramine degradation is shown in Figure 18-1. Such enzyme malfunction, inhibition, or absence possibly has its ultimate cause in gene damage or mutation more fully described in the following paragraph. It is possible that the migraine syndrome may be yet another example of an "inborn error of metabolism." The nature of the hereditary factor in migraine has recently been reemphasized.[6]

Recent reports establishing a relationship between migraine and the oral contraceptive, especially those of higher estrogenic content suggests a role for estrogen in susceptible women.[2] A number of women taking the oral contraceptive with no prior history of headaches, have had episodes of head pain. It is well known that enzyme function is strongly influenced by hormones. If migraine is a heritable disease, it is probable that multiple alleles are involved in the genetic inheritance of this condition.

Phenotypic expression of a gene, or its mutant, is the result of the actions of the gene in its particular environment. The environment may enhance or modify the effects of the gene in a sequence of events resulting in phenotypic expression. Such phenotypic expression of a gene

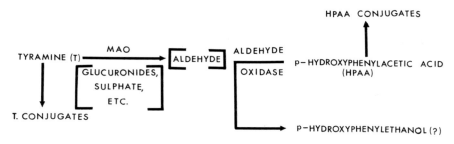

Fig. 18-1. The present understanding of the general metabolism of amines with tyramine used as an example.

depends in part upon neighboring genes and in part upon metabolic substances, hormones, nutrition, and other environmental factors. Brain and kidney cells are phenotypically different but genetically identical. Obviously genes have different effects in different tissue environments.

Migraine headaches may be the result of genetic differences or non-lethal gene mutations which result in different rates of degradation of certain vasoactive molecules. This deficiency of degradation may be enhanced by local metabolic products and materials such as estrogen. The latter allows expression of the enzyme abnormality and correlates with the greater incidence of migraine headaches in females and headache occurrence after exogenous estrogens. It has long been known that migraine attacks usually diminish in severity and number after menopause. A reverse situation applies to cluster headache migraine, which has a much higher incidence in men. This would involve a gene mutation at a different site on the same gene or gene sequence elaborated in the foregoing discussion. This second type of mutation would produce an aberrant enzyme more sensitive to male than female hormones, or female hormone metabolites.

It is probably significant that all of the agents effective in migraine prophylaxis are strong serotonin antagonists. An example is methysergide. Why this is significant awaits explanation.

The problem of migraine headaches and the role of food allergy will be undertaken. This postulated cause and effect relationship has been present since 1919 when first mentioned by Pagniez, Vallery-Radot, and Nast.[8] This mechanism has been subsequently championed by Rinkel[11] and many others. Vaughan's publications[15] are examples of these views. Based essentially on a clinical history of attacks following certain foods, skin tests to these foods were done and it was concluded that food hypersensitivity was relevant in seventy percent of migraine patients. About one half of these patients reported some relief on an elimination diet. It is interesting to see that lists of offending foods compiled by several authors have striking similarity (i.e., wheat, milk, eggs, chocolate). It is even more interesting to observe that many of the foods on these lists are of high tyramine content and known to be a cause of tyramine headache.[12] Today there remain many physicians who believe food hypersensitivity is a cause of migraine headache.

Unger proceeded a step further in an experiment attempting to link an allergen with migraine attacks.[14] He described the production of migraine attacks in one patient by feeding allergens which gave positive skin tests. He then failed to produce an attack in this same subject after administering harmless extracts alleged to be the offending allergen. An article published in 1970 by Unger [18] indicates he still supports this viewpoint.

The reports correlating food allergy and migraine have omitted a critical experiment. The alleged food offenders have not been administered in suitably controlled studies. Such experiments have subsequently been carried out by Wolff,[18] Loveless,[7] and Walker.[11] All of these controlled studies indicate there is no predictable relationship between disguised offending foods and occurrence of migraine. Many difficulties exist in interpreting skin tests, especially to foods. This problem has been discussed in Chapter 14. In young children, when the gastrointestinal tract is most permeable to food allergens, the occurrence of migraine is uncommon when compared with adults. Finally, the work of Kallós [7] should be considered. Carefully selecting a small group of patients having migraine in addition to urticaria, rhinitis, and asthma associated with specific allergen hypersensitivity, he produced true migraine headaches by parenteral injection of these allergens. They differed only in that phase I or preheadache phenomena were absent. He proceeded to show that with headache induction, rhinitis and/or asthma were always present. The naso-pulmonary symptoms were then prevented on subsequent occasions by prior administration of antihistamines, but the headaches occurred regardless. Kallós reversed the experiment and gave ergotamine prior to parenteral allergen administration and blocked the headache but not the occurrence of nasal and bronchial symptoms. This information makes it very difficult to equate the basic reaction mechanisms of migraine headaches and allergic hypersensitivity. Such material supports IgE or antibody mediation of urticaria while indicating the headaches are caused by a different mechanism. It is much more likely that migraine mechanisms similar to the tyramine headache model will adequately explain the diverse factors of the migraine syndrome. Consideration of atopic or antigen-antibody reactions of allergic nature as an important factor seems destined to be minimized as a causative factor in the headache syndrome. Such explanations or opinions become progressively tenuous when considering the above factors.

There are some foods which cause some headaches in some individuals Again using the tyramine headache as a model, it appears easier to explain these headaches as "food idiosyncrasy" rather than a "food allergy" or atopic reaction. The difference between idiosyncrasy, or metareaction as it is called more recently, and allergic reaction, has long been distinguished in pharmacology. Individuals with atropine sensitivity or idiosyncrasy are an example. Possibly food-induced headaches are another.

In conclusion, many aspects of migraine and allergic responses are shared. Attacks are paroxysmal with edema and hyperemia, in both. They are probably mediated, at least in part, by proteins or their breakdown products and relieved by vasoconstrictor substances. However, these responses show marked dissimilarities. Cellular infiltrations are absent in migraine; antihistamines have no effect in migraine; responses to adrenal steroids are different; and lastly, no controlled evidence exists that histamine or food allergens specifically cause migraine headaches.

There are "purists" who prefer to limit the use of the term migraine to head pain which begins and remains unilateral throughout the attack. There is no objection to such a precise use of the term except that it creates useless subdivisions of overlapping headache syndromes. It seems preferable to include them all in one general class called migraine syndrome and its variants with the understanding that they have similar vascular mechanisms and clinical phenomena.

ATYPICAL MIGRAINE EQUIVALENTS

Mention should be made of a group of poorly understood head pains referred to by Wolff as cephalalgias and atypical neuralgias.[18] They maintain some of the characteristics of migraine but also carry features of the typical facial neuralgias. The several types included here are sphenopalatine ganglion or Sluder's headache, occipital neuralgia, vidian neuralgia, atypical facial neuralgia, carotidynia, autonomic faciocephalalgia, and lastly, cluster headache or Horton's cephalalgia. This last type, cluster headache, receives more detailed consideration below. They all depart from the typical facial neuralgias in the following ways: (1) pain is rarely limited to fifth or ninth cranial nerve distribution; (2) pain is not reduced or ablated by section of the fifth or ninth cranial nerves; (3) pain is steady, diffuse, and aching lasting from hours to days in contrast to short severe paroxysms characteristic of trigeminal neuralgia, (4) they do not have "trigger zones"; (5) these pains occur in a younger age group with women predominating; (6) pain is not precipitated by cold drafts or food ingestion, swallowing, etc. common in *tic douloureaux;* (7) vasodilators increase the intensity of pain in these cephalalgias while vasoconstrictors diminish pain as they do in migraine syndrome. The reverse holds in the facial neuralgias. None of these cephalalgias appear to be immunologically mediated, particularly IgE mediated. Further details of these atypical head pains can be found in Wolff's elaborations.[19]

CLUSTER OR HISTAMINE HEADACHE

It is doubtful that histamine headache (Horton's headache, cluster headache) warrants being classified as other than a variant of migraine. This type does carry several distinguishing features, but the symptomatic spectrum of migraine is adequately diverse to accommodate this type. It is predominant in males, frequently of extreme severity, has predilection for the same side, with sudden onset and sudden departure. There is marked parasympathetic reaction of the conjunctiva, nasal mucosa, and malar blood vessels on the affected side. The attacks are rarely over two hours' duration. They occur as clusters of attacks over days to weeks and then remit entirely for periods of short to long duration. Phases I and III of the classical migraine syndrome are usually not present. Horton named these headaches "histamine headaches" because of the ability to induce this type of headache in some patients with parenteral administration of 0.35 mg. histamine base.[3] He suggested an unusual sensitivity to histamine. It was subsequently shown by Horton that alcohol can often duplicate this phenomenon. More recently experiments of Kunkle using spinal fluid from patients in the immediate posthead-ache phase indicate that an acetylcholinelike substance is released, not histamine.[5, 6] This strongly implicates parasympathetic discharge over the seventh cranial nerve. Horton went on to suggest a histamine de-sensitization technique as an approach to treatment. However, Wolff reports that several controlled studies failed to furnish support for this technique.[18]

Treatment

Both migraine and cluster headache are reduced or relieved by ergotamine compounds. Both types appear reduced by pretreatment with methysergide. Both types of headache have symptom variants that grade into each other, and each can vary widely in one person.

Treatment of these vascular headache types devolves about two aspects: headache relief and headache prevention. If a food is implicated (usually suggested by the patient who often has long experimented with elimination diets), it is appropriate to withdraw the food or group of foods and after several weeks reintroduce them. Certainly if headaches cease upon withdrawal and recur with repeated reintroduction, these foods should be eliminated. It remains difficult to escape the feeling that "food coincidence," as opposed to food allergy or idiosyncrasy, plays a major role in headache induction and relief. If a patient comes to suspect or implicate a given food or group of foods as the cause of headache or numerous other medical maladies, it is very difficult to relieve him of this notion. All people are suggestible, some more than others. If a suspect food is knowingly ingested, headaches seem to promptly ensue; if this food is avoided, the patient at least seems to believe the attacks are fewer or less severe. Most physicians have observed this phenomenon. The earlier cited works of Loveless [7] and Walker [17] are relevant here. It is the responsibility of the physician to work with the patient, help him understand his problem, and prevent increasing avoidance of a wide variety of nutrients which do not actually result in amelioration of headaches but which could result in a bizarre, nutritionally deficient diet.

Aspirin and rest will relieve most of the milder migraine headaches, but for the moderate to severe typical migraine or cluster-type headache, the only nonnarcotic drugs effective in relief are the ergot compounds. These have the advantage of both oral, parenteral, and rectal suppository forms of administration. The latter is a significant factor when considering the frequent occurrence of nausea with these headaches. Ergotamine is effective in migraine reduction or relief in 70 to 80 percent of these cases. The oral form is much more effective if taken early in the attack—during the prodrome or phase I before arterial dilatation has occurred. More drug is required and still often fails if taken orally during phase II. The rectal suppositories or parenteral injections are more often effective in phase II, though not invariably. Orally, 1 to 2 mg. are usually taken at the beginning of the attack and 1 mg. orally every hour thereafter until a maximum of six tablets has been taken, nausea and vomiting occur, or the headache is relieved, whichever occurs first. Ergotamine is always contraindicated in arterial occlusive disease of any type and during pregnancy. There are several commercial preparations available in the 1-mg. size. The suppositories contain 2 mg. of ergotamine. Dehydroergotamine for parenteral use comes in 1-mg. vials.

Methysergide appeared to be an excellent agent for migraine prevention. It effectively relieved 70 to 80 percent of moderate to severe migraine attacks and could be taken orally but had to be taken continuously. Methysergide is a potent serotonin inhibitor. Although effective, methysergide infrequently causes serious side effects. There is arterial constriction in some patients with leg cramping and arterial insufficiency. This must be checked for carefully and frequently. It has been associated with retroperitoneal fibrosis in occasional cases. The mechanism of this reaction has not yet been elucidated. Urinary tract obstruction can result from this retroperitoneal inflammation. Fortunately, the number of cases has been small.

SINUS HEADACHE

This section is designed to explore briefly the interrelation of headaches and allergic disease of the nasal and paranasal structures. The classical question of whether patients with allergic nasal disease experience increased "sinus headaches" seems better understood since the observations of Proetz [9] and many experiments of Wolff. Proetz reported a patient whose maxillary sinus mucosa was stretched from normal thickness to about 1 cm. within several hours during the course of an asthmatic attack. By chance, she had her sinuses filled with lipoidal just before her accidental contact with the offending allergen. Serial x-rays revealed this immense change, but, significantly, the patient was totally unaware of any change in her sinuses.

It can be seen from the figures presented below that obstruction or pressure on the sinuses is of itself inadequate to stimulate sinus pain or headache of any significance. This should remain true from any cause of noninfectious sinus obstruction or pressure whether of allergic or other origin. Mucous secretions cannot be trapped in sinuses without encouraging bacterial invasion and infection. The issue that has gone unappreciated is that sinus inflammation rarely occurs without simultaneous inflammation and engorgement of adjacent nasal structures. Whether obstruction of nasal cavities or sinus orifices lead to an increase of infectious sinusitis has not been conclusively determined. Many patients carry nasal polyps and swollen nasal membranes for years without sinus infections or frequent headaches.

Description

The term sinus headache has traditionally been assigned to headaches associated with sinus disease. Despite this ongoing conception, Wolff has conclusively demonstrated that headaches originating in nasal and paranasal structures are fairly uncommon.[19] When headaches did occur, they were always deep, dull, aching, and nonpulsating. They rarely caused nausea or vomiting and seldom rivaled migraine attacks in intensity. Acute sinus disease usually gave rise to headaches of greater intensity than did chronic sinus inflammation, but still was seldom severe.

It has been shown that location of sinus headache is predominantly related to the nasal region that is most diseased. Disorders of the superior nasal structures cause pain in the front and top of the head and between the eyes. Diseases of the middle and inferior nasal areas cause headache in the zygomatic and temporal areas and in the teeth and jaws. No one has shown that diseases of the paranasal sinuses underlying the above areas provides any significant contribution to this pain.

Wolff developed a useful system for the experimental study of pain. The structures shown in Figures 18-2 to 18-6 were pressed upon by a probe and stimulated by an insulated faradic current electrode. Pain was graded from 1 plus—a barely discernible discomfort, to 10 plus—an intolerable pain. The faradic current intensity used was that which elicited 1-plus pain when applied to the tongue.

From Wolff's series of experiments it was apparent that there are four areas of major pain sensitivity in the nasal and paranasal structures. They are the turbinates, the ostia, the nasofrontal ducts, and the superior nasal areas. These four areas contribute by far the greatest number to any so-called sinus headaches.

Etiology

The pathophysiology and cause of pain from disease of the nasal structures has led to much controversy. Again, Wolff and colleagues brought order to this debate. Variations in venous pressure, sinus exudates, negative and positive sinus air pressure, vasomotor changes, and nasal mucosal irritants were all considered and investigated. It was apparent that sinus inflammation rarely occurs without concurrent inflammation of the nasal structures. The only exception was that due to periapical abscess. From the available evidence the only conclusion to be drawn was that inflammation of the turbinates, the ostia, the nasofrontal ducts, and superior nasal structures caused nearly all of the pain issuing from sinuses or paranasal structures. All other factors served only to aggravate this basic underlying prerequisite. Such inflammation served mainly to lower the pain threshold to all of these other factors which in themselves were simply inadequate stimuli. This inflammation usually occurs through secondary infection resulting from recent upper respiratory infection, sinus engorgement with obstruction, chemical irritants like tobacco smoke, or neoplastic invasion. Even the extreme mucosal swelling and nasal obstruction of allergic rhinitis or its ultimate "tour de force," the nasal polyp, are inadequate to generate sinus headache. An underlying infection or inflammation of one or more of the four critical areas of the nasal cavity must precede the pain.

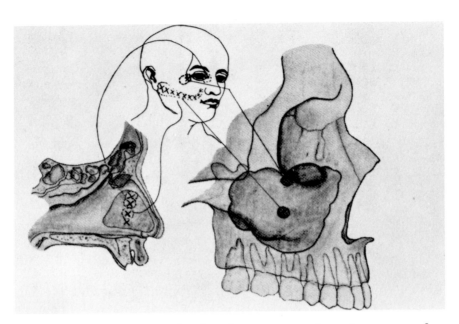

Fig. 18-2. The points stimulated on the septum are shown by crosses and on the lateral wall of the maxillary sinus by cross-hatched circles. The areas in which pain of 1 to 2 plus intensity was felt are indicated by crosses within an outline on the small head above. Note that widely separated stimuli cause pain to be felt in the same areas.

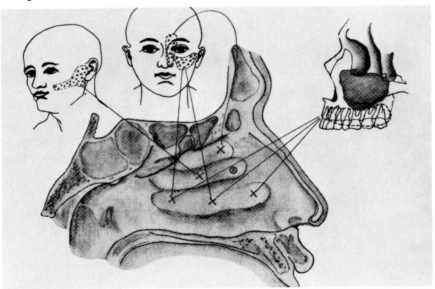

Fig. 18-3. The points stimulated on the turbinates are indicated by crosses, from which lines lead to the indicated areas in which pain of 4 to 6 plus intensity was felt.

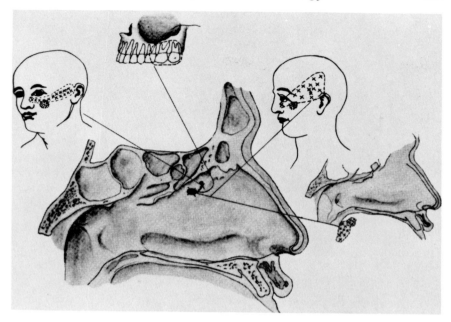

Fig. 18-4. Large crosses indicate stimulation of the ostium of the maxillary sinus. Lines lead to the areas indicated by small crosses in which pain of 6 to 9 plus intensity was felt. A dotted circle over the zygoma indicates the area of erythema and hyperalgesia that long outlasted stimulation of the ostium.

Treatment

In contrast to migraine headaches, nearly all "sinus headaches" can be relieved by aspirin or codeine, at least temporarily. Such headaches are often preventable if prevention of conditions leading to secondary infection are undertaken soon after aggravating nasal factors appear, i.e., sinus exudates and allergic mucosal obstruction.

Local treatment for reduction and ablation of sinus headaches includes hot compresses or a heating pad and careful use of nasal sprays or drops. Such use should rarely exceed four times daily for four days. Rebound phenomena of the nasal mucosa can occur rapidly with any type of local decongestant spray and become a greater problem than the original inciting cause for use. Local insertion of procaine tampons for five minutes between the two lower turbinates, the ostia, and/or nasofrontal duct quickly relieves nearly all sinus headaches temporarily. It should be understood, without saying, that cocaine should never be used, though it was a very effective treatment of such headache and nasal discomfort in a bygone era. Its only justifiable use in the nose

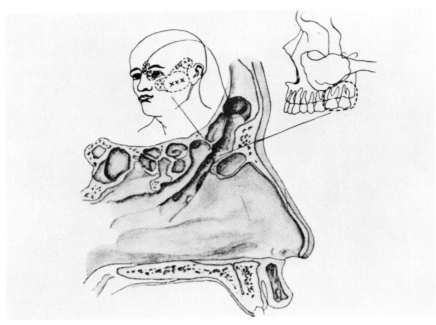

Fig. 18-5. Lines lead from the points stimulated in the nasofrontal duct to the areas in which pain of 5 to 7 plus intensity was felt. On stimulation of the inner wall of the frontal sinus minimal pain or no more than ½ plus intensity was felt only in the area indicated directly over the sinus.

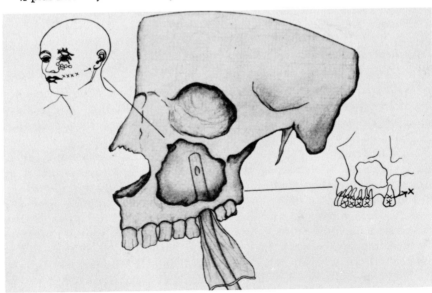

Fig. 18-6. The thin rubber balloon is shown in the maxillary sinus. The areas are indicated in which pain was felt when positive pressure was applied to the walls of the sinus for prolonged periods.

today is as a local anesthetic tampon preparatory to sinus puncture and drainage. Polyps should always be removed if they create total obstruction of the nose or sinus ostia resulting in recurrent sinusitis and if adequate control of the inciting allergic condition has been obtained i.e., desensitization or drug control.

Systemic measures used to control these headaches are the following. Analgesics of aspirin or codeine type are usually adequate for temporary pain relief. Sympathomimetics of the ephedrine or phenylpropanolamine class serve to reduce nasal congestion and edema without excessive "drying effect" on the mucosa. They are usually taken in standard tablet form and many brand names are available. Antihistamines are effective in much the same manner as sympathomimetics but often cause an uncomfortable "drying effect" upon the entire respiratory system. If severe exudation is present, as in hayfever, this is not objectionable. The almost universally present infection of nasal structures, causing the inflammation, usually requires an antibiotic for control. Choice of the antimicrobial should be made after results are obtained from a local culture. A broad spectrum agent may be started after the culture while results are awaited. Very occasionally, sinus drainage may be required.

REFERENCES

1. Barolin, G. S., and Sperlich, D.: Migraine families—a contribution to the genetic aspect of migraine. Hemicrania, 2:1, p. 15, 1970.
2. Carroll, J. D.: Migraine and oral contraception. Hemicrania, 1:4, 1970.
3. Horton, B. T.: Medicine symposium: head and face pain. Trans. Am. Acad. Ophth. Otolaryng., Sept.-Oct.: 23, 1944.
4. Kallós, P., and Kallós-Deffner, L.: Allergy and migraine. Int. Arch. Allerg., 7:367, 1955.
5. Kunkle, E. C., and Anderson, W. B.: Dual mechanisms of eye signs of headache in cluster pattern. Trans. Am. Neurol. Ass., 85:75, 1960.
6. Kunkle, E. C., Pfeiffer, J. B., Jr., Wilhoit, W. M., and Hamrick, L. W., Jr.: Recurrent brief headache in "cluster" pattern. Trans. Am. Neurol. Ass., 77:240, 1952.
7. Loveless, M.: Milk allergy: a survey of its incidence: experiments with a masked ingestion test: allergy for corn and its derivatives: experiments with a masked ingestion test for its diagnosis. J. Allerg., 21:489, 1950.
8. Pagniez, P., Vallery-Radot, P., and Nast, A.: Thérapeutique préventive de certaines migraines. Presse méd., 27:172, 1919.
9. Proetz, A. W.: Sudden allergic reactions localized in the antrum, Ann. Otol., 39:87, 1930.
10. Riley, H. A.: Migraine. Bull. Neurol. Inst., New York, 2:429, 1932.
11. Rinkel, H. J.: Considerations of allergy as factor in familial recurrent headache. J. Allerg., 4:303, 1933.

12. Smith I., Kellow, A. H., and Hanington, E.: A clinical and biochemical correlation between tyramine and migraine headache. Headache, *10*:43, 1970.
13. Tretyakova, K. A., and Fets, A. N.: Total blood serotonin concentration in patients with migraine during and between attacks. Hemicrania, *1*:4, p. 14, 1970.
14. Unger, L., and Cristol, J. L.: Allergic migraine. Ann. Allerg., *28*:3, 1970.
15. Vaughan, W. T.: Allergic migraine, JAMA, *88*:1383, 1927.
16. Vaughan, W. T.: Analysis of allergic factor in recurrent paroxysmal headaches. Trans. Ass. Am. Psycns., *49*:348, 1934.
17. Walker, V. B.: Report to the Ciba foundation conference on migraine. London, 1960.
18. Wolf, A. A., and Unger, L.: Migraine due to milk: feeding tests, Ann. Int. Med., *20*:5, p. 831, 1944.
19. Wolff, H. G.: Headache and Other Head Pain. ed. 2. p. 227. Oxford University Press, New York, 1963.

MENIERE'S DISEASE

John D. Holloman, M.D.

Meniere's disease is a syndrome of undetermined etiology consisting of hearing loss, tinnitus, and vertigo. As in other problems of unknown origin, allergy has often been suggested as a cause. It is the intent of this chapter to review certain aspects of the disease, the evidence for allergic mechanisms and other possible explanations for its occurrence.

Despite the recent progress made in other areas of otology, precise understanding and specific therapy of Meniere's disease has not been achieved. Review of the material presented at the International Symposium on Meniere's Disease in October, 1967, demonstrates how many different theories of pathogenesis and how many modes of treatment remain. This should not be surprising if it is recalled that Meniere, writing in 1861, was often unclear about the characteristics of this disorder. He did provide an improved classification for this disease, from "apoplectiform cerebral congestion" to a disorder of the labyrinth.

Allergic or immunologic mechanisms are often postulated for diseases of unknown etiology. If the autoimmune reactions can be omitted here, it is relevant to review Chapter 2 on reaginic and IgE antibody mechanisms and evaluate how strongly they support the facts known about Meniere's disease.

What is Meniere's disease and the symptom complex by which it is recognized? It is easy to understand Meniere's lack of clarity when noting the variable clinical course and long periods of dormancy which often accompany this disease. Three symptoms occur at some point in its history: (1) an early low-tone deafness, usually reversible after onset; (2) tinnitus, often accompanied by a sense of cranial fullness or pressure; and (3) vertigo, usually of the true rotational type and frequently associated with nausea and vomiting.

Many temporal bones have been removed at autopsy from patients with Meniere's disease of both long and short duration. The striking feature observed in most of these specimens is the enormous distention of the endolymphatic system with distortions, herniations, and rupture of its various anatomic portions.[3] These observations have led to the synonym for Meniere's disease of endolymphatic hydrops. However, is this engorgement of the endolymphatic spaces the cause of symptoms or simply a concurrent event? Guinea pigs and cats exhibit no behavioral changes while undergoing progressive endolymphatic hydrops after destruction of the endolymphatic sac. In addition, light microscopy has

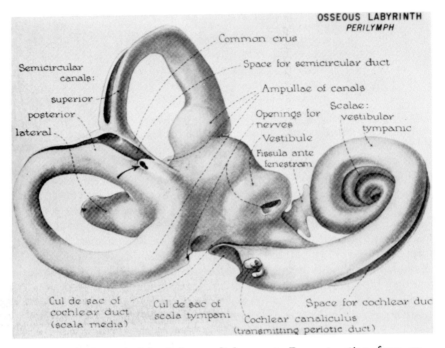

Fig. 18-7. Osseous labyrinth: medial aspect. Reconstruction from an otological series. Wisconsin Collection, series undetermined. The proximal part of the vestibular aqueduct is indicated by an arrow. The lumen of the labyrinth (for the perilymph) is modeled as a solid. The sulci represent the parts of the cochlea and the semicircular canals occupied, in the fresh state, by the cochlear duct and the semicircular ducts (compare with Fig. 18-8).

failed to demonstrate any changes in the human sense organ that could explain hearing loss. The normal anatomical structures which are being discussed are shown in Figures 18-7 and 18-8. By contrast, the microscope does reveal pathologic changes in the vestibular system which explain the vertigo. Recent evidence presented by Schuknecht from autopsy material shows rupture of the membranes of the endolymphatic system, usually of the ampullary or saccular walls.[3] This is presumably due to their great dilatation and engorgement. This allows the endolymph to cascade into the contracted perilymphatic space. Sudden rupture could lead to sudden positional change of the cupula and utricular macula thus accounting for sudden vertigo.

There are marked differences in the ionic composition of endolymph and perilymph (Fig. 18-9). Since it is commonly accepted that perilymph is the source of endolymph, obviously some structure must

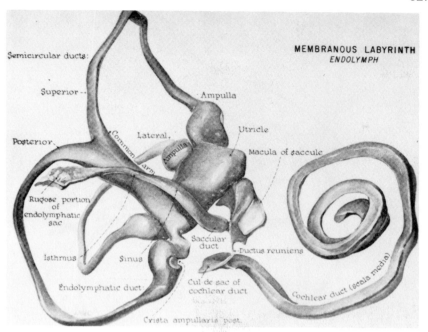

Fig. 18-8. Membranous labyrinth: medial aspect. Reconstruction from an otological series. Infant, 6 months old. Wisconsin Collection, series 121. The lumen of the duct-system (for the endolymph) is modeled as a solid. Only the proximal part of the endolymphatic sac is included in the reconstruction.

actively maintain the large sodium-potassium gradient between the two compartments. Current indications are that Reissner's membrane is important in maintaining high potassium concentration of endolymph.

The variations in ion concentration between endolymph and perilymph could explain the hearing loss in addition to the vestibular symptoms. If rupture of the endolymphatic system occurs, the entrance of high potassium content fluid into the perilymph could result in paralysis of the vestibular nerve. Such a theory has been submitted by Dohlman.[1] The release of a portion of endolymph into a markedly diminished perilymph is probably toxic to sensory function.

One thing appears certain from the pathologic observations described above. Endolymphatic hydrops or engorgement must result from either overproduction or diminished absorption of endolymph. It is reasonable to assume that by whatever process this hydrops occurs, it leads either directly or secondarily to the anatomic or chemical changes in the inner ear that result in Meniere's disease. The cause of the hydrops is unknown.

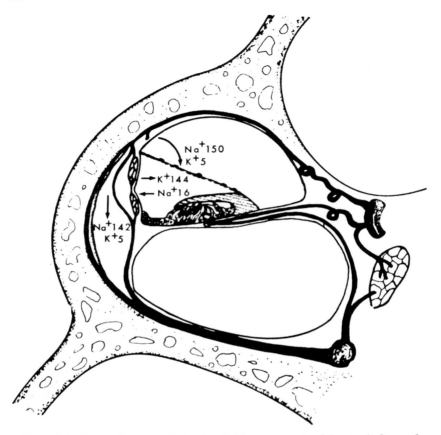

Fig. 18-9. Ion exchange within the fluids as conceived by Naftalin and Harrison. Perilymph is the source of endolymph; the ionic content of endolymph is controlled by the stria vascularis promoting the build-up of potassium. A breakdown of this mechanism could produce fluid imbalance.

Since this disease, like serous otitis, migraine headache, and several others of uncertain etiology, is often suspected to be allergic in origin, a definition of what is meant by immediate-type allergy is necessary for further consideration of the possible relationship. Allergic hypersensitivity or "atopic reactivity" involves the interaction of an external allergen or hapten with an induced antibody of special characteristics called reagin, described in detail in Chapter 2. This reaginic antibody-antigen interaction is known to release mediator substances which are capable of effects ranging from minor skin reactions to major systemic anaphylaxis. These substances in primates are histamine, slow-reacting substances, and possibly various kinins.

Our understanding of this system was advanced by Ishizaka when he demonstrated that IgE, a new class of immunoglobulin, contained most of the reaginic activity in man.[2] It now appears that all normal humans have some small amount of IgE. Allergic patients with extrinsic asthma or atopic dermatitis have a larger amount. Reaginic antibodies in these patients can be demonstrated by skin testing. Such antibodies correlate well with inhalant allergy but correlate poorly with Meniere's disease. Such facts make it difficult to support foods as an allergic cause of Meniere's symptoms. In addition, labyrinthine symptoms correlate poorly with inhalant symptoms of allergy.

Certainly people with cutaneous reactions of urticaria or angioedema to some foods like strawberries and tomatoes, will rapidly respond to ingestion but still give a negative skin test to the extract of the offending food. Such a situation can be explained in two ways. Either the reaction is not mediated by reagin or the offending polypeptide or polysaccharide antigens which are absorbed after digestion differ from those of the challenging food extracts that are used for skin testing. To consider Meniere's disease as a symptom complex of allergic origin, several problems are encountered. As yet, no study has been made of the immunoglobulins in the labyrinth or its fluids. Allergic interactions occurring outside the labyrinth but exercising pathologic effects therein have no support. The established respiratory and systemic allergic reactions either due to inhalant or food allergens do not produce symptoms of Meniere's disease. For example, clearly defined inhalant allergic rhinitis and asthma or cutaneous and anaphylactic reactions to ingested foods are not associated with Meniere's disease.

Statements supporting an allergic hypothesis for this disease are tenuous. Anecdotes relating the occurrence of labyrinthine symptoms with recurrent ingestion of specific foods or inhaled dusts and molds are reported. Withdrawal of the specific ingestants or inhalants, or desensitization to them, is then reported as alleviating the attacks. Carefully controlled studies of such cases are not available. Cautious physicians who deal with food factors relating to the many parameters of health are aware of the extreme suggestibility of many people regarding dietary influence upon daily subjective state. Only a double blind study could resolve such an argument, and that is practically impossible with food. Controlled reintroduction of a suspect food in an alleged susceptible patient may help provide information, but caution is still advisable. Iatrogenic enthusiasm is probably more effective in symptom relief than iatrogenic food restriction.

Of interest are the similarities shared by both Meniere's disease and migraine headache. Both are episodic and run similar courses of exacerbation and remission. They have a similar variety of apparent triggering factors, often centering on the same foods. There may be some true relation to food in these diseases in which foods appear related to symptoms. This could be a form of idiosyncrasy or metareaction as it is more recently called. This form of biologic reaction has long been known and described in pharmacologic textbooks. It is not an immunologic but rather a pharmacologic reaction. Atropine hyperreactivity in susceptible individuals is an example. It is more logical to explain some of the food related symptoms of migraine and Meniere's disease on this basis than on an immunologic one, though even the pharmacologic one is probably seldom involved.

Endocrine dysfunctions and their relation to Meniere's disease should be noted. Most commonly discussed are the hypothyroid and hypoadrenal states. Close investigation of such literature often reveals a diagnosis based on clinical impression rather than on cases with definitive laboratory diagnosis. Administration of hormones have not altered the disease state in most cases.

The direction of the most hopeful outlook for better understanding and treatment of this disease may be the studies involving factors influencing shifts of ions and possibly larger molecules across the various membranes and compartments of the labyrinth. Active and passive transport and metabolic factors involved are only beginning to be understood. It is possible that the labyrinthine membranes share metabolic characteristics in common with kidney tubules. Perhaps some of the same investigative techniques utilized in nephrology can be utilized for Meniere's disease.

Current methods of treatment can be reviewed briefly. The material presented in this chapter should make it obvious that whether the treatment is medical, surgical, or both, it will remain controversial. More distressing are the reports on both medical and surgical therapy which reveal about the same results in relieving vertigo.

The surgically destructive procedures of the inner ear all relieve vertigo but also result in total hearing loss of the involved ear. This requires careful preoperative consideration in a disease with a marked propensity to become bilateral. The newest surgical method of repetitive sacculotomy and cryosurgery of the horizontal canal appears encouraging but needs long-term evaluation. Vertigo remitted while hearing was maintained in a majority of patients.

Medical therapy should be centered upon a sodium restriction program and long term diuretics. Hormone replacement, vitamins, or the restriction of foods other than those high in sodium content have no potential usefulness in therapy.

REFERENCES

1. Dohlman, G.: The mechanism of secretion and absorption of endolymph in the vestibular apparatus. Acta Otolaryng., 59:275, 1965.
2. Ishizaka, K. and Ishizaka, T.: Identification of IgE antibodies as a carrier of reaginic activity. J. Immun., 99:1187, 1967.
3. Schuknecht, H. F.: Correlation of pathology with symptoms of Meniere's disease. *In* Otolaryngologic Clinics of North America, Symposium on Meniere's Disease. Philadelphia, pp. 433-440. W. B. Saunders, 1968.

HYPERSENSITIVITY PNEUMONITIS

Jordan N. Fink, M.D.

Most of the hypersensitivity diseases in man involving the respiratory tract take the form of asthma or rhinitis, and are largely due to the release of pharmacologic mediators by the antigen-antibody reaction. The antibody participating in this reaction is most likely IgE and is fixed to specifically reactive cells. Recent evidence, however, has indicated that allergic respiratory reactions may take forms other than those mentioned above, and that additional immunologic processes (possibly involving precipitating antibody, circulating antigen-antibody complexes, or even cellular mechanisms, as found in delayed hypersensitivity) may play a role. Although asthma and rhinitis occur most often in individuals with atopic backgrounds, the diseases to be discussed in this section can be seen in both atopic and nonatopic patients. The disorders may be grouped under the general term of hypersensitivity pneumonitis, although they are sometimes referred to as extrinsic allergic alveolitis. These diseases occur as a reaction to the inhalation of a variety of organic dusts and may present in several clinical forms, probably depending on the immunologic responsiveness and intensity of exposure of the patient to the offending dust.

ETIOLOGY

Almost any inhaled organic dust can cause sensitization and the subsequent development of a hypersensitivity pneumonitis; a list of antigenic materials associated with these disorders is shown in Table 18-1. The sizes of all of these inhaled particles are not known, but they must be no larger than 3 to 5 micra to reach the terminal airway passages where the lesions seem to be initiated. The dusts may be derived from animal proteins as in pigeon breeders' disease where the inhaled proteins are contained in dried avian droppings. In pituitary snuff taker's disease, the offending material is the pituitary powder containing bovine or porcine proteins. The inhalation of vegetable dusts contaminated with fungi also cause hypersensitivity reactions such as farmer's lung, bagassosis, and mushroom picker's disease. In these disorders, the inhaled dusts from the moldy vegetation are contaminated with thermophilic actinomycetes such as *Micropolyspora faeni* or *Thermoactinomycetes vulgaris,* which have been shown to cause sensitization and subsequent disease. These organisms are ubiquitous in nature and grow best at temperatures of 45° to 60°C; such temperatures commonly occur in decomposing hay, and sugar cane or mushroom compost. The spores are less than 1 micron in size and thus are able to reach the terminal airways where they can evoke an immunologic reaction without invading the tissue. Recently, thermophilic actinomycetes have also been shown to contaminate heating or air conditioning systems of commercial or residential buildings, and certain individuals living or working in those environments developed a hypersensitivity pneumonitis.[2, 9, 12, 17]

The inhalation of other than thermophilic fungi may also result in a hypersensitivity pneumonitis. This has been described in workers removing the bark from maple logs and inhaling the spores of *Cryptostroma corticale,* in woodworkers exposed to redwood dust which contains *Graphium sp.* of mold, in individuals working in cheese factories in which *Penicillium caseii* spores may be inhaled, and in brewers working in malt factories where spores of *Aspergillus clavatus* may be present. Recent evidence further suggests that a similar pneumonitis may occur in workers exposed to the enzyme of *Bacillus subtilis* used in detergent manufacturing. It is likely that the list of inhaled organic dusts resulting in a hypersensitivity pneumonitis will grow as exposure to new antigens increases.

TABLE 18-1
Sensitivity Materials in the Hypersensitivity Pneumonitides

ETIOLOGY	DISEASE ENTITY	ANTIGENIC MATERIAL INHALED	ANTIGEN
Induced by serum proteins	Bird breeder's lung Pituitary snuff taker's lung	Avian dust Pituitary powder	Avian proteins Bovine or porcine proteins
Induced by micro-organisms	Farmer's lung Bagassosis Mushroom picker's lung Pneumonitis due to contaminated air conditioner or heating system	Moldy hay Moldy sugar cane Mushroom compost Dust from furnace or air conditioner	*Micropolyspora faeni* or *Thermoactinomycetes vulgaris* *Micropolyspora sp.*
	Maple bark disease	Moldy maple bark	*Cryptostroma corticale*
	Sequoiosis Suberosis Cheese washer's lung Paprika splitter's lung Malt worker's lung	Redwood dust Mold cork dust Cheese particles Paprika dust Malt dust	*Graphium sp.* Moldy cork dust *Penicillium caseii* *Mucor stolonifer* *Aspergillus clavatus*
Probably similar disease	Smallpox handler's lung Enzyme worker's lung	Smallpox scab dust Enzyme dust	? *Bacillus subtilis*

Certainly other factors, in addition to the presence of an organic dust in the environment, must play a role in the development of a hypersensitivity pneumonitis in the exposed individual. The frequency and extent of exposure and the immunologic reactivity of the host will most likely influence the response to the dust, as should other factors such as ciliary transport mechanisms and alveolar phagocytosis.

CLINICAL FEATURES

The clinical manifestations of these respiratory disorders may present in a number of forms depending upon the immunologic response to the inhaled antigen, the antigenicity of the dust, and the frequency and intensity of exposure. In general, the manifestations of these illnesses are similar regardless of the organic dust inhaled, and the hypersensitivity pneumonitides may be considered as a syndrome with a spectrum of clinical features, even though each specific disease may be due to a different organic dust. The atopic individual may demonstrate typical bronchospasm or rhinorrhea immediately following inhalation of the dust, and this reaction may be followed hours later by the clinical features of a hypersensitivity pneumonitis. The nonatopic patient, on the other hand, will respond only with the late type reaction characteristic of these disorders.

The Acute Form

Probably the most common and most easily recognized form of a hypersensitivity pneumonitis follows intermittent exposure to a specific organic dust. Within 4 to 6 hours of exposure the sensitized patient develops respiratory and systemic symptoms of cough, dyspnea, fever, chills, myalgia and malaise resembling a systemic viral or bacterial infection. These symptoms may persist for 8 to 12 hours, but the patient recovers spontaneously only to experience a recurrence of symptoms with reexposure. Numerous attacks may be associated with weight loss and anorexia. Between the acute attacks the individual often feels quite normal. Clinical examination of the patient during an attack reveals an acutely ill, dyspneic patient with prominent bibasilar, moist rales. Although the patient appears to recover within a few hours, the rales may persist for a few days.

During the attack, laboratory studies usually demonstrate a leukocytosis with the white count as high as 25,000. Eosinophilia is unusual but may be as high as 10 percent. Often, levels of the immunoglobulin IgG are elevated, but in some patients all of the major immunoglobulin classes are increased.

Pulmonary function studies done during the asymptomatic period of the acute form of a hypersensitivity pneumonitis are usually normal. However, measurable changes occur 4 to 6 hours after exposure to the offending antigen. There is reduction in vital capacity, decrease in gas transfer across the alveolar wall, as measured by diffusing capacity, and decreased pulmonary compliance. Some patients also demonstrate decreased expiratory flow rates and one second forced vital capacity indicating airway obstruction. Chest x-rays may show fine nodular densities and peripheral infiltrations suggestive of interstitial as well as alveolar involvement (Fig. 18-10). With avoidance of exposure to the offending materials or therapy with corticosteroids, all symptoms disappear, and abnormal laboratory tests return to normal. Continued intermittent exposure to the offending organic dust, however, may lead to more permanent pulmonary function and x-ray abnormalities associated with progressive respiratory insufficiency.

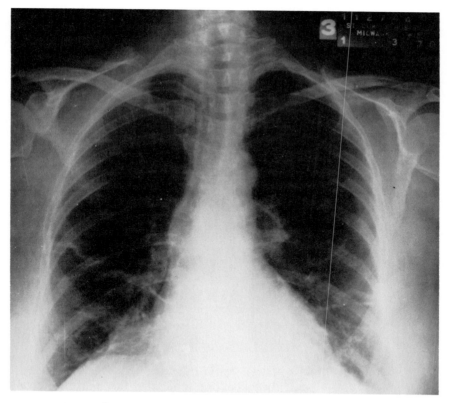

Fig. 18-10. Chest x-ray of patient with a hypersensitivity pneumonitis due to the inhalation of thermophilic actinomycetes contaminating her furnace humidifier.

Subacute Form

Some individuals have a more insidious type of disease with rare acute attacks. These individuals are usually exposed to small amounts of antigen over long periods of time (for example, lovebird or parakeet fanciers). The symptoms resemble those of a progressive bronchitis with dyspnea, chronic productive cough with scanty sputum, anorexia, fatigue and weight loss. Laboratory studies usually demonstrate pulmonary function abnormalities of progressive restriction, diffusion defect, and increased stiffness of the lung. Chest x-rays may show fibrosis or in some cases may be normal. These patients are often diagnosed as having chronic bronchitis, idiopathic pulmonary fibrosis, Hamman-Rich syndrome, or recurrent episodes of influenza. Although the clinical and laboratory abnormalities respond to corticosteroids or prolonged avoidance of exposure to the offending dust, the response is much less prompt than in the acute form. If fibrosis is present, the pulmonary function abnormalities may be irreversible.

Chronic Form

In some cases of the hypersensitivity pneumonitides, chronic irreversible lung damage may occur. This may take the form of irreversible fibrosis and pulmonary insufficiency and is seen in long standing cases of farmer's lung and in individuals keeping parakeets, budgerigars or lovebirds. These individuals may develop irreversible pulmonary function abnormalities of restriction, diffusion defects and "stiff" lungs which do not respond to corticosteroids. Lung biopsies from these patients have demonstrated interstitial fibrosis with granulomas, as well as thickening of alveolar walls.

In a few patients with farmer's lung, pigeon breeders' disease or bagassosis, pulmonary function tests have shown persistently marked elevation of the residual volume, diminished flow rates, and loss of pulmonary elasticity, suggestive of emphysema. Histologic examination of these lungs has revealed obstructive bronchiolitis with distal destruction of alveoli. Such patients do not usually respond to corticosteroids or avoidance of exposure, even if this is pursued for prolonged periods.

IMMUNOLOGIC FEATURES

The characteristic immunologic feature of these disorders is the presence of precipitins against the offending antigen in the sera of affected individuals (Fig. 18-1). These antibodies may usually be demonstrated by gel diffusion techniques using the patient's serum and the suspected antigen. Immunoelectrophoresis has shown these antibodies to be of the IgG class. A few patients have low titers of precipitins, and it may be necessary to concentrate their serum to detect the antibodies, but relatively high titers of these antibodies have been seen in the sera of most symptomatic patients studied. A significant percentage of asymptomatic individuals exposed to the same antigen may also have precipitins, but of lesser titer. Thus, the finding of precipitins must be considered in the light of the clinical history when the diagnosis is considered.

Skin tests with suspected thermophile antigens have been shown to be unreliable because of nonspecific-irritation type reactions. In the disorders due to inhalation of serum proteins such as pigeon breeders' disease, however, skin tests may be of value. Both immediate wheal and flare and late (4 to 6 hour) skin reactions may be observed. The immediate reactions are the same type as seen with the common inhalant allergens, but the late reactions resemble the Arthus phenomenon indicative of a vasculitis due to a precipitin-antigen reaction. The late reaction begins with variable edema and erythema of the injected area; it can progress to central necrosis, but it usually subsides in 24 hours unless necrosis has occurred. Histologic examination of biopsies of such skin reactions have demonstrated lesions consistent with Arthus reactions with a vasculitis consisting of polymorphonuclear and plasma cell infiltration of the area. This type of late reaction may also be occurring in the lung after antigen inhalation, but as yet there is no clear evidence to prove that precipitating antibody participates in the genesis of hypersensitivity pneumonitides.

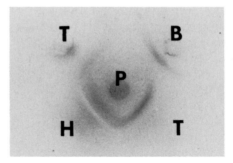

Fig. 18-11. Immunodiffusion studies of serum of patient (P) in Fig. 18-10 against thermophilic antigens (T) bagasse (B), and moldy hay (H).

X-RAY FEATURES

The hypersensitivity pneumonitides cannot be distinguished radiographically from other nonimmunologic interstitial disorders. Roetgeno-

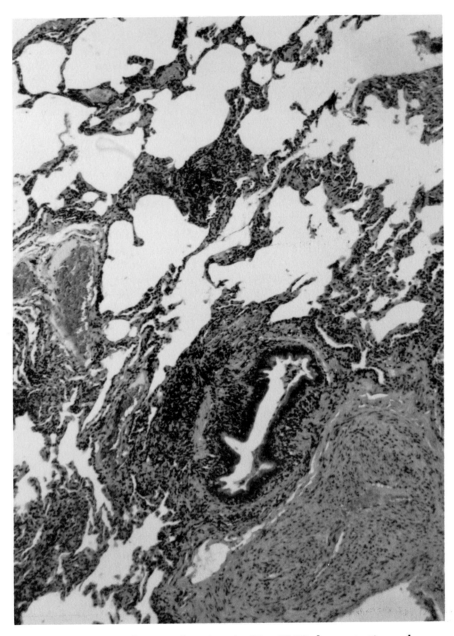

Fig. 18-12. Lung biopsy of patient in Fig. 18-10 demonstrating a lymphocytic interstitial pneumonitis with early granuloma formation. ×250

grams may be normal or may show recurrent interstitial nodular infiltrations, or fibrotic changes, depending on the stage of the disease.

PATHOLOGIC FEATURES

The histologic features of the lung in the hypersensitivity disorders
depend upon the stage of the disease at the time of biopsy (Fig. 18-12).
In early stages of farmer's lung, bagassosis, mushroom picker's disease,
and some of the hypersensitivity pneumonitides due to other than
thermophilic fungi, the alveolar walls are infiltrated mainly with lymphocytes. Plasma cells and histocytes containing foamy cytoplasm may also
be seen within the alveolar spaces. Later, the interstitium becomes
infiltrated with mononuclear cells and scattered giant cell granulomata.
In still later stages, fibrosis of these areas occurs and an organizing
bronchiolitis obliterans may be seen.

In biopsied cases of pigeon breeders' disease, similar interstitial and
alveolar granulomatous and infiltrative changes may be found. In addition, foamy macrophages, possibly derived from alveolar macrophages,
may be found in the interstitial areas as well as within the alveoli.
The interstitial position of these foam cells may be unique for pigeon
breeders' disease, as this feature has not been described in the other
hypersensitivity pneumonitides.

Bronchiolitis obliterans can be observed with peripheral destruction
of alveloi in some chronic cases of farmer's lung, bagassosis or pigeon
breeders' disease. The interstitial and intra-alveolar infiltrate in these
cases is less distinctive, and the foam laden macrophages are less frequent than in the other forms of the disorder.

DIFFERENTIAL DIAGNOSIS

The diagnosis of a typical case of a hypersensitivity pneumonitis can
usually be made by the evaluation of the environmental history, appropriate laboratory and serologic studies, and a trial of avoidance and
reexposure where possible. The more insidious and progressive forms of
a hypersensitivity pneumonitis may be difficult to diagnose. Chest x-ray
and pulmonary function abnormalities of other interstitial pulmonary
disorders such as chronic eosinophilic pneumonia, the collagen-vascular
diseases, lymphogenous spread of carcinoma, desquamative interstitial
pneumonia, and sarcoid may be similar. The finding of extrapulmonary
involvement (such as generalized lymphadenopathy or abdominal or-
ganomegaly) probably rules out a hypersensitivity pneumonitis. At
times, however, a lung biopsy may be necessary to make a definitive
diagnosis. Biopsy may also be necessary to differentiate these disorders
from the diffuse idiopathic pulmonary fibrosis known as the Hamman-

Rich syndrome, which clinically resembles the fibrotic stage of the hypersensitivity pneumonitides.

Controlled Exposure to Antigens

On occasion the patient may be cautiously exposed to the suspected antigen and his reaction carefully observed. This may be done during an asymptomatic period by allowing the farmer to enter his barn or the pigeon breeder to enter his coop. The patient should then be brought to the hospital and observed frequently over the next 8 hours for symptoms or signs of a hypersensitivity pneumonitis.

Some reactions may be diagnosed by careful inhalation exposure to nonirritating sterile extracts of the suspected antigen, athough less desirable than observation after natural exposure. With dilute extracts, previously shown not to induce any changes in normal individuals, minimal abnormalities in pulmonary function tests or a rise in temperature of a few degrees 4 to 6 hours after exposure may clarify the diagnosis. Corticosteroids should be available for use in these cases to abort severe attacks inadvertently induced.

PATHOPHYSIOLOGY

The mechanisms responsible for the development of a hypersensitivity pneumonitis have not yet been clarified. The precipitating antibody so characteristic of this group of diseases may be a result of exposure to antigen rather than the cause of the disease. The Arthus reaction or vasculitis characteristic of precipitating antibody-antigen complexes is absent in lung biopsies examined until now. However, the Arthus reaction has been described as an acute immunologic reaction. The result of a chronic Arthus reaction on the lung parenchyma, that is, prolonged deposition of complexes, utilization of complement, chemotaxis of polymorphonoclear cells and release of lysosomal enzymes is not known.

The lesions of the hypersensitivity pneumonitides are more consistent with a delayed or tuberculin type of reaction. Such lesions, however, have been described by Germuth in the lungs of rabbits following injection of antigen at doses equivalent to antibody. It is thus apparent that further studies will be necessary before the immunologic sequences involved in the production of lesions is known; perhaps several different mechanisms will be found to play a role in the etiology of these diseases.

THERAPY

As in all other allergic disorders, the prime mode of therapy should be avoidance of the offending antigen once it is known. Since many of these disorders are occupational, the use of masks with filters capable of removing the antigen, appropriate ventilation of working areas, or even changing of occupations may be necessary.

Drug therapy may be needed in the acute or subacute forms of these disorders when avoidance cannot be carried out immediately. Although antihistamines or bronchodilators have no effect on the symptom pattern, the patients usually respond to the administration of corticosteroids. Moderate doses of these drugs may be necessary for prolonged periods, along with avoidance, to determine if reversibility of the clinical abnormalities is possible. Hyposensitization should be avoided, since toxic immune complexes may be formed when the injected antigen combines with the precipitating IgG and systemic vasculitis or serum sickness may result.

REFERENCES

1. Avila, R., and Villar, T. G.: Suberosis. Respiratory disease in cork workers. Lancet, *1*:620, 1968.
2. Banaszak, E. F.; Thiede, W. H., and Fink, J. N.: Hypersensitivity pneumonitis due to contamination of an air-conditioner. New Eng. J. Med., *283*:271, 1970.
3. Barboriak, J. J.; Sosman, A. J., and Reed, C. E.: Serologic studies in pigeon breeders' disease. J. Lab. Clin. Med., *65*:600, 1965.
4. Bringhurst, L. S., Byrne, R. N., and Gershon-Cohen, J.: Respiratory disease of mushroom workers. J.A.M.A., *171*:15, 1959.
5. Buechner, H. A., Prevatt, A. L., Thompson, J., and Butz, O.: Bagassosis —a review with further historical data, studies of pulmonary function and results of adrenal steroid therapy. Amer. J. Med., *25*:234, 1958.
6. Campbell, J. M.: Acute symptoms following work with hay. Brit. Med. J., *2*:1143, 1932.
7. Cohen, H. I., Merigan, T. C., Kosek J. C., and Eldridge, F.: A granulomatous pneumonitis associated with redwood sawdust inhalation. Amer. J. Med., *43*:785, 1967.
8. Cross, T., Maciver, A. M., and Cacey, J.: The thermophilic actinomycetes in moldy hay. J. Gen. Microbiol., *50*:351, 1968.
9. Dickie, H. A., and Rankin, J.: Farmer's lung: an acute granulomatous interstitial pneumonitis occurring in agricultural workers. J.A.M.A., *167*:1069, 1958.
10. Emanuel, D. A., Wenzel, F. J., Bowerman, C. I., and Lawton, B. R.: Farmer's lung. Clinical pathologic and immunologic study of twenty-four patients. Amer. J. Med., 37:392, 1964.
11. Emanuel, D. A., Wenzel, F. J., and Lawton, B. R.: Pneumonitis due to *Cryptostroma corticale* (maple-bark diesase). New Eng. J. Med., *274*:1413, 1966.
12. Fink, J. N., Sosman, A. J., Barboriak, J. J., Schlueter, D. P., and Holmes,

R. A.: Pigeon breeders' disease. A clinical study of a hypersensitivity pneumonitis. Ann. Intern. Med., *68:*1205, 1968.

13. Fink, J. N., Banaszak, E. F., Thiede, W. M., and Barboriak, J. J.: Interstitial pneumonitis due to hypersensitivity to an organism contaminating a heating system. Ann. Intern. Med., *74:*80, 1971.

14. Flindt, M. L. H.: Pulmonary disease due to inhalation of Bacillus subtilis containing proteolytic enzyme. Lancet, *1:*1177, 1969.

15. Hargreave, F. E., Pepys, J., Longbottom, J. L., and Wraith, D. G.: Bird breeder's (farmer's) lung. Lancet, *1:*44, 1966.

16. Norris-Evans, W. H., and Foreman, W. H.: Smallpox handler's lung. Proc. Roy. Soc. Med., *56:*274, 1963.

17. Pepys, J., Longbottom, J. L., and Jenkins, P. A.: Vegetable dust pneumoconiosies. Immunological responses to vegetable dusta and their flora. Amer. Rev. Resp. Dis., *89:*842, 1964.

18. Pepys, J., Jenkins, P. A., Lachmann, P. J., and Mahon, W. E.: An iatrogenic auto-antibody: Immunological responses to pituitary snuff in patients with diabetes insipidus. Clin. Exp. Immun., *1:*377, 1966.

19. Pepys, J.: Hypersensitivity disease of the lungs due to fungi and other organic dusts. *In:* Monographs in Allergy. No. 4. Basle, S. Karger, 1969.

20. Rankin, J., Kobayashi, M., Barbee, R. A., and Dickie, M. A.: Pulmonary granulomatoses due to inhaled organic antigens. Med. Clin. N. Amer., *51:*459, 1967.

21. Reed, C. E., Sosman, A., and Barbee, R. A.: Pigeon breeders' lung. J.A.M.A., *193:*261, 1965.

22. Riddle, H. F. V., and Grant, I. W. B.: Allergic alveolitis in a malt worker. Thorax, *23:*271, 1968.

23. Salvaggio, J. E., Buechner, H. A., Seabury, J. H., and Arquembourg, P.: Bagassosis I. Precipitins against extracts of crude bagasse in the serum of patients with bagassosis. Ann. Intern. Med., *64:*748, 1966.

ALLERGIC BRONCHOPULMONARY ASPERGILLOSIS

Raymond G. Slavin, M.D.

Pulmonary disease due to circulating antibody is prominent among immunologic diseases. We have previously referred to Type 1, IgE mediated bronchial asthma (see Chap. 7) and Type 3, Arthus, precipitating antibody mediated pulmonary hypersensitivity (see Chap. 18). We will now deal with a disease, allergic bronchopulmonary aspergillosis, in the pathogenesis of which both nonprecipitating reaginic antibody and precipitating antibody are probably involved.

Pulmonary aspergillosis has been recognized for many years in several different forms. In one form there is actual invasion of the tissues with resultant bronchitis, pneumonia and possible systemic spread. This form is seen most often in patients whose resistance is compromised either by severe underlying disease or by the use of antibiotics, marrow depressing drugs or immunosuppressive agents. In a second and more common form, local growth of the organism occurs without invasion of tissues. This is the familiar aspergilloma, or fungus ball, and occurs as a secondary complication of an anatomical abnormality such as a cavity or cyst. The third type of pulmonary disease due to *Aspergillus* was first described in 1952[3] and was designated allergic bronchopulmonary aspergillosis. The essential features of this syndrome are episodes of wheezing with low grade fever, expectoration of characteristic brown plugs, transient pulmonary infiltrates, and eosinophilia of the blood and sputum. Since the initial description, reporters from England[1,5] and the United States[4,6] have associated allergic aspergillosis with positive immediate wheal and erythema skin reactions and with precipitins to aspergillus extracts.

There are compelling reasons for devoting special attention to this disease. First is the fact that allergic aspergillosis is being recognized more frequently. In addition, other related organisms such as helminthosporium, alternaria or candida may cause a similar clinical picture. Second, by a separate discussion of this disease, we emphasize the importance of broadening the physician's knowledge of antibody mediated pulmonary disease beyond simple IgE mediated bronchial asthma. Finally, by the proper recognition of the disease, appropriate therapeutic measures can be taken which may prevent the development of bronchiectasis and pulmonary insufficiency. There is little question that many instances of allergic aspergillosis have been identified erroneously as the "PIE" syndrome (pulmonary infiltrates and eosinophilia) or Löeffler's pneumonia. Detecting the cause of these entities is necessary for proper therapy and a satisfactory clinical result.

CLINICAL AND LABORATORY CHARACTERISTICS

The vast majority of patients with allergic aspergillosis are atopic and have a past history of bronchial asthma. Wheezing and low grade fever are uniform. The patient frequently notes the production of golden-brown mucous plugs. Occasionally there is a clear-cut history of exposure to a heavy concentration of fungi as in a compost pile.

Serial chest x-rays are necessary to appreciate the transient and migratory pulmonary infiltrates. Mucus plug impaction with subsequent collapse of a lobe is a common finding. The bronchiectasis which so often follows allergic aspergillosis is quite characteristic. The involvement is of the proximal part of the bronchial tree rather than the distal part. Thus, one will see a localized saccular type of bronchiectasis at the site of a previous segmental pulmonary infiltrate, with normal peripheral filling. The nature of the dilatation suggests a direct local toxic action resulting from the presence of the fungus.

Eosinophilia of blood and sputum is always seen, the range in the peripheral blood being from 10 to 50 percent. Sputum culture will generally be positive for *Aspergillus.* Although the species most often identified is *fumigatus,* others such as *niger, flavus, nidulens, terreus* and *clavatus* are sometimes seen. *Aspergillus fumigatus* is ubiquitous and has been identified in many diverse sources. Because it is pervasive in air samples, the fungus is probably inhaled and expectorated by a large part of the population. Since it is a common contaminant of sputum and may be present at times in the respiratory tract without harmful effects, the mere culture of A. *fumigatus* from sputum cannot by itself be taken as proof that it is the cause of clinical manifestations. The presence of well-preserved mycelia is much better evidence of active disease. Careful examination of the previously mentioned mucus plug will usually reveal numerous eosinophils and septate hyphae imbedded in mucus and fibrin debris. The demonstration of intact cytoplasm in the mycelia indicates viability and growth rather than mere contamination. The mycelia found in association with aspergilloma are empty and appear dead.

Lung biopsy shows chronic interstitial granulomatous pneumonitis with many eosinophils and giant cells. The pulmonary function abnormality is predominantly airway obstruction. Because the involvement is largely peribronchial without involvement of the alveoli, one does not find signs of restrictive lung disease such as decreased compliance or impairment of gas exchange.

IMMUNOLOGIC FEATURES

The presence of skin sensitizing antibody to Aspergillus is manifested by the development of a positive immediate wheal and erythema reaction to an aspergillus skin test and is an essential finding in allergic aspergillosis. The antibody appears to be a typical IgE reaginic antibody and can be passively transferred to the skin of man and monkey and systemically to the monkey.[7]

In most patients a "dual" skin test reaction is seen. Several hours after the complete abatement of the wheal and erythema reaction, edema and erythema begin at the skin test site, reaching a peak at 24 hours and subsiding completely by 48 hours. Biopsy of the late skin reaction site shows a picture compatible with an Arthus reaction.

Precipitating antibody, generally of the IgG class, directed against aspergillus antigen is found in most cases of allergic aspergillosis. The precise role of the precipitating antibody to Aspergillus in the pathogenesis of allergic aspergillosis has been somewhat controversial. It has been pointed out that over 90 percent of patients with aspergilloma have precipitating antibody to Aspergillus and yet they do not develop wheezing, pulmonary infiltrates or eosinophilia. The combination of the allergic skin sensitizing antibody and the precipitating antibody would seem to be necessary for the complete picture of allergic aspergillosis. The recent demonstration of the successful serum transfer of pulmonary lesions from man to monkey lends credence to the importance of precipitating antibody in the pathogenesis of the disease.[2] Passive transfer of serum from a patient with allergic aspergillosis to a monkey followed by aerosol challenge with aspergillus antigen resulted in the development of pulmonary lesions in the monkey consistent with the human donor's illness. Transfer of serum containing only skin sensitizing antibody caused no pulmonary lesions.

TREATMENT

Corticosteroids have been shown to dramatically decrease the pulmonary infiltrates of allergic aspergillosis and have been used in this disease to lessen the allergic reaction and reduce airway obstruction to enable more rapid expectoration of remaining antigen. The best results have been seen when the course of corticosteroid therapy was continued over a two- to three-month period. When exacerbations result or if the response to corticosteroids is not satisfactory, one might consider aerosolization of amphotericin B, if the organism is sensitive to the drug.[7] Hyposensitization with aqueous extracts of Aspergillus is not recommended because of the adverse local and systemic effects.

CONCLUSION

It appears that a low index of suspicion and errors of omission account for the paucity of reports of allergic aspergillosis in the United States. Septate hyphae may be missed on the sputum smear, transient pulmonary infiltrates may not be appreciated or skin-sensitizing and precipitating antibodies may not be investigated. With the proper appreciation of the clinical and laboratory characteristics of this disease, it and related conditions may be recognized sooner and proper therapy instituted at the earliest possible time.

REFERENCES

1. Campbell, J., and Clayton, Y. M.: Bronchopulmonary aspergillosis: a correlation of the clinical and laboratory findings in 272 patients investigated for bronchopulmonary aspergillosis. Amer. Rev. Resp. Dis., 89:186, 1964.
2. Golbert, T. M., and Patterson, R.: Pulmonary allergic aspergillosis. Ann. Intern. Med., 72:395, 1970.
3. Hinson, K. F. W., Moon, A. J., and Plummer, N. S.: Bronchopulmonary aspergillosis: a review and a report of 8 new cases. Thorax, 73:317, 1952.
4. Patterson, R., and Golbert, T. M.: Hypersensitivity disease of the lung. Univ. Mich. Med. Cent. J., 34:8, 1968.
5. Pepys, J., Riddel, R. W. Citron, K. M., Clayton, Y. M., and Short, E. I.: Clinical and immunologic significance of aspergillus fumigatus in sputum. Amer. Rev. Resp. Dis., 80:167, 1959.
6. Slavin, R. G., Stanczyk, D. J., Lonigro, A. J., and Broun, G. O., Sr.: Allergic bronchopulmonary aspergillosis—a North American rarity. Amer. J. Med., 47:306, 1969.
7. Slavin, R. G., Million, L., and Cherry, J.: Allergic bronchopulmonary aspergillosis: characterization of antibodies and results of treatment. J. Allerg., 46:150, 1970.

PSYCHIATRIC ASPECTS OF ALLERGIC DISEASES

Thomas M. Golbert, M.D., Roy Patterson, M.D., and
Raymond G. Slavin, M.D.

The diseases described in this book are considered to be within the broad category of allergic problems. Many have definite evidence that they are IgE mediated. The others have clinical manifestations similar to the IgE (immediate type, reaginic)-mediated diseases. All of these diseases, except anaphylaxis, have been classified by some physicians as primarily the result of psychiatric factors.

The approach to the etiology and management of these diseases, as described in this book by a variety of authors, is based on the premise that they are not primarily psychiatric in origin. This section reviews certain opinions which have stressed psychogenesis of the allergic diseases. These previous theories are refuted, and the role of psychiatric factors in allergic diseases is presented from the viewpoint of physicians who constantly treat patients having these clinical problems.

PREVIOUS THEORIES

Some authors have considered all of the allergic diseases to be of psychosomatic etiology.[21] Most psychological and psychiatric studies of allergic diseases have attempted to establish a psychosomatic etiology for asthma. Other studies have implied psychogenesis for urticaria, eczema, and allergic rhinitis. Vasomotor rhinitis is a nonimmunologically mediated disease having clinical characteristics similar to reagin (IgE)-mediated perennial allergic rhinitis. Vasomotor rhinitis is considered a psychosomatic disorder by some.[29]

Urticaria

Urticaria has been related, by previous theories, to repressed weeping; the allergic and psychological states of frustrated longing for dependent passive love complement each other.[18] Champion et al.[6] reviewed 554 consecutive cases of chronic urticaria and angioedema. They concluded that psychological factors were contributory in 25.4 percent but were never the sole cause. The cause was determined in 79 percent. The authors indicated that acute urticaria is mainly reagin (IgE)-mediated disease.

547

Eczema

Numerous psychological factors and personality traits have been related to eczema. These include suppression of anger, repressed hostility toward members of the famiy, exquisite sensitivity, above average intelligence, emotional immaturity, cutaneous erotization, sexual difficulties with self-punishing inclinations, and feelings of inadequacy, inferiority, and lack of self-confidence. Separation anxiety may become a matrix for the symptoms. Separation may involve approval, status, or love. These patients are said to react with unexpressed rage followed by guilt. The erotization of the skin was considered to be a diffuse sexual immaturity by which these patients "seek the maternal care and close contact given them in infancy." [16]

Family interaction with the eczematous patient has been considered. The mother may perceive the rash as a blemish which reflects upon her care. She may generate anxiety, anger, hostility, and shame. The patient may use the rash to serve his own emotional needs. Scratching the skin could be used to keep the mother close and involved, as a means of expressing hostile and aggressive needs of the patient, or as a method of controlling or punishing himself or the mother.[11, 27] These reactions occur at a subconscious level.[27]

Parents of some eczematous *infants* are said to be emotionally distant from each other and from the infant. They apparently fear damaging their infants, and the rash is perceived as evidence of the child's defect. Feelings of guilt and revulsion are aroused.[11]

Parents of eczematous *preschool children* may tend to overstimulate and overmanipulate the child's skin. This is suggested to be a covert expression of hostility to the child or an attempt to receive and give erotic gratification. Finally, the parents have been characterized as having a need to inhibit their children's assertiveness and to infantilize them.[11]

A controlled evaluation of psychotherapy as an adjunct to dermatological management of adult onset eczema was recently reported.[5] The results suggested that psychotherapy may be beneficial in some highly motivated patients with overt psychological disturbance which preceded the rash by less than one year. Eczema is an organic illness which can create emotional problems in the patient or his family. The emotional problems may aggravate the illness.[27]

Allergic Rhinitis

A personality study of patients with hay fever suggested dominant characteristics of self-absorption, dreaminess, and overweening ambition.[28] Psychoanalytic studies suggested that repressed olfactory sexual curiosity remained a source of conflict and constant nasal irritation.[18]

A psychiatric review concluded that these hypotheses probably represent an oversimplification of the problem. The role of allergens has been established more clearly than the precise role of psychological factors.[29]

Vasomotor Rhinitis

The phylogenetic origin and anatomic structure of the nose have provided the basis for much of the psychosomatic theory related to vasomotor rhinitis. The nose is a sexual organ and contains erectile tissue around the turbinates. This is innervated by sympathetic fibers from the superior cervical and sphenoidal ganglia. Nasal hypersensitivity of minor degree accompanies menstruation, pregnancy, and erotic activity. Hypersensitivity increases and produces symptoms when these functions are associated with conflict. Some authors have suggested that swelling of the turbinate mucosae, mucous secretions, and obstruction may accompany feelings of humiliation, frustration, and resentment. Most cases probably involve varying proportions of psychological stimuli and local irritative, physical, and biochemical stimuli.[29]

Asthma

Theories of Psychosomatic Etiology of Asthma. Asthma has been psychodynamically characterized as a repressed cry, an attempt to satisfy unresolved dependency.[18] The asthmatic patient and his mother theoretically have a close but ambivalent emotional relationship. The "separation anxiety" is mobilized with the fear of separation or loss of love from the mother, father, sibling, or other significant person in the patient's life. Rejection is the significant influence, but variable degrees of introjection or overprotection occur.[19] The "typical" asthmatic has a dependent relationship to an overprotective parent, usually the mother.[7]

The adult asthmatic was proposed to be an individual heavily predisposed to respiratory and "other psychosomatic illness." The patient was allegedly a product of an unstable childhood with an ambivalent mother who either neglected or smothered the child. The reaction was somatized instead of expressed in behavior or neurotic symptoms. The psychodynamics were holding in, suppression, and repression. If psychological symptoms supervened, they usually were of depression and introjection. This somatization continued into adulthood.[7]

Patients with asthma reportedly have a high incidence of fear of water or dreams utilizing water symbolism. All patients with these dreams had previous frightening experiences with water, but the data have been interpreted as unconscious conflicts relating to the patient's desire for reunion with the mother reflected in intrauterine fantasies.[10] A more reasonable interpretation has been offered: the reality experiences of water as a destructive or hostile force initiated the fears in susceptible individuals.[29]

Unconscious psychosexual conflict has been blamed for precipitating acute symptoms.[7, 10, 29] Adult sexual temptation may arouse feelings of guilt or revive infantile conflicts. Hostility developed in response to oral frustration extended into the genital development, resulting in a concept of sexuality as something hostile and sadistic. These patients repress all obvious interest in sex.[10] Demands of female asthmatic patients for pills and injections have been interpreted as a genital effort to manipulate male physicians into gratifying needs which were not gratified at an infantile oral level.[7]

The psychodynamics of the asthma symptoms were theoretically an unconscious attempt by the patient to protect himself, regressively, from loss of maternal love. The patient attempts to be united projectively or introjectively with the ambivalently regarded mother. The patient rejects these wishes and the depriving aspects of the mother. Sadistic impulses directed against the mother and the consequent feelings of guilt and anxiety date from early infancy.[29]

Characterizations of "Asthmatic Personalities." Asthmatic children are stereotyped as emotionally insecure, having an intense need for parental love and protection. They have been said to display these characteristics by clinging to their mothers in a self-centered, quiet, and repressed manner. Although they are usually intelligent, their performances are impaired by anxiety. They have considerable latent aggressiveness.[7]

The adult asthmatic reportedly conceals the basic childhood pattern by various defense mechanisms. The resulting characteristics are described as "clingers, do-gooders, withdrawers, aggressive deniers, and beseechers." [7]

The "clingers" retain the anxiety tendencies from childhood. They are described as lacking self-confidence and suppressing their feelings, particularly those which may threaten the dependent relationship with the parent or parent substitute.

The other personality types and the development of defense mechanisms result from the conflicts attending the fear or fact of separation from the mother:

The "do-gooders" attempt to satisfy their needs by ostentatiously helping others. They seek love and esteem by projecting their own needs onto the world.

The "withdrawers" deny their underlying insecurity and withdraw into a philosophical calm. The previously active drive for parental affection is replaced by self-satisfying activities.

The "aggressive deniers" attempt masking their insecurity by engaging in stressful situations. These patients are frequently provocative or aggressive in sexual, vocational, or social situations.

The "beseechers" have persistent needs to confess to a parent figure. The wheezing dyspnea in these patients has been likened to the inhibited cry of the deserted child.[10]

Asthmatogenic Parent. The theoretical psychodynamics and stereotyped personality descriptions of the patient with asthma have a corollary in the parent. This is characterized as the rejecting or unloving parent. Three forms are described: overt hostility and neglect, perfectionism, and compensatory overprotection.[18]

The theory of engulfment and domination is an extension of both the concepts of rejection and overprotection. The allergic patient is engulfed and dominated. Insecurity and dependency are perpetuated. The patient is rejected when parental needs are unsatisfied.[1]

Psychological studies have been interpreted to suggest a tendency for parents of asthmatic children to endorse punitive, authoritative, and restrictive attitudes.[24]

CRITICAL EVALUATION OF PREVIOUS THEORIES

Most of the psychiatric theories of asthmatic patients are supported only by descriptive personality studies and psychological treatment of relatively few patients who were referred to psychiatrists for management of specific psychiatric disorders. These reports are anecdotal and testimonial[18] and presuppose psychosomatic etiology for the asthma. Allergy management was usually in progress, and many authors indicated that the asthma had improved before psychiatric consultation.

The psychosomatic theories of urticaria, eczema, allergic rhinitis, and vasomotor rhinitis are based largely on studies of asthmatic patients. Psychopathology can be caused by the allergic disease or can coexist without any etiological relationship to the allergic disease.[30] The coexistence of allergic and psychiatric disorders can aggravate severity and complicate management of both.[8]

The incidence of concomitant psychopathology among children with asthma is similar to that of children with other disorders.[12, 19] This suggests that the psychiatric disorder is secondary to the asthma or due to unrelated factors.[12]

Emotional factors and the personality of asthmatics have been reviewed.[15] No association was demonstrated between (1) emotional stress and a history of infantile eczema or (2) acute or chronic emotional stress and likelihood of asthma becoming continuous. Psychological stress was rarely the dominant etiological factor, but it was recognized as an aggravating influence in some cases. A specific personality structure in asthma does not exist.

The original psychopathological concepts have not been confirmed.[15] Asthma symptoms are not a form of repressed crying.[22] Asthmatic patients are not different from normals or from patients with bronchitis [20] by psychological and psychophysiological studies. Numerous reports have evaluated parent-child relationships. No consistent association with variables of the family situation and variables of the patient's asthma can be determined.[15] In comparisons of psychological variables, parents of asthmatic children were not different from parents of children with congenital or other diseases [3, 9] or mothers of nonasthmatic children.[23] Purcell *et al.* suggested that a more passive father might provoke less anxiety for a relatively handicapped child.[23]

SUMMARY STATEMENT

Patients with allergic diseases are heterogeneous with respect to personality, psychodynamic characteristics, and parent-patient relationships. Generalizations regarding the entire spectrum or even individual syndromes cannot be made. The concepts of asthmatic personalities, asthmatogenic psychodynamics, and asthmatogenic parents are not supported by scientific studies. These diseases should not be considered to be psychosomatic in origin. Emotional problems in the patient and the family can result from allergic diseases, or pre-existing emotional problems can be aggravated. Emotional problems can aggravate the allergic disease.

PRACTICAL APPROACH TO PSYCHIATRIC FACTORS IN ALLERGIC DISEASES

The diseases discussed in this book are of three general types: (1) immediate-immunologically mediated (Type I, IgE, reagin-mediated), (2) other immunologically mediated (types II, III, or IV) varieties, or (3) nonimmunologically mediated disorders having clinical characteristics similar to the immunological ones. Vasomotor rhinitis and infective or intrinsic asthma are examples of the third category. None is considered to be of psychiatric origin. Variable degrees of psychiatric participation and interrelationship with organic factors occur.[8] The emotional complications of allergic disease are determined by the patient's personality and emotional conflicts, the severity of the disease, and the impact of the disease on the life style of the patient and his family. The multiple factors in the pathogenesis of allergic diseases include the state of sensitization, current allergen exposure, infection, environmental irritants, weather, heredity, neuroendocrine factors, and psychic influences. Reciprocal interaction renders each factor susceptible to the influence of others. Symptoms precipitated by allergen exposure or infection can aggravate emotional problems. Similarly, psychic influences may cause increased susceptibility to allergens or other factors, resulting in symptoms.[8]

Psychophysiologic Considerations

Altered immunological reactivity is the primary element in allergic diseases. This probably is not changed by psychological or central nervous system influences.[8] However, these influences may alter the expression of immunological reactivity.

Autonomic Nervous System. An imbalance of the autonomic nervous system has been considered. A relative increase in parasympathetic activity may account for hyperreactivity of the airways to diverse stimuli.[13] Blockade of beta adrenergic receptors is another proposed mechanism for increased airway reactivity; the enzyme adenylcyclase is decreased with these changes.[25] Bronchospasm can result from bronchial reflex arcs mediated through vagal pathways.[26] Airway resistance can be increased in the asthmatic patient by various stimuli. These include coughing, hyperventilation, and inhalation of cold air or irritants such as citric acid. Emotions such as anger, but not implying psychogenesis or "asthmatic personality," can also increase airway resistance. This response can be inhibited by atropine, suggesting a vagal pathway.[17]

SPECTRUM OF RELATIONSHIP OF PSYCHIATRIC FACTORS TO ALLERGIC DISEASE

Background

Various reports have examined the relationship of "allergic potential" and psychiatric disturbance in patients with asthma. Block *et al.* suggested more evidence for psychopathology in patients of low allergy potential and in their mothers than in the group with high allergy potential.[4] Purcell *et al.* extended these findings to the patients and both parents.[24] Hirt *et al.* showed no correlation between high or low allergy potential and psychopathology.[14]

Allergy potential was expressed as a score. Variable points were assigned for family history of allergic diseases, personal history of collateral allergy, cutaneous reactivity, and whether the disease was seasonal or perennial. Patients with scores above the median or mean were assigned to the high allergy potential group. The low allergy potential group consisted of patients whose scores were below the median or mean. Psychopathology was determined by psychological tests and expressed as a mean score or a total score for each group.

The incidence of psychopathology within each group was not determined and may be of equal or greater importance than the mean scores on psychological tests. Psychopathology was presumed to have a causal relationship to the asthma. The possibility that psychopathology resulted from, or existed coincidentally to the asthma, at least in some individuals, was not assessed.

Seasonal asthma due to pollen allergy was not distinguished from perennial asthma. These entities often have different clinical courses, and they probably have different incidences of psychopathology. Psychopathology existing among patients with seasonal pollenosis probably differs from that existing among patients with perennial asthma. These differences could be obscured by combining the two groups.

Allergic Diseases Having Little or No Psychiatric Relationship

Seasonal Asthma or Rhinitis Due to Pollen Allergy. Patients with simple seasonal pollenosis asthma or allergic rhinitis have not been studied as a single group relative to psychopathology. They have relatively brief symptoms the same time each year. Specific allergenic etiology is easily demonstrated, and response to hyposensitization is usually excellent. The incidence of psychopathology in patients with seasonal allergic asthma and rhinitis appears similar to that in the general population. The psychopathology which occurs in this group seems coincidental and unrelated to the allergic disease.

Potential Psychiatric Relationship with Allergic Diseases

Psychiatric Effects of Allergic Diseases. Depression frequently accompanies symptoms of allergic disease.[18] Patients may become depressed by chronic symptoms of asthma, urticaria, eczema, or even rhinitis. This depression is usually based on inability to work, attend school, or participate in athletic or other activities.

Significant allergic symptoms, such as asthma, are frightening, particularly to children.[18] The dyspnea of asthma frequently causes anxiety.[20] Recurrent hospitalizations may reinforce anxiety.

Financial Stress. Chronic diseases in general create a cumulative financial burden on the patient and his family. This occurs from doctors' fees, cost of drugs, hospital expenses, loss of vocational or academic productivity, and increased premiums for health insurance, disability insurance, and life insurance. Patients with asthma often are refused insurance protection, or they are offered policies which exclude pre-existing diseases. These economic problems are potential causes of depression, anxiety, guilt, or hostility.

Disease State Affected by Psychiatric Factors. Two of the most common causes of therapeutic failure in patients with allergic respiratory diseases are smoking and pets.

Smoking is initiated, at least in part, by social and cultural pressures to conform. The habit is perpetuated by physiologic addiction to nicotine. Emotional factors apparently determine the quantity of smoking, many occasions for excessive smoking, and certain forms of compulsive smoking. Some smokers have masochistic neuroses, and the outward sign—such as the cigarette—is an oral "pacifier." [29] Patients offer various excuses for continuing smoking. Patients who continue to smoke contribute significantly to the severity of the disease, particularly of the lower respiratory tract, by their emotional inability to terminate this habit.

Some patients are sufficiently allergic to animals that retention of the animal in the home constitutes a serious threat to maintenance of health. Retention of pets may be a decision of the patient or the family. When the disease is sufficiently severe, such refusal to complete appropriate therapy may indicate lack of judgment or maturity, or, in some cases, a more significant psychiatric abnormality.

Special Problems of Children with Asthma. Parents sometimes overreact to the child with asthma and impose excessive restrictions. The child needlessly may be prohibited from participating in athletics or other physical activities. Unnecessary absenteeism from school may result from unreasonable concern over minor symptoms.

Parents may correlate asthma symptoms with the psychiatric factors. The emotional aspects may be misinterpreted as causal. Significant symptoms may be ignored and appropriate treatment deferred. The potential significance of asthma may not be realized by some parents. Spontaneous remission occurs in some patients, and "outgrowing" allergic disease is a popular concept. Appropriate allergy management is postponed or avoided.

The child with asthma may disrupt some aspects of family life. This can result from the economic impact of therapy, elimination of pets, and interference with vacations. Vocational plans for teenage patients might sometimes be altered because of potential occupational exposure.

Circumstances of Predominant Psychiatric Factors and Secondary Allergic Factors

Allergic diseases sometimes coexist with neurosis or psychosis. Many patients reject the psychiatric diagnosis and attribute all of their symptoms to "allergy." The significance of minimal cutaneous, nasal, or respiratory manifestations can be exaggerated.

Minimal complaints or previous significant disease sometimes are used to manipulate the patient's personal or family life. An example is the asthmatic with minimal disease who consciously or subconsciously hyperventilates. Some asthmatics may induce symptoms by voluntary exercise or cough.[8] Patients with eczema have been observed to inflict lesions as a method for personal gain.[27] Operant conditioning has been studied, but its rule in allergic diseases remains speculative.

PRACTICAL CLINICAL APPROACH

Management of allergic diseases requires individualization of care. Appropriate allergy treatment and assessment of psychiatric factors must be established for each patient.

Few patients with allergic diseases require psychiatric consultation. Emotional factors in the vast majority can be managed by the allergist or the primary physician—family practitioner, internist, or pediatrician. This physician must be aware of basic principles of psychosomatic medicine.

Supportive Therapy

The patient requires adequate education regarding the disease, objectives of therapy, and methods of relieving acute symptoms. The availability of theophylline or the doctor may be emotionally quieting to a patient even though additional medication may never be used. Symptoms of emotional origin must be distinguished from those of allergic etiology. The psychogenic symptoms will not improve with allergy management and may require another approach. The patient must have confidence that his requirements for care shall be fulfilled.

Reassurance

Reassurance must be appropriate and realistic. Cure should not be promised if only amelioration is possible; the prognosis should be discussed candidly. The patient should know that allergic diseases are not forms of emotional expression, but emotions can aggravate or precipitate mild or moderate symptoms. Iatrogenic psychopathology and stigmatizing interpretations regarding parental responsibility should be avoided.[8]

Psychiatric Consultation

Psychiatric consultation is indicated when remedial or intractable emotional problems exist. Some circumstances have been described: (1) families with severe psychopathology or deep-seated conflicts, (2) families harboring resentment of the patient because of the illness or other reasons, (3) patients with a personality disorder or neurotic symptoms, whether coincidental, secondary, or aggravating to the allergic disease, and (4) families who use the physical symptoms as devices for their own neurotic needs.[11]

The allergist or general physician must recognize the need for psychiatric consultation and properly prepare the patient and the family. This referral can be beneficial only if the patient and the family accept its necessity and are willing to cooperate with the therapist. They must also be reassured that the referring physician will continue the medical management.

SUMMARY

Allergic diseases are not of psychosomatic origin, but coexisting emotional problems and allergic disease aggravate each other. Various psychiatric disorders may be coincidental or secondary to the chronic disease. Most psychiatric factors can be successfully managed by the allergist or primary physician. Some require psychiatric consultation.

REFERENCES

1. Abramson, H. A.: Some aspects in the psychodynamics of intractable asthma in children. *In* Schneer, H. I.: The Asthmatic Child. New York, Hoeber, 1963.
2. Aitken, R. C. B., Zealley, A. K., and Rosenthal, S. V.: Psychological and physiological measures of emotion in chronic asthmatic patients. J. Psychosom. Res., *13:*289, 1969.
3. Block, J.: Parents of schizophrenic, neurotic, asthmatic, and congenitally ill children. Arch. Gen. Psychiat., *20:*659, 1969.
4. Block, J., Jennings, P. H., Harvey, E., and Simpson, E.: Interaction between allergic potential and psychopathology in childhood asthma. Psychosom. Med., *26:*307, 1964.
5. Brown, D. G. and Bettley, F. R.: Psychiatric treatment of eczema: a controlled trial. Brit. Med. J., *2:*729, 26 June, 1971.
6. Champion, R. H., Roberts, S. O. B., Carpenter, R. G., and Roger, J. H.: Urticaria and angioedema. A review of 554 patients. Brit. J. Derm., *81:*588, 1969.
7. Edgell, P. G.: Psychiatric approach to the treatment of bronchial asthma. Mod. Treat., *3:*900, 1966.
8. Falliers, C. J.: Psychosomatic study and treatment of asthmatic children. Pediat. Clin. N. Am., *16:*271, 1969.
9. Fitzelle, G. F.: Personality factors and certain attitudes toward child rearing among parents of asthmatic children. Psychosom. Med., *21:*208, 1959.
10. French, T. N. and Alexander, F.: Psychogenic factors in bronchial asthma. Psychosom. Med. Monograph, *4.* Washington, D.C., National Research Council, 1941.
11. Friedman, D. B. and Selesnick, S. T.: Clinical notes on the management of asthma and eczema. Clin. Pediat., *4:*735, 1965.
12. Graham, P. J., Rutter, M. L., Yule, W., and Pless, I. B.: Childhood asthma: a psychosomatic disorder? Some epidemiological considerations. Brit. J. Prev. Soc. Med., *21:*78, 1967.

13. Hahn, W. W.: Asthma: psychophysiologic considerations. Pediat. Digest, 9:65, June, 1967.
14. Hirt, M., Goldberg, R., and Bernstein, I. L.: Interaction of personality variables and allergic predisposition in asthma. Psychosomatics, 9:340, 1968.
15. Kelly, E. and Zeller, B.: Asthma and the psychiatrist, J. Psychosom. Res., 13:377, 1969.
16. Knight, J. A.: Psychodynamics of the allergic eczemas. Ann. Allerg., 25:392, 1967.
17. Luparello, T. J., McFadden, E. R., Jr., and Bleecker, E. R.: Psychologic factors and bronchial asthma. Laboratory model for investigation. New York J. Med., 71:2161, 1971.
18. McGovern, J. P. and Knight, J. A.: Allergy and Human Emotions. Springfield, Ill. Charles C Thomas, 1967.
19. Neuhaus, E. C.: A personality study of asthmatic and cardiac children. Psychosom. Med., 20:181, 1958.
20. Oswald, N. C., Waller, R. E., and Drinkwater, J.: Relationship between breathlessness and anxiety in asthma and bronchitis: a comparative study. Brit. Med. J., 2:14, 1970.
21. Pierloot, R. A. and Van Roy, J.: Asthma and aggression. J. Psychosom. Res., 13:333, 1969.
22. Purcell, K.: Critical appraisal of psychosomatic studies of asthma. New York J. Med., 65:2103, 1965.
23. Purcell, K., and Clifford E.: Binocular rivalry and the study of identification in asthmatic and nonasthmatic boys. J. Consult. Psychol., 30:388, 1966.
24. Purcell, G., Muser, J., Miklich, D., and Dietiker, K. E.: A comparison of psychologic findings in variously defined asthmatic subgroups. J. Psychosom. Res., 13:67, 1969.
25. Reed, C. E.: Beta-blockade and allergy. A progress report. *In* Serafini, U., Frankland, A. W., Masala, C., and Jamar, J. M.: New Concepts in Allergy and Immunology. Proceedings of the VII International Congress of Allergology. Amsterdam, Excerpta Medica, 1971.
26. Simonsson, B. G., Jacobs, F. M., and Nadel, J. A.: Role of autonomic nervous system and the cough reflex in the increased responsiveness of airways in patients with obstructive airway disease. J. Clin. Invest., 46:1812, 1967.
27. Vaughan, V. C.: Emotional undertones in eczema in children. J. Asthma Res., 3:193, 1966.
28. Wittkower, E.: Studies on hay-fever patients. J. Ment. Sci., 84:352, 1938.
29. Wittkower, E. D. and White, K. L.: Psychophysiologic aspects of respiratory disorders. *In* Arieti, S.: American Handbook of Psychiatry. vol. 1. New York, Basic Books, Inc., 1959.
30. Zealley, A. K., Aitken, R. C. B., and Rosenthal, S. V.: Psychopathology in bronchial asthmatic patients. Scot. Med. J., 15:102, 1970.

THE WHEEZING INFANT

Howard Melam, M.D.

Asthma in the first two years of life, the period of infancy, is not uncommon. It has been reported that 22 percent of children who developed asthma during their first ten years of life had onset of their symptoms in the first year and 17 percent in the second.[1] The diagnosis of asthma in infancy may be difficult to make. In older children and adults, the characteristic findings on physical examination during an asthmatic episode consist of expiratory wheezing and a prolonged expiratory phase of respiration. These episodes are usually recurrent with complete clearing between attacks.

In contrast, an infant, under 6 months of age, with asthma may present with: (a) relatively characteristic wheezing, a prolonged expiratory phase of respiration and musical rhonchi or (b) coarse expiratory and inspiratory rhonchi and rales with an associated cough. The infant usually has a respiratory infection in addition, which may be responsible for the major physical findings. After 6 months of age the physical findings of asthma in the infant become more typical of those found in the older child and the adult.

The approach to the infant with suspected asthma begins with a complete history. Detection of the presence of other atopic diseases may be of value. These include a history of eczema or rhinitis in the older infant. Colic, feeding difficulties and bowel disorders, although occurring more frequently in the atopic individual, may have causes other than allergy. Documentation of parents or siblings with eczema, rhinitis, asthma or urticaria may provide supportive evidence as to the allergic status of the infant.

If the infant's wheezing is due to asthma, it should be intermittent by history. Bronchodilators such as epinephrine should rapidly reverse the wheezing state if it is not complicated by dehydration or infection. A history of continuous wheezing should alert the investigator to a nonallergic cause of the infant's illness.

The strongest evidence that the respiratory distress is due to an allergic cause is the observation that an inhalant or food will definitely precipitate an attack. However, this observation is rarely made in infancy, and often infection is the most prominent precipitating factor associated with asthma in this age group.

559

The next diagnostic approach in the evaluation of an infant with suspected asthma is a complete physical examination. Special attention should be directed to the child's growth and development, nutritional status, upper respiratory and lower respiratory systems and cardiovascular system. As discussed, in the early months of life it may be difficult to make a diagnosis of asthma by auscultation of the chest. Even if wheezing is not present the diagnosis of asthma has not been excluded.

Certain studies should be done to aid in making the diagnosis of asthma and to exclude other diseases. Nasal smears should be examined for eosinophilia. However, this test is less reliable in infants for several reasons. Nasal eosinophilia may be a transient feature of the secretions of otherwise normal infants.[7] Because of the frequent occurence of associated upper respiratory infections, nasal eosinophils may be replaced by polymorphonuclear leukocytes in nasal exudate. A blood eosinophilia of greater than 4 percent may be suggestive of allergy.[2] Attempts to measure pulmonary function are usually fruitless, as are attempts to examine sputum.

Although skin tests are usually negative under 2 years of age, the application of a selected number of skin tests is indicated in an infant having repeated respiratory difficulty. These tests, if positive, may provide information as to the atopic nature of the patient. If the infant gives positive reactions to certain food antigens, the physician is provided with possible allergens to evaluate further by diet or environmental manipulation.

Other studies of value in evaluating the infant are skin test for tuberculosis, chest x-ray, white blood cell count and differential, and sweat electrolytes. Examinations which may be necessary in selected cases to exclude diseases other than asthma include barium swallow, bronchoscopy, bronchography and quantitative immunoglobulins.

In making the diagnosis of asthma in an infant it is important to rule out other common or uncommon conditions which can mimic asthma. Among the common conditions would be bronchiolitis, aspirated foreign body and cystic fibrosis.

BRONCHIOLITIS

Bronchiolitis is an acute respiratory illness in infants. The respiratory syncytial virus has been identified as the most frequent cause, but other agents both bacterial and viral may be responsible.[4] The illness in the infant may start as mild rhinitis and then progress to involve the lower respiratory tract. The infant becomes tachypneic, irritable, anxious, and sometimes develops respiratory failure and cyanosis. Examination of the chest reveals shallow, rapid respiration, nasal flaring, and inter-costal retraction. The chest is resonant to percussion. On auscultation, there may be expiratory wheezes, coarse rhonchi, rales and diminished breath sounds. Chest x-rays show hyperaerated lungs with flattened diaphragms. Treatment consists of hydration, correction of acidosis and humidified oxygen. Debate continues as to the value of antibiotics, bronchodilators and corticosteroids, but most observers believe they do not alter the course of the patient with bronchiolitis uncomplicated by other disease. In infants with severe respiratory failure mechanical ventilation has been successfully employed.

It is often very difficult to differentiate between asthma and bronchi-olitis in early infancy. Family and patient history of atopy, causal rela-tion to extrinsic allergens, eosinophilia and other factors discussed earlier in this chapter are helpful in making a diagnosis of asthma. The infant with asthma has more frequent attacks of respiratory distress which also are usually of quicker onset than in bronchiolitis. Unless the asthma-tic infant is dehydrated or has a superimposed lower respiratory in-fection he will respond favorably to bronchodilators. The infant with bronchiolitis does not respond to these drugs.

An association between bronchiolitis and asthma has been recorded by several observers. It is estimated that 25 to 30 percent of infants who develop bronchiolitis will later go on to have asthma.[3, 8]

ASPIRATED FOREIGN BODY

Aspiration of foreign bodies is unusual before 8 to 10 months of age, when the infant begins to crawl. At times the observant parent may be suspicious that aspiration has occurred. A history of sudden explosive coughing is suggestive of foreign body aspiration. Unilateral wheezing is a helpful finding but most often the wheezing is bilateral. If the foreign body is opaque, a chest x-ray will identify it. If the object is nonopaque, inspiratory and expiratory x-ray films, which are difficult to obtain in infants because of lack of cooperation, may reveal unilateral air trapping. Absence of other evidence of atopy by laboratory studies, family history or previous history of allergic problems helps exclude asthma and may indicate the possibility of aspiration. Failure to have complete clearing of cough or wheezing with bronchodilators is sus-picious of aspiration. Often the diagnosis of foreign body aspiration can only be made by bronchoscopic examination of the infant. This should be done whenever the possibility of aspiration of foreign body exists. It is important that this diagnosis be made before the infant develops such complications as atelectasis or abscess.

CYSTIC FIBROSIS

Cystic fibrosis is a disease of the exocrine glands. The disease is inherited as a Mendelian recessive. The major clinical manifestations involve the respiratory and gastrointestinal systems, although other organs of the body are affected. The basic defect in cystic fibrosis is presently unknown.

Pulmonary disease is present in almost all patients. Highly viscous mucous secretions cause bronchial and bronchiolar obstruction. Obstructive emphysema and bronchiectasis usually develop. Respiratory symptoms may first appear weeks, months or years after birth. The initial symptom is often a nonproductive cough. This is followed by signs and symptoms of airway obstruction and secondary infection.

The diagnosis of cystic fibrosis should be considered when an infant has pulmonary disease, evidence of malabsorption, a family history of cystic fibrosis and sweat chloride concentration of greater than 50 mEq/liter.

Respiratory allergy occurs coincidentally in about 16 percent of patients with cystic fibrosis.[5] Both diseases should be treated appropriately. Treatment of the pulmonary complications of cystic fibrosis includes control of infection, adequate hydration, physical therapy including postural drainage and aerosol therapy. Treatment of respiratory allergy is discussed elsewhere in this text.

Other conditions which may be confused with asthma in infancy include laryngeal stridor, mediastinal masses and aberrant blood vessels compressing the respiratory tract. These conditions can be excluded by history, physical examination and chest x-ray, or they may require more detailed evaluation.[6]

Often it is impossible to make a diagnosis of asthma when the infant is first seen. At times the disease must evolve over a period of time before the allergic nature of the infant's respiratory distress becomes clinically evident. The parents should be instructed to note any association between foods or inhalants and the precipitation or increase in severity of the infant's respiratory symptoms.

If the disease is severe a period of diet manipulation is indicated. It is best to start with a milk substitute formula for 1 week and then add new foods every several days, watching for an increase in symptoms. If the infant's medications and diet have not been altered and he improves when out of the home only to develop symptoms again at home, an inhalant allergen should be suspected. Under these circumstances it is worthwhile to attempt to reduce the patient's exposure to pollens, spores, dust and animal danders.

The infant should be continually reevaluated with repetition of necessary studies, including skin tests, as indicated. With patience and perseverance the diagnosis of asthma can usually be made. Those patients whose respiratory distress is solely of an infectious nature usually improve and have less difficulty as they grow older. In the other patients the relationship between extrinsic allergens and their disease eventually becomes evident.

REFERENCES

1. Bray, G. W.: The asthmatic child. Arch. Dis. Child., 5:236, 1930.
2. Buffum, W. P.: The diagnosis of asthma in infancy, J. Allerg., 25:511, 1954.
3. Eisen, A. H., and Bacal, H. L.: Relationship of acute bronchiolitis to bronchial asthma. Pediatrics, 31:859, 1963.
4. Holdaway, D., *et al.*: The diagnosis and management of bronchiolitis. Pediatrics, 39:924, 1967.
5. Kulczycki, L. L., *et al.*: Respiratory allergy in patients with cystic fibrosis. JAMA, 175:358, 1961.
6. Nelson, W.: Textbook of Pediatrics. ed. 9. Philadelphia, W. B. Saunders, 1969.
7. Speer, F.: The Allergic Child. New York, Harper & Row Rev., 1966.
8. Wittig, H. J., and Glaser, J.: Relationship between bronchiolitis and childhood asthma. J. Allerg., 30:19, 1959.

THERAPEUTIC MEASURES OF UNCERTAIN VALUE

Bernard Hess Booth III, M.D.

Though allergic rhinitis and extrinsic asthma have long been recognized as distinct disease entities, only within the last few years has any significant information become available regarding the pathophysiologic mechanisms responsible for these diseases. As a consequence, until very recently, therapy for these illnesses was empirically derived and tested.

Numerous problems confront any investigator who attempts to evaluate the efficacy of a therapy for either allergic rhinitis or asthma. Both illnesses are highly variable, and patients do not have a uniform prognosis in regard to morbidity or mortality. Consequently, spontaneous improvement in symptoms can easily be attributed to concomitant therapy that really had no effect on the illness.

Many factors that are not related to the primary immunologic etiology of these illnesses can affect their clinical manifestations. Infections, inhaled irritants, fatigue, and emotional problems are variable factors that may affect the clinical course of the illness independently or cumulatively. The degree of significance of any one factor may vary greatly from patient to patient. Control of these variables represents a formidable obstacle to investigators studying the efficacy of a therapy.

Any chronic illness, particularly one like asthma, with its high morbidity and potentiality of a fatal attack can influence the objectivity of the patient and even his physician. It is therefore not surprising that the efficacy of some therapies has not been proven. Failure to clearly demonstrate efficacy of a treatment in all patients does not necessarily mean that the therapy is not efficacious in some patients.

It is important however for physicians to remain critical of all claims of therapeutic effectiveness. Sincere and honest individuals have been certain that honey, licorice, lemon juice, Chihuahua dogs, Persian cats, and various talismans have had beneficial effects on their own allergic disorders or those of others. It is appropriate for physicians to listen to these stories with sympathy and understanding. It is imperative however that physicians not accept these testimonials as scientific evidence.

Some treatments have been widely used even though their value has not been unequivocally demonstrated. Some evidence suggests that certain of these treatment modalities may be effective. Theoretical considerations make it seem likely that others are effective. Some treatments have no sound theoretical basis and all reports of their efficacy are anecdotal.

564

BACTERIAL VACCINE

Numerous studies have been performed to determine the efficacy of bacterial vaccines in the treatment of asthma. A superficial survey of the literature might indicate that there have generally been favorable results (Table 18-2). However more critical evaluation of these studies produces doubt regarding the efficacy of this treatment. Only six studies appear to have made any significant effort to control the results with double blind technique. The majority of the studies that utilized acceptable methodology appear to show that bacterial vaccine has no real effectiveness.

Frankland studied 184 adults and children with infectious asthma.[5] The patients were randomly divided into two groups. One group received placebo injections of carbo-saline. The second group received a mixture of autogenous and mixed stock vaccine. Fifty-eight percent

TABLE 18-2
Bacterial Vaccine Therapy in Asthma *

| AUTHOR | | NO. OF PATIENTS | | IMPROVEMENT RATE—% |
		TREATED	IMPROVED	
Banks	(1934)	143	114	80
Benson	(1933)	94	74	79
Bergqust	(1955)	122	84	69
Carmalt-Jones	(1909)	52	34	75
Frankland	(1955)	100	58	58
Helander	(1958)	228	161	70
Rackemann	(1923)	131	77	59
Rogers	(1921)	40	34	85
Stevens	(1939)	53	50	94
Thomas	(1924)	62	56	87
Thomas	(1933)	300	213	71
Voorsanger	(1929)	66	42	64
Walker	(1919)	178	117	60
Wilmer	(1933)	150	114	76
Johnstone	(1959)	50	48	80
Aas	(1963)	15	12	80
Fontana	(1965)	15	7	47
Barr	(1965)	22	10	45 †
Mueller	(1969)	62	47	75

* Modified from Helander, E.: Bacterial vaccines in treatment of bronchial asthma. Acta Allerg.; *13:*47, 1959.

† Were better than matched control—45% were worse and 10% were the same as control on symptom scale.

improved following vaccine therapy, and 52.2 percent improved after placebo therapy.

Helander studied 228 adults.[11] Sixty-eight percent of the patients improved after vaccine therapy while 62 percent improved after physiological saline. Johnstone studied 118 asthmatic children.[14] All of these children were felt to have clinical sensitivities to inhalant antigens in addition to episodes of wheezing with respiratory infections. The control group received hyposensitization to all inhalant allergens to which they reacted on skin testing. The vaccine-treated group received concomitant hyposensitization to inhalant antigens. Eighty percent of the vaccine-treated patients had fewer episodes of asthma after treatment and 91 percent of the control group had fewer episodes after treatment. The criteria for selecting these patients were different from those used in other studies, and the results may not be directly comparable. Most other studies selected patients who had wheezing only during infections and who had negative skin tests to other antigens. This in no way negates the value of the study, but it must be noted that different situations were being evaluated.

The study of Barr and associates also utilized patients who had clinical sensitivities to multiple antigens, in addition, their asthma was aggravated by infection.[1] They studied 22 pairs of patients who were matched as closely as possible with respect to age, sex, race, severity and duration of disease, pulmonary function studies and x-ray evidence of sinusitis. They all continued their immunization against other antigens. The vaccine-treated patients were significantly better when the number of prescriptions for inhalers were considered. Though there appeared to be some minimal improvement when symptom scores, emergency room visits, vital capacities, maximum expiratory flow rates, steroid tablets and asthma tablets were evaluated, none of these differences were statistically significant. These authors interpreted their data as suggesting that the vaccine was effective.

The same year Fontana and associates studied 41 children who had asthma only with respiratory infections.[4] All 41 were treated for 1 year with placebo then were divided into two groups one of which received the placebo while the second group received the vaccine for 1 year. No difference could be determined in the number of asthma tablets or the number of antibiotics between the two groups either before or after the treatment. Of the group that received the vaccine, 46 percent had fewer episodes of wheezing the second year. Seventy-three percent of the placebo group had fewer episodes of wheezing during the second year. Forty percent of the treated group had more infections the second year while only 20 percent of the placebo group had more infections. This completely double blind study which allowed each patient to function as his own control as well as comparing him to a control group failed to demonstrate any benefit from the vaccine.

Mueller and Lanz selected a very similar group of patients for study.[17] Only 14 patients were studied in a double blind manner. Nine received vaccine and 5 received placebo. The average number of infections each year remained the same in both groups but the treated patients had fewer episodes of wheezing with infections. On this evidence and that from an uncontrolled study the authors felt the vaccine might be effective.

The available literature certainly offers no convincing evidence that bacterial vaccine is effective or ineffective. If there is some benefit from therapy with bacterial vaccine, it is so subtle that it cannot be easily appreciated.

GAY'S SOLUTION

Asthma has been treated using a mixture of Fowler's solution, tincture of digitalis, sodium phenobarbital and potassium iodide (Gay's solution). There is only a limited amount of information that allows a judgment concerning efficacy.[6, 7, 10] The efficacy or toxicity of the mixture has been assumed to be due to the potassium arsenite in the Fowler's solution.

Gay's report concerns 1,128 patients who were treated from 2 to 7½ years with this solution. This was not a drug study but an evaluation of his experiences with the treatment. Eighty percent of these patients were treatment failures elsewhere. Thirty percent (337) of the patients had toxic reactions that were attributed to arsenic. These reactions were: mild edema, 175; pigmentation, 79; keratosis, 17; erythema, 1; and exfoliation, 1. In addition, 35 percent of the patients had swelling of the salivary glands or acneiform lesions that were attributed to the potassium iodide in the solution. Eighty percent of these patients reported that they were greatly improved. Only 5 percent reported that they were unimproved. These appear to be highly favorable results in a group of patients who had been treatment failures elsewhere. However, these results are difficult to evaluate for numerous reasons. There was no control group of patients, and no double blind technique was involved. All treatment results were determined by questionnaire; consequently, the parameter determined was whether or not the patients thought they were better. Most significantly, only patients who had taken Gay's solution 2 years or longer were included in the statistical analysis. All patients had been informed that the solution contained arsenic and could be toxic. It seems reasonable to assume that few patients would have persisted in taking arsenic for over 2 years unless they thought they were better. In addition, the classification of the type of asthma treated cannot be determined. All of these patients were treated by Gay who firmly believed in the efficacy of this solution and who, in addition, stressed the value of the simpler forms of psycho-therapy. Reassurance, common sense, the art of the practice of medicine and the lifting of restrictions that were unpleasant to the patient were considered important to Dr. Gay and may ultimately have had much to do with his patient's improvement.

Hartner and Novitch reported the only other large group of patients treated with Gay's solution.[10] In an uncontrolled study 25 steroid-dependent patients with severe asthma were treated and eight (32%) had dramatic improvement and were taken off steroids. Subsequently a double blind control study was performed with 31 patients. Seven of the 18 patients (39%) who received the solution containing potassium arsenite had dramatic improvement, and steroids were stopped; in addition, six (33%) had definite evidence of improvement, though steroids could not be completely discontinued. Only two of the 12 patients receiving solutions that did not contain the arsenic had any improvement. Consequently 72 percent of the arsenic patients had improvement while only 17 percent of the placebo-treated patients had improvement. The number of patients with toxic reactions was not given, but three patients had iodide rashes, three patients had salivary swelling, six patients had gastrointestinal symptoms, three patients had pigmentation, one had hyperkeratosis and one had a serum sickness-like illness. This study seems to suggest that Gay's solution is effective and may be the treatment of choice for some patients with intractable asthma.

All other reports concerning the use of Gay's solution deal with reports of arsenic toxicity secondary to its use. Even in these unfavorable reports, there is some presumptive evidence of its efficacy. Three case reports of toxicity also report clinical improvement in the patient's asthma when the arsenic was started and difficulty controlling asthma when the arsenic was stopped.[18, 19, 22] Hansen-Pruss reported 17 cases of treatment failures however, and four of the cases had severe cutaneous or hepatic reactions attributed to arsenic.[9]

In summary, the available literature suggests that this solution has been of benefit to patients with asthma. It clearly indicates that toxicity has occurred from its use. If it is effective, no logical reason for this pharmacologic action has been given. For these reasons its routine use should not be recommended. Further careful and critical evaluation of this form of therapy might be reasonable.

HISTAMINE INJECTIONS

One article reports the efficacy of histamine therapy in cases of cold urticaria and associated anaphylaxis; arteriosclerosis of the central nervous system associated with severe dizziness, vertigo and depression; "allergic" arthritis and optic neuritis; bilateral retrobular neuritis; the pain of acute gout; a penicillin reaction; diffuse arterial disease with angina pectoris and occlusive arterial disease of the left lower extremity; a right hemiparesis and aphasia resulting from a cerebral vascular accident; recurrent corneal ulcers; histamine cephalgia; Meniere's disease and locomotor ataxia associated with lightning pains and morphinism.[13] All were felt to have favorable responses. Other reports concern its use only in histamine cephalgia.[8, 12] Theoretical reasons advanced to explain possible therapeutic efficacy have never been impressive. Increasing knowledge of immune mechanisms as well as increased knowledge of the physiological actions of histamine have cast further doubt on the entire procedure.

ANERGEX

An alcoholic extract of poison oak (Anergex *) has been used to treat all allergic syndromes. Several reports appeared stating that it was efficacious in the treatment of asthma, seasonal and perennial rhinitis, eczema, gastrointestinal allergy, and excess pharyngeal mucus.[16, 20, 21] These reports not only did not employ a double blind technique but were also completely devoid of any control patients. Two studies utilizing a double blind technique failed to demonstrate any beneficial effect in patients with ragweed hayfever.[2, 3, 15]

Reports of the efficacy of Anergex are anecdotal; there is no valid theoretical reason for its use, and what reasonable evidence is available indicates that it is no more effective than placebo injections. Its use should be discouraged.

* Trademark, Lemmon.

REFERENCES

1. Barr, S. E., *et al.:* A double blind study of the effects of bacterial vaccine on infective asthma. J. Allerg., *36:*47, 1965.
2. Brown, E. B.: Report of the committee on drugs for 1962. J. Allerg., *34:*469, 1963.
3. Brown, E. B., Ipsen, J., and Papovits, C.: Use of poisonoak extract in ragweed hayfever. New York J. Med., *64:*2050, 1964.

4. Fontana, V. J., *et al.:* Bacterial vaccine and infectious asthma. JAMA, *193:*123, 1965.

5. Frankland, A. W., Hughes, W. H., and Garril, R. H.: Autogenous bacterial vaccine in treatment of asthma. Brit. Med. J., *2:*941, 1955.

6. Gay, E. D.: Chemotherapeutic agents and simple psychotherapy in the allergic state—survey of 1,128 cases. Mississippi Doctor, *33:*183, 1955.

7. Gay, S. F. and Gay, E. D.: The Gay treatment of asthma. Mississippi Doctor, *29:*142, 1951.

8. Hanes, W. J.: Histamine cephalgia resembling tic douloureux: differential diagnosis and treatment. Headache, *8:*162, 1969.

9. Hansen-Pruss, O. C.: Arsenic in the treatment of asthma. Ann. Allerg., *13:*1, 1955.

10. Hartner, J. G. and Novitch, A. M.: On evaluation of Gay's solution in the treatment of asthma. J. Allerg., *40:*327, 1967.

11. Helander, E.: Bacterial vaccines in treatment of bronchial asthma. Acta Allerg., *13:*47, 1959.

12. Horton, B. T.: The use of histamine in the treatment of specific types of headaches. JAMA, *116:*377, 1941.

13. ———: The clinical use of histamine. Postgrad. Med., *9:*1, 1951.

14. Johnstone, D. E.: Study of the value of bacterial vaccines in the treatment of bronchial asthma associated with respiratory infections. Pediatrics, *24:*427, 1959.

15. Kamin, S. H., Nastasi, L., Westlin, W., and Klein, A. H.: The treatment of allergy with extract of toxicodendron quercifolia: a controlled series. Pediatrics, *22:*887, 1958.

16. Lange, H. W. and Sheldon, R. W.: Nasal eosinophilia: response following anergex therapy. Eye Ear Nose Throat Mon., *38:*136, 1959.

17. Mueller, H. L. and Lanz, M.: Hyposensitization with bacterial vaccine in infectious asthma. JAMA, *208:*1379, 1969.

18. Pelner, L. and Waldman, S.: Toxic hepatitis caused by prolonged inorganic arsenic intake: studies on liver dysfunction. New York J. Med., *51:*2511, 1951.

19. ———: Toxicity of arsenic as used in the treatment of asthma. JAMA, *150:*1511, 1952.

20. Ravito, J.: Non-specific therapy in allergy: a further report. Am. Pract. Digest Treat., *7:*1447, 1956.

21. Reynolds, M. R.: Allergy in children: simplified management. Arch. Ped., *79:*137, 1962.

22. Silver, A. S. and Wainman, P. L.: Chronic arsenic poisoning following use of an asthma remedy. JAMA, *150:*584, 1952.

DIETARY PROPHYLAXIS IN INFANCY

Howard Melam, M.D.

Controversy continues concerning the prophylactic dietary management of potential allergy in infants. Some physicians believe that allergic syndromes in children can be prevented by avoidance of certain foods in early infancy. Johnstone and Glaser [6] studied 91 infants who were offspring or siblings of one or more individuals with one or more atopic disorders and, therefore, considered to be potentially allergic. These infants were kept on a diet free of cow's milk for up to 9 months after birth.

Potentially allergic infants on the dietary prophylactic regimen developed one quarter as many major respiratory allergies as their siblings and a nonrelated control group. In addition, the incidence of atopic eczema was four times greater in the siblings than in the diet-restricted study group.

Johnson and Dutton [7] in a later prospective study were unable to establish that prophylactic feeding of soybean milk lessened the incidence of eczema. However, they did show that there was a lower incidence of bronchial asthma and perennial allergic rhinitis in children on prophylactic dietary restrictions.

Other investigators [9, 10, 11] have challenged the foregoing interpretations concerning the value of dietary prophylaxis in preventing allergic disease. A positive family history of allergy was documented in more than 30 percent of infants studied by Mueller, *et al.*[11] They contend that if cow's milk were to be omitted from the diets of these infants, it would result in a large number of infants being placed on a milk free diet to prevent milk allergy in a few.

The following discussion takes into consideration these conflicting opinions as to the value of dietary prophylaxis in infancy.

The food of choice for all infants is breast milk because of convenience, lower cost and low antigenicity. Allergy to human breast milk has not been clearly established. The nonallergenicity of breast milk was demonstrated experimentally by Hederstedt and Heijkenskjöld.[5] Grulee and Sanford [4] reported that the incidence of eczema in formula fed infants was seven times greater than in breast infants while Kimball and Jorgenson [8] in another study reported the incidence to be eight times greater.

Reactions to breast milk are usually the result of substances ingested by the mother which are then transferred in the breast milk to the infant. This was demonstrated in passive transfer experiments carried out by Donnelly.[1] Serum of a patient sensitive to egg white was passively transferred to a normal subject. The injection of breast milk from a mother who had eaten an egg into the transfer site resulted in a positive skin reaction.

Since the intestinal mucosa of an infant is not well developed and is presumably more permeable to food proteins than in a more mature individual, substances ingested by the mother and transmitted in her milk may infrequently cause sensitization and clinical symptoms in an infant. If this should occur, the diet of the mother should be restricted to avoid foods such as chocolate, nuts and eggs, which are important food allergens.

Recently, there has been an increase in the number of mothers who want to breast feed their infants, reversing the trend of many years. Societies have been formed to encourage this practice. Family physicians, pediatricians and allergists should advise mothers of newborns to breast feed their infants when possible, because of the benefits to the infant.

If a mother is unable to breast feed an infant, a breast milk substitute must be used. In the great majority of infants this may be one of many cow's milk formulas which have been modified in various ways to reduce curd tension, to increase digestibility and/or to reduce the solute load to the infant's immature kidneys.

It may be justifiable to avoid cow's milk if the infant is potentially allergic; for instance, the offspring of highly allergic individuals with histories of difficulties during infancy or the baby whose siblings had allergic manifestations during infancy. Cow's milk is probably the leading cause of allergic reactions due to food in infancy and childhood. The incidence of cow's milk allergy has been reported at between 1 and 7 percent of the pediatric population.

Potentially allergic infants, as described above, may be started on a soybean formula instead of cow's milk. These preparations were formerly unpalatable and often resulted in diarrhea and skin irritation. About 15 percent of patients studied by Glaser and Johnstone [2] had to have this formula discontinued because of these difficulties.

Newer, more palatable forms of soybean milk have been introduced which have apparently significantly reduced these problems (Neo-Mull-Soy,* Isomil †). Long-term nutritional and growth studies of children given soybean formulas have not revealed any deficiencies.

In certain infants where sensitivity to soybean milk is suspected or

* Trademark, Borden, Inc.
† Trademark, Ross Laboratories.

the preparation cannot be tolerated, substitute formulas with lamb base, poi or amino acids derived from the enzyme digestion of casein (Nutramigen † have been used successfully.

In the large majority of infants who are not considered to be potentially allergic, solid foods may be added according to the recommendation made in accepted texts of pediatric nutrition.

The introduction of the solid foods to the diet of the potentially allergic infant should be done cautiously. Infants have immature digestive systems; the likelihood of absorbing undigested food products which may sensitize the baby is increased. For at least the first 3 months of life, and most likely even longer, the nutrition supplied by milk or a formula substitute, and supplemental vitamins is entirely adequate. After this period of time, solids may be slowly introduced into the diet. When a potentially allergic infant is started on solid foods, he should first be given small amounts which can then be gradually increased in quantity. New foods should not be introduced at the same time but should be given at intervals of at least 4 days. This will help eliminate confusion as to the cause of a food sensitivity should it develop. Mixed foods in the form of cereals, dinners or deserts are contraindicated until the infant has been introduced to each item separately.

Cereals should be the first category of foods started, and this may be done at 3 months of age. While sensitivity to cereal grains is not as common as sensitivity to milk, it does occur.[3] Because all grain cereals are grass seeds, they are antigenically related. If an infant is sensitive to one cereal he may have cross-sensitivity to others. Rice is probably the least antigenic cereal because of its low protein content. Poi, which has been used for centuries in Hawaii, has certain advantages as a cereal substitute in early infancy. It is derived from taro and is unrelated to cereal grains grown in the continental United States. However, because of its taste it is sometimes difficult to get infants to accept poi as part of their diet. Following the introduction of cereal grains, the infant may then be given certain noncitrus fruits, vegetables, and finally meats at intervals of approximately 1 month.

Eggs, fish, wheat, citrus, nuts, chocolate and coca should be withheld from the diet of a potentially allergic infant for the first 9 to 12 months. When egg is introduced into the diet it should be done gradually. Egg yolk is given before egg white because the yolk is considered to be less antigenic. The infant may be given one fourth of a hard boiled egg yolk the first time. This should then be increased until the infant is getting a whole hard boiled egg yolk. Hard boiled eggwhite is then started in the same manner.

† Trademark, Mead Johnson Laboratories.

Most infants who have been on a soybean milk or lamb base formula may be taken off between 6 and 9 months of age. The change to cow's milk should be gradual and not abrupt.

Final conclusions as to the value of dietary prophylaxis cannot be made until further well controlled studies are performed. Each physician caring for a potentially allergic infant must weigh the possibility of preventing allergic manifestations against the difficulty of dietary prophylaxis. The arguments for and against dietary prophylaxis as a means of preventing allergic manifestations in infancy must be adequately discussed with the parents. Without the parents' complete understanding of the problems involved and their full cooperation no program of infant care will succeed. The recommendations discussed in this article can be carried out without great inconvenience to mother or infant and may be of benefit to the potentially allergic infant.

REFERENCES

1. Donnelly, H. H.: The question of elimination of foreign protein (egg white) in women's milk. J. Immun., *19:*15, 1930.
2. Glaser, J., and Johnstone, D. E.: Prophylaxis of allergic disease in the newborn infant. J. Allerg., *25:*447, 1954.
3. Glaser, J.: The dietary prophylaxis of allergic disease in infancy. J. Asthma Res., *3:*199, 1966.
4. Grulee, C. S., and Sanford, H. N.: The influence of breast and artificial feeding in infantile eczema, J. Pediat., *9:*223, 1936.
5. Hedenstedt, S., and Heijkenskjöld, F.: Intravenous milk infusion in children. Ann. Allerg., *22:*76, 1965.
6. Johnstone, D. E., and Glaser, J.: Use of soybean milk as an aid in prophylaxis of allergic disease in children. J. Allerg., *24:*434, 1953.
7. ———: Dietary prophylaxis of allergic disease in children. New Eng. J. Med., *274:*715, 1966.
8. Kimball, E. R., and Jorgensen, I. H.: A pilot study of the advantages of breast feeding. AMA Convention, Chicago, Ill. June 11-15, 1956.
9. Lowell, F. C., and Schiller, I. W.: Substitution of soybean milk for cow's milk in allergic infants. JAMA, *154:*262, 1954.
10. ———: It is so—it ain't so. J. Allerg., *25:*57, 1954.
11. Mueller, H. L., Weiss, R. J., O'Leary, D., and Murray, A. B.: The incidence of milk sensitivity and the development of allergy in infants. New Eng. J. Med., *268:*1220, 1963.

CORTICOSTEROIDS IN THE TREATMENT OF ALLERGIC DISEASES *

Phillip L. Lieberman, M.D.

Because corticosteroids are effective agents in the treatment of the allergic diseases they have gained wide usage. Indeed, it is difficult for the recently-trained physician to imagine an era when corticosteroids were not available. Over the past two decades, much has been learned about the pharmacology of these agents and the indications and contra-indications for their use. This chapter will deal with some of these observations.

GENERAL COMMENTS

Regardless of the disease in question, the corticosteroid drug administered, or the route of administration, certain generalities concerning corticosteroid therapy should be considered. Because of the well-documented side effects of these agents, the dose should always be maintained at the lowest level that will keep the patient comfortable and allow him to pursue his daily activities.

Corticosteroid therapy should only be initiated when more conservative measures have not adequately controlled symptoms. This is especially true for oral or parenteral administration. The physician therefore is charged with the responsibility of maintaining all other forms of therapy before and during treatment with corticosteroids. For example, a patient should never be receiving corticosteroids for asthma without the concomitant administration of bronchodilators, antibiotics as necessary, etc.

Frequent attempts to lower the dose and eventually discontinue corticosteroids should be made. This entails close observation of the patient and a constant reevaluation of the case. The initiation of corticosteroid therapy does not condemn the patient to a lifetime of such treatment. Steroid therapy does not in itself produce steroid dependency. In other words, the initiation of corticosteroids in asthma, for example, will not alter the illness so as to make the patient forever dependent on corticosteroids for relief. Brief courses of corticosteroids are commonly employed successfully in this and other allergic diseases.

* The author wishes to thank Dr. William E. Rosenberg and Dr. Tom Wood for their aid in preparing this section.

MECHANISMS OF ACTION

The exact mechanisms of action of corticosteroids in allergic disease is unknown. A detailed discussion of these mechanisms is beyond the scope of this chapter. However a few of the postulated mechanisms will be briefly mentioned.

Glucocorticoids clearly reduce inflammation. They exert their antiphlogistic effects through numerous pathways. They can reduce capillary permeability and inflammatory edema by maintaining the integrity of the capillary wall.[1] It has been suggested that cortisol has a stabilizing effect on the basement membrane and intracellular cement of capillaries to account for this reduction in permeability.[44] Lysosomal membranes are stabilized in vitro by the addition of corticosteroids.[43] Thus release of inflammatory substances within the lysosomes is prevented. It therefore appears that corticosteroids reduce inflammation by maintaining the integrity of the capillary wall and stabilizing cell membranes.

Corticosteroids seem to have little effect on histamine metabolism. They do not alter the in vitro release of histamine from leukocytes of sensitive individuals subsequent to antigen challenge or antagonize histamine at the target organ.[29] They may, however, interfere with the reaccumulation of histamine in the tissue after discharge.[16, 39] The failure of corticosteroids to effect histamine release or inhibit histamine effect at the target organ probably accounts for their negligible effect on the wheal and flare reaction of the immediate reacting skin test. This is of clinical significance in that it is not necessary to discontinue corticosteroids prior to skin testing.

In large doses, using animal models, corticosteroids have been shown to inhibit the primary and, to a lesser extent, the secondary immune response.[34] Such inhibition is probably insignificant in man on the usual dose of corticosteroids employed to treat allergic diseases. Improvement in symptoms occurring after steroid therapy occurs too rapidly to imply a role for decreased antibody synthesis. In addition IgE levels appear to remain unchanged after corticosteroid therapy.[19]

There is a complex relationship between corticosteroids and catecholamine physiology and metabolism. Corticosteroids, in pharmacologic doses, seem to potentiate certain effects of the vasoactive catecholamines.[35] The precise mechanism involved in this potentiation is unknown. It is postulated, however, that corticosteroids may either increase the receptivity of the beta receptor or support the action of cyclic AMP.[15] This theory is not consistent with evidence obtained in histamine release studies in vitro. In this system in vitro, which is adenyl cyclase-dependent, steroids have no effect.

In summary, no conclusive statement may be made concerning the mechanism of action of corticosteroids in the allergic diseases. None-theless the most attractive hypothesis involves the ability of cortico-steroids to maintain the integrity of cell membranes and the micro-vascular wall.

TOPICAL CUTANEOUS CORTICOSTEROIDS

Corticosteroids applied to the skin are useful in atopic dermatitis and contact dermatitis. They are usually of little benefit in acute, severe, contact dermatitis, such as that caused by poison ivy, where systemic corticosteroids may be required, depending on the extent of the lesion.

Topical corticosteroids have gained wide usage in these dermatoses because of their effectiveness, safety, and ease of administration. Nevertheless, when prescribing these preparations, the physician faces several practical problems ranging from mild inconveniences to po-tentially serious side effects. These agents are expensive if used ex-tensively; there is a delivery problem when the lesions are generalized; there are over 200 preparations available, making selection of individual preparations difficult; and finally, adverse side effects can occur.

The problem of expense as well as that of delivery (in generalized dermatitis) can usually be solved by diluting commercially available agents in a hydrophilic ointment base.[3] Most cases of atopic dermatitis do not require the 0.025%, 0.1% or 0.5% corticosteroid strengths that are commercially available. Therefore a proper dilution in hydrophyl-lic ointment, U.S.P., will still provide an effective concentration while markedly reducing the cost of therapy. In addition, the ointment itself is valuable for its moisturizing effect. Two sample prescriptions are as follows:

1

        0.1% Betamethasone valerate cream   15
        Hydrophilic ointment U.S.P.
                  To make   150
    Label: 0.01% Betamethasone valerate cream
    sig: Use liberally on skin, rub in well

2

        0.1% Triamcinolone acetonide cream   15
        Hydrophilic ointment U.S.P.
                  To make   150
    Label: 0.01% Triamcinolone acetonide cream
    sig: Use liberally on skin, rub in well

These diluted preparations are safe, efficacious and relatively inexpen-sive. The patient should be told to apply them frequently. A tube of full strength medication should also be available for periodic, acute exacerbations and for localized areas not controlled by diluted corticosteroid agents.

The problem of choice of commercial preparations can be puzzling to a physician who uses these agents only occasionally. Fortunately, objective evaluation of the effect of cutaneous corticosteroids is now available both by a bioassay method [27] and by controlled clinical trials.[37] The more commonly used agents have been evaluated by these methods. Table 18-3 lists some of these preparations. They are listed in rough

TABLE 18-3
Topical Corticosteroid Preparations *

GENERIC NAME	BRAND NAME	PREPARATION	PARABEN PRESERVATIVE IN CREAM
Fluocinonide	Lidex	Cream 0.1%	No
Betamethasone valerate	Valisone	Cream 0.1% Ointment 0.1%	No
Fluocinolone acetonide	Synalar	Cream 0.01% 0.025% 0.2% (synalar HP) Ointment 0.025%	Yes
Triamcinolone acetonide	Kenalog Aristocort	Cream 0.1% 0.025% Ointment 0.1% 0.025%	(Kenalog) Yes (Aristocort) No
Flurandrenolide	Cordran	Cream 0.025% 0.05% Ointment 0.025% 0.05%	Yes

* Preparations are listed in order of their potency (starting with Fluocinonide) as determined by the McKenzie assay system.

order of potency according to their effectiveness (Lidex being the most potent) as judged by the McKenzie assay system.[27] This system is an in vivo assay of the cutaneous vasoconstrictive potency of topical corticosteroid compounds.

In addition to the agents cited in Table I, hydrocortisone cream or ointment is also available in 0.125%, 0.25%, 0.5% and 1.0% strengths. This preparation, although much less effective than those cited in the table, is less expensive and is generally effective in the treatment of atopic dermatitis or contact dermatitis.

Several practical points will aid in the administration of cutaneously applied corticosteroids. The patient should be instructed to apply liberal amounts frequently. The preparations should be rubbed into the skin as well as possible, although this is more difficult with the ointment base. Thickly applied layers are both inconvenient and unnecessary. Absorption can be increased and effectiveness improved with occlusive dressings applied overnight. This can be accomplished by employing plastic film wraps such as Glad Wrap, Saran Wrap, etc. This principal is also applied in flurandrenolide tape (Cordran tape), which may be used in small areas, where its expense does not prohibit its use. It must be remembered that occlusive dressings also increase the incidence of adverse side effects.[20]

Side Effects and Adverse Reactions. In general, adverse effects of cutaneously applied corticosteroids are minimal. Using dilute preparations in hydrophilic ointment, they are extremely rare. Local adverse reactions have been reported as follows: burning sensations, itching, irritation, dryness, folliculitis, acneiform eruptions and hypopigmentation. In addition, skin atrophy, secondary infection, maceration, and striae can occur. The latter complications are more frequently associated with the use of occlusive dressings. Contact dermatitis can develop to the vehicle or the preservative used. Paraben preservatives are known to cause this type of complication. Table 18-3 lists those preparations with parabens. If such a reaction does occur a preparation not containing parabens should be substituted.

Adrenal suppression may occur following extensive generalized use of cutaneous corticosteroids.[20] Although such incidences are rare they are a complication to be considered when topical corticosteroids are used extensively. Finally, these agents may exacerbate cutaneous fungal, viral, and bacterial diseases. They may be contraindicated in the presence of such lesions.

Topical Nasal Corticosteroid Therapy

Corticosteroids applied topically to the nasal mucosa can be used effectively in the treatment of allergic and vasomotor rhinitis and rhinitis medicamentosa. They are also useful in the control of nasal polyps [12] of both allergic and nonallergic etiology, and in the treatment of serous otitis media, where eustachian obstruction may be aggravated by upper respiratory allergies.[22]

Corticosteroids may be applied to the nasal mucosa using an aerosol spray of dexamethasone sodium phosphate (Decadron Turbinaire *). The aerosol cartridge contains the equivalent of 15 mg. dexamethasone. Each spray delivers the equivalent of .084 mg. dexamethasone. There-

* Trademark, Merck Sharp & Dohme.

fore 12 sprays deliver the theoretical maximum of 1.0 mg. of dexamethasone. The cartridge is filled to deliver approximately 170 such sprays.

Therapy with this aerosol is indicated only over relatively short periods of time such as during a well-defined pollen season, as a 4- to 6-week trial for reducing nasal polyps, or during the 1- to 3-week period required to reverse the nasal mucosal inflammation of rhinitis medicamentosa. This form of topical steroid treatment should be considered an adjunct to routine allergic therapy and should not substitute for other forms of management. It should be remembered that the anti-inflammatory actions of topical steroids are slow in onset. The patient should be told that he will not obtain immediate relief of symptoms with the aerosol, and that it is not to be used without specific medical advice. This is especially important in the patient with rhinitis medicamentosa who is being weaned from topical vasoconstrictor drugs.

A suggested dosage regimen for allergic rhinitis, nasal polyposis or rhinitis medicamentosa is shown in Table 18-4.

TABLE 18-4
Tapering Dosage Regimen for Dexamethasone Nasal Spray °

2 sprays in each nostril—q.i.d. (16 sprays /day)—for one week	followed by
2 sprays in " " —t.i.d. (12 sprays /day)—for one week	followed by
1 spray in " " —q.i.d. (8 sprays /day)—for one week	
1 spray in " " —t.i.d. (6 sprays /day)—for 4 days	followed by
1 spray in " " —b.i.d. (4 sprays /day)—for 3 days	

° In children this dosage regimen should be altered according to the size and age of the child.

Side Effects and Adverse Reactions. Although topical nasal corticosteroids can be used with relative safety it is important to note that systemic absorption occurs and can result in adrenal cortical suppression.[10] The degree of suppression is usually minimal, and normal function usually returns a few days after cessation of therapy.[30] Topical nasal corticosteroids should not be used in the presence of viral and fungal nasal disease or ocular herpes simplex, and they should be used with caution in any case where there is a contraindication to the use of systemic corticosteroids.

Topical Ocular Corticosteroids

Topical ocular corticosteroid administration is useful in atopic allergic conjunctivitis, vernal conjunctivitis and certain cases of uveitis. It is very effective in atopic conjunctivitis. Nevertheless the possible complications of topical ocular croticosteroid therapy are numerous and potentially grave Their use can result in permanent blindness in cases of herpes simplex conjunctivitis or other forms of corneal ulcers. In addition, they can precipitate open angle glaucoma and dispose to the formation of posterior subcapsular cataracts. For these reasons they should be administered only under the close supervision of an ophthalmologist.

Topical Bronchial Corticosteroids

Topical bronchial corticosteroids are of little value in the treatment of asthma. Although they may be somewhat effective, they are readily absorbed and therefore can cause all the side effects associated with systemic administration. [11, 25, 31] For this reason systemic administration, where the dose is more easily controlled, is preferable to topical bronchial therapy.

SYSTEMIC CORTICOSTEROIDS

Systemic corticosteroids are effective in all the diseases in which topical preparations can be used and are also of benefit in certain diseases in which topical compounds are of little value. Their advantages over topical preparations are their greater effectiveness and the greater accuracy with which their actual dosage can be controlled. The disadvantage to their use is the greater incidence and severity of adverse side effects. Corticosteroids may be administered systemically by the oral, intravenous, or intramuscular route.

Oral Administration

Oral preparations are useful in the symptomatic relief of numerous allergic diseases. They are highly effective agents in allergic contact dermatitis, atopic dermatitis, serum sickness, allergic rhinitis and asthma. Because of their well-known side effects, their safest use is in the acute, self-limited diseases such as serum sickness or poison ivy dermatitis. They should be used with caution in any chronic disease and should never be instituted in such cases unless all other forms of therapy have proven ineffective.

Allergic contact dermatitis, seasonal allergic rhinitis, and serum sickness are examples of diseases in which a brief course of corticosteroid therapy is relatively safe and generally very effective. Steroids are indicated in allergic contact dermatitis and serum sickness if the disease is extensive or the symptoms severe. The initial dose should be moderately high (the equivalent of 30 to 40 mg. of prednisone) and can be rapidly tapered. In most instances, one to two weeks of therapy is sufficient. In cases of allergic rhinitis, steroids may be indicated at the peak of a particular pollen season. A two- to three-week course of therapy once or twice a year would be a reasonable regimen in patients with severe seasonal exacerbations. Corticosteroid therapy should not replace other allergic management in this disease, and corticosteroids should not be administered chronically for relief of rhinitis.

Oral corticosteroids are also effective in the more prolonged allergic diseases of atopic dermatitis and asthma. In the former illness they are only very rarely, if ever indicated, such as when the disease is extremely extensive and cannot be reasonably controlled by other measures. Even in such cases they are best used only intermittently, for exacerbations of the disease.

Before corticosteroids are used in asthma, all other forms of therapy should be instituted and continued. If these measures have failed to produce adequate control for maintenance of function, corticosteroids are indicated. Failure of other forms of therapy should be considered to have occurred only under circumstances in which the patient's survival is threatened or when he is unable to perform necessary daily tasks. Examples of these types of situations are the patient who experiences multiple hospital admissions, is missing many work days or school days, or is unable to do housework or care for her children. If such a situation does exist, it is best to attempt to control the patient with short courses of corticosteroids during exacerbations of the illness. This should be accomplished with moderately high initial doses (equivalent to 30 to 50 mg. prednisone daily) followed by a slow tapering. The tapering should not be accomplished as rapidly as in allergic contact dermatitis. It is often necessary to treat for one to two months before steroids can be discontinued.

If short courses of therapy are not effective, chronic daily or every-other-day therapy should be instituted. The latter is preferable in regard to adrenal suppression [17] and especially in regard to the prevention of linear growth retardation in children. Alternate-day therapy appears to be beneficial in decreasing the severity of the other side effects of steroid administration. However, the effectiveness of alternate-day therapy in this regard is difficult to assess. Another advantage of the alternate-day regimen is that it is less suppressive to fever and causes less white count elevation. Thus two parameters useful to the physician in determining the presence of inflammation remain intact. Finally the alternate-day regimen may make it less difficult to discontinue corticosteroids in patients who have been on long-term maintenance, since there is less adrenal-pituitary axis depression. Therefore, if possible, the entire dose should be given on alternate days in the morning. It must be remembered that alternate day therapy is not to be used initially during the acute attack. It is only a maintenance form of administration. Initiation of therapy should be accomplished with daily administration. An alternate-day regimen is then instituted when the acute symptoms have been alleviated. The transition from daily to alternate-day treatment is often difficult, especially if the patient has been on daily doses for several months. And, in the author's experience, some patients do not do well even on repeated attempts to make this transition. Regardless of the schedule of administration, the patient should be maintained on as low a dose as will provide adequate control. Most patients can be maintained on a dose ranging between 7.5 mg. and 15 mg. of prednisone daily (15 to 30 mg. q.i.d.), although some patients require much more.[23] Some patients seem to require much larger mean doses on alternate-day therapy than on daily therapy, especially during the transition from the latter to the former.[18]

Dosage increments may be necessary to control asthma during acute exacerbations such as those precipitated by infection. Increments should be initiated with relatively high doses followed by slow tapering as described above.

The complications of chronic steroid administration are well known. Fluid retention, weight gain, peptic ulcer disease, hypertension, osteoporosis, reactivation tuberculosis, increased capillary fragility, cataract formation, diabetes mellitus, psychosis, growth retardation, and exogenous Cushing's syndrome are some of the more common adverse effects. Nevertheless, the incidence of severe, life-threatening or debilitating complications is low in the average asthmatic requiring a mean dose of 5 to 15 mg. prednisone daily. Most untoward effects are related to weight gain and fluid retention.[23] In the vast majority of cases, the degree of severity of the complications does not require cessation of therapy and is not comparable to the morbidity which would ensue if the corticosteroids were discontinued.

Certain difficult problems frequently arise in patients who are on chronic corticosteroid therapy. The pregnant patient, the patient requiring surgery, and the patient with a known peptic ulcer all require special consideration when they are taking corticosteroids.

Corticosteroid administration during pregnancy seems to entail little risk to the mother.[26, 36, 41, 42] * Although experimental data obtained in animals suggests a higher incidence of fetal malformation, death and prematurity,[2, 13, 14, 24] epidemiologic data in humans is sparse and controversial.[4, 26, 36, 41, 42] At this time it would appear that there is a slight increase in fetal morbidity when the mother is taking corticosteroids. However, the risk is probably not as grave as that which would occur if severe asthma with its associate hypoxemia were not controlled.

* Personal communication, Roy Patterson, M.D.

It would therefore appear that the safest course would be to keep the pregnant asthmatic on as low a dose of corticosteroids as possible while maintaining her relatively free of symptoms. The majority of patients with asthma who become pregnant can be managed with routine therapy without corticosteroids. Those patients who have demonstrated severe asthma prior to becoming pregnant and have required corticosteroids for control prior to pregnancy should not have these agents suddenly decreased or discontinued. Fetal anoxia due to severe asthma is a potentially greater risk than low dose maintenance with prednisone. The patient must be followed closely and with the minimal dose which will keep her reasonably comfortable.

General surgery for an asthmatic taking corticosteroids should only be done when the patient is as free of symptoms as possible. Therefore it is often desirable to increase the steroid dose a few days prior to the operation if the patient is symptomatic. Doses of corticosteroids large enough to maintain the absence of symptoms should be continued through surgery and during the immediate postoperative period. The acute operative morbidity due to bronchospasm and its pulmonary consequences is of much more concern than that due to brief, high dose corticosteroid treatment.

Any patient who has been receiving corticosteroids chronically must be assumed to have a suppressed adrenal response to stress. Therefore, the asthmatic on corticosteroids should be given adequate amounts of steroids before, during, and immediately after surgery. When the patient is unable to take oral medication, cortisone acetate may be given intramuscularly the day before and after surgery until oral intake is resumed. Hydrocortisone or methyl prednisolone may be given intravenously during the procedure. The dose of these drugs is dependent on the dose of corticosteroids the patient was requiring prior to the procedure.

The patient with known peptic ulcer disease who needs corticosteroids does not represent an insoluble therapeutic problem. Although it is widely held that oral corticosteroid administration predisposes patients to peptic ulcer disease,[21, 40] much of the data supporting this point of view has been tabulated from studies concerning patients with chronic diseases other than asthma, such as rheumatoid arthritis. When data limited to asthmatics is reviewed, the frequency and severity of ulcer disease during steroid administration is somewhat less striking, especially in regards to the severity of complications such as gastrointestinal bleeding. Nevertheless, there does appear to be a definitely increased incidence of ulcer related complaints in asthmatics on long-term steroid therapy.[23] The most reasonable approach to this problem would be to initiate or continue steroid therapy with simultaneous ulcer treatment. If the patient is hospitalized, and high doses of steroids are needed, regular milk and antacids may be given. If the patient is ambulatory he should be instructed to be alert to gastrointestinal symptoms, and ulcer therapy should be started if such symptoms occur.

The choice of oral preparations is of relatively little importance except in regards to the duration of action of the preparations when the patient is on alternate-day therapy. Longer acting drugs such as betamethasone, dexamethasone, triamcinolone or paramethasone may produce adrenal suppression even on alternate-day therapy. It is also noteworthy that certain commercial preparations contain tartrazine (yellow No. 5), an aniline dye used as a coloring agent. These preparations are Decadron * (dexamethasone), Deronil † (dexamethasone), and Paracort ‡ (prednisone). In sensitive persons this dye can in itself cause asthma [7] as well as urticaria [28] and anaphylactoid purpura.[9]

In summary, the long-term use of oral corticosteroids is indicated only in those cases in whom all other forms of therapy have failed. Such use is associated with well-known adverse effects, but these effects are not, in the vast majority of patients who are controlled with minimal or moderate doses, of grave consequence. They consist mainly of fluid retention and its sequellae. Alternate-day therapy is preferable to daily therapy, and vigorous attempts should be made to maintain a patient on an alternate-day regimen. It should be noted, however, that most patients require every-day therapy initially and are switched to alternate-day treatment only after symptoms are controlled. Regardless of the regimen of administration, frequent attempts should be made to decrease the dose and the patient should be maintained on the lowest dose that will allow him to continue his functional role in society. Tapering of the dose must be done slowly. A 2.5 mg. to 5 mg. drop of the daily dose each week is a reasonable regimen to follow. During acute exacerbations of the disease and during respiratory infections the dose must be raised. In such acute situations it is best to err on the side of giving too much rather than too little.

Intravenous

Intravenous corticosteroids are used in status asthmaticus, anaphylaxis and during surgery on an asthmatic who has been taking corticosteroids. In both instances it is best to be certain the amount administered is adequate. In status asthmaticus, a rigid dosage regimen of intravenous corticosteroids has not been established. Recommendations range from at least 200 to 300 mg. hydrocortisone over the first 24 to 48 hours [40]

* Trademark, Merck Sharp & Dohme.
† Trademark, Schering.
‡ Trademark, Parke, Davis.

to a dose adequate to keep plasma-11-hydroxycorticosteroids at a level of 150 μg. per 100 cc.,[8] which would require 2500 to 3000 mg. in 24 hours in a 70-kilogram man. The morbidity associated with high dose administration of corticosteroids to asthmatics over a two to three day period is minimal. Hypokalemia seems to be the only side effect of major significance.[8] Because of this low incidence of complications as compared with the risk of death in status asthma, a high dose regimen seems preferable. It is worth noting that the onset of action of intravenous corticosteroids is not immediate. A delay of several hours may exist before a therapeutic effect is achieved. Thus steroids are not to be depended upon to afford immediate relief in any allergic disorder. This is especially important in dealing with anaphylaxis.

Intramuscular

Intramuscular corticosteroids are of use in two instances. Intramuscular cortisone acetate is useful in the surgical preparation of an asthmatic who has been on prolonged corticosteroid administration. Sustained action intramuscular Depo-medrol * is occasionally used for chronic treatment under circumstances in which oral agents cannot be used. Such a circumstance exists in patients unable to understand or follow directions. Depo-medrol can also be useful in rare instances when the physician suspects that the patient is doing poorly because of an intentional but covert refusal to take on oral preparation. If Depo-medrol is substituted for the oral preparation over a two week period, and the patient improves, the suspicion may be well grounded.

The disadvantage of the depot preparation is that there is no way to determine the exact daily dosage because the sustained release mechanism does not assure an equal amount of corticosteroid release each 24-hour period. In practice the physician usually multiplies the ideal daily dose by 7 and administers this amount of Depo-medrol each week. Unfortunately this does not guarantee an even and equal release each hour.

Whenever intramuscular Depo-medrol or any corticosteroid preparation is administered the physician has certain responsibilities to the patient. He should inform the patient of the fact that he is taking a corticosteroid preparation and of the hazards involved in this form of therapy.

The Use of ACTH

In most, if not all, instances, corticosteroid administration is preferable to ACTH administration in the treatment of allergic disease. The dose is more easily controlled with corticosteroid administration. In addition

* Trademark, Upjohn.

anaphylactic reactions to ACTH have occurred in both children and adults.[5, 32, 38] Although the risk of anaphylaxis is probably small, it must be considered whenever the drug is administered to an atopic individual.

It has been suggested that ACTH be used to stimulate the adrenal gland when long-term corticosteroid therapy is being discontinued. Although this approach appears rational it has been shown to be of little benefit in rheumatoid patients on long-term corticosteroid therapy.[38] Paradoxically, ACTH administered for this purpose may result in increased pituitary-adrenal suppression.[38] Gradual reduction in corticosteroid dosage without ACTH administration can be accomplished without risk of hypocortisolism. Thus there appears to be little reason for employing ACTH in the treatment of allergic diseases.

REFERENCES

1. Benditt, E. P., Schiller, S. W., and Dorfman, A.: Influence of ACTH and cortisone upon alteration in capillary permeability induced by hyaluronidase in rats. Proc. Soc. Exp. Biol., 75:782, 1950.
2. Blackburn, W. R., Kaplan, H. S., and McKay, D. G.: Morphologic change in the developing rat placenta following prednisone administration. Am. J. Obstet. Gynec., 92:234, 1965.
3. Blank, H.: Clinical trials, a scientific discipline. J. Invest. Derm., 37:235, 1961.
4. Bongiovanni, A. M. and McPadden, A. J.: Steroids during pregnancy and possible foetal consequences. Fertil. Steril., 11:181, 1960.
5. Buytendijk, H. and Maesen, F.: Comparative skin tests with animal and synthetic corticotrophin in patients hypersensitive to animal corticotrophin. Acta. Endocrin., 47:13, 1964.
6. Carter, M. E. and James, H. J.: An attempt at combining corticotrophin with long term corticosteroid therapy. An. Rheum. Dis., 29:409, 1970.
7. Chafee, F. H. and Settipane, G. A.: Asthma caused by F D and C approved dyes. J. Allerg., 40:65, 1967.
8. Collins, J. V., Clark, T. J., Harris, P. W. R., and Townsend, J.: Intravenous corticosteroids in treatment of acute bronchial asthma. Lancet, 2:1047, 1970.
9. Criep, L. H.: Allergic vascular purpura. J. Allerg., 48:7, 1971.
10. Czarny, D. and Brostoff, J.: Effect of intranasal betamethasone-17—valerate on perennial rhinitis and adrenal function. Lancet, 2:188, 1968.
11. Dennis, M. and Itkin, I. H.: Effectiveness and complications of aerosol dexamethasone phosphate in severe asthma. J. Allerg., 35:70, 1964.
12. The Drug Committee of the Research Council of the American Academy of Allergy: A double-blind labeled study of dexamethasone nasal

aerosol vs placebo in the treatment of nasal polyposis. J. Allerg., *41*:10, 1968.

13. Fraser, F. C.: 2nd Int. Conf. Congenital Malformations. International Medical Congress, New York, 1963.

14. Fraser, F. C. and Fainstat, T. D.: Production of congenital defects in the offspring of mice treated with cortisone. Pediatrics, *8*:527, 1951.

15. Friedman, N., Exton, J., and Park, C. R.: Permissive effect of glucorosticord on the stimulation of gluconeogeneisis by glucagon and epinephrine: role of cyclic adenylate. Fed. Proc., *27*:625, 1968.

16. Goth, A., Allman, R. M., Merrit, B. C., and Holman, J.: Effect of cortisone on histamine liberation induced by Tween in the dog. Proc. Soc. Exp. Biol., *78*:848, 1951.

17. Harter, J. A., Redd, W. J., and Thorn, G. W.: Studies on intermittent corticosteroid dosage regimen, New Eng. J. Med., *269*:591, 1963.

18. Harter, J. G.: in Steroid Therapy, a clinical update for the 1970's published by Medcom Inc., 1970.

19. Johansson, S. G. O., Bennich, H., Berg, T., and Hogman, C.: Some factors influencing the serum IgE levels in atopic diseases. Clin. Exp. Immunol., *6*:43, 1970.

20. Keipert, J. A.: Percutaneous absorption of Topical Corticosteroids in Infancy and Childhood. Med. J. Aust., *1*:119, 1021-1025, 1971.

21. Kirsner, J. B., Kassriel, R. S., and Palmer, W. L.: Peptic ulcer: review of the literature pertaining to the etiology, pathogenesis and certain clinical aspects. Adv. Intern. Med., *8*:41, 1956.

22. Lecks, H. I., Kravis, L. P., and Wood, D. W.: Serous otitis media: reflections on pathogenesis and treatment. Clin. Pediat., *6*:519, 1967.

23. Lieberman, P., Patterson, R., and Kunske, R.: Complications of long term steroid therapy for asthma. (submitted for publication Sept. 1971.)

24. Liggins, G. C.: Premature parturition after infusion of corticotrophin or cortisol into foetal lambs. J. Endocrin., *42*:323, 1968.

25. Linden, W. R.: Adrenal suppression by aerosol steroid inhalators. Arch. Intern. Med., *113*:655, 1964.

26. McAllen, M.: Long term side effects of corticosteroids. Respiration (Supplement), *27*:250, 1970.

27. McKenzie, A. W. and Stoughton, R. R.: Method for comparing percutaneous absorption of steroids. Arch. Derm., *86*:608, 1962.

28. Madden, S.: Urticaria following betamethasone. J.A.M.A., *192*:368, 1965.

29. Norman, P. S. and Lichtenstein, L. M.: Allergic rhinitis: clinical course and treatment. *In* Samter, M., ed.: Immunologic Diseases, Boston, Little Brown, 1971.

30. Norman, P. S., Winkenwerder, W. L., Agbayani, B. F., and Migeon, C. J.: Adrenal function during the use of dexamethasone aerosols in the treatment of ragweed hay fever. J. Allerg., *40*:57, 1967.

31. Novey, H. S. and Beall, G.: Aerosolyzed steroids and induced Cushing's syndrome. Arch. Intern. Med., *115*:602, 1965.

32. Perkoff, G. T., Jager, B. V., and Tyler, F. H.: Complications in the man-

agement of Cushing's syndrome, including anaphylactic reactions to intravenous adrenocorticotrophin after subtotal adrenalectomy. J. Clin. Endocrin., *15*:362, 1955.

33. Radermecker, M. and Rose, B.: Bronchial asthma: clinical course and treatment. *In* Samter, M., ed.: Immunologic Diseases, p. 889. Boston, Little Brown, 1971.
34. Raffel, S.: Immunity. ed. 2. New York, Appleton-Century-Crofts, 1961.
35. Ramey, E. R. and Goldstein, M. S.: The adrenal cortex and the sympathetic nervous system. Physiol. Rev., *37*:155, 1957.
36. Rees, H. A. and Williams, D. A.: Long term steroid therapy in chronic intractable asthma. Brit. Med. J., *1*:575, 1962.
37. Rosenberg, E. W., Fluocinonide: preliminary evaluation of a new topical corticosteroid. (In press)
38. Rosenblum, A. H. and Rosenblum, P.: Anaphylactic reactions to adrenocorticotropic hormone in children. J. Pediat., *64*:387, 1964.
39. Schayer, R. W., Smiley, R. L., and Davis, K. L.: Inhibition by cortisone of the binding of new histamine in rat tissues. Proc. Soc. Exp. Biol., *87*:590, 1954.
40. Spiro, H. M.: Stomach damage from aspirine, steroids, and antimetabolites. Am. J. Dig. Dis., *7*:733, 1962.
41. Walsh, S. P. and Grant, L.: Corticosteroids in the treatment of chronic asthma. Brit. Med. J., *2*:796, 1966.
42. Warrell, D. W. and Taylor, R.: Outcome of the foetus of mothers receiving prednisone during pregnancy. Lancet, *117*:1968.
43. Weissman, G. and Themos, L.: The effect of corticosteroids upon connective tissue and lysosomes. Rec. Progr. Hormone Res., *20*:215, 1964.
44. Zarem, H. A. and Zweibach, B. W.: Microcirculatory effects of cortisol. Protective action against Na_4 EDTA damage. Proc. Soc. Exp. Biol., *118*:602, 1965.

TREATMENT FAILURES IN ALLERGIC DISEASES

INTRODUCTION

The initiation of any standard therapeutic regimen for treatment of allergic diseases, is expected to result in significant clinical improvement. The degree of improvement depends on the type of clinical problem. For example, significant improvement may be expected with a full therapeutic regimen used for extrinsic (atopic) asthma. Clinical control of disease—but control to a lesser degree than in extrinsic asthma—may be expected in cases of "intrinsic" asthma. The detection of an environmental antigen and its complete avoidance may be followed by a disappearance of symptoms (considered a clinical cure) if the atopic problem was the result of a single sensitivity. In most cases of chronic allergic disease, the results of therapy are rarely this dramatic and the patient and his physician must be satisfied with control of symptoms rather than a cure. In certain cases, the results of therapy appear inadequate, either to patient or physician, or both. When this situation occurs, the clinical problem must be reevaluated to determine whether the diagnosis is correct and the treatment appropriate. In certain cases the interpretation of a clinical result as a treatment failure is inappropriate, since the result may actually be the best that can be accomplished with current therapeutic regimens. In this situation it is a matter of attitude, and the patient and physician must recognize the problem and discuss the results which are reasonable to attain. This section discusses "treatment failures" in three common clinical problems: asthma, urticaria and rhinitis.

TREATMENT FAILURES IN ALLERGIC RHINITIS

Roy Patterson, M.D.

Objective clinical evaluation of the severity of allergic rhinitis is possible to some extent on the basis of nasal examination. In most cases, the evaluation of clinical severity and the degree of improvement subsequent to therapy is dependent on the subjective interpretation by the patient. The chronicity of symptoms, the long intervals between episodes of recurrent seasonal pollenosis, geographic changes, age changes and variation between pollenation seasons are only some of the variables that make long term evaluation of progress difficult. In spite of these difficulties, it is generally possible to evaluate patients with allergic rhinitis and determine whether the expected improvement as a result of therapy has occurred. In those cases in which the patient does not report the expected improvement, the following may be considered as possible explanations.

False Expectations

In treating cases of allergic rhinitis due to environmental antigens that cannot be completely removed or avoided, the complete control of symptoms by symptomatic and immunologic control may not be possible. The objective of therapy is control and improvement of symptoms. If the patient expects symptoms to disappear completely—as the result of inadequate information by his physician or misinformation from other laymen—he may actually have significant clinical improvement at the same time he is informing his physician that there is inadequate improvement.

The treatment of seasonal pollenosis with immunotherapy may be followed by limited improvement the first season, but subsequent seasons may show increasing improvement and, in these cases, some patience is advised. These problems may be prevented by adequately explaining to the patient at the outset what he may expect from allergic therapy.

Presence of Significant Allergens

One of the most significant causes of poor results of treatment are inadequate control or recognition of allergens. Examples include the introduction to the environment of allergens unknown to the physician. These are commonly cats or dogs, but gerbils, guinea pigs, rats, mice and birds may be highly significant factors. These animals may be introduced after therapy is started or may not have been eliminated because the physician did not consider them significant. Occasionally, a patient will conceal from the physician that he has retained or introduced a pet to the environment. Animal-sensitive patients may suffer symptoms upon moving into a dwelling previously occupied by individuals who had pets.

A new sensitivity may develop while therapy is in progress, particularly in children. This may be to an animal in the environment or to an aeroallergen.

Rhinitis Medicamentosa

This topic is discussed in the chapter on allergic rhinitis. It may appear during therapy of a patient who was not using vasoconstrictive nose drops during initial evaluation and so was not warned about the danger of chronic use. Occasionally the nose drops will be prescribed by a different physician and the patient feels this implies safety and does not inform the allergist of their use.

Vasomotor Rhinitis

Vasomotor rhinitis has also been discussed in detail elsewhere. This nonimmunologic, hyperreactive state of the nasal mucosa is differentiated without too much difficulty from allergic rhinitis by the usual allergic history and skin tests. Diagnostic and therapeutic problems arise in those cases of rhinitis in which the predominant cause of symptoms is the result of nonallergic vasomotor rhinitis but where the patient has positive cutaneous reactions to inhalant allergens. It is occasionally not recognized that both nonallergic vasomotor rhinitis or nonallergic "intrinsic" asthma can be the major or entire cause of symptoms in the presence of such cutaneous reactivity.

A marked increase in vasomotor rhinitis may occur during pregnancy, and, in the patient whose previous diagnosis was allergic rhinitis, may lead to further allergic investigations for allergens that are not contributing to the increase in symptoms.

Nasal Polyposis

Polyps may recur or occur for the first time during the course of a regimen of allergic therapy. Since this is generally unexpected, the diagnosis may not be made unless a thorough nasal examination is done.

Smoking and Other Irritants

Persistent irritation resulting from chronic, excessive use of tobacco —with or without the association of increased bacterial infection of the nasopharyngeal region—may be a cause of significant symptoms in patients. Other irritants, including air pollution, may be significant in certain patients. The effect of the latter in individual patients may be difficult to determine.

Sinusitis

Chronic sinusitis in the presence or absence of nasal polyposis may contribute to persistent nasal symptoms.

Wrong Allergen

Occasionally it is not recognized that the major allergen for certain patients during the warm seasons may be mold antigens. The initial diagnosis of pollenosis may have appeared logical because of history and cutaneous reactivity suggestive of these antigens when actually mold, animal danders or house dust antigen are more important but were not diagnosed or treated adequately.

Failure of Environmental Control

Patients with rhinitis due to house dust may initiate a dust control program at the beginning of an allergy program but subsequently ignore these precautions. The use of plastic covers for mattress and pillows and other relatively simple dust control measure will aid this clinical problem.

Nasal Deformities

At times, structural deformities of the nasal passages may be sufficiently severe that the marked alteration in air flow may contribute to the symptoms of rhinitis. In these cases, surgical correction may be considered.

Symptomatic Control

The patient with significant allergic rhinitis requiring symptomatic control with antihistamines, sympathomimetic amines or both may be taking these in inadequate dosage. Patients who have relief of symptoms with an antihistamine may find that it becomes less effective with prolonged use. In this case, substitution of an antihistamine of a different class should be attempted as discussed in the chapter on allergic rhinitis.

Inadequate Immunotherapy

The degree of effectiveness of long term immunotherapy appears dependent on the dose of antigen administered. Adequate doses of antigen may not have been achieved because of inability of the patient to tolerate them, irregularity of patient visits, or inexperience of the physician managing the treatment program. In certain patients it is possible that the doses of antigen administered may increase the nasal symptoms, although this is uncommon in the absence of marked local reactions.

Other Possible Explanations for Treatment Failures in Cases of Allergic Rhinitis

Rarely, a wrong diagnosis explains the failure to improve clinically. For example, a patient's chronic sinusitis may be diagnosed as allergic rhinitis. A rare condition causing rhinorrhea is a puncture in the cribiform plate of the ethmoid bone with cerebrospinal fluid appearing as nasal secretions. This condition is the result of head trauma with a skull fracture or a sharp object in the nose. Recognition is essential as surgical repair can prevent meningitis.

The initiation of reserpine for the management of hypertension may result in significant nasal congestion. This medication may be started by another physician unknown to the allergist. Hypothyroidism may be accompanied by nasal symptoms and could be a possible correlation with poor treatment results. Patients may move from one area to another and have an increase in symptoms because pollen concentrations vary in different geographic areas. Finally, certain patients may have poor results to an adequate treatment regimen and must be classed as treatment failures.

TREATMENT FAILURES IN ASTHMA

Angelo E. Falleroni, M.D.

NATURAL COURSE OF ASTHMA

A discussion of the treatment failure of asthma must first include what is known regarding the natural course of the disease. Since there are multiple factors known to cause or precipitate asthmatic symptoms in the susceptible individual, it may be difficult to accurately prognosticate the course and severity of symptoms in every patient. Furthermore, the exact genetic, medical, immunologic and pharmacophysiologic factors responsible for making asthmatic symptoms more resistant to the present modes of therapy continue to remain unknown. Despite the above inadequacies of our knowledge, clinical studies available have allowed certain generalizations to be made about the natural course, severity and treatment resistance of asthma.

A widely held misconception is that most asthmatic children will eventually outgrow their disease. As a result many asthmatic children are denied proper evaluation and therapy in the misguided expectation that their disease will be ameliorated with the mere passage of time. Long term studies have shown that only 20 to 25 percent of asthmatic children have remissions of their disease without specific therapy. Another misconception is that asthma is solely a psychosomatic symptom complex thus rendering it a high position on the list of neurotic syndromes. Such a narrow attitude assuredly results in improper treatment for many asthma sufferers and often engenders a bilaterally negative doctor-patient relationship.

Patients with predominately allergic (extrinsic) asthma have the best prognosis. In part, this is probably a reflection of our better understanding of etiology and of the availability of relatively specific therapy. Indeed, studies in children have shown improvement to the extent of complete relief of symptoms in 70 to 75 percent. However, for children whose onset of asthma is within the first two years of life, or in whom eczema is also present, the prognosis is less favorable. The severity of symptoms in childhood appears to be another indicator of prognosis; those patients with more severe childhood symptoms have a poorer outlook. Asthma in early childhood (below age 10) is twice as prevalent in males, and the most severe cases are predominately males. In the teen and adult years the sex incidence becomes equal. The reasons for these age-sex variations of incidence and severity remain unknown.

In nonallergic (intrinsic) asthma the prognosis is variable, but generally less favorable than that of allergic asthma. The basic etiologic mechanisms in this type of asthma continue to remain unknown. Although infection of the respiratory tract appears to be a significant precipitating factor in some patients, it is by no means the only cause. Most of these patients are adult onset asthmatics or children below the age of three. With appropriate medical management many of these patients will be significantly improved, but to expect complete cessation of symptoms is unrealistic.

The asthma associated with nasal polyposis and aspirin sensitivity has the least favorable prognosis. It is within this group that a significant number of patients have resistant symptoms and severe, life-threatening episodes of asthma.

WHAT CONSTITUTES A TREATMENT FAILURE

When one considers the many factors, known and unknown, which account for the varied clinical expressions of the asthmatic state, it becomes difficult to define treatment failure with concise and absolute criteria applicable to every patient. While in one patient the clinical response to a planned treatment regimen may be considered a failure, in another an identical clinical status may be considered a good treatment response. It is advised, therefore, that after a thorough evaluation the physician should attempt to formulate an expected treatment response for each patient. It is also wise to inform the patient (or the parents) of the tentative prognosis with a candid discussion of what can and what cannot be expected with the proposed treatment plan. In this context, treatment failure of asthma can simply be said to exist when objective improvement is less than expected or when no objective improvement occurs.

When confronted with a treatment failure a complete and thorough reevaluation is mandatory. The extent of this reevaluation should be determined by the individual clinical situation and, to a certain degree, by the extent of the original evaluation. During the course of treatment other interim developments may occur; some of these can adversely affect the treatment response while others may require additional therapy. Results of the reevaluation in conjunction with relevant clinical data observed during the treatment course may also suggest that a treatment failure indeed does not exist but rather the original optimistic prognosis was erroneous.

TREATMENT FAILURE REEVALUATION

What will be presented here is an approach to the treatment failure reevaluation. It is not intended as a review of the diagnosis or treatment of asthma, but certain of these aspects will be considered only as related to treatment failure. Reevaluation should basically answer the following questions:

1. Is the condition definitely asthma?
2. Is there another coexistent illness which can aggravate asthma or make it more resistant to therapy?
3. Is the drug therapy being used adequate?
4. Is allergy management, when indicated, appropriate and adequate?
5. Are nonspecific aggravating factors adequately controlled?

The Accuracy of the Diagnosis

The essential criterion for the diagnosis of asthma is objective evidence of reversible obstruction to expiratory air flow. In the patient considered a treatment failure, reversible airway obstruction must be documented. Spirometric studies before and after epinephrine administration or isoproterenol inhalation are commonly used to determine reversibility. It must be remembered, however, that with moderately severe symptoms, these maneuvers are less effective in completely reversing airway obstruction. Repeat spirometry during an asymptomatic period or after a four- to five-day course of corticosteroids (in suppressive doses) may better reflect the extent of reversibility.

Wheezing dyspnea is a common feature of all the conditions which may be misdiagnosed as asthma. Most of these conditions have more resistant bronchopulmonary symptoms and a graver prognosis than does asthma. Other more specific therapy may be required for amelioration of symptoms. In evaluating the treatment failure patient, the physician must seek out signs and symptoms which may suggest these conditions and then plan an appropriate laboratory investigation when indicated.

Table 18-5 lists various conditions known to mimic asthma and others in which asthmatic symptoms may occur. Chronic bronchitis probably represents the most common disease misdiagnosed as asthma. The presence of slight to moderate eosinophilia favors the diagnosis of asthma, but pulmonary function study is required to differentiate the two conditions. Irreversible airway obstruction and moderately decreased diffusion capacity are typical findings for chronic bronchitis. Interestingly, a few patients with homozygous alpha$_1$ antitrypsin deficiency have asthmatic type symptoms and were previously diagnosed as having asthma. Vithayasai and Hyde [4] have recently reported a 37 percent incidence of heterozygous alpha$_1$ antitrypsin deficiency in 19 children with severe chronic atopic asthma. Bronchiectasis is another bronchial condition often diagnosed as asthma. These patients have repeated bronchial infections, produce copious amounts of sputum and often have significant hemoptysis. Bronchography is required to document this diagnosis.

Obstructing lesions (or foreign body obstruction) of the larynx and tracheobronchial tree are well-known conditions which often simulate asthma.[2] Clinical clues which may suggest these obstructions include repeated bronchopulmonary infections, stridor, inspiratory wheezes, localized wheezing or wheezing which may vary with change of body position. A prior history of endotracheal intubation or tracheostomy in a patient with wheezing should suggest tracheal stenosis as a possible cause. Laboratory investigations helpful in diagnosing these conditions are x-ray study of the neck with soft tissue technique, laminograms of the tracheobronchial tree and inspiratory flow spirometry. If a central airway (larynx and trachea) lesion is fixed, inspiratory and expiratory flow will be equally compromised. When the lesion is variable, (airway is able to respond to transmural pressure), changes in flow pattern will depend on whether the lesion is intra or extrathoracic. An extrathoracic variable lesion will result primarily in a decreased inspiratory flow and with intrathoracic variable lesions there will be a predominante decrease in

expiratory flow. The $\dfrac{FEV_1}{FIV_1}$ ratio can be used as an indicator of this flow relationship.* Normally this ratio is 0.85 to 1.0. With a fixed lesion, since both inspiratory and expiratory flow are decreased, the ratio remains normal. A variable extrathoracic lesion will usually result in a ratio greater than 1 because of the predominate decrease in inspiratory flow. The presence of decreased MVV with a normal FEV_1 or MEFR also suggests the presence of a variable extrathoracic lesion. With a variable intrathoracic lesion the $\frac{FEV_1}{FIV_1}$ ratio is usually lower than normal (0.5 or lower), but in this situation the ratio would not be helpful in differentiating asthma, since asthma itself is associated with a decreased ratio. When clinical and laboratory data suggest the possibility of an obstructive airway lesion, bronchoscopy must be performed for diagnostic and possible therapeutic purposes.

Pulmonary embolus is usually not a serious consideration when one is concerned with the chronic treatment failure patient, but it should be considered as a possible cause of acute refractory episodes. Definitive diagnosis depends on pulmonary angiographic study. Perfusion lung scan study will characteristically show areas of decreased perfusion, but it must be remembered that acute asthma without emboli may also result in similar abnormal perfusion defects.

With common findings of nocturnal wheezing and dyspnea, decreased exercise tolerance, amelioration with aminophylline and even epinephrine, it would be expected that congestive heart failure may be confused with asthma. Some differential clinical features occurring with congestive heart failure include hypertension, angina, arrythmias, gallop rhythm, heart murmurs, fine basilar rales, hepatomegaly and edema. The diagnosis is documented by cardiomegaly, increased circulation time, and the subsequent improvement of symptoms with digitalis and diuretics.

In those treatment failure patients in whom the course is marked by numerous respiratory infections serious consideration must be given to the possibilities of cystic fibrosis (CF) and immunoglobulin deficiency. There is an increasing number of CF patients in whom the diagnosis was first made in the second or third decade of life. Most of these patients had been previously diagnosed as asthmatic. These patients probably represent formes frustes of the disease with mainly pulmonary involvement. An elevated sweat chloride establishes the diagnosis. Immunoglobulin levels in asthmatics are usually normal or elevated, but patients with hypo- or dysgammaglobulinemia may present with re-

* FEV_1 – forced expiratory volume in first second
  FIV_1 – forced inspiratory volume in first second
  MVV – maximal voluntary ventilation
  MEFR – mid-expiratory flow rate

peated respiratory infections and wheezing. Some patients with IgA deficiency may be allergic,[3] and thus some of these patients may have coexistent allergic asthma.

In a few patients with precipitin-mediated pulmonary reactions, i.e., bird fancier's disease and *B. subtilis* enzyme allergy, asthmatic type symptoms may occur, and an erroneous diagnosis of asthma can be made. Although precipitin-mediated reactions should be considered, it probably represents a rare cause of treatment failure in the chronic asthmatic.

Severe and resistant asthmatic symptoms may be associated with the vasculitis group of diseases. This group consists of various clinical syndromes ranging from asthma with Löeffler's syndrome, (eosinophilia, fever and pulmonary eosinophilic infiltrates), to the more serious and often fatal conditions of Churg's allergic granulomatosis and polyarteritis nodosa. During the active phase of the vasculitis, asthma may become more severe but it may antedate or even remain quiescent for years before the onset of vasculitis. In every treatment failure asthmatic the possibility of an associated vasculitis must be considered. Findngs which may suggest the condition are hypertension, eosinophilia, pulmonary infiltrates, fever, neuritis, elevated sedimentation rate, hematuria, proteinuria and skin lesions which may be purpuric, maculopapular or ulcerative. Skin, muscle or lung biopsy are often necessary to establish the diagnosis.

Hiatal hernia is a rare cause of wheezing. In this condition wheezing probably results from aspiration of gastric contents, but it is possible that large hernias may cause bronchospasm by reflex mechanisms. These patients will usually have associative gastrointestinal symptoms. Upper GI and esophageal x-ray study will establish the diagnosis.

Asthma may be a rare presenting feature of Addison's disease.[1] The mechanism of asthma is unclear; these patients may represent latent asthmatics in whom the decrease in endogenous corticosteroids will induce overt bronchospasm.

Other Coexistent Conditions

Theoretically any of the conditions listed in Table 18-5 may coexist with asthma and account for more severe or resistant symptoms. With most of these conditions, wheezing dyspnea usually represents a symptom of the underlying disease process, not asthma. However, in conditions such as bronchitis, bronchiectasis, cystic fibrosis and dysgammaglobulinemia asthma may coexist. A complete clinical, medical, allergy and laboratory evaluation is necessary, not only to document the presence of both conditions, but also to determine the severity of the coexisting illness so that a more accurate prognosis can be formulated.

TABLE 18-5

Conditions which may simulate asthma	Conditions in which asthmatic symptoms may occur

1. Bronchopulmonary diseases:
  Bronchitis-emphysema
  Bronchiectasis
  Bronchiolitis
  Bronchial obstructing lesions
  Laryngotracheal lesions
  Foreign body
  Extrinsic tracheobronchial obstruction:
    thyroid tumors; lymph nodes;
    thymoma
  Precipitin mediated lung disease:
    bird fancier's disease; pulmonary
    aspergillosis; organic dusts;
    B. subtilis enzymes
  Loeffler's pulmonary eosinophilia
2. Congestive heart failure
3. Hypo- or dysgammaglobulinemia
4. Cystic fibrosis
	1. Pulmonary emboli
	2. Polyarteritis nodosa
	3. Churg's allergic granulomatosis
	4. Carcinoid syndrome
	5. Hiatal hernia
	6. Addison's disease

Furthermore, in certain of these conditions asthma may be an important etiologic factor. For example, in a few patients with predominately intrinsic asthma and frequent bronchial infections, irreversible pulmonary damage may result. Usually the irreversible component is less than that seen in bronchitis and emphysema. Another example is the bronchiectasis that may occur in patients with allergic bronchopulmonary aspergillosis. This disease occurs in patients with extrinsic asthma, and it is characterized by increased wheezing, expectoration of brownish mucus plugs, pulmonary infiltrates, eosinophilia (pulmonary and peripheral), and elevated serum IgE levels. Without specific treatment (i.e., coricosteroids and/or amphotericin), bronchiectasis may result.

Some patients with resistant asthma have moderately severe paranasal sinus disease. With proper medical or surgical treatment of the sinuses, asthma may improve. The exact mechanism by which this coexistent condition aggravates asthma is not known.

Adequacy of Drug Treatment

A review of drug therapy is necessary in the patient considered a treatment failure. In patients with chronic symptoms, round-the-clock use of oral bronchodilators has proved superior to using them only when symptoms occur. Although it is practical to use the many available combinations of ephedrine, theophylline and expectorants, the recommended doses of these combinations may not be sufficient for some patients. A better response may result with one and one half to two times the recommended dose. A recent clinical study [5] of asthmatic children showed that the improved response from high dose combination therapy resulted from the high dose of theophylline alone (7 to 10 mg./kg. every 6 to 8 hours). No significant side effects were noted with this dose. Round-the-clock therapy with maximum tolerable doses of theophylline should be used in patients with severe and chronic symptoms. The danger of theophylline toxicity must be kept in mind continuously.

In view of the known side effects of corticosteroids, a general reluctance to use them is well warranted, but they remain the most effective group of drugs for the treatment of asthma. To advocate their use in every case of asthma is not advised, but to categorically avoid their use in every child or adult with asthma is unjustified. Considering the significant morbidity and mortality of severe asthma, corticosteroids are especially indicated in those treatment failure patients in whom incapacitating symptoms persist despite maximum doses of round-the-clock bronchodilators. For chronic maintenance therapy, side effects are markedly reduced by using short-acting preparations every other day with the total dose given in the morning.

Another aspect of drug therapy which may be related to the problem of treatment failure is the overuse of aerosolized isoproterenol. The recommended dose of these aerosols is one to two sprays every 4 to 6 hours, but many patients tend to overuse them. It has been well established that in approximately 40 to 50 percent of patients the overuse of aerosols will perpetuate symptoms and when discontinued marked improvement occurs. A patient can be considered to be overusing the aerosol if 20 to 30 ml. is used within a two-week period. The chapter on treatment of asthma contains a thorough discussion of the hazards of aerosol overuse.

Adequacy of Allergy Management

Allergy treatment includes two basic features: environmental control of certain allergens and hyposensitization to those allergens which cannot be controlled. In those patients in whom allergy management has not proved effective, a complete reevaluation is necessary to determine the adequacy of treatment as well as the accuracy of the presumed extrinsic (allergic) etiology of symptoms.

Environmental review must include the home, the nature of hobby activities and the place of occupation. Occasionally it may be worthwhile for the physician to personally inspect the home or place of occupation. Less than optimal control of house dust and molds may be an important factor contributing to treatment failure. The continued presence of a pet is another important cause of resistant symptoms. Many households today may contain a variety of pets which are allergen sources; cats, dogs, birds, hamsters, gerbils, guinea pigs, rats, mice and monkeys are a few examples. It is possible that at the onset of treatment allergy to a pet may not have existed, but with continued exposure the patient may become sensitized. Without making it known to the physician, some patients may acquire a pet after noting initial improvement with treatment.

Unsuspected occupational allergen exposure must also be considered in the treatment failure patient. Amelioration of symptoms when absent from work may indicate a clinically important occupational allergen. Asthmatic symptoms may result from exposure to organic dusts as may be seen in workers of castor or coffee bean factories and detergent (*B. subtilis*) factories. Another example is grain dust exposure in grain elevator workers. Inhalation of wheat flour may elicit asthma in bakers. Animal dander exposure may be an important factor in zoo workers, slaughterhouse employees and veterinarians. Patients who are gardeners may note seasonal symptoms that may suggest pollen sensitivity but in fact result from mold inhalation. Platinum salts rarely cause asthma; it has been seen in platinum refinery workers and chemists. Factory workers exposed to toluene diisocyanate may develop severe asthmatic symptoms. This compound is used in the production of polyurethane foam and plastics. It is felt that this compound when inhaled may form a haptene conjugate which is immunogenic. Other low molecular weight substances known to cause asthma include tannic acid and phenylmercuric compounds.

Food allergy is rarely a cause of asthma, and consequently it maybe overlooked as a possible cause. In the treatment failure patient this possibility must be investigated. A discussion of food allergy and its evaluation is found in Chapter 14.

The success of hyposensitization therapy depends to a great extent upon the amount of antigen administered. High dose therapy gives the best results. Optimal maintenance dose levels of antigen should range from 0.25 to 0.50 ml. of a 1:50 w/v (weight by volume) concentration of the aqueous antigen preparation. Some treatment failures may be due to an insufficient antigen dose. In others optimal dose therapy cannot be achieved because of large local or systemic reactions.

In contrast to the above statements it must be remembered that hyposensitization therapy itself may induce symptoms and result in what appears to be a treatment failure. Increased symptoms within 24 hours after the injection with gradual waning within the next few days may suggest this possiblity. Often these changes in symptoms are subtle and the patient will not correlate them with the injections. The observations of increased symptoms after beginning hyposensitization or the return of symptoms after a period of improvement may also suggest that hyposensitization may be causing symptoms. It is important to remember that the absence of local reactions at the injection site does not preclude the possibility of systemic symptoms. A temporary cessation of therapy should document whether or not hyposensitization is contributing to increased symptoms. If clinical improvement results, treatment should continue with lower, more tolerable doses.

During the course of treatment a patient may become sensitized to new allergens. At the onset of treatment he may have had seasonal symptoms secondary to pollens, and later he may begin to develop perennial symptoms from dust, dander or molds. The opposite sequence may also occur. These clinical changes would superficially suggest a treatment failure. Repeat skin testing may aid in detecting these changes in sensitivity, and when appropriate, these new antigens should be added to the hyposensitization therapy.

There are chronic atopic asthmatics who have continuing severe symptoms and in whom no apparent improvement results from an adequate hyposensitization regimen. Many of these patients require chronic maintenance corticosteroid therapy. The original allergy evaluation suggested an allergic etiology because of positive skin tests to inhalants and accordingly hyposensitization therapy was instituted. In evaluating their course in retrospect, with consideration of severity, corticosteroid dependence and the poor response to hyposensitization, it appears that some of these patients are intrinsic asthmatics and the positive skin tests were clinically insignificant. It is evident that more accurate and sensitive methods of allergy evaluation are needed to depict this type of patient.

Adequacy of Control of Nonspecific Factors

Asthmatics who smoke cigarettes cannot be expected to respond optimally to any treatment modality. This is especially true for the chronic asthmatic. Some improvement will certainly occur if the severe chronic asthmatic stops smoking.

Occupational exposure to irritating dust, fumes, odors and vapors may account for treatment failure in some patients. The use of face masks may be helpful, but if it can be documented that these substances are producing significant symptoms a change of occupation may be required.

The physician should attempt to gain some insight into the emotional makeup of the treatment failure patient. Although emotional or psychiatric factors are rarely causative in treatment failure, the possibility must not be overlooked. When there is suggestive clinical evidence of emotional disturbance, psychiatric evaluation and treatment may be helpful. The presence of psychoneurosis or psychosis may indirectly cause treatment failure. Because of these associative illnesses the patient may have an unrealistic attitude toward his asthmatic state. He may be un-cooperative or unable to follow instructions or take medicines as instructed. Continuation of symptoms would then appear to represent treatment failure when in fact it does not exist.

TRUE TREATMENT FAILURE

In some treatment failure patients, a thorough and judicious reevaluation, as outlined above, will reveal no treatable or untreatable cause for the refractory nature of symptoms. A number of these patients will function well and lead normal lives with maintenance corticosteroid therapy of minimal or moderate doses. Other patients require doses of corticosteroids that are massive, and the complications of corticosteroid therapy become a serious concern. These patients may benefit from a period of evaluation and treatment in a hospital specialized in the care of the chronic intractable asthmatic.

REFERENCES

1. Green, M., Lim, K. H.: Bronchial asthma with Addison's disease. Lancet, *1*:1159, 1971.
2. Miller, D. R., Hyatt, R. E.: Obstructing lesions of the larynx and trachea: Clinical and physiologic characteristics. Mayo Clinic Proceedings, *44*:145, 1969.
3. Nell, P. A., Ammann, A. J., Hang, R., Stiehm, R. E.; Familial selective IgA deficiency. Pediatrics, *49*:71, 1972
4. Vithayasai, V., Hyde, J. S.: Personal communication.
5. Weinberger, M. N., Bronsky, E. A.: Oral bronchodilator therapy in asthmatic children; a critical evaluation. J. Allerg. Clin. Immun. [Abstract #87], *49*:1972.

SUGGESTED READING

Pepys, J.: Hypersensitivity diseases of the lung due to fungi and organic dusts. New York, S. Karger, 1969.

Case Records of the Massachusetts General Hospital (Case 5-1971-Polyarteritis Nodosa). New Eng. J. Med., *28*:262, 1971

Freeman, S. O., Krupey, W.: Respiratory allergy caused by platinum salts. J. Allerg., *42*:233, 1968.

Johnston, T. G., *et al.*: Bronchial asthma, urticaria and allergic rhinitis from tannic acid. J. Allerg., *22*:494, 1951.

Mathews, K. P.: Immediate type hypersensitivity to phenylmercuric compounds. Am. J. Med., *44*:310, 1968.

Scheel, L. D., Josephson, A.: Immunological aspects of toluene diisocyanate (TDI) toxicity. Am. Indust. Hyg. A. J., *25*:179, 1964.

TREATMENT FAILURES IN URTICARIA

Jordan N. Fink, M.D.

Failure to bring urticaria under control in a given patient is probably more common in the chronic than the acute form. The latter often remits spontaneously, while the chronic type often continues to plague both the patient and his physician. When this occurs, the physician should reevaluate the case and attempt to discover, if possible, why his efforts have not provided the patient with relief.

The misdiagnosis of urticaria is quite unlikely, since the lesions are distinctive and are usually not mistaken for other disorders. In order to be certain of the diagnosis, however, direct observation of the patient should be carried out at a time when the lesions are prominent. If the patient cannot accurately describe his lesions and no direct observation has taken place, urticaria may be mistaken for multiple insect bites, erythemas associated with viral or bacterial infections, or other toxic eruptions. Inadequate diagnosis of urticaria is probably more common in treatment failure, and is usually due to the physician not eliciting an adequate history.

The most common cause of urticaria is related to the use of drugs, and therefore a complete and thorough drug history must be obtained in every case. Specific questions should be asked regarding the use of aspirin, sedatives, birth control pills, laxatives, vitamins, and suppositories. Sometimes showing the patient a list of proprietaries containing aspirin may be rewarding. If salicylate ingestion is suspected but denied by the patient, determining a blood level may be useful. Patients often do not remember all of the drugs they use, and it may take several interviews before the complete history is obtained. Asking a question such as "What do you put in your mouth besides food?" may be helpful.

Failure to thoroughly elicit and evaluate a food history may also play a role in the adequate diagnosis of urticaria. It is often difficult to correlate temporally the ingestion of a food with the onset of an attack of urticaria. It may be necessary to ask the patient to keep a careful and accurate food diary, listing the time, amount and type of food ingested, and the time and duration of the attack. The physician must then, of course, attempt to correlate the attacks with a specific food or group of foods. This means he may have to spend considerable time in evaluating the patient's diary.

The correlation of skin reactivity with food allergy is usually low. If there are skin reactions to certain foods, however, the physician should consider eliminating the foods temporarily from the diet in an attempt to control the urticaria. It should be emphasized that the lack of skin reactivity to food antigens does not always rule out food allergy, and elimination diets are warranted in cases where food allergy is suspected. In addition to elimination diets, the physician may use a provocative diet, giving large amounts of the suspected food(s) in hopes of evoking an episode of urticaria. Again, accurate records must be kept so that the appropriate correlation may be made.

Since urticarial lesions can be present in other diseases, the failure to completely exclude other diseases may also be reason for treatment failure. Disorders such as underlying infections (viral and bacterial), collagen diseases (especially) lupus erythematosus, and carcinomas must be considered and evaluated and, when discovered, appropriately treated if possible. Other forms of urticaria such as the cholinergic type associated with heat and exercise, or urticaria resulting from physical agents, must also be carefully considered when treatment appears to be inadequate. Again, a carefully taken history and the use of some specific tests such as intradermal injection of methacholine, light or ice cube application, may often reveal the reason for the apparent failure of therapy.

Treatment failure in cases of urticaria may also often be the result of inadequate medical management on the part of the physician. The physician must be certain he knows each drug which the patient may be taking. He must make the patient aware that proprietaries such as aspirin vitamins and laxatives are drugs and may have to be avoided. Again, a thorough and carefully taken history is most important.

In cases of food allergy, the patient may not have been properly instructed in the elimination diet. Often the patient will have to read the labels on each item of food bought to be certain it does not contain the suspected antigen. Cross-reacting food or whole food families may have to be eliminated, and the physician should be aware of the relationships between such foods and food families.

The inadequate management of urticaria may also be due to the inadequate use of therapeutic drugs. A several days' to two weeks' trial of the maximum tolerated dose of a drug should be attempted before that drug is abandoned or before other drugs are added. Hydroxyzine may be given safely in doses as high as 400 mg. per day with only a mild sedative effect in most patients. Ephedrine and its related compounds may be used for a short time in doses causing mild nervousness or slight tachycardia. Combinations of these two drugs may be of benefit to the patient, not only in controlling his symptoms but in counteracting each others' side effects. In addition to these useful drugs, the physician may find it necessary to add other drugs or combinations of drugs to the treatment regimen. Again, an adequate and thorough trial of the therapy should be tried before it is modified.

Finally, a frequent cause of treatment failure in urticaria is the failure of the physician to recognize and explain the inability to demonstrate extrinsic factors in many cases of hives. It has been estimated that in from 50 to 75 percent of the cases of urticaria, no cause can be determined. This frustration on the part of the physician, as well as his patient, must be taken into consideration when cases of chronic urticaria are present and yield only minimally to therapy.

DIAGNOSTIC PROBLEMS IN ALLERGY PRACTICE
EOSINOPHILIA

Bernard Hess Booth III, M.D.

A review of some of the illnesses that have been associated with eosinophilia contradicts the commonly held belief that an increase in circulating eosinophils indicates that a patient must be allergic (see list below). Indeed the vast number of illnesses associated with eosinophilia has prompted some to say that eosinophilia is of no diagnostic significance.[8] However, although eosinophil counts are almost never diagnostic, they can be of great clinical use.

Conditions Associated with Eosinophilia

1. Idiosyncratic drug reactions
2. Malaria
3. Cat-scratch fever (nonbacterial regional lymphadenitis)
4. Primary pulmonary coccidioidomycosis
5. Pulmonary aspergillosis
6. Phycomycosis
7. Toxoplasmosis
8. Balantidiosis
9. Dermatomyositis
10. Polyarteritis nodosum
11. Post-irradiation
12. Post-splenectomy
13. Wegener's granulomatosis
14. Erythema multiforme (Stevens-Johnson syndrome)
15. Sarcoidosis
16. Systemic mastocytosis
17. Whipple's disease
18. Incontinentia pigmenti (Bloch-Sulzberger syndrome)
19. Hodgkin's disease
20. Reticulum cell sarcoma
21. Lymphosarcoma
22. Other solid malignant tumors
23. Allergic pulmonary alveolitis Bagassosis

34. Familial hypokalemic periodic paralysis
35. Parasitic infestations
    A. Nemathelminthes (roundworms)
       1. Trichinella spiralis
       2. Enterobius vermicularis
       3. Hookworm (Necator americanus)
       4. Ascaris lumbricoides
       5. Trichuris trichiura
       6. Strongyloides stercoralis
       7. Dracunculus medinensis
       8. Onchocerca volvulus
       9. Angiostrongylus cantonensis
       10. Mansonella ozzardi
       11. Wuchereria bancrofti and malayi
    B. Platyhelminthes (flatworms)
       1. Cestoda (tapeworms)
          a. Taenia saginata
          b. Taenia solium
          c. Echinococcus granulosus
          d. Hymenolepis nana
          e. Diphyllobothrium latum
       2. Trematoda (flukes)
          a. Clonorchis sinensis

608

Farmer's lung
Pigeon breeder's disease
Allergic pulmonary
  aspergillosis
Probably others
24. Pernicious anemia
25. Folic acid deficiency
26. Chronic lymphocytic leukemia
27. Chronic myelocytic leukemia
28. Myelofibrosis
29. Multiple myeloma
30. Macroglobulinemia
31. Heavy chain disease
32. Pan-pituitary insufficiency
33. Adrenal insufficiency

b. Opisthorchis felineus
c. Fasciolopsis buski
d. Fasciola hepatica
e. Paragonimus
  westermani
f. Schistosoma
  japonicum
g. Schistosoma
  haematobium
h. Schistosoma mansoni
36. Eosinophilic gastroenteritis
37. Allergic rhinitis
38. Atopic eczema
39. Extrinsic asthma
40. Hypereosinophilic syndromes

After many years of intensive investigation and continuous speculation, most of the fundamental questions regarding the function of eosinophils remain unanswered. Clearly, they are not simply neutrophils with peculiar staining properties because they do respond differently to many apparently nonspecific stimuli. The number of circulating eosinophils fluctuates widely from day to day not only in patients with many different illnesses but also in normal individuals. Both adrenergic and cholinergic drugs have been reported to affect circulating eosinophils. Circulating eosinophils are definitely decreased by epinephrine and other catecholamines and β-adrenergic blockade can be accompanied by a significant rise in circulating eosinophils.[9]

Circulating eosinophils drop dramatically in response to adrenal corticosteroids, and this response has been the basis for a test of adrenal cortical function. Though the response is clearly present, the mechanism by which these hormones affect the regulation of circulating eosinophils remains unknown. A decrease or disappearance of circulating eosinophils has been attributed to bacterial infections by some [11]; others have reported an increase due to infections.[13] It is probably reasonable to assume that both responses can occur in different situations.

The wide number of nonspecific factors that affect eosinophils obviously can and does limit the clinical value of eosinophil counts. There is evidence from multiple sources that eosinophils do appear after immediate-type allergic reactions in various species. What function the eosinophils perform at the site of such reactions remains undetermined. Archer extracted and identified a substance from the eosinophils of horses that functioned as an antihistamine.[1] Similar results have not been obtained with human eosinophils. It was once thought that eosinophils contained large amounts of histamine and brought this to the reaction site.[13] However, basophils are the only circulating white cells in man that have a significant histamine content. It has been proposed that eosinophils remove histamine from the site of a reaction by detoxifying it or by transporting it to another site to be detoxified.[14,15] No clear evidence has confirmed this concept.

Some information is available concerning the mechanism that attracts eosinophils to these reaction sites. When lung tissue was removed after anaphylaxis and implanted into the peritoneal cavity of a nonsensitive guinea pig recipient an eosinophilia occurred.[10,12] The nature of this eosinophil chemotactic factor has now been further elucidated.[7] In guinea pigs it can be extracted from lung tissue after anaphylaxis. It has an estimated molecular weight of 500 to 1000 and is not related to histamine, SRS-A, bradykinin, serotinin or the prostaglandins. In these experiments the activity did not seem to be complement dependent.

From a practical clinical standpoint we know only that immediate-type hypersensitivity reactions probably release a factor that can affect the distribution of eosinophils. Other pharmacological and hormonal factors also influence the distribution of eosinophils. Despite much speculation, the function of eosinophils remains unknown.

A slight elevation of circulating eosinophils is nonspecific and should be viewed in the same manner as clinicians view other nonspecific laboratory abnormalities. An elevated erythrocyte sedimentation rate or a slightly elevated total white count is not specific for any one illness. Similarly, an eosinophilia of 3 to 15 percent is not specific but indicates the need for a careful history and physical examination.

Elevations of circulating eosinophils greater than 20 percent, particularly if the increase is persistent, necessitate a more thorough evaluation aimed at ruling out specific entities. The first step in evaluating eosinophilia of this degree is to stop all drugs the patient is taking. Skin and muscle biopsies should then be studied for evidence of polyarteritis. Stool and tissue specimens should be examined repeatedly for parasites.

In regard to parasite-related eosinophilia, some points are of practical significance. Protozoan parasites are neither as large nor as biologically complex as the helminths. Parisitism with protozoa probably does not present the host with the number and variety of antigens that helminthic parasitism does. Consequently, protozoal infestations such as amebiasis are not routinely associated with eosinophilia, although almost all helminthic infections are usually associated with significant eosinophilia.

Of all helminthic infections the ones that are most commonly associated with eosinophilia are strongyloides and trichinella. The trichinella skin test consequently may be of some value if it is negative. A positive test has less value because skin reactivity can persist for many years after the illness has become quiescent.

Serological tests for many different parasites have been evaluated. These tests utilize indirect hemagglutination, gel diffusion and fluorescent antibody techniques. Their clinical usefulness at the present time is limited, and they will probably lack any specificity until a large number and variety of very complex parasitic antigens have been carefully defined and characterized. Until these tests become specific enough to clarify these clinical problems, the best course is to continue to observe the patient and to repeatedly examine stool and tissue specimens. The clinical problem is made more complex because nonhuman helminths such as *Angiostrongylus, Toxocara,* and *Gnathostoma* can occasionally pass through human tissue. Though incapable of causing a true infestation, they may elicit a significant eosinophilia.

Patients may have persistent eosinophilia associated with an occult malignancy. Eosinphilia is most commonly associated with malignancies of the lymphoma group but can be present with almost any type of malignancy. A general medical evaluation would include appropriate laboratory and x-ray studies and must frequently be followed by lymph node biopsy and examination.

If these evaluations are negative, the patient should be observed. Rarely he will develop one or more symptoms characteristic of a group of illnesses called the hypereosinophilic syndromes.[6] These syndromes may represent a continuum of disease with multiple gradations of clinical expression (Table 18-6).

Löeffler's syndrome was initially the name given to a benign illness of short duration characterized by transient pulmonary infiltrations, low fever and peripheral eosinophilia. Similar clinical patterns have been described after the use of some drugs.[5] It is apparent that this syndrome is similar to and overlaps a syndrome characterized by a chronic eosinophilic pneumonia.[2] In these patients the pulmonary lesions, which histologically consist of pneumonic foci with many eosinophils, are extensive, persistent and progressive. In addition, the patients have a severe illness with high fever, night sweats, weight loss, and severe dyspnea. Though an increase in circulating eosinophils is usual it has not been a constant feature. Cardiac involvement is not a feature. In contrast to the other hypereosinophilic syndromes, the response of chronic eosinophilic pneumonia to corticosteroid therapy has been excellent.

Löeffler's endocarditis refers to a similar illness that, in addition to the pulmonary infiltrates and marked circulating eosinophilia, is characterized by increasing cardiac disability. It is generally progressive and fatal. The myocardium and endocardium have cellular infiltrations in which there are many eosinophils.

Eosinophilic leukemia or disseminated eosinophilic collagen disease

TABLE 18-6
The Hypereosinophilic Syndromes

Current terminology	Loeffler's disease; pulmonary infiltration with eosinophilia syndrome	Loeffler's endocarditis parietalis fibroplastica	Eosinophilic leukemia; disseminated eosinophilic collagen disease
Extent of involvement	Eosinophilia with pulmonary involvement	Eosinophilia with cardiopulmonary involvement	Eosinophilia with generalized involvement
Symptoms — Frequent	Asymptomatic; malaise, fever, cough	Malaise, fever, cough, dyspnea, weight loss	Malaise, fever, sweats, cough dyspnea, chest pain, weight loss
Symptoms — Occasional	Dyspnea	Pruritus	Pruritus
Signs — Frequent	None; transitory rales, sinus tachycardia	Sinus tachycardia, arrhythmias, cardiomegaly, murmurs, rales, edema	Sinus tachycardia, arrhythmias, cardiomegaly, murmurs, rales, edema, hepatosplenomegaly
Signs — Occasional		Hepatosplenomegaly	Lymphadenopathy
Laboratory findings — Hemogram	Mild leukocytosis and eosinophilia	Mild to moderate leukocytosis and eosinophilia	Moderate to marked leukocytosis and eosinophilia, progressive anemia
Marrow	Data scant (eosinophilic hyperplasia reported)	Data scant (eosinophilic hyperplasia when reported)	Marked granulocytic hyperplasia with eosinophilia
Chest x-ray	Transient infiltrates	Cardiomegaly, pulmonary infiltrates	Cardiomegaly, pulmonary infiltrates, pleural effusion
Electrocardiogram		Usually abnormal but nonspecific	Usually abnormal but nonspecific (Arrhythmias, ST-T changes)
Pathology — Lungs	Eosinophilic bronchitis and bronchopneumonia, granulomas, arteritis	Passive congestion, fibrosis, eosinophils	Passive congestion, granulomatous vasculitis, infiltrates of eosinophils
Heart	Normal	Hypertrophy, mural thrombi, subendocardial fibrosis	Hypertrophy, mural thrombi, focal necrosis, fibrosis, infiltrates of eosinophils
Liver and spleen	Normal	Occasionally enlarged with eosinophilic infiltrates	Hepatosplenomegaly with infiltrates of mature eosinophils
Course	Self-limited	Generally progressive	Generally progressive
Prognosis	Recovery	Often fatal	Generally fatal

From: Hardy, W. R., Anderson, R. E.: The hypereosinophilic syndrome. Ann. Int. Med. 6:1227, 1968.

refers to a syndrome characterized by gradual onset of cardiac and pulmonary signs and symptoms such as tachycardia, cardiomegaly and dyspnea. Initially few pulmonary infiltrates are seen on chest x-ray. This is followed by hepatosplenomegaly, cough, fever, weight loss, arrhythmias, cardiac murmurs and refractory congestive heart failure. The patients progressively deteriorate and death occurs in 1 to 3 years. There is a persistent, eosinophilic leukocytosis. The bone marrow shows marked hyperplasia of the eosinophilic series but no evidence of abnormal maturation. All normal marrow elements seem to be present and normal in appearance. At autopsy the heart is markedly enlarged with mural thrombi. The myocardium and endocardium as well as the liver, spleen and most other organs are infiltrated with large numbers of morphologically mature eosinophils. The use of the term leukemia to describe this syndrome may or may not be correct. Certainly there is a marked clinical difference between this syndrome and other myelocytic leukemias. There is an orderly maturation of the myeloid series in the bone marrow without hypoplasia of the remaining elements. The cells in the peripheral blood remain mature, and there are no blastic crises. The Philadelphia chromosome abnormality that is seen in chronic myelogenous leukemia has been demonstrated only once in patients with this disorder.[4] Since it does not respond to the therapeutic regimens used for other myelocytic leukemias, it may be inappropriate to consider it a leukemia. On the other hand, it does represent a hyperplasia and proliferation of a particular leukocyte and it is associated with an ominous prognosis. If it can be demonstrated that it responds to conventional antileukemic therapy, then there would be practical value in conceptually considering it to be a leukemia. However, at the present time there is no evidence that corticosteroids, radiotherapy and myelosuppressive agents alter the clinical course. Only one patient seems to have responded to an antihistamine.[6]

REFERENCES

1. Archer, R. K.: The Eosinophilic Leukocytes. Oxford, Blackwell, 1963.
2. Carrington, C. B., *et al.*: Chronic Eosinophilic pneumonia. New Eng., J. Med., *280*:787, 1969.
3. Code, C. F.: The mechanism of anaphylactic and allergic reactions: An evaluation of the role of histamine in their production. Ann. Allerg., 2:457, 1944.
4. Gruenwald, H., Kiossoglou, K. A., Mitus, W. J., and Dameshek, W.: Philadelphia chromosome in eosinophilic leukemia. Amer. J. Med., 39:1003, 1965.
5. Hailey, F. J., Glascock, H. W., Jr., and Hewitt, W. F.: Pleuropneumonic reactions to nitrofurantoin. New Eng. J. Med., *281*:1087, 1969.

6. Hardy, W. R. and Anderson R. E.: The hypereosinophilic syndromes. Ann. Int. Med., *6:*1220, 1968.
7. Kay, A. B., Stechschulte, D. J., and Austen, K. F.: An eosinophilic leukocyte chemotactic factor of anaphylaxis. J. Exper. Med., *133:*602, 1971.
8. Kirk, R. C.: The causes of eosinophilia. Int. Clin. I, *5:*219, 1942.
9. Koch-Weser, J.: Beta adrenergic blockade and circulating eosinophils. Arch. Int. Med., *121:*255, 1968.
10. Parish, W. E. and Coombs, R. R. A.: Peripheral blood eosinophilia in guinea pigs following implantation of anaphylactic guinea pig and human lung. Brit. J. Haemat., *14:*425, 1968.
11. Samter, M. and Czarny, P.: Immunological Diseases. p. 379. Boston, Little, Brown, 1971.
12. Samter, M., Kofoed, M. A., and Pieper, W.: A factor in lungs of anaphylactically shocked guinea pigs which can induce eosinophilia in normal animals, Blood, *8:*1078, 1953.
13. Sheldon, J. M., Lovell, R. G., and Mathews, K. P.: A Manual of Clinical Allergy. chap. 3. Philadelphia, W. B. Saunders, 1967.
14. Vaughn, J.: The stimulation on the eosinophil leucocyte. J. Path. Bact., *64:*91, 1952.
15. ———: The function of the eosinophil leucocyte, Blood, *8:*1, 1953.

PRURITUS

Isaac Weiszer, M.D.

Pruritus or itching is an unpleasant cutaneous sensation which provokes the desire to scratch. It may be associated with many skin diseases (symptomatic pruritus) or it may occur without any visible evidence of a somatic disease of the skin (essential pruritus). Essential pruritus may be local or general. Generalized pruritus may be due to physiological or psychologic factors or it may be associated with an underlying systemic disorder.

In this section, we will discuss some general aspects of itching and focus on the patient who presents with generalized pruritus without any visible evidence of a skin disorder. Such a patient presents a diagnostic challenge to the internist, allergist or dermatologist and requires a thorough medical evaluation to rule out the presence of an underlying disorder.

PATHOPHYSIOLOGY

The sensation of itching can be elicited only from the outermost portion of the skin and the palpebral conjunctiva. It may be a sensation in its own right or it could be a specialized type of pain. Itching is detected by free nerve endings and networks in the epidermis and upper dermis. There are itch points (low threshold areas where less stimulus causes itching) which seem to correspond to sites in which nerve endings are assembled in large numbers. Experiments with cowhage spicules show that itching can be elicited in the epidermis under the horny layer, at the epidermal-dermal junction and in the upper dermis. Itching does not occur on the stratum corneum, deep dermis or in denervated areas. Complete removal of the epidermis decreases or stops itching under many circumstances.[3]

Stimuli for itching are many and variable. Changes in skin temperature, rough clothing, dryness of the skin, many diseases of the skin and internal organs, application to the skin surface of mechanical, chemical, electrical and thermal stimuli, as well as systemic administration of drugs and allergens may result in pruritus.[2]

The first chemical substance recognized as an important mediator for itching was histamine. When histamine is introduced into the most superficial layers of the skin, such as by pricking, it causes itching, but

615

when injected intradermally, it produces pain. Histamine liberators cause itching and are inhibited by antihistamines. Histamine causes the triple response of Lewis as well as pruritus. Antihistamines will abolish the triple response but not always the pruritus.

Proteolytic enzymes, such as trypsin, papain, mucunain (produced by mucuna pruriens, the cowhage plant) cause pruritus. Kallikrein causes pruritus when injected intradermally. These substances will usually cause pure pruritus without edema and erythema.

A *postulated scheme* for the mechanism of pruritus could be as follows: Injury and cell damage release kinases, which activate proteases. These act on a protein substrate to release polypeptides or histamine. The latter act on nerve endings to cause itching.

Pruritus is conducted chiefly over unmyelinated C fibers. From the nerve ending, it is thought that the impulse goes to the dorsal horn of the spinal cord, to the opposite anterolateral spinothalamic tract, to the thalamus, then via the internal capsule to the sensory area of the posterior central gyrus. These nerve pathways also serve pain sensations.

Secondary factors that increase pruritus are heat, vasodilatation and emotional irritability. Cooling and vasoconstriction, as produced by epinephrine and ephedrine, reduce itching. It is said that atopic patients have a lowered itch threshold and are generally more "itchy" than their normal counterparts.

ETIOLOGY

Symptomatic pruritus, or itching secondary to a somatic skin disease, is a common accompaniment of atopic dermatitis, contact dermatitis, urticaria, some drug eruptions as well as other skin conditions. Localized pruritus, such as pruritus ani and vulvae, can usually be explained on a local, physical basis after evaluation.

Essential pruritus or itching without a demonstrable skin condition is the presenting complaint of many patients. The patient is usually middle-aged or elderly and factors such as dry skin, cold weather, air-conditioning and aging skin may be responsible for the itching. Psychological factors can cause and often do aggravate pruritus.

Pruritus associated with an underlying disorder may be the presenting manifestation of that disorder or may be one of other features. Some of the systemic conditions in which pruritus may occur are listed on page 618.

Generalized Allergic Reaction

Pruritus may be the first manifestation of human anaphylaxis. It may also occur with drug reactions, either by an immunologic mechanism or by histamine release on a nonimmunologic basis.

Pregnancy

Pruritus is a farily common manifestation of the last trimester of pregnancy. Hormonal alterations and hepatobiliary stasis are thought to be causative factors. The itching usually subsides after delivery.

Liver Disease

Patients with obstructive jaundice may suffer from generalized itching. Drug-induced intrahepatic biliary obstruction and primary biliary cirrhosis may be heralded by generalized pruritus. The pruritus of liver disease appears to be related to the serum and skin levels of retained bile acids. Surgical relief of biliary obstruction or use of cholestyramine reduces serum bile acid levels and reduces itching. Terminal hepatocellular failure impairs synthesis of bile acids and also results in improvement of the pruritus.

Renal Disease

Pruritus in kidney disease usually is associated with uremia, and dialysis relieves the itching in some cases.

Diabetes Mellitus

Pruritus vulvae is a common presenting complaint in diabetes. Generalized pruritus is occasionally present. When it occurs, it does not appear to be related to the severity or duration of the diabetes, control of glycosuria is said to improve the itching.

Other Endocrine Disorders

Both hyperthyroidism and hypothyroidism have been associated with pruritus, with improvement of the itching when the underlying condition was treated. Hyperparathyroidism, secondary to chronic renal failure, is associated with a generalized pruritus, which is relieved dramatically within hours after parathyroidectomy. This would imply a relationship between the itching and high levels of circulating parathormone.

Malignancy

Pruritus, often severe and continuous, occurs in about 30 percent of patients with Hodgkin's disease. It may occur long before any other manifestations of the disease are evident or may have its onset at any time during the course of the disease. Itching is less frequent in lymphosarcoma and reticulum cell sarcoma. Early mycosis fungoides may be associated with severe itching. Patients with polycythemia vera may have pruritus, usually episodic in nature precipitated by a hot bath or exposure to cold.

Carcinoma of the stomach, pancreas, breast, lung or prostate may have pruritus as a manifestation, often up to a year before the cancer becomes detectable. Removal of the tumor results in relief of the itching and recurrence may be manifested by recurrence of the pruritus.

In a series of 34 patients evaluated because of generalized pruritus, a systemic disease was found in 17 (50 percent). The following dieases were found: reticuloendothelial malignancy (6 patients); another malignancy (3 patients); renal insufficiency (4 patients); liver disease (2 patients) and diabetes (2 patients).[4]

CLINICAL EVALUATION

A searching history and complete physical examination are mandatory in the evaluation of the patient presenting with generalized pruritus. The history will help to establish in more detail the characteristics of the pruritus, and detect the presence of associated symptoms.

Inquiry should be made about the location, time of occurrence and severity of the itching. Is it constant, recurrent or intermittent? Does it interfere with sleep or work? What is the quality of the itching, as perceived by the patient? It may be described as burning, prickling, stinging or itching. Pruritus is often more pronounced at night, due to the absence of other distracting stimuli and vasodilation. It may be difficult from the characteristics of the pruritus to establish an etiology, but, in general, pruritus which is generalized and severe suggests an underlying disorder. Pruritus occurring at a particular time suggests a specific cause (winter pruritus due to dry skin or itching on exposure to a particular allergen). Is there any associated skin rash?

Does the patient present with pruritus as the chief complaint or is the pruritus only one of several symptoms? Are there associated systemic symptoms such as weight loss, fever, generalized malaise, jaundice, pain? Are there symptoms pointing to a specific organ system, such as respiratory, cardiovascular or gastrointestinal? A review of systems should be done, so as not to miss associated symptoms that the patient may not volunteer. Was the patient exposed to a specific allergen? Did he travel out of the country (parasites)? Is there a past history of liver disease or kidney disease? Is there a family history of diabetes? The physician should search for clues suggesting any of the conditions listed below:

Some Systemic Conditions Associated with Pruritus

Infestation
    Trichinosis
    Echinococcus
    Onchocerciasis

Allergic Reaction
> Drug
> Insect
> Contactant

Pregnancy

Liver Disease
> Intra- and extrahepatic cholestasis
> Primary biliary cirrhosis

Kidney Disease
> Uremia

Diabetes

Endocrine Disorders
> Hyperthyroidism
> Hypothyroidism
> Hyperparathyroidism, secondary to chronic renal failure

Neurologic Disorders
> Herpes zoster, pre-eruptive stage
> Tabes dorsalis

Malignancy
> Lymphoma
>> Hodgkin's
>> Lymphosarcoma
>> Reticulum-cell sarcoma
>> Mycosis fungoides
> Polycythemia vera
> Carcinoid syndrome
> Carcinoma
>> Stomach
>> Lung
>> Prostate
>> Pancreas
>> Breast

The physical examination may reveal skin lesions and findings of other conditions. The skin lesions may be primary, with the pruritus as a secondary feature (as in atopic dermatitis) or the skin lesions may be secondary to the scratching. Scratches and excoriations may be sufficiently severe to result in exudation of serum and crust formation. Scars may result. Rubbing of the skin produces erythema, lichenification and hyperpigmentation. Alopecia may be present. Shiny or bevelled nails may be present. There may be secondary pyogenic infection or secondary contact dermatitis if sensitizing topical agents are used.

LABORATORY TESTS

Laboratory tests which may be useful in evaluation of the patient with generalized pruritus include:

Laboratory Tests in the Evaluation of Pruritus

Complete blood count
Erythrocyte sedimentation rate
Urinalysis
Blood urea nitrogen
Fasting and postprandial blood sugars
Glucose tolerance test
Liver function tests
Protein-bound iodine, tri-iodothyronine uptake, radioactive iodine uptake
Calcium, phosphorus, alkaline phosphatase
Heterophile agglutinin
Chest x-ray

Other tests may be suggested by the history and physical examination, such as upper and lower GI series in search for internal malignancy, examination for ova and parasites, urinary excretion of 5-hydroxyindolacetic acid for carcinoid syndrome, bone marrow aspiration, etc.

Tissue biopsies may be performed if suggested by the clinical and laboratory evaluation of the patient. Skin biopsy may reveal mycosis fungoides. Lymph nodes, liver or other tissues found at surgery may be biopsied with elucidation of the diagnosis.

In the work-up of the patient with pruritus, it is important to periodically reevaluate the situation if initial evaluation is negative. The underlying systemic process may not manifest itself for six months to one year after the pruritus and the patient who had been labeled as having psychogenic pruritus may well be harboring an internal malignancy.

TREATMENT

As always in the practice of medicine accurate diagnosis is the first principle of good treatment. Treatment of the underlying condition associated with the pruritus will sometimes dramatically relieve the itching (see section on etiology).

Symptomatic therapy is also important. Topical therapy is aimed at soothing inflamed skin and replacing missing natural oils. Bath oils and lotions, such as Alpha-Keri,* may be useful for dry skin. Baths at comfortable temperature may be soothing. Hot water has been recommended in the treatment of severe pruritus and the mechanism seems to be replacement of the itch stimulus by a pain stimulus. Antipruritic lotions usually contain menthol, calamine, phenol and topical steroids. It is important here to avoid contact sensitizers.

Systemic therapy of pruritus usually consists of antihistamines, but may also include sedatives and tranquilizers. Diphenhydramine may be very useful. Hydroxyzine, chlordiazepoxide, diazepam or barbiturates may be helpful.

* Trademark, Westward Pharmaceuticals.

REFERENCES

1. Beeson, P. B. and McDermott, W.: Cecil-Loeb Textbook of Medicine. ed. 13. Philadelphia, W. B. Saunders, 1971.
2. Keele, C. A.: Chemical causes of pain and itch. Ann. Rev. Med., *21*:67, 1970.
3. Lewis, G. M. and Wheeler, C. E.: Practical Dermatology. ed. 3. Philadelphia, W. B. Saunders, 1969.
4. Rajka, G.: Investigation of patients suffering from generalized pruritus, with special references to systemic diseases. Acta Dermatovener., *46*:190, 1966.
5. Rook, A., Wilkinson, D. S. and Ebling, F. J. G.: Textbook of Dermatology. vol. 2. Philadelphia, F. A. Davis, 1968.
6. Winkelman, R. K. and Muller, S. A.: Pruritus. Ann. Rev. Med., *15*:53, 1964.

Index

Numerals in italics refer to illustrations and tabular material concerning the subject.

Plates illustrating allergenic plants appear between pages 118 and 119.
Color plates illustrating cutaneous drug reactions appear between pages 314 and 315.

general rules in, 338
severity of, 331
symptoms of, 327-328, 331, 419
treatment of, 334-336, 335
Anaphylotoxin, 215
Anderson Sampler, in mold studies, 110
Anemia(s), aplastic, drug-induced, 428-429
transfusions in, 460
hemolytic, auto-immune, 9
drug-induced, 427, 428
Coombs-positive, 10
oxidant drug idiosyncrasy and, 401-402
transfusions in, 460
immunohemolytic, drug-induced, 426, 428
tests in vitro in, 440
penicillin in, 426
Anergex, in allergic disease, efficacy of, 569
Anesthesia, in surgery in asthma, 287
Anesthetics, local, alternatives to, 474-476
antigenic grouping of, 475
toxic reactions associated with, 474-475
vasovagal reactions associated with, 475
Angiitis, necrotizing, Type III reaction in, 17
Angio-edema. *See* Edema, angioneurotic
Angiosperms, 97-98
Animal(s), as cause of therapeutic failure, 555, 602
dander of, allergy to, treatment of, 296-297
as allergen, 111
as antigen, 69-70
models of allergy, 49-50
saliva of, 111
Antacids, drug absorption and, 397-398
Anthemideae, pollen of, 102-103
Antibacterial agents, allergic reactions associated with, 471-473
Antibiotics, in asthma, 252-253, 275
in atopic dermatitis, 389-390
macrolide, allergic reactions associated with, 471
in asthma, 263-264
in sinus headache, 523-524
in status asthmaticus, 280
Antibody(ies), allergens and, 37
in allergic patients, 51
in allergy, 32
antigluten, in nontropical sprue, 372-373

biologic activity of, 42
blocking, 32, 44-45
measurement of, 40-41
in atopic patients, 51
production and activity of, studies of, 53-54
blocking activity of, 44-45
complement fixation and, 42-43
complement-fixing, in Type II reactions, 5, 9
cytotropic activity of, 43-44
homocytotropic. *See* Reagin(s)
IgE. *See* Immunoglobin(s), IgE
IgG. *See* Immunoglobulin(s), IgG
mastocytropic. *See* Reagin(s)
measurement of, 39-45
nature of, 32-36
production of, antigens in, 37
plasma cells in, 38
ragweed-binding, production and activity of, studies of, 53-54
reagin. *See* Reagin(s)
skin-sensitizing. *See* Reagin(s)
Anticholinergics, in asthma, 268
drug absorption and, 398
in gastrointestinal allergy, 370
side effects of, 370
Anticoagulants, displacement of, 398
warfarin, metabolism of, drugs accelerating, 399
Anticonvulsants, lymphadenopathy associated with, 432-433
Antidepressants, in asthma, 268
Antigen(s), airborne, 67-70, 92-94
antibody complexes, activities of, in Type III reactions, 13-14
in mediator release, 47-49
-antibody reaction, drugs for intervention in, 58
in antibody production, 37
avoidance of, 293-294, 336
B, of timothy grass, 90-91
characteristics of, general, 67-70
D, of timothy grass, 91
E, of ragweed, 89-90, 89
in immunotherapy, 296-298
choice of, 181-182
mixture of, related, 297
unrelated, 297-298
K, of ragweed, 89
in pollen, 88
Antihistamines, in allergic rhinitis, 175, 178
in anaphylaxis, 334-335
in asthma, 268
classes of, properties of, 176
clinical use of, 176-177